3RD EDITION

BEVERLEY TAYLOR
STEPHEN KERMODE
KATHRYN ROBERTS

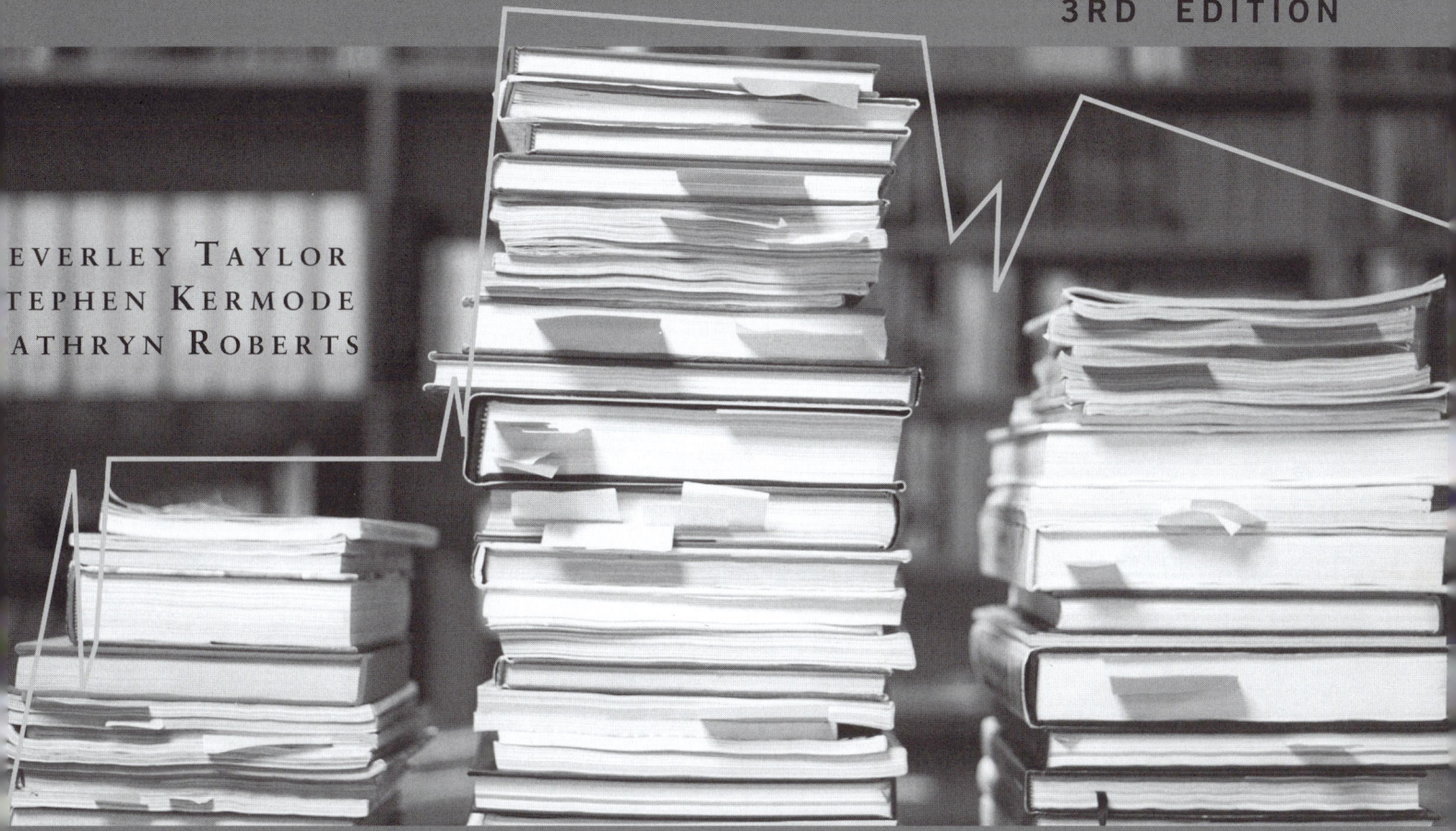

RESEARCH IN NURSING AND HEALTH CARE: EVIDENCE FOR PRACTICE

THOMSON

Australia · New Zealand · Canada · Mexico · Singapore · Spain · United Kingdom · United States

THOMSON

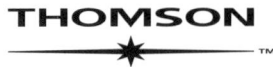

Level 7, 80 Dorcas Street
South Melbourne, Victoria
Australia 3205

Email: highereducation@thomsonlearning.com.au
Website: www.thomsonlearning.com.au

First published in 1998
Second edition published in 2002
This edition published 2006
10 9 8 7 6 5 4 3 2 1
10 09 08 07 06

Copyright © 2007 Nelson Australia Pty Limited.

National Library of Australia
Cataloguing-in-Publishing data

> Taylor, Beverley J. (Beverley Joan), 1951–.
> Research in nursing and health care: creating evidence for practice.
> 3rd ed.
> Includes index.
> ISBN-10 0 17 012315 4.
> ISBN-13 978 0 17 012315 0.
>
> 1. Nursing – Research – Australia. 2. Nurses – Research – Australia. I. Kermode, Stephen. II. Roberts, Kathryn L. (Kathryn Louise), 1943–. III. Title.

610.73072094

Publishing manager: Michael Tully
Publishing editor: Elizabeth Vella
Project editor: Kate McGregor and Louise Powell
Developmental editor: Benjamin Cocks
Production controller: Ruth Coleman
Text designer: MAPG
Cover designer: Olga Lavecchia
Editor: Anne Molvaney
Indexer: Neale Towart
Cover image by Getty images
Typeset in Sabon 11/13pt by KGL Chennai
Printed in China by China Translation Printing Services

This title is published under the imprint of Thomson.
Nelson Australia Pty Limited ACN 058 280 149 (incorporated in Victoria) trading as Thomson Learning Australia.

The URLs contained in this publication were checked for currency during the production process. Note, however, that the publisher cannot vouch for the ongoing currency of URLs.

FOREWORD

The fact that I have been invited to write the foreword to the third edition of this text symbolises its success as a resource for students and practitioners of nursing – and the commitment of the authors to refine and update this resource. I was very pleased to have had the opportunity to write the foreword for the first and second editions of this book; I am even more pleased to have been invited to introduce this third edition.

As international interest in basing practice on the best available evidence continues to accelerate, systematic reviews of evidence for nursing and health care practices increasingly highlight the gaps in an evidence base for practice. Thus, the need for high-quality, large-scale research in nursing and health has never been greater and recognition of this need is growing in the health care industry. For example, nursing research has, until recently, been the province of a small cadre of nurses, and being a nursing researcher or a nursing scientist was largely considered to be of peripheral interest to 'real' nurses struggling in the 'real' world to deliver complex care in demanding work environments.

The first and second editions of this book played a crucial role in developing research-mindedness and research activity in Australian nursing. Drawing on feedback from readers, the authors have made substantial revisions to strengthen the content. This third edition expands its view internationally and into multidisciplinary health research and evidence-based practice. I congratulate the authors on their continuing work in dispelling the myths that surround research through writing in a way that is accessible and enjoyable. More importantly, this text offers clear and practical advice on both using research and on doing research. I recommend this edition to those who teach or practise nursing or any other health care practices, and to students of those practice disciplines, who will shape health care practice for the future.

Alan Pearson

CONTENTS

Foreword   iii
Preface   xiv
About the Authors & Dedication   xv
Acknowledgements   xvi

Chapter 1: Research in nursing and health   1
              by Beverley Taylor and Kathryn Roberts

Chapter objectives   1
Introduction   2
'Doing' collaborative research   3
Practice and research in health professions   4
Overview of research paradigms   5
Evidence-based practice   10
The relationship between research, practice and theory   13
What is a theory?   14
Using nursing and health models and theories in research   16
How to use a conceptual framework in a research project   23
Summary   24
Main points   24
Case study   25
Multiple choice questions   26
Review topics   27
Online reading   28
References   28

Chapter 2: Computers in nursing and health research   33
              by Stephen Kermode, Beverley Taylor and Kathryn Roberts

Chapter objectives   33
Introduction   34

Using computers in research   34
Databases and managing literature   37
Ways your computer can help you do research   42
Summary   47
Main points   48
Case study   48
Multiple choice questions   49
Review topics   50
Online reading   51
Reference   51

Chapter 3: The research question   52
            by Beverley Taylor and Kathryn Roberts
Chapter objectives   52
Introduction   53
Finding research problems: sources and strategies   54
Criteria for selecting problems   58
Stating the problem/question/purpose of the study   62
The process   63
Stating an hypothesis and identifying variables
in quantitative research   63
Defining an area and identifying intentions in
qualitative research   65
Summary   66
Main points   67
Case study   68
Multiple choice questions   68
Review topics   70
Online reading   70
References   71

Chapter 4: Reviewing the literature   72
            by Beverley Taylor and Kathryn Roberts
Chapter objectives   72
Introduction   73
Why review the literature?   73

Identifying relevant literature   74
Possible resources   76
Types of literature sources   77
Useful sources of literature   77
Selecting literature   81
Acquiring your own collection of information   82
Reading and documenting the information   83
Critiquing individual reports   85
Putting it together   93
Summary   94
Main points   94
Case study   95
Multiple choice questions   95
Review topics   97
Online reading   97
References   97

Chapter 5:   Ethics in nursing and health research   98
by Beverley Taylor and Kathryn Roberts

Chapter objectives   98
Introduction   99
Historical examples of unethical research conduct   99
Codes of ethics and research ethics guidelines   101
Human research ethics committees   102
Protecting the rights of human participants   104
Ethical aspects of research in special cases   119
Research ethics in health practices   123
Scientific misconduct   124
Reading a research report: ethical considerations   125
Summary   125
Main points   126
Case study   126
Multiple choice questions   127
Review topics   128
Online reading   129
References   129

Chapter 6: Obtaining approval and support for your project   131
    by Stephen Kermode, Beverley Taylor and Kathryn Roberts

Chapter objectives   131
Introduction   132
The research proposal   132
Funding   164
Obtaining informal approvals   164
Summary   165
Main points   165
Case study   166
Multiple choice questions   167
Review topics   168
Online reading   169
References   169

Chapter 7: Quantitative research designs   172
    by Stephen Kermode and Kathryn Roberts

Chapter objectives   172
Introduction   173
Major types of research design   173
Validity in scientific research   177
Reliability in scientific research   181
Types of experimental design   182
Summary   194
Main points   194
Case study   195
Multiple choice questions   195
Review topics   197
Online reading   197
References   198

Chapter 8: Quantitative methods   199
    by Stephen Kermode and Kathryn Roberts

Chapter objectives   199
Introduction   200
Choosing a setting   200
Defining the population   201
Sampling   202

Quantitative methods of obtaining data   208
Summary   236
Main points   236
Case study   238
Multiple choice questions   239
Review topics   240
Online reading   241
References   241

Chapter 9: Quantitative data collection and management   244
by Stephen Kermode and Kathryn Roberts
Chapter objectives   244
Introduction   245
Preparing for data collection and management   245
The process of data collection   251
Management of data and products of analysis   256
Pilot Study   261
Summary   263
Main points   263
Case study   264
Multiple choice questions   265
Online reading   266
References   267

Chapter 10: Quantitative data analysis   268
by Stephen Kermode and Kathryn Roberts
Chapter objectives   268
Introduction to data   269
Quantitative data analysis   271
Introduction to probability and hypothesis testing   280
Want to learn more about statistics?   298
Summary   298
Main points   299
Case study   299
Multiple choice questions   300
Review topics   301
Online reading   302
References   302

Chapter 11: Determining the clinical relevance of quantitative findings 303
by Stephen Kermode and Kathryn Roberts

Chapter objectives 303
Introduction 304
Preparation 304
Data reduction and summaries 304
Interpreting descriptive findings 305
Findings of association and difference 305
Summary 313
Main points 314
Case study 314
Multiple choice questions 315
Review topics 316
Online reading 317
References 317

Chapter 12: Qualitative interpretive methodologies 318
by Beverley Taylor

Chapter objectives 318
Introduction 319
Research as a means of generating knowledge 319
Defining epistemology and ontology 320
Some common qualitative theoretical assumptions 321
Differences between quantitative and qualitative research 321
Postmodern influences on contemporary epistemology and ontology 323
Differences between interpretive and critical qualitative methodologies 325
Postmodern alternatives for qualitative methodologies 325
Creating flexible approaches to methodologies 327
Combining qualitative methodologies 329
Grounded theory 330
Phenomenology 336
Ethnography 342
Historical research 347
Summary 351
Main points 352
Case study 353
Multiple choice questions 354

Review topics   355
Online reading   355
References   356

Chapter 13:   Qualitative critical methodologies and
                  postmodern influences   363
                  by Beverley Taylor
Chapter objectives   363
Introduction   364
Common qualitative critical theoretical assumptions   365
Critical methodologies compared with poststructuralism   366
Poststructuralism compared with postmodern thought   367
Action research   369
Feminisms   374
Critical ethnography   380
Research discourse reflecting postmodern influences   383
The co-author's postscript to postmodernism   384
Summary   385
Main points   385
Case study   386
Multiple choice questions   387
Review topics   388
Online reading   389
References   389

Chapter 14:   Qualitative methods   393
                  by Beverley Taylor
Chapter objectives   393
Introduction   394
Differentiating between methods, processes and methodologies   394
Choosing congruent methods   396
Using methods alone or in combination   397
Research contexts and participants   399
'Rigour' in qualitative research   400
Methods that may be used in qualitative research   405
Summary   427
Main points   427
Case study   430

Multiple choice questions   430
Review topics   432
Online reading   432
References   433

Chapter 15:   Qualitative data collection and management   437
                  by Beverley Taylor
Chapter objectives   437
Introduction   438
Forms of qualitative data   438
The usefulness of qualitative data   439
Postmodern possibilities   440
Preparing for data collection   441
Strategies for collecting the data   443
Use of computers in qualitative data collection and management   448
Summary   450
Main points   450
Case study   451
Multiple choice questions   452
Review topics   453
Online reading   454
References   454

Chapter 16:   Qualitative data analysis   455
                  by Beverley Taylor
Chapter objectives   455
Introduction   456
Approaches to analysing qualitative data   456
Other methods of text analysis   468
Computer systems that manage qualitative data   473
Examples of completed qualitative analyses   475
Adjust analytic methods with a rationale   477
The analysis of images as qualitative data   478
Summary   478
Main points   478
Case study   480
Multiple choice questions   480
Review topics   482

Online reading   482
References   483

Chapter 17:   Interpreting qualitative findings   486
                  by Beverley Taylor

Chapter objectives   486
Introduction   487
Differentiation between analysis and interpretation   487
Qualitative research findings as relative interpretations   490
Qualitative findings in relation to methodological approaches   491
Qualitative interpretive and critical categories of
interpretive processes   492
Processes for synthesising qualitative interpretive
and critical results   494
Summary   502
Main points   502
Case study   504
Multiple choice questions   504
Review topics   506
Online reading   506
References   507

Chapter 18:   Disseminating the findings   509
                  by Beverley Taylor, Stephen Kermode
                  and Kathryn Roberts

Chapter objectives   509
Introduction   510
The research report   511
The written report   512
Presenting a report at professional meetings   546
Writing for a wider audience   551
Summary   553
Main points   554
Case study   555
Multiple choice questions   555
Review topics   557
Online reading   557
References   557

Chapter 19: Using research in practice and education   559
          by Beverley Taylor and Kathryn Roberts

Chapter objectives   559
Introduction   560
Research and practice   560
Research and education   561
Getting research into practice   562
Problems with clinical guidelines   565
Educating evidence-based clinicians   569
Summary   572
Main points   572
Case study   573
Multiple choice questions   574
Review topics   575
Online reading   576
References   576

Glossary   578
Answers to multiple choice questions   586
Index   587

PREFACE

When the first edition of this book was published in 1998, for the first time students were able to access a research text written by Australian nurse-researchers. The success of the first edition reflected the warm reception of the Australian nursing context and content. The second edition was published in 2002 and Bev Taylor and Kathryn Roberts continued the use of Australian nursing research examples, with equal space devoted to quantitative and qualitative research approaches.

This edition welcomes Stephen Kermode as a co-author, who was invited to undertake the rewriting of Kathryn's chapters. Kathryn retired in 2004, but her name remains on this book in honour of her initial role as first author on two editions and the fact that some of her reworked content appears in this edition.

We have changed the title of this third edition to be more inclusive of other health professionals and in view of the international readership of the book. The content reflects a multidisciplinary approach to health research with research examples from nursing and other professional health care groups.

This edition is as user-friendly as ever, and we have continued the main points and the use of student exercises in the form of practical exercises in the text, case studies, multiple choice questions and review topics. We have also incorporated reviewer feedback in a greater emphasis on evidence-based practice, postmodernism and updated information suitable for undergraduate, honours and postgraduate students.

We hope that the third edition will also be well received.

Bev Taylor
Stephen Kermode
Kathryn Roberts

ABOUT THE AUTHORS

Beverley Taylor (PhD) is Professor of Nursing, School of Nursing and Health Care Practices, Southern Cross University, Lismore campus, New South Wales.

Stephen Kermode (PhD) is Associate Professor of Nursing, School of Nursing and Health Care Practices, Southern Cross University, Lismore campus, New South Wales.

Kathryn Roberts (PhD) was formerly Professor of Nursing at Northern Territory University. She retired from full-time academic work in 2004.

DEDICATION

This book is dedicated:

by Bev Taylor, to the memory of Wili Callan, PhD, for his unceasing spirit of inquiry;

by Stephen Kermode, to all the students of research methods I have taught, for pushing me to find better ways to help them learn;

by Kathryn Roberts, to Ron Roberts, for his mentorship, editorship and, most of all, his love;

and by all of us, to all of the nurses and professional health carers everywhere, who have undertaken research for the purpose of advancing the knowledge base of their discipline.

ACKNOWLEDGEMENTS

The authors and publishers would like to gratefully credit or acknowledge the following for permission to reproduce copyright material:

Blackwell Publishing for extract from McCallin, A.M., 2003. 'Research: Designing a grounded theory study: Some practicalities'. *Nursing in Critical Care* vol.8, no.5, 203–210 (this extract p.205), with permission from Blackwell Publishing. Commonwealth of Australia for extracts: *National Statement on Ethical Conduct in research Involving Humans* © Commonwealth of Australia, National Health & Medical Research Council 2001, *National Statement on Ethical Conduct in research Involving Humans*. © Commonwealth of Australia, reproduced by permission. Elsevier for extracts, reprinted from: Young, A., Gebhardt, S., et. al. 2001 *Connections: Nursing Research, Theory and Practice*, Mosby, St. Louis, 2001; Clifford, C., & Clark, J. (eds) 2004 *Getting Research into Practice*, Elsevier Churchill Livingston; Davies, P., ©2005, 'Changing policy and practice' in *Evidence–Based Practice: A Primer for Health Care Professionals* 2nd ed., Dawes, M., Davies, P., Fray, A., Mant, J., Seers, K., Snowball, R., 2005. Elsevier Churchill Livingston, Edinburgh, pp 223–240. All with permission of Elsevier. *International Journal of Mental Health Nursing* for extract reprinted from McCann, T.V. and Clark, E., 2003 "A grounded theory study of the role that nurses play in increasing clients willingness to access community mental health services', *International Journal of Mental Health Nursing* vol.12, no.4. pp 279–287. *International Journal of Nursing Practice* for extract 'Reasons for attending and not attending a support group for recipients of implantable cardioverter defibrillators and their carers'. Reprinted from: Williams, A. et. al. *International Journal of Nursing Practice*. Vol 10, No.3, pp 127–133. *International Journal of Nursing Practice* for extracts, reprinted from: Juntunen A., Nikkonen M., Janhonen S. 2002, 'Respect as the main lay care activity among the Bena in Ilembula village in Tanzania'. *International Journal of Nursing Practice*. Vol. 8, No.4, pp 210–220; Yuginovich, T. 2000, 'More than time and Place: using historical competitive research as a tool for Nursing', Vol. 6, pp 70–5; Watson, J. et. al. 2002 'Evaluation of the extended role of the midwife: the voices of midwives'. *Nursing Inquiry* for extracts, reprinted from: Harding, P. 2003 'Shape shifting discourses of anorexia nervosa: reconstituting psychopathology' *Nursing Inquiry* Vol. 10. No.4, pp 209–217; Meyer, D & de Oliveira, D. 2003, 'Breastfeeding policies and the production of motherhood: a historical – cultural approach' Vol. 10 No. 1, 11–18; Rankin J, 2003, 'Patient satisfaction: knowledge for ruling hospital reform – an institutional ethnography' Vol.10 No.1, pp 57–65; Jervis, L.

(2002), Working in and around the 'Chain of command' power relations among nursing staff in an urban nursing home', vol. 9, No. 1 pp 12–23. Princeton University Press for extract from Rosenau, Pauline M. *Post-Modernism and the social sciences* © 1992 Princeton University Press. Reprinted by permission of Princeton University Press. Royal College of Nursing Australia for extract, reprinted from Langridge, M. & Ahern, K. 2003. 'A case report on mixed methods in qualitative research' *Collegian*, vol.10, no.4, pp 32–36, with the permission of Royal College of Nursing, Australia. Sage, London for extracts, reprinted from: Atkinson, P. Coffey, A., Delamont, S. Lofland J., & Lofland, L. (eds) 2001 *Handbook of Ethnography,* Sage, London. Thomson Learning for extract McMullin E. 1987, 'Alternative approaches to the philosophy of science', in *Scientific Knowledge, Basic issues in the Philosophy of Science* 1st edition by Kourany, © 1987, reprinted with permission of Wadsworth a division of Thomson Learning: www.thomsonrights.com.

Every attempt has been made to trace and acknowledge copyright holders. Where the attempt has been unsuccessful, the publisher welcomes information that would redress the situation.

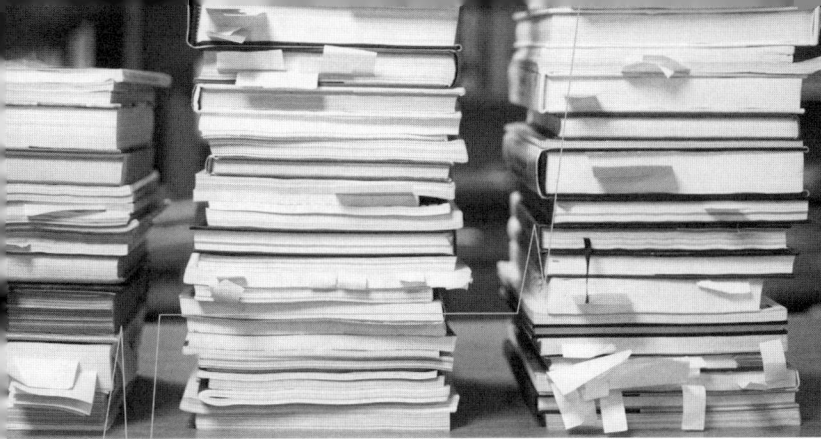

CHAPTER 1

RESEARCH IN NURSING AND HEALTH

CHAPTER OBJECTIVES

The material presented in this chapter will assist you to:

- appreciate the value of collaborative research within the multidisciplinary health team
- describe the research paradigms
- distinguish between quantitative and qualitative research processes
- understand postmodern influences on 'shifting paradigms' in research
- describe evidence-based practice
- describe the relationship between research, practice and theory.

Introduction

This research text is the third edition of a book written originally for nurses and using mainly Australian research projects. This edition seeks to broaden its focus into health generally and thereby take in the interests of other health professionals, such as doctors, nurses, physiotherapists, speech therapists, nutritionists, occupational therapists and so on. The research examples are taken from a wide range of international projects reported in peer-reviewed professional journals. At times the text will focus on nurses and nursing, but on the whole it will attempt to be inclusive of all health professionals.

Research literally means 'looking carefully again'. In the simplest interpretation of the word, when researchers undertake projects, they are searching again for new or adapted knowledge to inform them about areas of interest, so they can begin or add to a body of knowledge. Clifford (2004, p. 14) suggests that the 'word "research" implies a cyclical process with the notion that we search out information and then, in the light of our new knowledge, search again, i.e. re-search'. Whether quantitative, qualitative, or a combination of these two main approaches to inquiry, research is systematic in its approach to finding and adapting knowledge.

Research can be either basic or applied. **Basic research** develops fundamental knowledge and tests theory. Studies of clients' health states, their ability to care for themselves, and their perceptions of phenomena pertaining to health and illness are cases in point. An example is the study seeking evidence of rehabilitation in nephrology nursing (Pryor, Stewart & Bonner 2005). **Applied research** concerns the application of knowledge to specific situations. It addresses problems, such as the best way to practise health care. A warning to complementary practitioners of the risk of hypersensitivity pneumonitis associated with handling exotic mushroom varieties is an example of applied research (Rao et al. 2005).

Health professions claim that their practices are based on research (Clifford & Clark 2004; Courtney 2005; Dawes et al. 2005). However, their claims need to be justified. For example, even though nursing strives to be a research-based profession, it still does not conduct enough research, nor heed and apply research findings in its spheres of practice, education and management, to be fully research-based. There is also a time-lag between development and implementation of research, and **theory** derived from research is not immediately applied to the everyday work, concerns and issues of clinical nursing practice.

This chapter introduces some fundamental ideas relating to research in nursing and health. The importance of collaborative, multidisciplinary research is emphasised, as is the nature of health care professions and why research is integral to their practice. Research **paradigms** are identified as quantitative or qualitative and the three major categories of research used in this book are introduced – empirico-analytical, interpretive and critical. Quantitative research and **qualitative research** processes are described, including postmodern influences on research and the current tendency towards shifting paradigms.

Evidence-based practice (EBP) is described in terms of definitions, origins, criteria for judging levels of evidence, and how to get research into practice. Research is linked with theory in a reciprocal relationship within the theoretical framework of a study. This chapter describes the nature of theory and presents some theories of nursing and health that can be applied to other health care professions, especially in using a theoretical framework in all stages of the research project.

'Doing' collaborative research

Nurses and other health professionals from various disciplines can participate in research in various ways. At an independent level, a researcher may conduct the whole project alone, but this takes a considerable amount of training, preferably to the doctoral level. At an interdependent level, a researcher may participate in a research project in collaboration with other researchers. Interdependence implies that the researcher makes a contribution to the conceptualisation, implementation, evaluation and dissemination of the project (Downie et al. 2001). At a dependent level of participation, a researcher may be a **data** collector for another researcher's project but not make a significant contribution to the conceptual part of the project.

Nursing and health research provide many opportunities to collaborate with other researchers in a multidisciplinary team. They share common interests in people, the environment and health, so there is a great deal of scope for collaboration in projects that have a specific focus or that cover a range of domains (Dalton et al. 2003). It may be possible to set up collaborative projects in which disciplinary groups cooperate in projects with other health care researchers, or with people from other disciplines that could adopt a health focus, such as environmental science or education.

Health professionals working in practice, administration and education have opportunities to collaborate with other researchers on research projects. For example, a group of clinicians working within the same ward or unit may have a specific practice question they wish to pursue. Also, they may work across various wards or units in the same health care facility, or collaborate on a larger project that requires more research participants and the expertise of multiple researchers.

Health care requires the expertise of many workers qualified in different fields of practice, such as doctors, nurses, physiotherapists, speech therapists, nutritionists, occupational therapists and so on. The complexity of human problems when body dysfunction is present means that the overall needs of patients are often best met by multidisciplinary teams in hospitals and community organisations. Many research questions that can directly benefit patient care can be raised within such multidisciplinary teams.

Researchers with a background in human sciences, such as sociology, psychology and education, may be invaluable sources of assistance and support for anyone undertaking nursing and health research. For example, a researcher skilled and experienced in reflective practice and critical perspectives for change may facilitate collaborative research projects with nurses or physiotherapists in their work settings (Byrne & Keefe 2002).

Research collaboration is possible between researchers in nursing and health, and researchers from other disciplines. It may take time, energy, opportunities and organisational skills before projects get under way, but the rewards can be many for respective disciplines and for the other people with whom they collaborate (Koopman, Benbow & Neary 2001).

Practice and research in health professions

Health care workers identify themselves as professionals, having moved in their practice evolution from occupational to professional status. Occupations become professions by attaining the credentials of professionalism. The ways in which an occupation is transformed into a profession vary, but are generally considered to entail a strong level of commitment; a long and disciplined educational process; a unique body of knowledge and skill; discretionary authority and judgement; active and cohesive professional organisation; and acknowledged social worth and contribution.

Goode (1966, in Freidson 1970) describes professions according to two core characteristics: 'a prolonged specialised training in a body of abstract knowledge' and 'a collectivity or service orientation', with autonomy for professional standards and education, licensing, legislation and freedom from lay evaluation and control. Freidson (1970), however, argues that the only truly important and uniform criterion for distinguishing professions from other occupations is the fact of autonomy – a position of legitimate control over work (1970, p. 82). He adds that professionalisation often requires the support of powerful groups within the social structure. Regardless of whether you agree with an emphasis on expert service or an autonomous power interpretation of professions, the underlying commonality is the need to maintain research activities to keep professional knowledge relevant and current.

Fundamental to the development of professional research is the tertiary education system, which promotes systematic inquiry and scholarship development. For example, in the first half of the twentieth century, nursing went through a phase in which service was paramount. There was almost no clinical nursing research during this period, the emphasis being on the improvement of nursing through better management. This reflected an industrial trend towards efficiency through the development of such strategies as the assembly line. In Australia, an academic period of nursing began in the 1950s, and still continues. The move of basic nursing education in the late 1980s into the tertiary education sector was an important influence on the development of Australian nursing research. Other health professions, such as medicine, have been educated in the tertiary sector much longer and this is reflected in the strong professional status of doctors as clinicians and the high priority of government support of biomedical research into health and illness.

Overview of research paradigms

A paradigm is a broad view or perspective of something. Some people may even say that a paradigm is a 'world view', so you can see that it is a comprehensive approach to a particular area of interest. The paradigm of a profession not only concerns the content of the professional knowledge, but also the processes by which that knowledge is produced (Cutcliffe & Goward 2000; Krasner 2001a & b; Malinski 2002).

Various approaches to doing research can be classified paradigmatically. For example, researchers may speak of quantitative or qualitative research, or they may refer to certain paradigms across all the possible kinds of knowledge that can be generated through research. A paradigmatic view provides overall, overarching categories, in which can be placed certain kinds of research and ways of knowledge generation and verification.

A student who is new to research will find that there is a lot of detail to be learnt about the various research approaches. This can be very confusing for novice researchers, who are trying to get an overview of the possibilities and problems confronting them. With this in mind, we have organised this book into distinct chapters that give information on quantitative and qualitative research. We have also maintained the **concept** of two forms of qualitative inquiry, to help sort out the differences in qualitative research methodologies. In Chapter 12 we have also described how the qualitative research methodologies differ from one another and from quantitative research.

The three major categories of research we have used to structure this book generate and verify empirico-analytical (quantitative), interpretive (mostly qualitative) and critical (mostly qualitative) forms of knowledge. In addition, researchers use the ideas of **postmodernism** in their research, but as this approach resists categorisation it will be dealt with outside the confines of a paradigm. These distinctions will be described in Chapters 12 and 13, but a brief introduction to them will be given in this chapter.

Science and empirico-analytical (quantitative) research

Traditional science has had a strong influence on research. Science is:

> a collection of propositions, ranging from reports of observations to the most abstract theories accounting for these observations . . . the end product of research, the careful statement in approved technical terms of something that has been empirically determined to be so, and perhaps also of a tentative explanation of why it is so (McMullin 1987, p. 3).

Science can also be thought of as being all the things that a scientist does that affect the scientific outcome in any way. These can include any influences on the scientist, whether or not the scientist is conscious of them (McMullin 1987). This definition incorporates the first definition. It allows scholars and philosophers to suggest that there is no such thing as a totally objective approach to science; that scientists impose their own values and beliefs upon their research.

Empirico-analytical research is interested in observation and analysis by the scientific method. The scientific method is basically a set of rules for how to do research that can be considered to be rigorous, in the sense that it can be shown to test something over and over again and be consistently accurate (reliability). It also shows that it is testing what it actually intends to test (validity) rather than other things that are there unnoticed (extraneous variables). To achieve this, the scientific method demands that research be as free as possible from the distorting influences of people, such as their ideas, intentions and emotions (subjectivity). In other words, research needs to show that due consideration has been given to achieving objectivity. This process is common to all disciplines that produce scientific knowledge, and has traditionally been regarded as the best way to build knowledge. The scientific method comprises both induction (a theory-building approach) and deduction (a theory-testing approach).

Another requirement of the scientific method is that the only research questions that can be legitimately asked are those that can be structured in ways that can be observed and analysed (by empirico-analytical means) and measured by numbers, percentages and statistics (quantified). This is why research using the scientific method is also referred to as empirico-analytical and/or quantitative research.

Empirico-analytical and/or quantitative researchers want to reduce things of interest to their most focused and smallest parts (reductionism) in order to study them. They do this based on an underlying assumption that there are cause and effect links between certain objects and subjects (variables). It is assumed that these cause and effect relationships have a far greater chance of being discovered if the variables in a study are carefully controlled and manipulated. Researchers take a great deal of care to design their projects to ensure that they are observing and analysing the effects of what they intend to study so that they can demonstrate to 'the scientific community' that the results are statistically significant. This means they try to confirm or dispute the degree of certainty they can place in cause and effect relationships through mathematical explanations.

Health professions have been identified as sciences because primarily they use the empirical method for their research inquiry. For example, nurses adopted the empirical scientific method because they believed that it was the best way of developing nursing knowledge and of promoting the acceptance of nursing as a valid discipline. The classification of any health profession as a science allies it to empirical science, especially when decisions about research funding and research ethics are concerned.

The quantitative research process

The steps of the scientific quantitative research process are (Moody 1990, p. 89):
- identifying the problem or phenomenon of interest
- explicating the linkage of the research question or problem to a theoretical framework
- formulating testable research questions or hypotheses
- designing the study
- refining the research questions/hypotheses and how the data will be collected
- specifying the sample/participants to be studied

- planning for data management
- collecting data
- analysing data
- interpreting the findings
- identifying conclusions
- making recommendations
- disseminating findings.

The quantitative research process is often iterative – that is, one moves back and forth between the steps rather than completing one phase entirely before going on to the next.

The quantitative research process attempts to find out scientific knowledge by the measurement of elements. This may be at four levels: description, in which elements of a phenomenon are counted; correlation, in which relationships of two or more elements are investigated; explanation, in which one element explains another; and prediction, in which the activity of one element can be predicted from that of another. This process uses an empirical method in which data are collected by means of our senses, primarily sight.

The quantitative research process may involve an inductive process, in which a lot of data are collected and described. For example, if you wanted to find out the average of some characteristic of people, you could go out and measure many people and calculate the mean. However, you would then have to test your findings to see if they hold up generally. You would do this by measuring a lot more people of varying kinds and seeing if most of the measurements fell near the average. Many quantitative designs involve testing relationships between phenomena, usually by proposing an hypothesis or statement about the relationship between the variables. Then data are gathered, findings analysed, and conclusions drawn about the findings.

Qualitative research

In this book we make a distinction between qualitative interpretive research and critical research. The principal difference is that interpretive forms are concerned mainly with creating meaning, while critical forms focus on causing socio-political change. Postmodern influences on research can be considered as extending combinations of qualitative interpretive and critical research, taking a highly eclectic view of knowledge generation and validation methods and processes.

Qualitative interpretive research

Qualitative research is interested in questions that involve human consciousness and subjectivity, and which value humans and their experiences in the research process. Qualitative research involves finding out about the changing (relative) nature of knowledge, which is seen to be special and centred in the people, place, time and conditions in which it finds itself (unique and **context**-dependent). Qualitative research uses thinking that starts from the specific instance and moves to the general pattern of combined instances (inductive), so it grows from the ground up to make larger statements about the nature of the thing being investigated.

Rather than starting with a statement (hypothesis), qualitative research begins a project with a statement of the area of interest, such as: 'This research will explore the nature and effects of multidisciplinary team relationships in intensive care units'. The measures for ensuring validity in qualitative research involve asking the participants to confirm that the interpretations represent faithfully and clearly what the experience was/is like for them. Reliability is often not an issue in qualitative research, as it is based on the idea that knowledge is relative and is dependent on all of the features of the people, place, time and other circumstances (context) of the setting. People are valued as sources of information and their expressions of their personal awareness (subjectivity) are valued as being integral to the meaning that comes out of the research. Rather than saying that something can be claimed to be statistically significant, qualitative research makes no claims to generate knowledge that can be confirmed as certain (absolute).

Interpretive research aims mainly to generate meaning. It tries to explain and describe, in order to make sense of things of interest.

Qualitative critical research

All the statements made for qualitative interpretive research apply to critical research, but there is a difference between the two in terms of their intention to bring about social and political change. Qualitative critical research overtly aims to bring about change in the status quo. By working collaboratively with participants as co-researchers to address research problems systematically, qualitative researchers try to find answers and use them to bring about change. These differences will be discussed further in Chapters 12 and 13. Essentially, interpretive research is about making meaning while critical research is about causing change.

Postmodern influences on research

The postmodern era has provided an eclectic extension to what we are naming in this book as qualitative interpretive and critical research. It is not possible to claim postmodernism as a third research paradigm in this book, as postmodern thinking questions many of the taken-for-granted assumptions about knowledge generation and validation in research, and so resists taking on the authority of a 'grand narrative'. Instead, we can discuss postmodern influences on research methods and processes. Postmodernism seeks to 'turn on their heads' cherished notions of the importance of author, text, subject, history, time, theory, truth, representation and politics (Rosenau 1992). Postmodernism requires researchers to redefine their basic assumptions, intentions and roles and to make adjustments to their present ways of viewing and doing research and practice. These influences will be discussed further in Chapters 12 and 13.

The qualitative research process

There are similarities in the processes for quantitative and qualitative research. All projects need a well-planned beginning; a careful middle section when the data are collected, analysed, and interpreted; and a thoroughly executed end stage in which the results are written up and disseminated. However, there are also differences between quantitative and qualitative research processes.

Qualitative research tends to define the word 'process' differently from the accepted dictionary usage, which is synonymous with a set of steps or methods. Qualitative research defines process as the 'how' of research, especially in relation to how the people in the research relate to one another. Therefore, there are some features of research processes that identify qualitative research projects as being different from quantitative research projects. The differences lie in the use of language, the degree of involvement and collaboration of the research participants, and the 'ownership' of the project. Quantitative researchers tend to refer to the people they have accessed in the research as subjects. By objective means, subjects are exposed to carefully prepared methods and instruments such as surveys, questionnaires, clinical trials and so on.

In contrast, qualitative researchers tend to refer to the people they have accessed in the research as participants. By means that value the participants' subjectivity, researchers claim to 'work with' participants when doing qualitative research projects.

There are variations in the degree of participant involvement in qualitative research. For example, critical forms of qualitative research pay far more attention to ensuring a high degree of research participant involvement and collaboration. This is evidenced by the tendency of many of the researchers who use critical methodologies to refer to participants as co-researchers. Critical researchers also try to minimise the effects of power differences between the researcher and the participants/co-researchers. Friendships that last throughout the life of the project and beyond may even develop between the people involved in the research.

In qualitative critical methodologies such as feminist and action research approaches, and those reflecting postmodern influences, there is a tendency for participants/co-researchers to have an influential voice in the overall conduct of the project. The project may run according to the wishes and directions of the group, which may develop a strong sense of joint ownership of the project. This sense of ownership may be reflected in the acknowledgement in the research report of all the people involved in its direction. Ownership may also manifest in the publication of jointly authored journal articles and the presentation of jointly prepared papers at professional conferences.

Shifting paradigms

There has been a recent shift of focus towards qualitative research and mixed methods research in nursing and other health professions (Bassett 2004; Cody 2000; Streubert-Speziale & Rinaldi-Carpenter 2003; Young Brockopp & Hastings-Tolsma 2003). However, research in the quantitative paradigm still dominates overall because it attracts major funding from governments and health research sponsors; and it is seen to be more effective in giving clear, concise and accurate answers to the causes, effects and treatment of human illnesses (Courtney 2005).

Although postmodernism resists being represented as a paradigm, it should be noted that it has an important effect on the present trends in shifting paradigms. Postmodern

the human condition &/or the medical condition.

thinking allows researchers to create highly imaginative research strategies to replace the rigid rules and methods that have been reflected in modernist (i.e. quantitative and qualitative) research projects. Affirmative postmodern influences encourage researchers to move from their reliance on the scientific method to be guided by their feelings, personal experience, empathy, emotion, intuition, subjective judgement, imagination, creativity and play (Rosenau 1992). The inclusion of these subjective elements constitutes a major departure from the rules of the scientific method reflected in quantitative research, and constitutes an extension of qualitative researchers' ideas about the role of relative and personal knowledge in their projects.

Evidence-based practice

Health professionals use their knowledge, skills and humanity in the service of making and keeping people well. Health care practice is complex and health professionals are responsible for giving the best possible care, based on sound knowledge and experience, which is tested and retested by reliable and valid research methods. This section deals with evidence-based practice (EBP), by describing definitions, origins, criteria for judging levels of evidence, and how to get research into practice.

Definitions

As the words imply, evidence-based practice is about basing current practice on research. Definitions abound for evidence-based practice, including that it is 'the conscientious, explicit and judicious use of current best evidence in making decisions about the healthcare of patients' (Sackett et al. 1997, p. 2) and that it also involves patients' values (Sackett et al. 2000). In nursing, French (2002) located more than 14 different definitions of evidence-based practice, with common elements being the need for the best evidence, expert clinical decision-making, and consideration of patients' needs and values.

Dawes (2005, p. 4) suggests that the simplest definition is that evidence-based practice 'aims to provide the best possible evidence at the point of clinical (or management) contact'. This definition begs the questions: What is the best possible evidence? Who judges it? How? Why? For whom? Under what circumstances? This section deals with these questions, and as you will see, it has to do with judgements about the merits of designs and results of research projects deemed capable of creating and establishing credible answers for clinical practice.

Origins

Evidence-based practice has been established in medicine for decades and it has more recently become the catchcry of allied health research and practice. Lockett (1997) traces the development of EBP to medical researchers in Canada, who wanted to ensure that medical practice was based on research evidence. Since that time, EBP has become firmly established in the USA, United Kingdom, Europe and southern hemisphere countries. Key EBP organisations in Australia and New Zealand are 'the National Institute of Clinical Studies (NICS): the Joanna Briggs Institute (JBI); the Centre for Evidence based Nursing-Aotearoa (CEBNA): and the New Zealand Guidelines Group' (Courtney et al. 2005, p. 9).

The worldwide spread of EBP has been attributed by Sackett et al. (1997) to the need for research-based clinical decisions, guidelines and protocols, and to the knowledge explosion in new journals in preference to textbook information. The online information format is favoured because it is a quick method of locating up-to-date resources that are often free of cost. Sources of EBP information are databases, such as Medline, CINAHL, Meditext, PsychINFO, the Australian Digital Thesis Program and the Conference Papers Index, and library holdings such as the Cochrane Library. These databases are described within the discussion of computers in Chapter 2.

The systematic review process

The evidence for EBP is gained by systematically searching for and analysing research reports accessed though databases and libraries. Pearson and Field (in Courtney 2005, p. 74) claim that the systematic review process for accessing and analysing research projects 'is a form of research'; indeed, it is frequently referred to as 'secondary research'. They describe the systematic review process as developing the review protocol, asking answerable questions, finding the evidence, appraising the evidence and judging the applicability of the evidence.

Developing the review protocol is akin to developing a research proposal because it includes undertaking a background literature review, formulating objectives and questions, and describing inclusion criteria, a search strategy for the literature, assessment criteria, data extraction and data synthesis (Pearson & Field, in Courtney 2005).

Asking answerable questions in relation to EBP is a skill that comes with experience, when clear and focused questions are posed based on the participants, activities or interventions, outcomes of interest and relevant studies. Pearson and Field (in Courtney 2005, p. 77) suggest that a 'well-formulated question will give direction to the search strategy to be pursued'.

Finding the evidence involves the logistics of the search, including the databases to be searched, the people to do the work, and the assistance anticipated from librarians. Finding the evidence also includes conducting the search, which is a complex and skilful undertaking performed by people experienced in the activity. Appraising the evidence is according to criteria for judging the levels of evidence (see the next section). Judging the applicability of the evidence involves getting the information into settings and establishing it in current practice (Pearson & Field, in Courtney 2005).

EBP criteria

The National Health and Medical Research Council (NHMRC) in Australia provides a guide for developing, implementing and evaluating clinical practice guidelines (NHMRC 1999). Table 1.1 indicates the levels of evidence that are favoured in creating EBP guidelines, from the highest, most valued Level 1 to the lowest, least valued Level 1V.

Table 1.1 Guidelines for the Development, Implementation and Evaluation of Clinical Practice Guidelines (NHMRC 1999)

Level 1	Evidence obtained from a systematic review of all relevant randomised controlled trials.
Level 11	Evidence obtained from at least one properly designed randomised controlled trial.
Level 111–1	Evidence obtained from well-designed pseudo-randomised controlled trials (alternate allocation or some other method).
Level 111–2	Evidence obtained from comparative studies with concurrent controls and allocation not randomised (cohort studies), case-control studies or interrupted time-series with a control group.
Level 111–3	Evidence obtained from comparative studies with historical control, two or more single arm studies or interrupted time-series without a parallel control group.
Level 1V	Evidence obtained from case series (either post-test or pre-test and post-test).

As you can see, the levels indicate the types of research that are deemed the best sources of information, and unsurprisingly, quantitative research methods dominate because of their fit with the generation and validation of biomedical science. Evidence-based practice grew out of the discipline of medicine and therefore it reflects biomedical values about what constitutes knowledge that can be valued and trusted.

The almost total absence of qualitative research data as evidence has been a source of critique of EBP and researchers have attempted to address this deficit. For example, Morse (2003) compiled a comprehensive list of questions as evaluation criteria, relating to relevance, rigour and feasibility, in the sequence of a research proposal. Accordingly, direct and answerable questions are posed about the research problem or question, investigator capability, and the research methods, context, design, analysis, timelines, budget, subjects, dissemination and outcomes. For instance, questions relating to the relevance of the research question/problem include: Is it a fascinating topic? Is it important to the substantive area? Does it make a significant contribution to the discipline topic and practice? In relation to the rigour of the research question/problem, questions include: Is the literature review comprehensive? Is the philosophical framework identified? In relation to the feasibility of the research question/problem, questions include: Is it doable? Does it have appropriate scope? By carefully answering these comprehensive questions relating to every aspect of a qualitative research project, it is possible to evaluate a project's worth in providing evidence for practice.

Other researchers have compiled lists for evaluating qualitative research evidence (Greenhalgh & Taylor 1997; Horsburg 2003; Whittemore, Chase & Mandle 2001). The Joanna Briggs Institute in Australia has compiled a hierachy of four levels of evidence, which is inclusive of qualitative research (Pearson 2002), and judges the merit of research according to feasibility, appropriateness, meaningfulness and effectiveness. You can view these criteria online at: www.joannabriggs.edu.au/pubs/approach.php#B

The relationship between research, practice and theory

Research is linked with theory in a reciprocal relationship. Research findings are 'incorporated into theory by human scientists … to describe, explain, predict and prescribe important aspects of our lives' (Greenwood 1996). Research can lead to the revision of existing practice theories through testing that theory using quantitative approaches. Conversely, research using qualitative methodologies, such as grounded theory, can lead to the development of useful theories for any health profession. Both approaches can lead to the development of knowledge in a health discipline.

Research into the health status of the client and professional practice can lead to the development of useful theories for health and nursing. Even if a research project concerns a basic procedure or phenomenon, it can lead to the development of theoretical knowledge (Byrne 2001; Diers 2004; Ziegler 2005). Deriving theory from research data is an inductive approach. Many instances of data are collected and then a theory is proposed that fits the observations. This approach is associated with qualitative research designs, such as grounded theory and phenomenology.

Theory can stimulate research when a researcher has ideas that are based in a theory. These ideas about the potential outcomes of the study form the framework of a study. The conceptual framework of a research study is like the skeleton of the body: it gives structure. This structure helps to plan the work, to know how the parts fit together, to know where to add parts, and to provide a place to attach the other parts. All parts of the research project are linked to the theory, thus forming a coherent whole. Using theory as a conceptual framework is a deductive approach that is associated primarily with quantitative research methodology.

Research can also answer questions about theory through theory-testing. For example, a researcher might decide to test one of the propositions of an existing theory against a new group of clients or in a health care situation in which previous research on that proposition has not been carried out. Theory-testing is a deductive approach associated primarily with quantitative research design.

Knowledge is transmitted primarily through scholarship in the discipline (Bjornsdottir 2001; Edwards 2002). For example, there are four types of scholarship in nursing: theoretical, clinical, teaching and research (Roberts 1996). These have been derived from Boyer's (1990) typology of integrative scholarship, which relates to theoretical scholarship; scholarship of application, which is clinical scholarship in nursing; scholarship of discovery, which is research scholarship; and teaching scholarship. Teaching, theoretical and clinical scholarship are not research scholarship in the sense of research as it has been defined above. They do, however, have a reciprocal relationship with research scholarship. They raise questions that are answered by research, and research in turn helps to build up that body of knowledge and, in turn, scholarship.

The unique perspective of each discipline is judged by its metaparadigm. The metaparadigm of a discipline comprises the fundamental ideas on which its knowledge is founded. Fawcett (1989, p. 5) explained that:

> The metaparadigm of each paradigm of each discipline . . . is the first level of distinction between disciplines. It is not unusual, however, to find that more than one discipline is interested in the same or similar concepts.

For example, there is consensus in the nursing literature on the metaparadigm of nursing. In relation to nursing's metaparadigm, Kemp (1983, p. 610) wrote that:

> . . . there is general agreement that the domain of nursing is person, environment, health, and nursing. By specifying the domain of nursing, research and practice should reflect common goals of providing nurses with knowledge within these four conceptual dimensions.

This means that knowledge that can be claimed to be unique to nursing is concerned directly with any or all of the four domains that represent the scope of nursing. Given that the domains are broad, this means there are many interpretations of what constitutes nursing knowledge, and by whom, how, and for what purposes. The broad range of knowledge in other health professions, and their common interests in health, people and environment mean that deeper and richer knowledge can be generated and tested over time, to continually improve health care.

In the following section, we explore some definitions of theory; consider the links between theory and research; discuss the use of major nursing and health theories in research; and explain specific ways in which a theoretical framework can be used in nursing and health research.

What is a theory?

A theory is an attempt to describe, organise or explain a phenomenon or group of phenomena of a discipline in a language appropriate to the discipline. Furthermore, models and theories organise our knowledge in an orderly, coherent way, thus providing a 'map' of the knowledge of the discipline (Marriner-Tomey & Raile Alligood 2002; Rothrock & Smith 2000; Smith 2001; Walsh 2000).

For example, theories of nursing and health describe and explain nursing and health. They define the practice of nursing and they deal with knowledge about health in humans. They may describe or explain the relationship between the nurse and the client. For example, Orem's Self-Care Deficit Nursing Theory states that nurses devise nursing systems to care for clients at different dependency levels (Orem 2001).

In order to understand the nature of a theory, it is necessary to understand its component parts and related terms, such as phenomenon, concept and model. A phenomenon is something that happens and that can be perceived directly by the senses, for example, electricity. A phenomenon may be visible; for example, lightning is a visible form of electricity. A phenomenon may also be invisible, for example, the electricity that runs through electrical wires is not visible. In human terms, a phenomenon may be an event or an experience that needs further explication to understand it better. For example, Taylor (1994, 2000) used phenomenology to explore the phenomenon of ordinariness in nursing.

A concept is an abstract generalised idea that describes a phenomenon or a group of related phenomena, for example, caring, blood pressure, or stress. Concepts range from the fairly concrete (e.g. 'photograph') to the more abstract (e.g. 'health'). A concept may be inferred from direct measurements, for example, central venous pressure may be measured directly using a manometer. A concept may also be inferred from indirect measurements such as measuring pain by means of visual analogue pain scales. A concept may also be explored through qualitative research methodologies. The major concepts in the discipline of nursing have been identified as nursing, person, environment and health. Very abstract concepts, for example 'well-being', are sometimes called constructs. Constructs such as energy fields may sometimes be identified through research.

A model is a structure that represents phenomena or concepts. A model may show the physical structure of what it represents, for example, a model aeroplane or a model of the solar system. However, a model may also use language to describe what it represents, in which case it is called a theoretical or conceptual model (Pearson et al. 2005). Young, Gebhardt and McLaughlin-Renpenning (2001, p. vii) expressed the importance of models well when they wrote:

> In any mature discipline, scholars, scientists and practitioners know the models that specify the phenomena and characteristics of the nature of the object or disciplinary focus. The also know the relationships between and among the phenomena of concern. They know the variables based on both universal and individual characteristics. They know what measures specific to phenomena are relevant and legitimate. They know how to use valid and reliable measures to ascertain the characteristics of the situation. They develop practice models that in turn enable practitioners to identify dimensions that are amenable to intervention or change.

Theories and models are generally considered to be at several different levels of complexity. The least complex level is a descriptive-level model, which identifies the major elements of a phenomenon by naming them. For example, Henderson's 14-needs model just lists the client's needs (Henderson 1966). The next level is a descriptive model that classifies its components by grouping them in meaningful categories. For example, all nursing diagnoses have been classified into 11 functional health patterns (Gordon 1982).

The next level of complexity of a model or theory is one in which the relationships between the concepts in the theory or model are shown. For example, the Neuman Systems Model shows the relationships between the core body structure and the lines of defence that surround it (Neuman 1995). The next level explains the relationships, or why the concepts are related. For example, in her Self-Care Deficit Nursing Theory, Orem explains the link between self-care, self-care demands and self-care agency (Orem 2001). The highest level is prescriptive-level theory, in which it is hypothesised that a certain intervention will result in a predictable outcome (Dickoff, James & Wiedenbach 1968). It is this level that promotes theory-testing. However, predictability may not be an issue for some research methods that emphasise induction.

Using nursing and health models and theories in research

The latter half of the twentieth century saw the development of a considerable number of models and theories of nursing and health. However, some of these attracted more research interest than others. The most-researched theories are those that contain concepts with sufficiently precise definitions to provide a useful research framework. There are two major groups of these: grand theories that are broad in scope and middle-range theories that are more restricted in scope (Liehr & Smith 1999). The former are used in researching broadly, whereas the latter have been used in specialty research. Many of these models and theories can be applied to other health professions, which share a common interest in providing care for people. For more information, the publication on the original theory should be consulted.

Grand theories

The grand theories most used for conceptual frameworks in studies listed in CINAHL are Orem's Self-Care Deficit Nursing Theory (Orem 2001), Levine's Conservation Model (Levine 1991), the Neuman Systems Model (Neuman 1995), Roy's Adaptation Model (Roy & Andrews 1991), and Rogers's Energy Fields Model (Rogers 1994).

Orem's self-care deficit nursing theory

Orem's model, called the Self-Care Deficit Theory of Nursing, was initially developed in the 1970s but it has continued to evolve and Orem's book is now in its fifth edition (Orem 2001). The model comprises three related theories: the theory of self-care, which describes and explains self-care; the theory of self-care deficit, which describes how clients need nursing; and the theory of nursing system, which describes and explains relationships necessary for nursing to take place.

The theory of self-care proposes that people will normally act in a rational way to care for themselves and their dependants. People can therefore develop and function optimally, be healthy and achieve a sense of well-being. In doing so, they meet requirements, or self-care requisites. These are of three types: universal, or those required by everyone regardless of their age; developmental, or those required at a particular stage in the person's development; and health deviation, or those relating to the person's state of health, or health care. Care requisites may be met through self-care, care of dependants or nursing care.

The theory of self-care deficit proposes that, at times, persons or their dependants will have a greater need for self-care than they can fulfil. This creates a self-care deficit or a need for care to be provided by an external source, such as a nurse or a social worker.

The theory of nursing system links the nurse and the client by proposing that nurses act to provide nursing care for people or groups of people who are unable to meet their own or their dependants' needs for self-care. The nursing systems that the nurse and client devise can be wholly compensatory, in which the nurse performs all care for the client; partially compensatory, in which the nurse and client share the care; or supportive–educative in which the nurse supports and educates the client.

Orem's theory has been used fairly extensively in nursing research in a broad range of topics (Eben et al. 1994). Orem has developed a complete set of assumptions and propositions, which are testable. Many doctoral theses based on her theory have been carried out and many research papers have been published that have been at some level based on her theory. Several tools have been developed to assess self-care and attitudes to self-care. These include Denyes's Self-Care Agency, Kearney and Fleischer's Exercise of Self-Care Agency, and Hanson and Bickel's Perception of Self-Care Agency (McBride 1991). In Australia, studies have been done on teaching self-care skills for headaches (Del Fante 1985), differing attitudes to self-care of hospital and community nurses (Yelland & Sellick 1988), and use of relaxation for the promotion of comfort and pain relief in clients with advanced cancer (Sloman et al. 1994). Sloman and colleagues used Orem's concept of self-care to conceptualise their study. They reasoned that patients experiencing severe cancer pain could use relaxation techniques and gain a degree of self-control. Participants were randomly assigned to three groups: one that received relaxation techniques, a group that received relaxation training and a control group that received no relaxation training. The researchers found that the patients who received relaxation training perceived that they were more relaxed. The study also found that there was a reduction in p.r.n. medication for those groups. The researchers concluded that the nurse could play a supportive–educative role in encouraging and teaching self-relaxation to cancer patients and thereby promote client self-care in accordance with Orem's theory. In the United Kingdom, a more recent study (Lauder 1999) explored the concept of self-neglect using Orem's theory.

Levine's conservation principles

Levine, one of the early nurse-theorists, developed her four Conservation Principles to provide a structure for teaching medical–surgical nursing (Artigue et al. 1994). The four principles are: conservation of energy, of structural integrity, of personal integrity, and of social integrity. The Principle of Conservation of Energy refers to balancing energy output and energy input to avoid excessive fatigue. The Principle of Conservation of Structural Integrity refers to maintaining or restoring the structure of the body by prevention of physical breakdown and the promotion of healing. The Principle of Conservation of Personal Integrity refers to the maintenance or restoration of the patient's sense of identity and self-worth. Finally, the Principle of Conservation of Social Integrity refers to the patient's status as a social being who interacts with others, particularly significant others (Levine 1990).

Levine's model views the person as a holistic being, able to adapt and preserve their integrity with the external environment. If any of these principles is altered, the person's health status is changed. The nurse acts therapeutically to help the client conserve energy and maintain integrity or adapt to changes in energy or integrity. When further adaptation cannot occur, the nurse supports the individual and family while care is needed.

Levine's model is undergoing a recent resurgence. It has been used as a conceptual framework in several studies. These include client-based studies such as one on fatigue in clients with congestive cardiac failure (Schaefer & Potylycki 1993). In Australia, Levine's framework has been used in two studies of boomerang pillows (Roberts et al. 1994; Roberts, Brittin & deClifford 1995). In the study of the effect of boomerang pillows on frail elderly women, a comparison of volumes before and after 10 minutes on a boomerang pillow showed that the lung volume was significantly lower after using the boomerang pillows. It was argued that the use of these pillows may lead to less conservation of energy in these women (Roberts, Brittin & deClifford 1995).

Roy's adaptation model

The Roy Adaptation Model views the individual as a system that constantly adapts in response to stimuli from its external or internal environment. Stimuli can be classed as focal immediate stimuli, contextual contributing stimuli, or residual background stimuli (Roy & Andrews 1991). Each person has a level of adaptation that can be tolerated with ordinary adaptive responses. The response can be positive if adaptation occurs in a way that contributes to the achievement of goals such as survival or growth, or ineffective if it does not. Each person has two mechanisms for responding to stimuli and controlling adaptation: the regulator or physiological mechanism, and the cognator or behavioural mechanism. Persons adapt in four modes. The physiological mode deals with physiological responses. The three psychosocial modes are the self-concept mode, which deals with psychic integrity; the role function mode, which deals with social roles; and the interdependence mode, which deals with interactions with other people.

Roy's model has been used extensively as a conceptual framework in many doctoral theses and published research studies in nursing research. The research studies have been carried out in the field of paediatric nursing, midwifery nursing, neonatal nursing and gerontological nursing. The emphasis on babies and children is not surprising as Roy developed her model originally for paediatric nursing. Roy's model was used in experiment to determine whether the effect of caregiving relatives' level of involvement in care increased their satisfaction with nursing home care (Toye & Blackmore 1996). The researchers found that it did not.

Neuman's systems model

Neuman's model views the client's system as consisting of the basic structure or core, surrounded by layers of defences, rather like the layers of an onion. The basic structure is the energy resources, comprising all basic variables that compose intrinsic human factors related to survival, such as genetic and ego structures, and regulation of body temperature.

The basic structure is immediately surrounded by the flexible lines of resistance, which represent the body's resources that help defend against stressors, for example, the immune system. Outside the flexible lines of resistance is the normal line of defence, which is a constant stability state for the individual who has adjusted to stressors. The outermost ring is the flexible lines of defence which is another shield against stressors or environmental forces that may alter the stability of the system. Stressors are of three types. Intrapersonal stressors are forces occurring within the individual, for example, negative emotions. Interpersonal stressors are forces that occur between one or more individuals, e.g. role expectations. Finally, extrapersonal stressors are forces occurring outside the individual, e.g. financial circumstances. The nurse uses prevention to intervene in the interaction of the client with stressors. Primary prevention occurs when a stressor is suspected or identified; secondary prevention occurs after symptoms from stress have occurred; and tertiary prevention occurs after the active treatment and leads back to primary prevention.

Neuman's model has also been used extensively in nursing research. Neuman (1995) reports that her model is one of the three most frequently utilised models for nursing research. It is used extensively for graduate students' research projects and has identified future study and practice impact (Louis 1995). Abstracts of many studies using the Neuman model are presented in Neuman's book (Neuman 1995). Many published clinical research studies and several doctoral theses have used the Neuman Systems Model as an organising framework. The studies have been in the areas of premature infants, high dependency nursing, pain, stress, anxiety and health promotion. These topics reflect the emphasis in Neuman's theory on stress and prevention.

Neuman herself has identified additional topics for further research using her model. She suggests that evaluation of primary preventive health education programs for school children, availability of alternative health care delivery services for clients, development of primary prevention programs for adults in the middle years of 40 to 60, and evaluation of multidisciplinary health promotion programs are appropriate contemporary issues for exploration and research with the Neuman model (Beckman et al. 1994). There does not as yet appear to be any published research by Australian nurse-researchers using the Neuman Systems Model.

Rogers's theory of unitary human beings

Rogers postulated that human beings are dynamic energy fields inseparable from their environmental energy fields. In Rogers's paradigm, the four major concepts are: energy fields, a universe of open systems, pattern, and pan-dimensionality (Daily et al. 1994). Rogers saw the fundamental unit of the living and the non-living as the energy field. A unitary human being is an energy field that is not limited by time and space. It is identified by its unique pattern and its characteristics cannot be predicted from knowledge of the parts. An environmental energy field is an energy field that is similar to a human energy field. Each person is a human energy field that incorporates its own specific environmental energy field. These form open systems that exchange energy with each other. Both fields are changing all the time. The pattern is seen as a wave and includes behaviours, qualities, and characteristics of the field. Rogers postulated three principles of homeodynamics: the Principle of Helicy, or the continuous variety of human and environmental field patterns; the Principle of Integrality, or the continuous mutual human–environmental field interaction and processes; and the Principle of Resonancy, or change from lower to higher frequency of the wave patterns as the person develops and becomes more complex (Daily et al. 1994).

Recent studies using Rogers's conceptual model as a base have been numerous, as have doctoral theses using Rogers's theoretical framework. Studies have concerned therapeutic touch, parental attachments, addictions, and perception of time. There does not appear to be any published research by Australian nurse-researchers using the Theory of Unitary Human Beings.

Middle-range theories and models

These theories and models include Leininger's Model of Transcultural Care (Leininger 1995), King's Theory of Goal Attainment (King 1981), Benner's Model of Skill Acquisition (Benner 1984), Watson's Theory of Human Caring (Watson 1979), Johnson's Behavioral Systems Model (Johnson 1990), Newman's Health as Expanding Consciousness (Newman 1994), Mercer's Maternal Role Attainment Model (Bee, Legger & Oetting 1994), Parse's Theory of Human Becoming (Parse 1992), Peplau's Model of Psychodynamic Nursing (Peplau 1991), and Becker's (1974) and Penders's (1982) Health Belief Model. There has been little research in Australia using these models.

Research using Leininger's Model of Transcultural Care as a theoretical framework has not been published widely (Alexander et al. 1994). However, in the USA many **cultures** have been studied as part of research into transcultural nursing and care (Alexander et al. 1994). This research has been slow to be funded because qualitative research has not been as successful in attracting funding as quantitative research. One would think that Leininger's model would be a very relevant one for studying people in such a multicultural society as Australia. However, the author could find only a few published research studies by one Australian nurse-researcher, Omeri, that used the Leininger model. These are studies of culture care of Iranian immigrants in New South Wales (Omeri 1997), and utilisation of culturally congruent strategies to enhance recruitment and retention of Australian Indigenous nursing students (Omeri 1999). In the study on Iranian immigrants, Omeri used Leininger's model to develop care that was compatible with the women's cultural beliefs.

King's (1981) Theory of Goal Attainment is a systems model that conceptualises the person as an open system interacting with the environment. The individual is seen as a personal system that is a part of a group. A group is an interpersonal system that is a part of a social system. These systems interact with each other. This theory has led to a small amount of nursing research. It has been used in a variety of studies overseas in which goal attainment was investigated (Ackermann et al. 1994). Areas of focus include adolescent health, women's health, cardiac rehabilitation, family health and nursing home clients.

Benner's Model of Skill Acquisition in Nursing has basically used research to uncover the knowledge embedded in clinical practice (Alexander & Keller 1994). Benner has stated that 'the lack of charting of our practices and clinical observations deprives nursing theory of the uniqueness and richness of the knowledge embedded in clinical practice' (Benner 1984, p. 2). This knowledge is central to the advancement of nursing practice and to the development of nursing science. Benner's model has been used as the theoretical framework in several research studies pertaining to specialist nursing education and clinical career ladders, including Alexander and Keller (1994).

Watson developed a model incorporating 10 carative factors that nurses should use. Watson and others have attempted to research the 10 carative factors of Watson's model (Barnhart et al. 1994), but this is difficult because of the abstract nature of the theory and the limitations of caring in the clinical setting, for example, brief encounters with clients. The theory was clinically validated by researchers using qualitative methodology (Barnhart et al. 1994).There have been several studies using Watson's Theory of Human Caring, primarily on clients' and nurses' perceptions of caring.

Johnson's Behavioral Systems Model proposes seven behavioural subsystems that classify human behaviour, including the biological subsystem and the achievement subsystem. The model has been used in several research studies on the visually impaired, cancer sufferers and the elderly. Furthermore, Derdiarian has developed and tested an instrument (Derdiarian 1988, 1991) and has tested the model in a research study (Derdiarian 1990).

Newman's Model of Health as Expanding Consciousness uses the concepts of movement, space, time and consciousness to depict health (Newman 1986). It has attracted a limited amount of research, perhaps because of its abstract nature. Newman herself has been developing a research methodology consistent with her theoretical paradigm (Newman 1994). Several researchers have undertaken studies about time, space and movement, particularly in the study of the elderly (Keffer et al. 1994).

In the specialist area of maternal–child health, Mercer's Theory of Maternal Role Attainment has been used in a few published studies in the maternal–child nursing area (Bee, Legger & Oetting 1994). The work of Mercer's predecessor, Rubin, was used as the theoretical rationale for a study by Barclay and Martin on episiotomy care in Australia (Barclay & Martin 1983). They argued that the theory of the attainment of the maternal role encompassed a phase of 'taking in' the stresses of labour and delivery and that the enjoyment of 'taking on' motherhood would be diminished by pain, including the pain of the episiotomy. Therefore, any midwifery interventions that could diminish the pain would enhance the 'taking on' of motherhood. In their study of treatment of the episiotomy wound, they compared the treatments of warm sitz bath, iced sitz bath and ray lamp against an untreated control group. While they found no difference in the groups with regard to healing and incidence of infection, they found that the group using an iced sitz bath perceived less pain than the other groups. They concluded that the use of iced sitz baths was more likely than the other methods to reduce pain, which was an important consideration in taking on the role of mother (Barclay & Martin 1983).

Parse's Theory of Becoming Human was developed using Rogers's model as a foundation, along with concepts from existential–phenomenological thought (Lee, Schumacher & Twigg 1994). Parse's model is very abstract and involves the notion that health is a lived experience in which humans structure meaning multi-dimensionally, move towards greater diversity, and reach beyond the self. Parse's model has been used for a growing body of research. Studies using Parse's methodology are qualitative in approach and phenomenological in nature. Parse has developed a research methodology that is congruent with her theory and the phenomenological research tradition (Parse 1995). Research using Parse's model appears to centre on the elderly and on the lived experience of human emotions such as grieving. Parse's theory has been used in several research studies concerned with the lived experience of health, being elderly, being unemployed or homeless, grieving, and laughter. In Australia, Professor John Daly has done research using Parse's methodology to study the lived experience of suffering (Daly 1995).

Peplau's Model of Psychodynamic Nursing identifies four phases of the nurse–client interaction and delineates such aspects of the role of the nurse as teacher and resource person (Peplau 1991). Peplau's model, developed originally in the 1950s, has been used as a conceptual framework in a limited amount of research over 30 years, mostly in psychiatric nursing (Brophy et al. 1994). The Peplau model is another that has undergone a revival in recent times, led by Forchuck in Toronto, Canada.

The Health Belief Model seeks to explain factors that influence people to take preventive 'health' action. It was originally developed and extended by Becker (1974). This model hypothesised that persons would generally not seek preventive care or health screening unless they had some relevant health motivation and knowledge, saw themselves as potentially vulnerable and the condition as threatening, were convinced of the value of intervention and foresaw few difficulties in undertaking the recommended action (Becker 1974). The Health Belief Model suggested that the likelihood of taking a recommended preventive health action was promoted by the perceived threat of the disease and the perceived benefits of preventive action but was inhibited by perceived barriers to preventive action. Perceived threat was affected by perceived susceptibility to the disease and the perceived seriousness of the disease. Modifying factors such as age, sex, personality and cues to action affected the perceived threat of the disease.

Becker and colleagues suggested that the original Health Belief Model was in need of modification in response to research findings. They developed the Preventive Health Behaviour Model. The Preventive Health Behaviour Model, despite its name, is really a model of prevention of disease. The Preventive Health Behaviour Model suggests that the likelihood of complying with individual 'health-related' behaviours could be predicted by motivation, value of illness threat reduction, and probability that the compliant behaviour would reduce the threat. These were moderated by modifying and enabling factors such as demographic variables, structural variables (e.g. cost), attitudes, interaction, and enabling variables such as experience.

In her 1982 book, *Health Promotion in Nursing Practice*, Pender proposed a modification of the Health Belief Model (Pender 1982). Pender proposed two phases in the model – the decision-making phase and the action phase. The decision-making phase comprises individual perceptions and modifying factors, and constitutes the perceived barriers and the cues to action. The perceived benefits of preventive action are moved to the individual perceptions sector of the model. The cues to action are moved to the action phase of the model.

The Health Belief/Preventive Health Behaviour model was used as a theoretical framework for a study by Agars and McMurray evaluating the effects of three different methods of breast self-examination (BSE) on nurses' personal BSE practice (Agars & McMurray 1993). The researchers used a pre-test/post-test design to follow three groups, using a BSE instruction booklet, a film and group discussion, and individual teaching. They found that each group had a significant improvement but the nurses given the film and discussion had the most improvement. The researchers found that barriers to action were more predictive of behaviour before the instruction and perceived susceptibility was more predictive after the instruction.

Pender also proposed the Health Promotion Model (Pender 1982), which represented a breakthrough in that she turned everything around – rather than preventing disease, the person was promoting health. The model was revised in her 1987 book (Pender 1987).

The Health Promotion Model uses the concept of perceived self-efficacy. The model was developed from an extensive review of health research. The central proposal of the model is that the individual has cognitive–perceptual (thinking and sensing) factors that are modified by situational, personal and interpersonal characteristics to result in the participation in health-promoting behaviours in the presence of a cue to action (Tillett 1994). The cognitive–perceptive factors have a direct effect on the decision, whereas the modifying factors have an indirect effect through the cognitive–perceptual factors. Pender's Health Promotion Model has been used as a theoretical framework for investigating the health-promoting activities of clients in all age groups.

How to use a conceptual framework in a research project

The theoretical framework is used in all stages of the research project. The first step in using a conceptual framework is to choose a theory or model that is suited to the research question. For example, if clients from another culture are involved, transcultural nursing may be the theory of choice. If stressors are involved, then the Neuman Systems Model would be appropriate. If independence is a major concept, then the Orem Self-Care Deficit Nursing Theory would be appropriate. However, it is inappropriate to stretch a theory to fit something for which it was not intended.

It is important to examine the relationship between the question asked and the theoretical framework. You should ensure that the question is congruent with the conceptual framework and that it is phrased in the language of the theory. You then state testable hypotheses, defining variables that have been derived from the concepts of the theory. You should define the variables in the theory in a way that is consistent with the theory. If there are relationships between the variables, you should state them in terms of the theory. You can use the conceptual model to help find and interpret the literature. The concepts and variables, defined in terms of the model, can be used as key words to retrieve and organise the literature. This will help you to select appropriate literature and exclude inappropriate literature.

The methodology of the study, including data analysis, should be congruent with the model. For example, Parse's model has its own suggested method of data analysis.

You can use the model as a guide to interpreting the findings and judging their significance. In writing up the report, you can use the model to provide a structure for organising the literature review, the presentation of the results and the discussion. If used appropriately, it leads to an integration of the parts of the study.

EXERCISE

Consider the conceptual frameworks presented in this section and decide which ones would help you best in your practice and research. Why do they suit you?

Now, create your own conceptual framework — it may be a 'hybrid' of an existing framework or it may be totally new. When you are ready, apply your conceptual model in your research project.

Summary

This chapter set the foundation for this research text by introducing some fundamental ideas relating to research in nursing and health. The importance of collaborative, multidisciplinary research was emphasised, as well as the nature of health care professions and why research is integral to their practice. Research paradigms were identified broadly as quantitative or qualitative and the three major categories of research used in this book were introduced as empirico-analytical (quantitative), interpretive (mostly qualitative) and critical (mostly qualitative). Quantitative and qualitative research processes were described, including postmodern influences on research and the tendency towards shifting paradigms.

Evidence-based practice (EBP) was described in terms of definitions, origins, criteria for judging levels of evidence, and how to get research into practice. Even though the overwhelming consensus is that EBP is essential for current practice, busy clinicians have many pressures competing for their attention. If they are to base their practice on recent research, there must be practical strategies put in place in the clinical context to ensure that EBP happens.

Research is linked with theory in a reciprocal relationship and these ideas about the potential outcomes of the study form the framework of a study. This chapter described the nature of theory and presented some theories of nursing and health that describe approaches to connecting theory to research and practice. Many of these models were created by nurses, but they can also be applied to other health care professions, especially in using a theoretical framework in all stages of the research project.

Main points

- Research is a systematic approach to finding and adapting knowledge, whether it is quantitative, qualitative, or a combination of these two main approaches to inquiry.

- Nursing and health research provide many opportunities to collaborate with other researchers in the multidisciplinary team.
- Various approaches to research can be classified paradigmatically such as quantitative and qualitative, and/or empirico-analytical (quantitative), interpretive (mostly qualitative) and critical (mostly qualitative).
- The quantitative research process attempts to find out scientific knowledge by the measurement of elements.
- Qualitative research processes involve finding out about the changing (relative) nature of knowledge, which is seen to be special and centred in the people, place, time and conditions in which it finds itself (unique and context-dependent).
- Postmodern thinking questions many of the taken-for-granted assumptions about knowledge generation and validation in research, and resists taking on the authority of a 'grand narrative'.
- There has been a recent shift in paradigms towards qualitative research and mixed quantitative and qualitative methods research in nursing and other health professions.
- Evidence-based practice bases current practice on research.
- A theoretical framework is used in all stages of the research project to give it structure.
- Research, practice and theory are linked in a relationship that connects knowledge generation and validation and applies it to solve practice problems and to create deeper insights into how people experience health disruptions, and how health professionals can give them the best possible care.

CASE STUDY

Wendy is an experienced Registered Nurse with a Masters qualification, who works as a diabetes educator in a large rural hospital. Over many years of practice, she has noticed that diabetics seem to view their disease processes and outcomes differently to the members of the multidisciplinary health team. In particular, Wendy has noticed that the multidisciplinary team discusses diabetes mellitus in terms of its risks and treatment, whereas people with diabetes speak of their lifestyles primarily and of diabetes as a secondary consideration. For example, last week Wendy was trying to impress upon Mrs White, an elderly woman, the importance of foot care, but all Mrs White wanted to talk about was how she would decorate her daughter's 21st birthday cake. This experience and other anecdotes made Wendy wonder whether diabetics and the health team are aware of one another's priorities, how their priorities might differ. She wonders what, if anything, could be done to improve communication between patients and the health team, to result in improved care practices.

Realising that her questions involved the expertise of the multidisciplinary team, Wendy decided to formulate a research proposal to present to them during a team meeting.

Can you help Wendy to brainstorm ideas for the project? Respond to the questions Wendy is putting to herself before she begins to write the proposal (with the help of Chapter 6 in this book).

1   What members of the multidisciplinary team could be involved in the research?
2   What clinical expertise can they offer?
3   What research paradigms are they likely to favour?
4   How can the research team ensure that their research provides the best evidence for practice?

Multiple choice questions

1   Multidisciplinary health team research involves:
    a   the use of quantitative research designs only
    b   all members collaborating in the project
    c   allied professionals gathering data for doctors
    d   a doctor as the named Chief Investigator

2   Occupations become research-based professions by:
    a   attaining the credentials of professionalism
    b   actively lobbying influential politicians
    c   undertaking tertiary education programs
    d   demonstrating years of practice experience

3   A broad 'world view' or perspective that provides a comprehensive approach to a particular area of interest is a:
    a   model
    b   concept
    c   theory
    d   paradigm

4   Empirico-analytical research is also known as:
    a   postmodern
    b   critical
    c   quantitative
    d   qualitative

5   Qualitative research is interested in questions that involve:
    a   cause and effect relationships
    b   consciousness and subjectivity

    c   control and measurement

    d   generalisation and prediction

6   Basing current clinical practice on the most recent and best research is known internationally as:

    a   practice-based evidence

    b   evidence-based practice

    c   basic practice evidence

    d   evidence for practice

7   For research to be taken up in practice it must be:

    a   enforced by researchers and developers

    b   deemed important by clinical managers

    c   accepted and established by clinicians

    d   approved by patients and their relatives

8   'Systematically developed statements to assist clinician and patient decisions about appropriate healthcare for specific clinical circumstances' are known as clinical:

    a   guidelines

    b   policies

    c   trajectories

    d   procedures

9   A theory is:

    a   a form of questioning and rejecting paradigmatic views, which requires researchers to redefine their basic assumptions, intentions and roles

    b   finding out about the changing nature of knowledge, which is seen to be special and centred in the people, place, time and conditions in which it finds itself

    c   an attempt to describe, organise or explain a phenomenon or group of phenomena of a discipline in a language appropriate to the discipline

    d   a means of systematically finding and adapting knowledge, whether it is quantitative, qualitative, or a combination of these two main approaches

10   In what stage(s) of a research project is a theoretical framework used? In:

    a   the data collection stage

    b   the proposal stage

    c   the write-up stage

    d   all stages

Review topics

1   Why is it essential for health professions to be active in research?

2   What research questions are best suited to a quantitative approach?

3   How do qualitative interpretive and critical approaches differ in their research intentions?

4 Does the evidence-based practice movement perpetuate the idea that quantitative research is superior to qualitative research? Discuss your position.

5 In what ways can nursing theories and models be applied to the research and practice of other health professionals?

Online reading

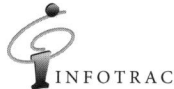

INFOTRAC® COLLEGE EDITION

When accessing information use the following keywords in any combinations you require to retrieve information relating to your health profession's areas of research:

➤ evidence-based practice
➤ models
➤ multidisciplinary research
➤ qualitative research
➤ quantitative research
➤ research paradigms
➤ theoretical framework
➤ theories

References

Ackermann, M., Brink, S., Clanton, J., Jones, C., Marriner-Tomey, A., Moody, S., Perlich, G., Price, D. & Prusinski, B. 1994, 'Imogene King: theory of goal attainment', in A. Marriner-Tomey (ed.), *Nursing Theorists and Their Work*, 3rd edn, C.V. Mosby, St Louis.

Agars, J. & McMurray, A. 1993, 'An evaluation of comparative strategies for teaching breast self-examination', *Journal of Advanced Nursing*, vol. 18, 1595–1603.

Alexander, J., Beagle, C., Butler, P., Dougherty, D., Robards, K., Solotkin, K. & Velotta, C. 1994, 'Madeleine Leininger: cultural care theory', in A. Marriner-Tomey (ed.), *Nursing Theorists and Their Work*, 3rd edn, C.V. Mosby, St Louis.

Alexander, S. & Keller, S. 1994, 'Patricia Benner: from novice to expert – excellence and power in clinical nursing practice', in A. Marriner-Tomey (ed.), *Nursing Theorists and Their Work*, 3rd edn, C.V. Mosby, St Louis.

Artigue, G., Foli, K., Johnson, T., Marriner-Tomey, A., Poat, C., Poppa, L., Woeste, R. & Zoretich, S. 1994, 'Myra Estrin Levine: four conservation principles', in A. Marriner-Tomey (ed.), *Nursing Theorists and Their Work*, 3rd edn, C.V. Mosby, St Louis.

Barclay, L. & Martin, N. 1983, 'A sensitive area', *Australian Journal of Advanced Nursing*, vol. 1, no. 1, 12–19.

Barnhart, D., Bennett, P., Porter, B. & Sloan, R. 1994, 'Jean Watson: philosophy and science of caring', in A. Marriner-Tomey (ed.), *Nursing Theorists and Their Work*, 3rd edn, C.V. Mosby, St Louis.

Bassett, C. (ed.) 2004, *Qualitative Research in Health Care*, Whurr Publishers, London.

Becker, M. 1974, 'The health belief model and sick role behavior', *Health Education Monographs*, vol. 2, 409.

Beckman, S., Boxley-Harges, S., Bruick-Sorge, C., Harris, S., Hermiz, M. & Steinkeler, S. 1994, in A. Marriner-Tomey (ed.), *Nursing Theorists and Their Work*, 3rd edn, C.V. Mosby, St Louis.

Bee, A., Legger, D. & Oetting, S. 1994, 'Ramona T Mercer: maternal role attainment', in A. Marriner-Tomey (ed.), *Nursing Theorists and Their Work*, 3rd edn, C.V. Mosby, St Louis.

Benner, P. 1984, *From Novice to Expert: Excellence and Power in Clinical Nursing Practice*, Addison-Wesley, Menlo Park, California.

Bjornsdottir, K. 2001, 'Language, research and nursing practice', *Journal of Advanced Nursing*, vol. 33, no. 2, 159–66.

Boyer, E.L. 1990, *Scholarship Reconsidered: Priorities of the Professoriate*, Carnegie Foundation for the Advancement of Teaching, Princeton, New Jersey.

Brophy, G., Carey, E., Noll, J., Rasmussen, L., Searcy, B. & Stark, N. 1994, 'Hildegard E Peplau: psychodynamic nursing', in A. Marriner-Tomey (ed.), *Nursing Theorists and Their Work*, 3rd edn, C.V. Mosby, St Louis.

Byrne, M. 2001, 'Linking philosophy, methodology, and methods in qualitative research', *AORN Journal*, vol. 73, no. 1, 209–10.

Byrne, M. & Keefe, M. 2002, 'Building research competence in nursing through mentoring', *Journal of Nursing Scholarship*, vol. 34, no. 4, 391–6.

Clifford, C. 2004, 'Introduction', in C. Clifford & J. Clark (eds), *Getting Research into Practice*, Churchill Livingstone, Edinburgh.

Clifford, C. & Clark, J. (eds) 2004, *Getting Research into Practice*, Churchill Livingstone, Edinburgh.

Cody, W. 2000, 'Paradigm shift or paradigm drift? A meditation on commitment and transcendence', *Nursing Science Quarterly*, vol. 13, no. 2, 93–8.

Courtney, M. (ed.) 2005, *Evidence for Nursing Practice*, Elsevier Churchill Livingstone, Sydney.

Courtney, M., Rickard, C., Vickerstaff J. & Court, A. 2005, 'Evidence based nursing practice', in M. Courtney (ed.), *Evidence for Nursing Practice*, Elsevier Churchill Livingstone, Sydney.

Cutcliffe, J. & Goward, P. 2000, 'Mental health nurses and qualitative research methods: a mutual attraction?', *Journal of Advanced Nursing*, vol. 31, no. 3, 590–8.

Daily, J., Maupin, J., Murray, C., Satterly, M., Schnell, D. & Wallace, T. 1994, 'Martha E Rogers: unitary human beings', in A. Marriner-Tomey (ed.), *Nursing Theorists and Their Work*, 3rd edn, C.V. Mosby, St Louis.

Dalton, L., Spencer, J., Dunn, M., Albert, E., Walker, J. & Farrell, G. 2003, 'Re-thinking approaches to undergraduate health professional education: interdisciplinary rural placement program', *Collegian*, vol. 10, no. 1, 17–21.

Daly, J. 1995, 'The lived experience of suffering', in R. Parse (ed.), *Illuminations*, National League for Nursing, New York.

Dawes, M. 2005, 'Evidence-based practice', in Dawes, M., Davies, P., Gray, A., Mant, J., Seers, K. & Snowball. R., *Evidence-Based Practice: A Primer for Health Care Professionals*, 2nd edn, Elsevier Churchill Livingstone, Edinburgh.

Dawes, M., Davies., P., Gray, A., Mant, J., Seers K. & Snowball, R. 2005, *Evidence-Based Practice: A Primer for Health Care Professionals*, 2nd edn, Elsevier Churchill Livingstone, Edinburgh.

Del Fante, A. 1985, 'Teaching self care skills for migraine and tension headaches', *Australian Journal of Advanced Nursing*, vol. 2, no. 3, 4–8.

Derdiarian, A. 1988, 'Sensitivity of the Derdiarian Behavioral System Model instrument to age, site, and stage of cancer: a preliminary validation study', *Scholarly Inquiry for Nursing Practice*, vol. 2, no. 2, 103–21.

Derdiarian, A. 1990, 'The relationships among the subsystems of Johnson's Behavioral Systems Model', *Image: Journal of Nursing Scholarship*, vol. 22, no. 4, 219–24.

Derdiarian, A. 1991, 'Effects of using a nursing model-based assessment instrument on quality of nursing care', *Nursing Administration Quarterly*, vol. 15, no. 3, 1–16.

Dickoff, J., James, P. & Wiedenbach, E. 1968, 'Theory in a practice discipline: part 1. Practice-oriented theory', *Nursing Research*, vol. 5, 415–35.

Diers, D. 2004, *Speaking of Nursing . . . Narratives of Practice, Research, Policy and the Profession*, Jones and Bartlett, Boston.

Downie, J., Orb, A., Wynaden, D., McGowan, S., Seeman, Z. & Ogilvie, S. 2001, 'A practice-research model for collaborative partnership', *Collegian*, vol. 8, no. 4, 27–32.

Eben, J., Gashti, N., Hayes, S., Marriner-Tomey, A., Nation, M. & Nordmeyer, S. 1994, 'Dorothea E Orem: self-care deficit theory of nursing', in A. Marriner-Tomey (ed.), *Nursing Theorists and Their Work*, 3rd edn, C.V. Mosby, St Louis.

Edwards, S. 2002, 'Nursing knowledge: defining new boundaries', *Nursing Standard*, vol. 17, no. 2, 40–4.

Fawcett, J. 1989, *Analysis and Evaluation of Conceptual Models of Nursing*, 2nd edn, F.A. Davis, Philadelphia.

Freidson, E. 1970, *Profession of Medicine: A Study of the Sociology of Applied Knowledge*, Harper and Row, New York.

French, P. 2002, 'What is the evidence on evidence-based nursing? An epistemological concern', *Journal of Advanced Nursing*, vol. 37, 250–7.

Gordon, M. 1982, *Nursing Diagnosis: Process and Application*, McGraw-Hill, St Louis.

Greenhalgh, T. & Taylor, R. 1997, 'Papers that go beyond numbers (qualitative research)', *British Medical Journal*, vol. 315, 740–3.

Greenwood, J. 1996, 'Nursing research and nursing theory', in J. Greenwood (ed.), *Nursing Theory in Australia: Development and Application*, Harper Educational Australia, Sydney.

Henderson, V. 1966, *The Nature of Nursing: A Definition and Its Implications for Practice, Research, and Education*, Macmillan, New York.

Horsburg, D. 2003, 'Evaluation of qualitative research', *Journal of Clinical Nursing*, vol. 12, no. 2, 307–12.

Johnson, D. 1990, 'The behavioral systems model for nursing', in M.E. Parker (ed.), *Nursing Theories in Practice*, NLN–PUBL 1990 #15–2350, National League for Nursing, New York.

Keffer, M., Hensley, D., Kilgore-Keever, K., Langfitt, J. & Peterson, L. 1994, 'Margaret A Newman: model of health', in A. Marriner-Tomey (ed.), *Nursing Theorists and Their Work*, 3rd edn, C.V. Mosby, St Louis.

Kemp, V.A. 1983, 'Themes in Theory Development', in N.L. Chaska (ed.), *The Nursing Profession: A Time to Speak*, McGraw-Hill, New York.

King, I.M. 1981, *A Theory for Nursing: Systems, Concepts, Process*, Delmar Publishers, Albany, New York.

Koopman, W., Benbow, C.-L. & Neary, N. 2001, 'The challenges to integration in health care research', *Axon*, vol. 22, no. 3, 12–15.

Krasner, D. 2001a, 'Qualitative research: a different paradigm – Part 1', *Journal of Wound, Ostomy and Continence Nursing*, vol. 28, no. 2, 70–2.

Krasner, D. 2001b, 'Qualitative research: a different paradigm – Part 2', *Journal of Wound, Ostomy and Continence Nursing*, vol. 28, no. 3, 122–4.

Lauder, W. 1999, 'Construction of self-neglect: a multiple case study design', *Nursing Inquiry*, vol. 6, no. 1, 48–57.

Lee, R., Schumacher, L. & Twigg, P. 1994, 'Rosemarie Rizzo Parse: man-living-health', in A. Marriner-Tomey (ed.), *Nursing Theorists and Their Work*, 3rd edn, C.V. Mosby, St Louis.

Leininger, M. 1995, *Transcultural Nursing: Concepts, Theories, Research and Practices*, 2nd edn, McGraw-Hill/Greyden Press, Columbus.

Levine, M. 1990, 'Conservation and integrity . . . Levine's conservation model', in M.E. Parker (ed.), *Nursing Theories in Practice*, National League for Nursing, New York.

Levine, M. 1991, 'The conservation principles: model for health', in K. Schaefer & J. Pond (eds), *Levine's Conservation Model: A Framework for Nursing Practice*, F.A. Davis Co., Philadelphia.

Liehr, P. & Smith, M. 1999, 'Middle range theory: spinning research and practice to create knowledge for the new millennium', *Advances in Nursing Science*, vol. 21, no. 4, 81–91.

Lockett, T. 1997, 'Traces of evidence', *Healthcare Today*, July/August, 16.

Louis, M. 1995, 'The Neuman model in nursing research: an update', in B. Neuman (ed.), *The Neuman Systems Model*, 3rd edn, Appleton & Lange, Norwalk, Connecticut.

Malinski, V. 2002, 'Research issues: nursing research and the human sciences', *Nursing Science Quarterly*, vol. 15, no. 1, 14–20.

Marriner-Tomey, A. & Raile Alligood, M. 2002, *Nursing theorists and their work*, 5th edn, Mosby, St Louis.

McBride, S. 1991, 'Comparative analysis of three instruments designed to measure self-care agency', *Nursing Research*, vol. 40, no. 1, 12–16.

McMullin, E. 1987, 'Alternative approaches to the philosophy of science', in J. Kourany (ed.), *Scientific Knowledge: Basic Issues in the Philosophy of Science*, Wadsworth Publishing Co., Belmont, California.

Moody, L. 1990, *Advancing Nursing Science through Nursing Research*, vol. 2, Sage Publications, Newbury Park, California.

Morse, J.M. 2003, 'A review committee's guide for evaluating qualitative proposals', *Qualitative Health Research*, vol. 13, 833–51.

National Health and Medical Research Council (NHMRC) 1999, A guide to the development, implementation and evaluation of clinical practice guidelines, Australian Government Publishing Service, Canberra.

Neuman, B. (ed.) 1995, *The Neuman Systems Model*, 3rd edn, Appleton & Lange, Norwalk, Connecticut.

Newman, M. 1986, *Health as Expanding Consciousness*, National League for Nursing, New York.

Newman, M. 1994, *Health as Expanding Consciousness*, 2nd edn, National League for Nursing, New York.

Omeri, A. 1997, 'Culture care of Iranian immigrants in New South Wales, Australia: sharing transcultural nursing knowledge', *Journal of Transcultural Nursing*, vol. 8, no. 2, 5–16.

Omeri, A. 1999, 'Using culturally congruent strategies to enhance recruitment and retention of Australian nursing students', *Journal of Transcultural Nursing*, vol. 10, no. 2, 150–5.

Orem, D. 2001, *Nursing: Concepts of Practice*, 6th edn, C.V. Mosby, St Louis.

Parse, R. 1992, 'Human becoming: Parse's theory of nursing', *Nursing Science Quarterly*, vol. 5, no. 1, 35–42.

Parse, R. 1995, 'Research with the human becoming theory', in R. Parse (ed.), *Illuminations*, National League for Nursing, New York.

Pearson, A. 2002, 'Nursing takes the lead: redefining what counts as evidence in Australian healthcare', *Reflections on Nursing Leadership*, Fourth quarter, 18–21.

Pearson, A. & Field, J. 2005, 'The systematic review process', in M. Courtney (ed.), *Evidence for nursing practice*, Elsevier Churchill Livingstone, Sydney.

Pearson, A., Vaughan, B. & FitzGerald, M. 2005, *Nursing Models for Practice*, 3rd edn, Butterworth Heinemann, Edinburgh.

Pender, N. 1982, *Health Promotion in Nursing Practice*, Appleton & Lange, New York.

Pender, N. 1987, *Health Promotion in Nursing Practice*, 2nd edn, Appleton & Lange, New York.

Peplau, H. 1991, *Interpersonal Relations in Nursing: a Conceptual Frame of Reference for Psychodynamic Nursing*, G Putnam's Sons, New York.

Pryor, J., Stewart, G. & Bonner, A. 2005, 'Seeking evidence of rehabilitation in nephrology nursing', *Collegian*, vol. 12, no. 3, 20–6.

Rao, J., Elborn, S., Millar, C. & Moore, J. 2005, 'Potential increased risk of hypersensitivity pneumonitis (HP) in complementary medicine practitioners associated with handling exotic mushroom varieties', *Complementary Therapies in Clinical Practice*, vol. 11, no. 2, 76–7.

Roberts, K. 1996, 'A snapshot of Australian nursing scholarship 1993–94', *Collegian*, vol. 3, no. 1, 4–10.

Roberts, K., Brittin, M., Cook, M. & deClifford, J. 1994, 'Boomerang pillows and respiratory capacity', *Clinical Nursing Research*, vol. 3, no. 2, 157–65.

Roberts, K., Brittin, M. & deClifford, J. 1995, 'Boomerang pillows and respiratory capacity in frail elderly women', *Clinical Nursing Research*, vol. 4, no. 4, 465–71.

Rogers, M. 1994, 'The science of unitary human beings: current perspectives', *Nursing Science Quarterly*, vol. 7, no. 1, 33–5.

Rosenau, P. 1992, *Post-Modernism and the Social Sciences: Insights, Inroads and Intrusions*, Princeton University Press, New Jersey.

Rothrock, J. & Smith, D. 2000, 'Selecting the perioperative patient focused model', *AORN Journal*, vol. 71, no. 5, 1030–2, 1034, 1036–7.

Roy, C. & Andrews, H. 1991, *The Roy Adaptation Model: The Definitive Statement*, Appleton & Lange, Norwalk, Connecticut.

Sackett, D.L., Richardson, W.S., Rosenbery, W. & Haynes, R.B. 1997, *Evidence-Based Medicine: How to Practice and Teach EBM*, Churchill Livingstone, New York.

Schaefer, K. & Potylycki, M. 1993, 'Fatigue associated with congestive heart failure: use of Levine's Conservation Model', *Journal of Advanced Nursing*, vol. 18, no. 2, 260–8.

Sloman, R., Brown, P., Aldana, E. & Chee, E. 1994, 'The use of relaxation for the promotion of comfort and pain relief in persons with advanced cancer', *Contemporary Nurse*, vol. 3, no. 1, 6–12.

Smith, M., 2001, 'Analysis and evaluation of contemporary nursing knowledge: nursing models and theories', *Nursing and Health Care Perspectives*, vol. 22, no. 2, 92–3.

Streubert-Speziale, H. & Rinaldi-Carpenter, D. 2003, *Qualitative Research in Nursing: Advancing the Humanistic Imperative*, Lippincott Williams and Wilkins Philadelphia.

Taylor, B. 1994, *Being Human: Ordinariness in Nursing*, Churchill Livingstone, Melbourne.

Taylor, B. 2000, *Being Human: Ordinariness in Nursing* (adapted and reprinted), Southern Cross University Press, Lismore, NSW.

Tillett, L. 1994, 'Nola J Pender: the Health promotion model', in A. Marriner-Tomey (ed.), *Nursing Theorists and Their Work*, 3rd edn, C.V. Mosby Co., St Louis.

Toye, C. & Blackmore, A. 1996, 'Satisfaction with nursing home care of a relative: does inviting greater input make a difference?', *Collegian*, vol. 3, no. 2, 4–6, 8–11.

Walsh, M. 2000, 'Chaos, complexity and nursing', *Nursing Standard*, vol. 14, no. 32, 39–42.

Watson, J. 1979, *The Philosophy and Science of Caring*, Little, Brown & Co., Boston.

Whittemore, R., Chase, S. & Mandle, C. 2001, 'Validity in qualitative research', *Qualitative Health Research*, vol. 11, 522–37.

Yelland, J. & Sellick, K. 1988, 'Community health and hospital-based nurses: differing attitudes to self-care', *Australian Journal of Advanced Nursing*, vol. 5, no. 2, 3–7.

Young, A., Gebhardt, S. & McLaughlin-Renpenning, K. 2001, *Connections: Nursing Research, Theory, and Practice*, Mosby, St Louis.

Young Brockopp, D. & Hastings-Tolsma, M. 2003, *Fundamentals of Nursing Research*, 3rd edn, Jones and Bartlett, Boston.

Zeitz, K. & McCutcheon, H. 2003, 'Evidence-based practice: To be or not to be, this is the question!', *International Journal of Nursing Practice*, vol. 9, no. 5, 272–9.

Ziegler, S. 2005, *Theory-Directed Nursing Practice*, 2nd edn, Springer Publishing Company, New York.

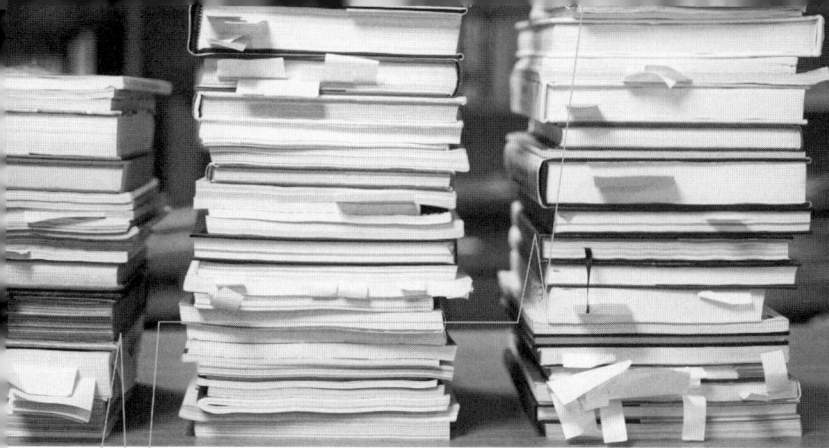

CHAPTER 2

COMPUTERS IN NURSING AND HEALTH RESEARCH

CHAPTER OBJECTIVES

The material presented in this chapter will assist you to:

- describe the basic structure and types of computers
- appreciate the need for attention to computer etiquette and legal aspects
- describe examples of indexes and how to use them
- examine means of copying and storing references
- describe ways in which computers can help you throughout the entire research project.

Introduction

This chapter describes basic computer structure and function, and the ways in which computers continue to be valuable tools in creating and storing research information. Practical hints are given on how to prepare and store files, access websites for literature and research interest group communication, and manage every step of the research process using computers. Exercises are also suggested to assist you in the practical application of the information.

Using computers in research

Computers have become an indispensable tool of the researcher. Even if you are not required to understand computers in order to carry out a research project, you will need to understand something about them if you are going to read research reports competently.

Researchers use computers in almost every phase of the research process. They use them as terminals to conduct a search of the literature and to download full text articles, to record data, and to analyse both qualitative and quantitative data; and as word processors to write the research documents and to compile bibliographies and lists of references. They even use them to design the posters with which they present their findings.

Computers have taken the hard labour out of some parts of the research process. For example, improved access to databases has simplified the identification of relevant literature. However, the use of computers has also complicated other parts of the research process, such as data analysis, as more sophisticated data analysis techniques have become the norm.

Structure of a computer

Computers are composed of innumerable components grouped into half a dozen structures: the keyboard, forgetful memory (RAM), never forgetful memory (hard disk or CD-ROM), portable memory (floppy disk), and the central processor (which takes messages from all the above and displays the result on the screen or printer or sends it to another computer linked by phone line).

What is important is how these components affect the user. The program you need to do your word processing or analyse your data will be either on your network or on the hard disk of your machine, or you may have to install it from a floppy disk or CD-ROM onto your hard disk. When you want to use the program, your central processor will grab parts of the program from the hard disk, stick bits of it into RAM, and 'run' the program. The more RAM you have, the bigger the pieces the central processor uses at any one time and the faster it will operate – up to a point. It will take the information you have keyed in initially (or stored in earlier sessions) and process it according to your instructions. As a prudent user, you will then ask the central processor to make a backup copy onto a floppy disk or CD, or your allocated memory area on the network. Next week, when the computer crashes because your cat chewed the power cord, you will not have to repeat the tedious process of rekeying in all your information.

EXERCISE

Locate how much RAM you have on your computer. Ask people how much RAM they had on the first computer they owned years ago. In what ways are computers different from how they were 15 years ago?

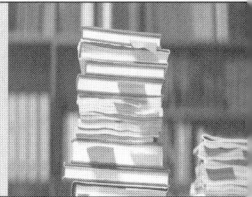

Types of computers

There are two kinds of computer: those that are hooked up to a network and those that are self-sufficient. It makes no difference whether your computer is Apple, IBM or IBM compatible: the value of what emerges from the machine depends totally on the integrity of the whole analytical process. If you are operating from a network, the choice of 'applications' (programs) available to you is probably so vast that your problem will be trying to choose the appropriate one or to find a simple version. If you are operating from your own personal computer your problem will be to choose 'software' (programs) that meets your needs and your wallet.

For the purpose of a typical research project, the basic entry-level computer these days will more than suffice. These machines have enough capacity to drive a respectable word processor and a sufficiently powerful statistical analysis program or qualitative software analysis program. To give examples without necessarily endorsing a particular product, we suggest that most basic word processor programs, such as Microsoft Word and ClarisWorks, and spreadsheet programs, such as Excel, Lotus123 or ClarisWorks, easily handle the basics of what will be discussed in this book. Such programs are usually supplied with the machine. Your word processor should be able to produce a neat research proposal or report and also have the ability to integrate graphics.

For quantitative data analysis, 'StatView' or a network version of Statistical Package of the Social Sciences (SPSS) will do anything and everything, all at once, but the interpretation is still up to the user. Here, you need the capability to draw up tables and graphs, fit regression lines, work out means, standard deviations, probabilities and Pearson correlation co-efficients and so forth, but do not worry – all will be revealed about these procedures in later chapters of the book!

For qualitative data analysis, software packages such as NUD*IST or N-Vivo or Ethnograph can be purchased that take all of the hard 'cut and paste' work out of the analysis. NUD*IST was developed in Australia and is very popular here. The NUD*IST package will analyse interviews containing many words, amounting to heaps of data.

In addition, voice-recognition programs are now beginning to be used to assist with audiotape transcription processes. This involves using the voice-recognition program to enter the data into the computer. The researcher listens to the audiotape recording and repeats it into the computer speaker, whereupon the program converts it into text. However, the technology is still not well-developed enough to make this a smooth process. Like any other program, learning the commands – which in this case can be voice-activated as well as keyboard- or mouse-activated – represents quite a lot of work. An evaluation of three different voice-recognition software programs showed that the IBM Via-Voice had a lower mean error rate than the Dragon Systems Naturally Speaking program (Devine, Gaehde & Curtis 2000).

Computers can now be used to assist with any part of the research process. However, you need to remember that no computer program substitutes for the thinking process.

Backing up

This section is not about reversing direction. It is about creating peace of mind by making duplicates of every computer file that you create. Every chapter ever written about the basics of handling documents on computer stresses the importance of backing up. This is undoubtedly because such chapters are written by people who have had some experience in the game. They may have all lost precious data. To summarise – you can never have too many backups. In the process of your research program, ask yourself: 'How much data can I afford to lose?' Think about the possibility of fire, power failure, hard disk failure, losing your briefcase with the only backup copy inside, or even theft. Even if your computer is insured and it can be replaced after theft, you cannot replace all the years of hard work you may have stored in it. Remember Murphy's (Sod's) Law: 'If anything can go wrong, it will'. Here's a corollary: 'It will go wrong at the worst possible time' – for example, the night before your assignment or thesis is due.

If what you are working on is not worth a dollar for the floppy disk (reusable almost indefinitely) or the two minutes it takes to copy it, then forget it. Even a document as simple as this chapter has been saved to disk every 10 minutes during composition and was copied to floppy disk and copied to the hard disk on another computer, all as a matter of course. You have been warned. Make an extra copy and store it in an independent place. You can consider emailing your working files to yourself from work to home or vice versa at the end of the day – they are then secure, off-site and easily retrievable; and the process is quick and inexpensive.

EXERCISE
Talk to researchers who have undertaken a PhD or large research project and ask them about the backing-up precautions they took to preserve data.

Computer etiquette

It is important when using a computer to be considerate of other researchers. One way that you can do this is to abide by the rules concerning access to your institution's machines. You should familiarise yourself with your institution's policies on the use of its computers.

Researchers often belong to a list such as 'NURSRES' whose members discuss research issues. When communicating by email, be courteous. If you belong to a list, familiarise yourself with the 'netiquette'. Most lists post out sets of guidelines to new people to help them fit in. Your fellow list members are unlikely to tolerate behaviour such as 'flaming' (destructive personal criticism). Failure to abide by the norms of behaviour on a list can lead to expulsion from the list by its owner or moderator.

Legal aspects

You should be aware of some of the **legal aspects** of communicating by electronic means. Some types of behaviour, such as defamation, can be a civil offence. A person has been sued in Australia for slandering a colleague by email. Remember that anything you distribute to a public email list can be treated as a publication.

It is also possible to commit a criminal offence when using email. Similar laws apply to email as apply to regular forms of communication, such as postal mail. Therefore, anything that is illegal to distribute through the postal system cannot legally be distributed by email. The data-handling rules concerning confidentiality and privacy of patient information also apply if the data are stored on a computer.

Supplying others with copies of software for which they need a licence is also illegal. It is as important to observe copyright regulations with regard to software. However, some software is free and distributed over the World Wide Web (WWW).

Databases and managing literature

This section describes literature **indexes**, and the mechanics of searching for and storing references, in preparation for considering the overall process of how computers can help you do your research.

Indexes

Literature is the main means by which research ideas are disseminated, debated and progressed. Each discipline usually has an index that lists the articles in most relevant journals by keyword headings. These may be cumulative indexes that do not necessarily publish abstracts, or they may be abstract indexes. Examples include Psychology Abstracts (known electronically as PsychLit), Sociological Abstracts, and ERIC (Education Resources Information Centre). There is even a dissertation index, Dissertation Abstracts International, which lists doctoral theses and has an electronic version. There are highly specific indexes such as CANCERLIT, which indexes all articles to do with cancer. The most useful index for nursing is CINAHL (Cumulative Index of Nursing and Allied Health Literature), which lists most nursing and health journals. MEDLINE, which indexes mainly medical literature but also indexes some nursing and health literature, can also be useful. The Health ROM indexes public health literature and has the full text of documents from organisations such as the NHMRC. You should ask the librarian to help you identify the most appropriate index, particularly if your topic is at all obscure. All of the relevant indexes can be accessed through a master index of databases such as FirstSearch. FirstSearch acts as a portal to the individual indexes and makes it easy to use more than one of them.

EXERCISE

Access the main index for your discipline. What other indexes may be useful for you as a researcher?

Indexes are usually a prime source of information because they index most journals that you will want to access and they are frequently updated. Articles are indexed by author and topic so you can find all articles by a particular author or authors. This can be useful if you know the authorities in the field. However, it is more likely that you will want to use the topic index to search for literature on a particular topic. In order to do this, you will need to use the keywords that you identified earlier. If you are having trouble finding information by using your keywords, it is useful to use the thesaurus function on the index. It will lead you to the exact keywords to use.

With the widespread use of computers, abstracting indexes are now exclusively on computer. Computer literature searches are effective because they are fast, accurate, current and comprehensive. They are flexible, since they allow searching by journal name and year of publication as well as by author and topic. You can exclude certain types of references, for example, non-research articles or those not written in English. You can also restrict the years of publication to those of interest to you.

With the arrival of Internet technology, the abstracting indexes are now accessible via the WWW. Modern libraries have switched over to this technology, with online computer terminal access to the databases. The databases can even be accessed from your home computer via your library web page if you are an authorised user.

Searching a database index is a fast, efficient process that you can do yourself. In addition, you can print out the results of your search, or even download it to your personal computer for printing or for inserting into an electronic reference manager. Furthermore, you can now download entire research articles from some databases and print them on your own printer. You can also have them emailed to you. You can learn details of how to use these specific methods by an orientation at your library.

There is also a growing amount of information available on the information super-highway, or 'infobahn', for example, reports by government agencies or position statements from client support groups. These can be accessed on the WWW by using programs such as Netscape. Powerful search engines such as LYCOS, YAHOO! and AltaVista will assist you to find information on any topic. It is possible to download documents to your own computer through these media. However, take care with information accessed from these sources because there is no guarantee as to its accuracy or quality, especially for research purposes. Unlike professional, refereed journals, which are subject to a peer-review process, there is no control over what is put up on the WWW.

The mechanics of searching

Essentially, the principle is that you enter the keyword or combination of keywords, and the database will list every article on that subject. For example, if you were searching for information on 'body position' and 'respiratory capacity', the search would turn up every article that had listed those two keywords. You can also search by author if you know a writer in the field. It is possible to narrow the search, for example, restricting the search to items written in English, research articles, or those from certain years only. Then, you can read through the list and mark those that you want to follow up. You can then print or download your list of marked items and go in one layer deeper, finding the abstract of each article if the index has it. Sometimes reading the abstract will rule out further searching for the article. Alternatively, you may wish to mark the reference as a key source that you must follow up. You can print each abstract separately, which gives you a very good beginning to your collection of material. You can also download the details, including abstracts, into an electronic reference manager.

EXERCISE

Spend some time becoming conversant with opening and using databases to explore their versatility in helping you access your research literature.

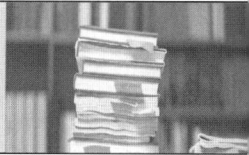

Filing your references

As your search progresses, you will build up a list of references, probably generated by a computer database and either printed as hard copy or saved onto a computer diskette for storage electronically. You may also have references from other sources, such as conference proceedings, that were not listed electronically, and which you have had to write by hand on cards or slips of paper. You need to file all references systematically. You will need to consider how you are going to organise these references. Only some of them will end up in your bibliography, but you need to keep track of all references obtained, even the useless ones. The larger the project, the more crucial it is to do this.

To organise these references, you will need some sort of filing system, which can be simple or sophisticated, cheap or expensive. Paper-based systems are the cheapest and simplest to use, but require double-handling of information. A simple, cheap system is a shoe box or plastic flip-top box with cardboard dividers and references written on pieces of paper or index cards. If you are using computer printout, separate it into individual references for filing and later assembly of relevant ones into a bibliography and put them in your filing box. Later you can assemble relevant references into a bibliography.

Much more sophisticated and efficient is the use of a word processing program on a computer. You can compile a 'library' of references which can be typed in, copied and pasted from the list of references in the electronic database, or downloaded electronically from a database. You are encouraged to use this type of system if you can because it allows you to keep a running reference system without having to write or type the details more than once.

The most technologically advanced method is to store documents electronically rather than in hard copy, but ensure that you have a backup. You can download the article directly into the computer or receive it by email if you have the authorisations from your library or you wish to pay for it. Alternatively, if you have a scanner and Optical Character Recognition

(OCR) software on your computer, you can scan your photocopied article for reading and storage. The scanner scans the entire document into the computer page by page. The OCR software then creates a word processor document on your computer that you can use as you wish, provided you obey the law. This technology is becoming more accessible and the price of scanners is decreasing. However, be warned that optical scanning technology is still not perfect and you may find you have to spend time correcting errors that the spellchecker finds on the transcribed copy. Advanced users of this technology use CD-ROM burners, which are also becoming cheaper, to store large volumes of information that they can then read from the CD-ROM. The inclusion of a CD-ROM reader as standard equipment in a computer has made this practicable. This system is obviously of great benefit as the information is then very portable from home to university and so forth. Imagine travelling around anywhere you choose with your laptop, writing your thesis or research report using your collection of references on CD-ROM and your reference manager program!

EXERCISE

What methods have you used for filing literature? What are the advantages and disadvantages of the methods described in this section?

Whatever method you use, it is usual to organise your references by author. You can use the universal 'find' facility of the word processor to find references on a particular topic in your word processor file. Once the details have been entered into your word processor, they can be cut and pasted into your reference list at the end of the word-processed report. Not only is this method more efficient, it is also more accurate because there is less opportunity to make typographical errors.

At the most complex technological end of reference management, there are computer programs such as EndNote and ProCite that allow you to keep a database of your references. You can create a 'library' of references or citations that you can insert into the word processor document of your assignment. You can keep a separate library for each topic or integrate all your references into one library. Figure 2.1 (opposite) shows you an EndNote library and Figure 2.2 shows you an individual entry of one reference into EndNote.

This system has three major advantages. First, it is efficient, since you have to enter an item into the library only once, regardless of how often you use it. Second, it is flexible, since you can insert and delete references easily and change the citation format with one command. Third, it is more accurate, since there is never a problem with mismatching citations in the document and the reference list(s). The more sophisticated programs have inbuilt capability to download items and abstracts from an electronic database, such as CINAHL, directly into your electronic library of references. This relieves you of the necessity of typing them in and eliminates transcription errors. Anyone doing a large research project would find such a program invaluable. The disadvantage is that it is relatively expensive.

There are two useful ways to organise the references: by topic or alphabetically by author. For larger projects, you may wish to have sections in your filing system in which to put items that you are obtaining on interlibrary loan or those that you find are not useful.

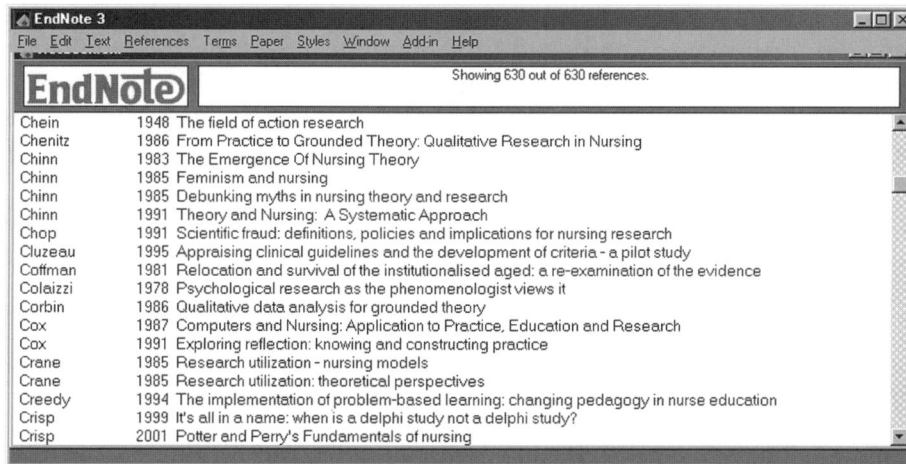

Figure 2.1 EndNote library

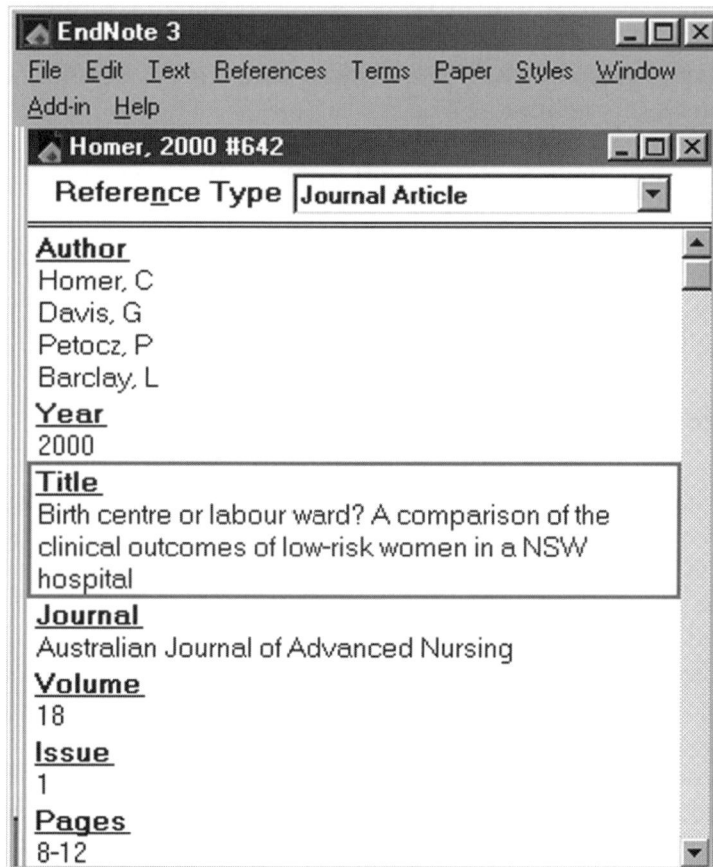

Figure 2.2 EndNote reference

Within these categories, you can still file items alphabetically by author. The author system is more useful since items may not always fit neatly into topics and referencing systems are usually author-based. Electronic systems normally index by author, but word-searching facilities enable you to retrieve items by topic. You will need to undertake lessons in how to run Endnote. These may be available through your organisation or a local distributor of the system.

Now that you have some general ideas about how to manage databases to retrieve literature and systems by which to copy and store it, it is time to consider some specific hints on how to get the best out of your computer at every step of the entire project.

Ways your computer can help you do research

Your computer will be your greatest ally when doing research, and it can be used at all stages of the research process – from working on your research question right through to producing the final write-up of your findings. The basic software on most computers is enough to carry out many research projects. Some projects, however, may require more sophisticated software. There is also a range of 'open source' or free software, which can be downloaded from the Internet to help you undertake research. If you know what you are looking for, this can be very helpful.

Preparing your proposal

Stage one in any research project is to prepare your research proposal. Most health research requires approval of an ethics committee, so it will be necessary to do a thorough job in putting the proposal together. There are a number of ways that you can use your computer to help in this area. Following are the most important points.

Performing a literature search

Chapter 4 explains the important issues involved in literature searches. In short, your computer can assist in focusing your research question, finding what research has already been done in your field of interest, and what kinds of research approaches have been used to address the problem in the past. It may even tell you if your research question is completely novel – an idea that has not previously been studied.

As mentioned previously, libraries have access to huge electronic databases of published research literature. In health research, the two most significant are Medline and CINAHL. Logging into these databases enables you to search all stored articles and books according to topic, author, keywords and a whole range of other options.

It is also useful to simply use one of the search engines available through your web browser. Search engines such as Google, LookSmart and Yahoo! can be used to look for published material in your area of interest. These can also be used to find definitions of key terms. In Google, for instance, you can type in 'define' followed by a space and the term you want defined, and it will search for definitions.

Finding an appropriate research instrument

Chapters 8 and 14 describe the issues associated with selecting approaches and instruments, which can be applied to your research question. Searching databases such as Medline and CINAHL can be useful to find what approaches and instruments may be available to you. It is also very useful to follow this up with a search using your search engine (Google, etc) to find sites that may give you access to more detailed information about these approaches or instruments.

There are sites, for instance, which specialise in one particular type of research, and which have resources and links attached to them, discussion forums and downloads available. If, for example, you were interested in grounded theory research, you would find a website available for the Grounded Theory Institute, including a specialist journal devoted entirely to this research approach.

It is also possible to find sites from which you can access specialist survey questionnaires, which can be used in your research. If, for example, you were interested in surveying the health of university students, you would find instruments that have been used extensively in the USA, which could be applied to the task. In preparing your research proposal for review by an ethics committee or a funding body, it is an advantage to use an established and well-validated instrument or approach.

Justifying your sample size

Chapter 8 describes the technical issues around selecting an appropriate sample size in quantitative research. When preparing a research proposal you will need to provide a clear rationale for the type and size of sample you have selected. In quantitative research there are specialist software packages that can help you determine what size sample you should use. Some of these are available for online calculations and some are open-source and available to be downloaded to your own computer.

Collecting your data

Once you are ready to commence the data collection stage of your research project you will find that your computer can be used in many ways. You can collect new data, extract existing data, and deliver data collection instruments through your computer. Following are examples of some of the common ways to do these.

Data mining

There are numerous web-based sources of data available to researchers. There are research organisations which make these available to other researchers for the purpose of conducting further research using these data. These organisations include the Australian Bureau of Statistics, the Australian Institute of Health and Welfare, the World Health Organisation, the Australian Social Science Data Archive, the National Center for Health Statistics (USA) and the Centers for Disease Control (USA).

EXERCISE

Locate any of the research organisations listed in this section. What kinds of information do they contain? How might this information be useful in your research?

Many researchers choose to 'mine' these databases in order to extract existing data, which can be used to answer their particular research questions. Many of these data sources are free, but some have to be purchased. There are numerous data warehouses available online. It is often a good idea to see what data already exists in these so that you are not wasting time, effort and money collecting data that may already exist.

Using email

Email is a very effective means of contacting potential participants for some research projects. It can be used to simply solicit interest in a project, or it can be used to actually deliver a survey questionnaire or establish a discussion forum for a project.

There are many online support groups for a whole range of health problems. If your research project is related to a particular disease or health problem, chances are that there is already an online support group established for sufferers of this problem.

EXERCISE

Inquire about the online support groups in your discipline that can help you in your research project. Join the group and involve yourself in the discussion.

The site administrator may allow you to make contact with the members of the group using their email list, thus allowing you to gather participants and also to deliver survey questionnaires. There are software packages, for example, Adobe Acrobat Professional, which will allow you to design an interactive form that can be attached to an email, completed by the recipient and returned to the sender. Simple forms can also be created in word processing software packages.

Conducting web-based research

One of the most cost-effective, time-effective and labour-effective means of conducting survey research is to do it online, by designing a survey questionnaire and placing it on a website.

There are various ways of doing this:

- Use a 'hosted' site on a fee-for-service basis. Do a Google (or similar) search on the term 'web based survey' and you will get dozens of commercial operators from which to choose. Some of them will let you do a free dry run with your survey using a small sample. You will need to be certain that the ethics committee approving your research will allow this. Ethics committees are usually very concerned about the security of the data that are collected, and may require you to have complete control over the database created by such research.

- Use a web-based survey package owned and operated by your own organisation. Many organisations now own and operate their own commercial survey packages for the purpose of market research, customer surveys and other research activities.
- Use a software package such as Adobe Acrobat Professional to design an online, interactive form and post it to a website.

Web-based research is very cost-effective because there are no postage, printing or telephone costs. You can deliver a hyperlink in an email message to the sample of participants you choose. When they click on the hyperlink it takes them straight to the survey site. There are no subsequent data entry costs as all responses are automatically loaded into a spreadsheet, which can be downloaded straight to your computer.

Managing and analysing your data

It is a good idea to plan in advance how you intend to store and handle your data. If you do this, you can enter and store it as you collect it. This not only saves time and effort, but also will significantly improve the analysis options and outcomes that your research produces. If you are faced with data in an unsorted and unstructured mass, then chances are that the process of 'making sense' of it will be seriously impeded. Following are some suggestions for using your computer to help store, handle and manage your data.

Handling qualitative data

There are databases designed specifically for storing and handling qualitative data. Software packages such as NUD*IST, Atlas/ti and The Ethnograph are useful for this purpose. It is also possible to use voice-recognition software to directly enter voice to computer, which eliminates the need for transcription. There is also a range of voice-recognition software packages. Such packages can be used to 'count text' to organise and link concepts and ideas and produce summaries of qualitative data.

Using spreadsheets

Every computer generally has a baseline spreadsheet package on it. Most commonly it is Microsoft Excel. If your data are quantitative you should enter and store them into a spreadsheet. It is a good idea to become familiar with the potential of your spreadsheet software, as it is generally capable of far more than most users are aware. If you examine the 'Paste Function' item in the Excel menu, for instance, you will find that it can produce a whole range of descriptive, inferential and epidemiological statistics. You may not need any more sophisticated software than this in order to complete all of your data analysis requirements. Excel is also capable of producing a range of graphs and tables from your data, which can be pasted directly into other documents.

Using specialist statistics software

If you are looking for sophisticated data analysis options to answer complex questions about quantitative data, you will need a specialist statistics software package. Such packages are essentially spreadsheet databases with far more complex analysis functions engineered into them. Most are fairly user friendly, although you will need to understand the particular functions you want them to perform in order to make sense of the output they provide you with. Packages such as SPSS, SAS, XLStat and EpiInfo are useful for such purposes. If you are a public health researcher, EpiInfo is particularly useful as it is a suite of programs, including word processing, data management and epidemiologic analysis. It allows forms design, data entry, geographical map-based output and a whole range of statistical analyses used in epidemiology.

Publishing and disseminating your findings

Once you have collected and analysed your data you will need to think about preparing the final report of your research. This may take the form of an article to be submitted to a journal, it may be a book or monograph, or it may be an in-house newsletter or bulletin for staff in your own organisation. No matter what the published outcome is, your computer will help you in this process. Following are some suggestions for using your computer to help you produce a good-quality research report.

Document preparation

The basic document preparation software is a word-processing application, which is available on all computers. Software packages such Microsoft Word can perform all of the functions necessary to produce a high-quality report. You will be able to cut and paste tables, graphs, charts, photographs and graphics into your report to enhance its appearance.

If you are presenting a manuscript for a commercial publisher you will need to pay close attention to their publication guidelines. They generally prescribe what size and style of font to use, the maximum length of the report and what to do with graphs, tables, charts and graphics. If you are self-publishing, you might consider allowing a desktop publisher to finish your document with a specialised desktop publishing application to give it a professional finish.

Reference management

All publishers have guidelines for including references and bibliographies in research reports. It is advisable to find out in advance which style they require you to use in your manuscript. Specialist reference managing software packages such as EndNote allow you to import reference details from other databases and also to enter them manually. The advantage of such applications is that they will automatically format your references according to the style parameters you require. It is a good idea when you first start on a research project to set up your reference database so that it is easy to manipulate and work with at the publication stage. There is nothing more frustrating than finishing your write-up and finding that you are missing important bibliographic details.

If you do not have access to a reference managing software package, you should collate your references as you go and keep them in a separate document so they don't accidentally become lost or unformatted. You should pick a recognised reference style and adhere to its conventions throughout your writing process. The most widely accepted styles are generally APA, Harvard and Vancouver. They differ across discipline areas, however. Science journals tend to be different to business journals, which differ from nursing journals. You can find the referencing requirements in any of these styles by doing a Google (or similar) search and logging on to any one of the many sites that describe them.

Presenting research findings at conferences

If it is your intention to present your research findings to an audience at a conference or seminar, you will need to prepare the presentation for delivery in an appropriate audiovisual software package. Probably the most commonly used package for this purpose is Microsoft PowerPoint. It runs as a slide show directly from your computer to a video projector. You can paste in text, graphics, photographs, sound and video. You can present it manually and run it while you talk along with it, or you can put it together so it runs automatically and at a prerecorded pace.

EXERCISE

Open PowerPoint and play with the possibilities of creating a slide show.

Summary

Using computers in research offers you amazing potential for managing the entire project. This chapter described basic computer structure and function, and showed how computers create and store research information. Practical hints were given on how to prepare and store files, access websites for literature and research interest group communication. Finally, practical advice was given on how to manage every step of the research process using computers.

Main points

- Researchers use computers in almost every phase of the research process.
- For quantitative data analysis, 'StatView' or a network version of Statistical Package of the Social Sciences (SPSS) will do anything and everything, all at once, but the interpretation is still up to the user.
- For qualitative data analysis, software packages such as NUD*IST, N-Vivo or Ethnograph help to analyse interviews containing 'mountains' of data.
- Backing up files creates duplicates of every computer file.
- It is important to remember etiquette when using a computer to be considerate of other researchers.
- Be aware of some of the legal aspects of communicating by electronic means, such as the risk of defamation and penalties for the illegal distribution of information.
- Each discipline usually has an index that lists the articles in most relevant journals by keyword headings.
- Indexes are usually a prime source of information because they index most journals and they are updated frequently.
- With the arrival of Internet technology, abstracting indexes are now accessible via the WWW, and modern libraries have online computer terminal access to the databases, which can also be accessed from home.
- To organise literature references a filing system is needed. This can include paper-based systems, computer printouts, word-processed bibliographies and computer programs, such as EndNote and ProCite.
- When preparing a research proposal, computers help with performing a literature search, finding an appropriate research instrument and justifying the sample size.
- When collecting data, computers help with data mining, using email and conducting web-based research.
- When managing and analysing data, computers help with handling qualitative data, using spreadsheets and using specialist statistics software.
- When publishing and disseminating findings, computers help with document preparation, reference management and presenting research findings at conferences.

CASE STUDY

You were introduced to Wendy in Chapter 1. Wendy is an experienced Registered Nurse with a Masters qualification, who works as a diabetes educator in a large rural hospital. Over many years of practice, Wendy has noticed that diabetics seem to view their disease processes and outcomes differently to the members of the multidisciplinary health team. Realising that her research interests involve the expertise of the multidisciplinary team, Wendy decided to formulate a research proposal to present to them during a team meeting. The team decided it was interested in how diabetics manage the everyday activities of living after initial adjustment to lower limb amputation. Being fairly inexperienced at using computers, Wendy asks you how she can make the best of using computers during the project. What will you tell Wendy about the usefulness of computers when:

- preparing a research proposal
- collecting data
- managing and analysing data
- publishing and disseminating findings?

Multiple choice questions

1   The part of a computer comprising the forgetful memory is the:
  a   CD-ROM
  b   RAM
  c   hard disk
  d   floppy disk

2   An example of a qualitative analysis package is:
  a   NUD*IST
  b   StatView
  c   SPSS
  d   Excel

3   PsychLit, Sociological Abstracts, ERIC, CANCERLIT, CINAHL and MEDLINE are all examples of:
  a   books
  b   software
  c   indexes
  d   backups

4   A scanner and Optical Character Recognition (OCR) software on your computer will allow you to:
  a   access research databases for literature searches
  b   analyse large amounts of qualitative research data
  c   download electronic references from a database
  d   'read' a photocopied article for perusal and storage

5   An example of an electronic reference management system is:
  a   EndNote
  b   OpCite
  c   LYCOS
  d   YAHOO!

6   Google, LookSmart and Yahoo! are examples of:
    a   research instruments
    b   computer nerds
    c   search engines
    d   refereed journals
7   When collecting research data, computers can help by:
    a   data 'mining'
    b   using email
    c   web-based research
    d   all of the above
8   A cheap, easy and effective means of entering, storing and analysing quantitative data is to use:
    a   specialist statistics software
    b   a Microsoft Excel spreadsheet
    c   Adobe Acrobat Professional
    d   SPSS, SAS, XLStat and EpiInfo
9   A high-quality report can be produced by using a word-processing application such as:
    a   Microsoft Word
    b   Excel
    c   EndNote
    d   Google
10   An audiovisual software package to prepare and present your research findings to an audience at a conference or seminar is Microsoft:
    a   Word
    b   Academic
    c   PowerPoint
    d   Office

Review topics

1   Describe the basic structure of a computer.
2   Explain how to access and use a research index.
3   Describe two ways of filing references assisted in some way by a computer.
4   Discuss how computers can help researchers perform a literature search.
5   Discuss three ways computers assist researchers in publishing and disseminating findings.

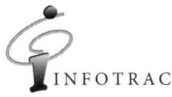

Reference

Devine, E., Gaehde, S. & Curtis, A. 2000, 'Comparative evaluation of three continuous speech recognition software packages in the generation of medical reports', *Journal of the American Medical Informatics Association*, vol. 7, no. 5, 462–8.

CHAPTER 3

THE RESEARCH QUESTION

CHAPTER OBJECTIVES

The material presented in this chapter will assist you to:

- identify people who can help you with finding research problems
- understand the usefulness of literature in finding research problems
- recognise how professional trends and research priorities influence the research area
- state the criteria for selecting research problems
- state a research problem and ask a specific research question
- refine the question, formulate an hypothesis and identify variables in quantitative research
- define an area and identify intentions in qualitative research.

Introduction

This chapter describes the formulation of a **research question,** including identifying the people, literature, professional trends and research priorities. In selecting **research problems** you will see that you need to consider factors such as the preparedness of the researcher, the difficulty, feasibility and legitimacy of the problem, and adequate resources to fund the project. This chapter also describes the process for stating a problem in quantitative and qualitative research. It differentiates between hypotheses and **variables** identification in quantitative research, and the definition and intention clarification process of a **research area** in qualitative research.

Many research projects begin with a research question that asks about a problem or issue and therefore guides the study. A clearly stated research question is essential for smooth progress through the project because it keeps the research interest in focus as it challenges, examines and analyses previous understandings while seeking new and/or amended knowledge.

EXERCISE

Write a sentence about a problem you would like to research in your health discipline. Write two questions related to that research problem.

Research problems and research questions are different, although the terms are sometimes used interchangeably. Generally, the research problem will be stated as a sentence, while the research question will be more specific and stated as a question. Sometimes, the research questions are not listed in the research report, but they are implicit in the data collection and analysis methods. For example, Fenwick, Gamble and Mawson (2003) examined the research problem of women's experiences of Caesarean section and vaginal birth after Caesarean. Although not stated as a research question, the main areas of inquiry were: What are women's experiences of Caesarean section? What are women's experiences of attempting to achieve a vaginal birth after Caesarean? These two main research questions were represented in more detail in a survey to 59 research participants containing 22 closed and open-ended questions, to which descriptive statistics and content analysis were applied as analysis methods. The researchers reported that six major factors were identified relating to the research problem and questions:

'(i) 'being supported' (ii) 'violated expectations' (iii) 'loss of control' (iv) 'health professionals' language, attitudes and care practices' (v) 'the labour experience and the cascade of interventions'; and (vi) 'surgical birth and separation from the baby' (Fenwick, Gamble & Mawson 2003, p. 10).

Beginners who are about to start a research project expect that it will be easy to find a problem to research. They are often surprised to discover that finding the right research problem can be one of the most difficult parts of the research process. The difficulties lie in the boundless number of potential research problems in health care fields and in recognising suitable research topics if you are not familiar with the research process and with previous research in the area.

Despite the difficulty in choosing a problem, a good research project clearly rests on the quality of the problem. In this chapter you will learn some sources of quantitative research problems, their criteria, how to state them, how to restate your problem as one or more hypotheses, and to identify the variables. You will also learn some sources of qualitative research problems, and explore defining an area and identifying objectives.

Finding research problems: sources and strategies
People

Your own interests are a source of research problems. You need to identify your interests and formulate a problem that reflects them, that is, a problem for which you really want to find the answer. You will be familiar with the territory and the terminology and thus be able to judge the relevance and significance of the problem.

Critical observation of practice will lead to problem formation. Just analysing the conversation in the tearoom may lead to ideas for research topics. In clinical practice, one often asks whether a particular approach is the best way to carry out an intervention. Why are procedures done a certain way? Are they based on scientific findings or on tradition or opinion? For example, how many minutes is the optimum time for handwashing before an aseptic procedure? Is the use of clean paper towels sufficient, or is it necessary to use sterile towels? You can also ask what factors encourage or discourage specific client outcomes, such as post-operative pain, and think about how you might measure the outcomes. You can listen to what your clients say or do not say during practice interactions.

Your own professional experience is a source of research problems. You can examine your own practice for observations or questions that you have asked. Look at what is happening and ask how it ought to be different. You can also ask questions about the nature and effects of phenomena and relationships in your profession. Ideas for research topics that come to you in the course of your experience are often more relevant and interesting to you than those that are remote. You may find that you have more enthusiasm for researching a problem that could have some impact on your own practice or practice setting. What has frustrated you at work? For example, St John et al. (2004, p. 211) used a case study approach to argue that 'there is a need to provide services that target community dwelling incontinence sufferers' using 'The Waterworx Model'. The researchers encouraged the use of the model to achieve greater client access, to decrease urinary incontinence and to improve client satisfaction in the community.

Your work manager, lecturer or supervisor may be a source of research problems. If you are doing an individual research project, you may find that your supervisor has a list of problems that you can tap into. In any case, your supervisor should be able to help you find a problem and discuss the implications of selecting that problem. Your supervisor will also help you to refine your general ideas into a more specific focus.

Your colleagues may be able to help you find a problem. Brainstorming with your friends and colleagues about problems they have encountered may help to clarify your ideas. Tuning into conversations on the Internet will also be a source of ideas. You can talk to colleagues at work, at professional meetings and at conferences, particularly research conferences. Listening to speakers at conferences, especially if they are leaders, can give you a feeling for the issues of the moment. The informal part of the conferences is fertile ground for the generation of new questions. Ideas and issues emanating from these situations can become research problems.

When you have identified an area of interest, talking to the expert clinicians in the field can lead you to research problems that they have identified. Such problems will probably be topical, relevant and worthwhile.

EXERCISE

In relation to the research problem and questions you listed in the previous exercise, make a list of all the people who could help you refine your ideas.

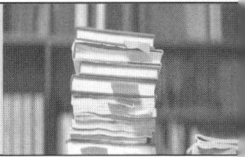

The research literature

The professional literature is a rich source of problems. Once you have examined your experience and identified your area of interest, look at the relevant research periodicals. Reading a study will often suggest ideas about how it could have been improved, and thus lead to ideas for further research. For example, Hsu et al. (2004) undertook a descriptive review of literature relating to health care staff knowledge of mental health. They determined that there

> is insufficient evidence within the literature to draw conclusions about staff knowledge levels in relation to mental health, however, the literature identified a link between continuing education, knowledge levels and staff attitudes to older people with mental disorders. Future studies are needed to investigate existing levels of mental health knowledge among health care staff in residential aged care and to identify and evaluate strategies to enhance their ability to provide care for this population (Hsu et al. 2004, p. 231).

Similarly, Street, Love and Blackford (2004) explored bereavement care in inpatient settings in Australia because the literature revealed that prior to the extension of services, 'service delivery was primarily located in community-based hospice or specialist palliative home care services' (p. 240). Changes in the system reported in literature inspired the researchers to undertake 88 semi-structured interviews with health care staff in relation to 'the provision of family-centered bereavement care in different Australian inpatient settings (p. 240).

Another source of inspiration can be the recommendations at the end of a research report. For example, Mathews, Tozer and Walker (2004, p. 251) described management responsibilities in the retirement village industry in New Zealand, and they concluded that:

> A more comprehensive survey is required, not only in order to investigate issues related to the distinctive nature of the industry, but also to better comprehend differentiating factors among the target group. Such a study would enable exploration of the impacts of the manager's role of such situational differences as the multi-purpose nature of each facility and the location and size of the facility.

This recommendation could lead the reader to plan a similar study that incorporates these recommendations in its design, by identifying the main research problem and listing specific research questions to cover the identified areas.

Sometimes, when reading through the literature, you will see certain research themes emerging. For example, professional journals may feature research undertaken in specific areas, such as in community health and aged care. Read the articles carefully and decide if you have a research interest you would like to pursue in these areas, especially if it would extend the research results already published in these professional journals.

The literature may also reveal a gap that needs to be filled. For example, Williams et al. (2004), who examined the reasons for attending and not attending a support group for recipients of implantable cardioverter defibrillators, were motivated because of a lack of Australian-specific information. They argued the need for further research by stating:

> Although previous research has provided insights into the distress that ICD insertion may cause to recipients and family members, most of this has been conducted in the United States of America (USA), using mainly quantitative methods. This type of research has not fully captured the full extent of recipients' and caregivers' perspectives, and consequently, information tailored to the Australian population of ICD recipients is limited (Williams et al. 2004, p. 128).

There may also be variations in findings that lead to the design of a study to settle the argument. For example, for some time now there has been a lot of research interest in falls in the elderly. O'Hagan and O'Connell (2005) noticed that the literature was contradictory in relation to causes of falls, such as the effects of gender and the time of day. Based on the contradictory results reported in the literature, the researchers examined the relationship between patient blood pathology values and patient falls in an acute-care setting. They undertook a 'retrospective audit of patient incident reports and medical records ... in an acute-care hospital for 220 patients who fell and did not fall' (O'Hagan & O'Connell 2005, p. 161). Hence, their idea for the research came from contradictory findings in the relevant literature.

The literature can also provide examples of studies that you may wish to replicate. Replication is repeating a study using the same methodology. Replication is generally considered to be desirable in order to verify existing findings and increase their validity by carrying out identical research with a variety of subjects in different settings. Hence, replication is most suited to quantitative research, because test and retest is encouraged, based on objective epistemological assumptions. Contrastingly, qualitative research does not favour replication, because its assumptions about knowledge are that it is relative and context-dependent, so there is no point trying to exactly replicate research into a human experience. Even so, qualitative researchers may opt to adopt many different approaches in exploring the same or similar research interests and phenomena, to achieve multiple layers of meaning that add to the richness of possibilities and insights.

However, there may be few quantitative studies published that replicate others, so the outcome is often a large number of small, unrelated studies with a limited generalisability of results. In quantitative research there is a need for more research that builds upon earlier research and addresses its limitations. Be aware, however, that originality is a requirement for research projects in many higher degrees. It is also important to realise that in some cases replication may not be seen as necessary or advisable. This is especially true if you are taking a qualitative approach, which assumes that people are unique in their respective contexts and that absolute replication is not possible. In such cases, the research would still need to be original, but not necessarily based on the research method used previously.

EXERCISE

In relation to the research problem and questions you have identified in the exercises in this chapter, access some literature through Infotrack to refine your problem/question/purpose even further.

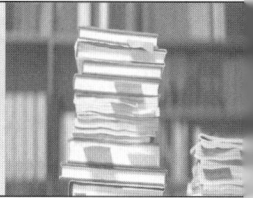

Professional trends

Major events that affect the profession can also be a source of research topics. By reading those columns of journals that deal with professional issues you can get advance warning of trends and use them to help you select a topic. One such event was the introduction of evidence-based practice worldwide. Unsurprisingly, books and journal articles directed towards members of the multidisciplinary health care team have focused on the importance of evidence-based practice (e.g. Dawes 2005; French 2002; Sackett et al. 1997). Accordingly, evidence-based practice lends itself well to research because it demands that the latest evidence from research be used in practical work in clinical situations. This means that there is a need to constantly examine ways of providing the best, most recent data and of ensuring that it finds its way into practice (e.g. Dowswell, Harrison & Wright 2001; Griffiths & Clark 2004; Zeitz & McCutcheon 2003). Other professional trends surface in professional journals from time to time, and research and scholarship ensures that they are thoroughly explored through critical debate and argumentation. Keep reading your discipline's journals to be in touch with the trends.

Identified research priorities

Research priorities that have been already identified are a useful source of problems. At a national level, governments that relay directives onto peak professional research bodies may set research priorities. For example, the Australian government may direct its health priorities to the National Health and Medical Research Council (NHMRC). In the United Kingdom the National Health Service (NHS) may inform the Medical Research Council of its research priorities. Given that the research priorities are government directives, it logically follows that funding is provided for research into these areas. Even though your research may be at a far more modest level, you can nevertheless become aware of your national research priorities and adapt a manageable project for your own research interests. In this way, even though you do not achieve large funding grants, your project can be published in professional journals that reflect the national research trends and priorities.

There are many sources of research problems if you remain open to the possibilities inherent in your work and look for them in your reading and discussion with colleagues. It is very important to get the right problem in terms of relevance, significance and feasibility. Spending time in the beginning can pay dividends by preventing the waste of time and energy involved in the selection of a problem that is unsatisfactory.

Criteria for selecting problems
The researcher

You, the researcher, must have the appropriate experience and skills to address the research problem. Frequently, research experience is related to qualifications. Beginning skills can be learned in undergraduate programs, although many undergraduate programs are now focusing on the preparation of research consumers rather than researchers. Advanced research skills are learned in research degrees, specifically honours, research masters and doctoral degrees. In advanced degrees you also begin to understand some of the assumptions that underlie the use of certain qualitative methodologies, for example, grounded theory, action research, and postmodern influences on critical feminisms.

An inexperienced researcher should select a problem that can use a simple design and instruments in quantitative projects, or a relatively uncomplicated methodology with congruent methods and processes in qualitative research. In both cases, the project for a new researcher should lead to 'easy' analytical processes, in which you are likely to experience a high degree of success and enjoyment. It is better to carry out a simple project well than do poorly in a complex one. Complicated designs requiring sophisticated measurement techniques and complex data analyses are best left to more experienced researchers. Obtuse methodologies with dense philosophies can wait until you are undertaking postgraduate research. If physical equipment is involved, or computer programs are necessary, you need to consider whether you have the technical expertise to run them.

You must have adequate knowledge of the general area you are preparing to research if you are to research it effectively. It is easier to research in an area with which you are familiar since you will already know the terminology and major ideas. For example, a physiotherapist would find it easier to do research in physiotherapy from a theoretical base of physiotherapist knowledge. Familiarity with relevant theories and concepts will assist you to plan research that is linked to theory. Knowledge of previous research in the area will also help you to select an appropriate problem to research.

You should research in an area that you are interested in and choose a problem for which you want to find the answer. This will help you to maintain enthusiasm for the project during the difficult periods. The interest factor is more important in a longer project than in a shorter one as it is more difficult to sustain interest over a longer period.

The problem

The problem selected should fall within the general area of your health discipline if it is to be considered research specific to that discipline. Be clear about what constitutes research in your discipline. Does this problem have a specific focus in your field, or is it common across the multidisciplinary spectrum? For example, a physiotherapist will need to ascertain where the boundaries lie between physiotherapy and medical research, and research in behavioural science. A rule of thumb is that if you have control over the decision-making in that area of practice, it is a suitable subject for research in your specific health care discipline. Research about client health is valid for many health disciplines. A good question to ask yourself is: 'How is this relevant to my profession?' The answer should show a link to your discipline's main foci. For example, in nursing, links can be made with nursing's major domain concepts of person, health, environment and nursing.

The importance of the research problem is also a consideration. For a beginning researcher, it need not be a problem that solves all of the important questions in the field. Nevertheless, it should be a question that is worth answering. Professional journals pay attention to significance for the specific discipline, particularly in the areas of clinical application. For example, the journal *Clinical Nursing Research* requires the author to address the question of clinical significance of the research. Since you are going to put a lot of time and effort into your study, you should select a topic that will produce findings of benefit to some person or group – the client, the health worker, the health care agency, the community or society. Will the answer to your research question have the potential to lead to improvements in client health, community health or practice? Will it lead to changes in protocols or policies in your institution? Will the study lead to the development of knowledge? Perhaps it will test a theoretical proposition or explore a new area of knowledge.

You should also consider feasibility, that is, whether the research can actually be carried out. By their very nature, some problems are difficult or impossible to research. For quantitative research you need to choose variables that can be measured using the current technology. For example, it would be impossible to assess neonates' attitudes to neonatal intensive care units, but you can collect data from their parents about their experiences. For qualitative research, the question needs to be stated broadly enough to permit a broad explanation of the phenomenon to be explored. It should also be aligned to the theoretical assumptions of how knowledge is produced through research. For example, Marquis, Freegard and Hoogland (2004) adopted an ethnographic view of family involvement in aged-care facilities, so they chose interviews to capture the culture of residential aged-care services.

Legitimacy is also a criterion. Just because a study can be carried out does not necessarily mean it should be. A research problem should not reflect a moral position. These areas involve religious beliefs, politics or ethics, so they are frequently value-laden. For example, 'Should nurses assist with euthanasia?' is not a suitable research topic because it is trying to answer a moral question, which is best answered by ethical debate rather than by research. This does not mean that value-laden, subjective areas cannot be researched. Many qualitative approaches value subjectivity and the researcher within the research process. It is a matter of eliminating the 'should' aspect of the question. Questions such as the above can be rephrased to something like 'What is the lived experience of nurses assisting with euthanasia?' or 'What are the attitudes to death of nurses who have assisted with euthanasia compared with those who have not?'

Research questions that show the researcher is biased and trying to prove a point are also unsuitable. For example, a research question such as 'Why are the graduates from University X incompetent?' indicates bias on the part of the researcher and is not a suitable research question. Such questions can frequently be rephrased, for example: 'What perception of their own competence is held by graduates of University X?'

Ethical standards are also a criterion. You should not proceed with any research project that involves harming or deceiving the subjects, coercing the subjects to participate, or exposing them to risks out of proportion to the benefits of the research. Any research project must comply with the ethical guidelines of the NHMRC and the relevant human research ethics committee(s) or it will not be approved. You can find further information about the ethics of research in Chapter 5.

EXERCISE

Review the work you have done in the exercises to refine your research problem/question/purpose. Critically analyse your decisions to see if the project is appropriate for your discipline, at the level of your research experience, feasible, legitimate, and able to be adequately resourced.

Resources

You need to be sure that you have sufficient time to carry out the project. A research project almost invariably takes longer than you expect. You need to make sure that the project itself will not consume more time than is available to complete it. You should consider the nature of the project. A collaborative process between the researcher and the participants, such as action research, will take longer than, say, a questionnaire. You should also consider the nature of the problem you are studying. For example, a study of client progress through a lengthy treatment would not be feasible if you only have one semester to carry out the project. You should also consider the time you can spend working on the project, and balance this with your other work and personal commitments. Finally, you should consider if data would have to be collected at a particular time of year or month and how that fits your schedule.

Money is also a consideration. Be sure that you can afford the project. Virtually every project has some cost attached. Some universities allocate money to students for research projects and may provide equipment such as computers and software. Hospitals may also have a research budget for focused clinical projects. However, they do not usually support the costs of expensive student projects. You should clarify at the outset the amount of financial support that will be provided. If the amount available from the university or health care facility, your own funds and other sponsors is not sufficient, you will need to rethink the project and scale it down to a more realistic level or choose another topic.

In deciding whether or not you can afford a project, consider its real costs, the budget available and the cost–benefit ratio. Before making a final decision, make a list of all projected expenses, including an adjustment for price rises. There will probably be costs for obtaining literature, including photocopying, computer searches, books and journal subscriptions. For carrying out the project, you may need stationery and other consumables such as printer cartridges. You may need to pay the participants in your project under conditions agreed to by an ethics committee. If you are doing a postal survey, postage (including return postage for questionnaires) will be a major cost. Printing questionnaires and self-addressed envelopes will also be significant costs, as will audiotapes if you are doing field research involving interviews. You may need to rent or purchase equipment such as tape recorders, video cameras, computers or instruments if they are not available through your institution. You may need to hire labour for data collection and management. If your project involves travel, you will have transportation, accommodation and possibly living costs to consider. You may also have communication costs such as telephone calls and faxes. For the data analysis stage, you may need to purchase computer software or hire specific services. For the writing-up stage, you will need more stationery and consumables. There is no such thing as free or no-cost research!

In selecting a problem, you must consider the people you will need to help you undertake the project. For example, there may be gatekeepers who can give or withhold permission to enter facilities for data collection. You will need to secure permission from gatekeepers before undertaking the project, at the problem formation stage. The gaining of administrative support is one of the highest priorities when beginning research in clinical settings. If you are employed in a clinical facility, you may need to negotiate with the authorities for the use of the facilities or for time off to carry out the project.

Availability of the people that you need to study for the research is an important consideration. Your being convinced of the value of your research does not mean that people will be queuing up to help you with it. Clinical research is notorious for subjects/participants disappearing. When you get out in the field you may find that you cannot locate enough people who meet the criteria for participating in your study, particularly if they are unusual. Potential participants may be geographically difficult to access, in the case of Aboriginal people in remote areas, or they may be hard to find, for example, illegal injecting drug users. Sometimes people may already be involved in other studies and will not have the time for involvement in two studies, or their participation in one study precludes their taking part in another. Even if potential participants are eligible, they may be unwilling to help, especially if there is any discomfort involved. Fear of unwanted consequences may make some people afraid of talking to a researcher on sensitive topics such as criminal behaviour or domestic violence. Sometimes people just do not trust a researcher, for example, elderly people may not be willing to sign a consent form because relatives have told them not to sign any documents.

There can also be procedural difficulties with accessing participants. For example, if the proposed participants are children, parental consent is required. The authorities and medical staff in the clinical facilities must agree that your study can take place. In addition, you will need to go through the appropriate channels for approval in your institution, such as your supervisor, the human research ethics committee, and all the other required committees.

Stating the problem/question/purpose of the study

It is normal for there to be a general statement of **research purpose**, or aim of the study. This is usually found near the beginning of the study and sets out concisely, in broad terms, what the study hoped to accomplish, or its goals and aims. Its purpose is to orient the reader to the study. For example, Griffiths and Taylor (2005, p. 112) make it clear that the aim of their project was:

> to describe the lived experience of acupuncture treatment, with specific objectives to: inform nurses of people's experiences of having acupuncture; give nurses the language to explain to patients the experience of having acupuncture; and create possibilities for offering acupuncture as an informed choice of treatment in nursing and health care.

The more specific problem or question that the study seeks to answer can be stated either as a declarative statement or a question. Stating it as a question helps you to clarify exactly what it is that you want to find out. For example, Fok and Tsang (2005, p. 192) examined the drug utilisation patterns of Hong Kong Chinese adults, so their objectives for the pilot study were:

- to develop a tool for collecting the patterns of drug use of Hong Kong Chinese adults
- to conduct a pilot study on the use of the tool and modify it, if necessary, for future development and use.

From these objectives we are left in no doubt that the researchers are in the beginning stages of a larger project and that they are setting the foundations for further extensive data collection.

One way of structuring a research question to ensure that it is as comprehensive as possible is to divide it into a stem, which is the 'who, what, when, where or why' part of the question, and a topic, which is what the question is about. You can draft the problem/question/purpose by making spontaneous responses to the questions: Who is involved in the research as participants? What is the area of interest? When is the research to be undertaken? Where is the research to be undertaken? Why is the research to be undertaken? Clear and direct answers to these simple questions will give you the basis of posing a research problem/question/purpose.

The process

The first step in formulating a research question is either to brainstorm topics or to make a list of potential topics, using the sources given earlier in this chapter. Write down your ideas on paper, a whiteboard or computer and play with them. Then select what seems to you the best idea and discuss it with colleagues, your supervisor or experts in the field. Evaluate the topic in terms of the criteria given previously, then narrow it down to a feasible topic. Finally, write a statement of purpose and then state your research problem as a question or set of questions. During this process you will be reading the literature to become an expert on the topic and this will help you with the formation of relevant research questions.

Once the research problem and its consequent question or questions have been formulated, you will need to refine them. Frequently, the initial question is too broad and beyond the limits of a feasible study, making it necessary to narrow down the problem until you have a research question that you can undertake. The narrowing-down process can relate to the topic or the setting for the research. You can narrow the topic by removing its less important parts. Alternatively, you can narrow the number of settings in which you will conduct the study, or the types of participants you include. It may be necessary to restrict the topic in several dimensions. Suppose you want to investigate the impact of managed care plans on nursing outcomes. To look at all kinds of care plans in all types of hospitals and for all types of clients would clearly be a lifetime's work, so you have to narrow down the topic to a few outcomes for one type of client in one type of hospital.

Stating an hypothesis and identifying variables in quantitative research

If you are undertaking quantitative research, once you have stated your problem you need to develop an **hypothesis** that will give you a working basis for investigation. Although stating an hypothesis might seem difficult at first glance, it is not. Basically, an hypothesis is only a statement of what the researcher thinks is going to be the outcome of the investigation. Another definition for hypothesis is that it is 'the formal statement of the expected relationship or relationships between two or more variables in a specified population' (Burns & Grove 2005, p. 159). We formulate hypotheses all the time, although we may not recognise them. For instance, we may say 'Every time I forget my umbrella it rains'. This could be restated as a research hypothesis: 'On the days when I forget to take my umbrella, it is more likely to rain than on days when I remember to take it'.

In a quantitative research project it is customary to formulate a formal research hypothesis that speculates about the relationship between two variables. In order to be an hypothesis it must state a possible relationship, and it must have at least two variables that enter into the relationship.

A variable, as its name suggests, is something that varies. In the example above there are two variables: whether I forget or remember my umbrella, and whether or not it rains. The variable that can be controlled by the researcher is called the independent variable. The variable that cannot be controlled by the researcher, or the variable that is hypothesised to be affected by the independent variable, is the dependent variable. It is helpful to think of the dependent variable as the outcome variable. In the example above, you could think of the weather as the dependent variable, and the remembering of the umbrella as an independent variable. However, this is not strictly correct as you are not manipulating your memory. In instances where the researcher does not control the independent variable, it is more correct to speak of research variables than of independent and dependent variables.

Research hypotheses can be stated as directional hypotheses, meaning that the researcher is speculating about the direction that the findings will take. In order to do this, the researcher must have some grounds for stating a direction. These can consist of a theoretical prediction, previous research findings or a logical argument.

Even when you express a directional hypothesis, it is usually converted to a null hypothesis because, in statistical analysis, it is customary to try to demonstrate that you reject the statement that there is no difference in the groups, rather than saying that there is a difference. This will be discussed further in Chapter 10.

Each hypothesis should be able to be tested, or it is not an hypothesis. Also, each hypothesis should deal only with one relationship and one set of variables. However, a study may have more than one hypothesis being tested.

Variables are, as stated above, the parts of an hypothesis that vary. They should be defined in terms of the concept that they measure. Variables should also be stated in terms of how they are going to be measured, which is not always stated in the hypothesis itself. For example, if you were going to measure blood pressure, you should state whether you are measuring it with a sphygmomanometer, or with a direct sensor in the blood vessel.

In a further example, Edwards et al. (2005, p. 169) reported on 'pilot study results from a randomized controlled trial to determine the effectiveness of a community-based "Leg Club" environment on improving the healing rates of venous leg ulcers'. A 'Leg Club' is a supportive social environment in which people with leg problems can meet and share information. The researchers' hypothesis was that 'clients who receive the Community Leg Club intervention will have improved ulcer healing rates compared to those who do not receive the intervention' (p. 171). To minimise high degrees of variation in variables, subjects were selected based on specific criteria, such as the location and severity of the ulceration, and then divided randomly into the intervention and control group. The details of the research are discussed in full in the research article. The researchers have made their research procedures as clear and transparent as possible to ensure that their research design and results are open to professional scrutiny and critique, to allow judgements relating to rigour. Many of these areas relating to quantitative research are described in Chapters 7 to 11 of this book.

To this point, this chapter has described some general ideas in stating a research problem/question/purpose and it has shed some light on the process for doing this, with particular interest in developing an hypothesis and identifying variables in quantitative research. As you may remember from Chapter 1, there are many differences in quantitative and qualitative research assumptions, methods and processes, so the next part of this chapter looks specifically at how to define an area and identify objectives in qualitative research.

Defining an area and identifying intentions in qualitative research

Qualitative research is based on particular assumptions about the nature of knowledge, such as the uncertain nature of 'truth' and claims to be 'truthful', how knowledge is generated and how it is judged to be trustworthy. For further information on the epistemological assumptions of qualitative research, turn to Chapters 1, 12 and 14. In tune with its epistemological assumptions, qualitative researchers would not deign to state an hypothesis or even try to anticipate the variables in a question about human experience. Rather, the beginning of a qualitative project begins most often with defining a research area and identifying research objectives. The reason for stating that a project 'begins most often' is that there is no 'hard and fast rule' in qualitative research, given that it varies so markedly through the various forms of qualitative interpretive and critical research. Added to these variations, postmodern influences give research an extremely relative quality that defies standard rules about beginning a project.

When defining an area for research, qualitative researchers typically begin with all of the preliminaries mentioned in this chapter, including exploring sources and strategies such as people, literature, professional trends and research priorities. They also consider the criteria for selecting problems, such as researcher readiness, what problem to select and the money needed to make the project manageable. However, at the point of stating the problem/question/purpose of the study, they can diverge in various directions according to the particular qualitative approach they are taking.

If researchers are taking a qualitative interpretive approach, such as an historical, grounded theory, ethnographic or phenomenological approach (see Chapter 12), the beginning part of the project may look fairly 'standard', in that there will be a clear statement of intent as to the general area to be explored and the specific aims or objectives to be fulfilled. For example, Fiveash and Nay (2004, p. 192) used a grounded theory approach in their research and stated clearly that 'the purpose of this study was to identify how healthcare clients achieve and maintain a sense of control over their health'. They also stated that they set out to 'verify [an] identified shortfall in the literature' (p. 193). Another example is research undertaken by Marquis, Freegard and Hoogland (2004, p. 179), who stated the 'purpose of this study was to discover the key factors influencing positive family involvement in aged care'. Both examples state broad intentions as an indication of what researchers are exploring. Unlike quantitative researchers, they do not state an hypothesis or list variables, because the research areas are unexplored and qualitative researchers are open to what might emerge during the project.

If researchers are taking a qualitative critical approach, such as an action research, feminist or critical ethnographic approach (see Chapter 13), the beginning part of the project may vary markedly. For example, action research often requires research participants to work with the researcher as co-researchers, and the problem/question/purpose of the project emerges within group processes as the research evolves collaboratively. The general objectives of the research to form an action research group to work on practice issues are revisited within the research group when the thematic concern (issue) has been identified. The following example shows you how the process evolves in an action research project.

Taylor (2001) reported on a project entitled: 'Identifying and transforming dysfunctional nurse–nurse relationships through reflective practice and action research'. The project aimed to facilitate reflective practice processes in experienced Registered Nurses (RN) in order to: raise critical awareness of practice problems; work systematically through problem-solving processes to uncover constraints; and improve the quality of care given by nurses in light of the identified constraints and possibilities. Twelve experienced female RNs working in a large Australian rural hospital shared their experiences of nursing during three action research cycles. A thematic concern of dysfunctional nurse–nurse relationships was identified, as evidenced in bullying and horizontal violence. The negotiated action plan was put into place and co-researchers reported varying degrees of success in attempting to improve nurse–nurse relationships. This project confirmed the necessity for reflective practice and continued collaborative research processes in the workplace to bring about a cultural change within nurses' collectives and in the places in which they work which weigh against mutual respect and cooperation in nurse–nurse relationships.

Even though the previous research project began with broad intentions to involve nurses in action research to improve their practice, the research participants decided on the direction of the project once it was under way. This means that qualitative researchers may 'facilitate' research processes and allow participants to direct the project according to their own needs; thus it becomes practical and useful for participants/co-researchers.

In research influenced by postmodern ideas there may be relatively little structure at the outset of the project. Researchers may state very broad intentions as a problem statement and thereafter leave the direction and flow of the project open to what might eventuate for the participants and the researcher. Therefore, we may see a research problem/question/ purpose being located anywhere along a continuum from a highly structured and objective quantitative approach of stating an hypothesis and variables, through the less structured and subjective forms of problem definition and statement of intentions in qualitative interpretive and critical research, to the extreme relativist and subjective forms of free form, open-ended research influenced by postmodern thinking.

Summary

This chapter described the formulation of a research question, including identifying the people, literature, professional trends and research priorities to help you. In selecting research problems you need to consider various factors, such as how prepared you are as a researcher, the difficulty, feasibility and legitimacy of the problem, and whether you have adequate resources to fund the project. This chapter also described the process for stating a problem in quantitative and qualitative research. In quantitative research you need to state an hypothesis and decide on variables. In qualitative research you must define an area and clarify your research intentions.

Main points

- A clearly stated research question is essential for smooth progress through the project, keeping the research interest in focus as it challenges, examines and analyses previous understandings, while seeking new and/or amended knowledge.
- Your own work interests are a source of research problems and critical observation of practice will lead to problem formation.
- The professional literature is a rich source of problems, because reading a study will often suggest ideas about how it could have been improved, and thus lead to ideas for further research.
- Evidence-based practice lends itself well to research because there is a need to constantly examine ways of providing the best, most recent data and of ensuring that it finds its way into practice.
- Even though your research may be at a fairly modest level, you can become aware of your national research priorities and adapt a manageable project for your own research interests.
- An inexperienced researcher is advised to select a problem that can use a simple design and instruments in quantitative projects, or a relatively uncomplicated methodology with congruent methods and processes in qualitative research.
- Frequently, the initial research question/problem/area is too broad and beyond the limits of a feasible study, making it necessary to narrow down the problem until you have a research question that you can undertake.
- If you are undertaking quantitative research, once you have stated your problem you need to develop an hypothesis that will give you a working basis for investigation.
- Variables are the parts of an hypothesis that vary, that should be defined in terms of the concept that they measure and stated in terms of how they are going to be measured.
- Qualitative researchers would not deign to state an hypothesis or anticipate the variables in a question about human experience. Rather, the beginning of a qualitative project begins most often with defining a research area and identifying research intentions/objectives.
- A research problem/question/purpose may be located anywhere along a continuum from a highly structured and objective quantitative approach of stating an hypothesis and variables, through the less structured and subjective forms of problem definition and statement of intentions in qualitative interpretive and critical research, to the extreme relativist and subjective forms of free form, open-ended research influenced by postmodern thinking.

Case study

Maxwell, aged 45 years, has been practising physiotherapy for 20 years and in that time, added to qualifications in physiotherapy, he has completed a Master of Business Administration. He is now at a point in his career where he is ready to contemplate PhD studies through his local regional university, which has professional and academic links with a large city teaching hospital and university. Before he approaches the university director of research, he needs to spend some time thinking about a possible research problem and associated questions. Although he had a traditional undergraduate education focusing on muscles and mobility, he is also interested in integrated forms of physiotherapy that are open to holistic models of health and wellness. As it has been some time since his last postgraduate studies experience, Maxwell realises that he must take a systematic approach to exploring the possibilities for deciding on his research problem.

Maxwell asks you for help in how to proceed. What will you advise him in relation to:

- locating sources and strategies
- deciding on researcher, problem and resource criteria?

Maxwell decides that he will adopt a quantitative approach to his project and that he is interested in the extent to which complementary therapies have influenced clients' help-seeking behaviours in attending 'orthodox' physiotherapist services. He suspects that the decline in attendance at his physiotherapy clinic may be due to clients preferring to seek naturopathic services and/or to self-medicate with herbal therapies.

1 How can he pose this research interest as an hypothesis?
2 Identify the dependent and independent variables in the hypothesis.

Multiple choice questions

1   A research problem will usually:
   a   be stated as a sentence
   b   be an explicit query
   c   state an hypothesis
   d   describe the participants

2   Which of the following people can influence your choice of a research problem:
   a   lecturers
   b   colleagues
   c   clients
   d   all of the above

3   A professional trend that could be an area for research:
   a   is specific to the discipline
   b   is common to all disciplines

c reviews disciplinary history

d has no disciplinary relevance

4 Which of the following is a legitimate research question?

    a Should health care workers become personally involved with clients?

    b Does frequent handwashing decrease cross-infection rates in hospitals?

    c Should health care workers support termination of pregnancy procedures?

    d Should clients who smoke be denied access to coronary bypass operations?

5 The first step in formulating a research question is to:

    a decide as soon as possible and access participants

    b brainstorm topics or make a list of potential topics

    c wait until someone assists you with possible ideas

    d narrow down the topic and the number of participants

6 Stating an hypothesis in quantitative research involves:

    a asking a question about what the researcher wants to know about the outcome of the investigation

    b making a broad statement about the research area and allowing participants to direct the investigation

    c asking people and reading literature to decide on the areas to be included in the investigation

    d making a statement of what the researcher thinks is going to be the outcome of the investigation

7 The variable that can be controlled by the researcher is called the:

    a dependent variable

    b extraneous variable

    c independent variable

    d outcome variable

8 In a research question, the stem identifies the:

    a hypothesis

    b variables

    c person or object being researched

    d relationship statement

9 Qualitative researchers do not state an hypothesis or try to anticipate the variables in a question about human experience because qualitative research:

    a does not have the credibility and rigour of quantitative research and therefore it cannot hope to achieve scientific standards of excellence

    b is based on particular assumptions about the nature of knowledge, such as the uncertain nature of 'truth' and how knowledge is generated and verified

    c is favoured by researchers, who do not understand mathematics, so they avoid statistics and undertake language-based approaches

    d is more progressive than quantitative research, in that it has moved with the times and made paradigmatic shifts towards postmodern thinking

10   A research problem/question/purpose:
   a   requires the clear statement of dependent and independent variables contained within an hypothesis, for it to have scientific legitimacy
   b   must define a broad area and identify intentions, leaving the direction and flow of the project to the co-researchers
   c   is unnecessary because postmodern thinking has freed up all research, allowing it to be highly relative, creative and evolutionary
   d   may be located anywhere along a continuum from quantitative approaches, to qualitative interpretive and critical approaches, to research influenced by postmodern thinking

Review topics

1   Differentiate between a research problem and a question.
2   Describe how people, literature, professional trends and research priorities can help you to decide on a research problem/area.
3   Discuss why funds, however small, are needed for research.
4   Discuss why a statement of aim or purpose is necessary at the beginning of a project.
5   Discuss how quantitative and qualitative research differs in stating research problems/questions/purposes.

Online reading

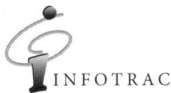

INFOTRAC

INFOTRAC® COLLEGE EDITION
When accessing information use the following keywords in any combinations you require to retrieve information relating to your health profession's areas of research and quantitative and/or qualitative research:

➤ hypotheses areas
➤ priorities
➤ problems
➤ purposes
➤ questions
➤ trends
➤ variables

References

Burns, N. & Grove, S. 2005, The *Practice of Nursing Research: Conduct, Critique, and Utilization*, 5th edn, Elsevier Sanders, St Louis.

Dawes, M. 2005, 'Evidence-based practice', in M. Dawes, P. Davies, A. Gray, J. Mant, K. Seers, & R. Snowball, *Evidence-Based Practice: A Primer for Health Care Professionals*, 2nd edn, Elsevier Churchill Livingstone Edinburgh.

Dowswell, G., Harrison, S. & Wright, J. 2001, 'Clinical guidelines: attitudes, information, processes and culture in English primary care', *International Journal of Health Planning and Management*, vol. 16, 107–24.

Edwards, H., Courtney, M., Finlayson, K., Lewis, C., Lindsay, E. & Dumble, J. 2005, 'Improved healing rates for venous leg ulcers: pilot study results from a randomized controlled trial of a community nursing intervention', *International Journal of Nursing Practice*, vol. 11, no. 4, 169–76.

Fenwick, J., Gamble, J. & Mawson, J. 2003, 'Women's experiences of Caesarean section and vaginal birth after Caesarean: a birthrites initiative', *International Journal of Nursing Practice*, vol. 9, no. 1, 10–17.

Fiveash, B. & Nay, R. 2004, 'Being active supports client control over health care', *Contemporary Nurse*, vol. 17, no. 3, 192–203.

Fok, M. & Tsang, W. 2005, 'The drug utilization patterns of Hong Kong Chinese adults', *Complementary Therapies in Clinical Practice*, vol. 11, no. 3, 190–9.

French, P. 2002, 'What is the evidence on evidence-based nursing? An epistemological concern', *Journal of Advanced Nursing*, vol. 37, 250–7.

Griffiths, M. & Clark, J. 2004, 'Managing the local agenda: Planning to get research/evidence-based care into practice', in C. Clifford & J. Clark (eds), *Getting Research into Practice*, Churchill Livingstone, Edinburgh.

Griffiths, V. & Taylor, B. 2005, 'Informing nurses of the lived experience of acupuncture treatment: a phenomenological account', *Complementary Therapies in Clinical Practice*, vol. 11, no. 2, 111–20.

Hsu, M., Venturato, L., Moyle, W. & Creedy, D. 2004, 'Mental health knowledge in residential aged care: A descriptive view of the literature', *Contemporary Nurse*, vol. 17, no. 3, 231–9.

Marquis, R., Freegard, H. & Hoogland, L. 2004, 'Influences on positive family involvement in aged care: an ethnographic view', *Contemporary Nurse*, vol. 16, no. 3, 178–86.

Mathews, M., Tozer, L. & Walker, R. 2004, 'Management responsibilities in the retirement village industry: a New Zealand study', *Contemporary Nurse*, vol. 17, no. 3, 251–60.

O'Hagan, C. & O'Connell, B. 2005, 'The relationship between patient blood pathology values and patient falls in an acute care setting: a retrospective analysis', *International Journal of Nursing Practice*, vol. 11, no. 4, 161–8.

Sackett, D.L., Richardson, W.S., Rosenbery, W. & Haynes, R.B. 1997, *Evidence-Based Medicine: How to Practice and Teach EBM*, Churchill Livingstone, New York.

St John, W., Wallis, M., James, H., McKenzie, S. & Guyatt, S. 2004, 'Targeting community-dwelling urinary incontinence sufferers: a multidisciplinary community-based', *Contemporary Nurse*, vol. 17, no. 3, 211–22.

Street, A., Love A. & Blackford, J. 2004, 'Exploring bereavement care in inpatient settings', *Contemporary Nurse*, vol. 17, no. 3, 240–50.

Taylor, B.J. 2001, 'Identifying and transforming dysfunctional nurse-nurse relationships through reflective practice and action research', *International Journal of Nursing Practice*, vol. 7, no. 6, 406–13.

Williams, A., Young , J., Nikoletti, S. & McRae, S. 2004, 'Reasons for attending and not attending a support group for recipients of implantable cardioverter defibrillators and their carers', *International Journal of Nursing Practice*, vol. 10, no. 3, 127–33.

Zeitz, K. & McCutcheon, H. 2003, 'Evidence-based practice: To be or not to be, this is the question!', *International Journal of Nursing Practice*, vol. 9, no. 5, 272–9.

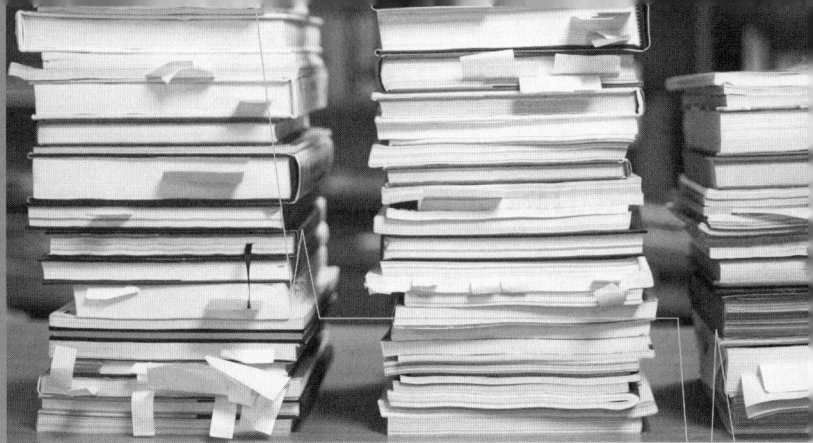

CHAPTER 4

REVIEWING THE LITERATURE

CHAPTER OBJECTIVES

The material presented in this chapter will assist you to:

- understand why you should review the literature
- locate possible sources of relevant literature
- set up an efficient system for keeping track of sources
- identify the literature that is pertinent to the project
- obtain the identified literature
- effectively read the literature that has been obtained
- extract the relevant information from the literature
- critique research reports
- set up an efficient system for dealing with references.

Introduction

The **literature** is the total body of writing that deals with the topic being researched. It comprises theoretical and research papers, together with any other relevant material. It may include books, articles in periodicals, conference proceedings, unpublished papers and personal communications from other researchers.

The term **review of the literature** has several meanings. In the sense of the act of reviewing the literature, it means to read, sort and analyse the work, putting it into some kind of order. It also involves critiquing individual research reports. These are the two senses of 'review of the literature' that we will deal with in this chapter. In the sense of the outcome of reviewing the literature, the phrase means that section of a paper, thesis or dissertation that presents an integrated evaluation of previous theory and research. How you go about writing a literature review will be dealt with in Chapter 6.

Beginning researchers often find the thought of dealing with the literature to be quite overwhelming, particularly when it is on a topic that has been well researched. It may seem an impossible task not only to read and understand all the literature, but to also critique it and organise it into a sensible framework. Nevertheless, it is essential to acquire, read and make sense of all relevant research on the topic. Researchers must understand the work that has gone before if they are to know how and where their study will fit into the overall work and add to the body of knowledge.

Why review the literature?

A beginning researcher may wonder why it is necessary to review the literature. It might seem more effective simply to decide what you want to research and then go and do it. However, reviewing the literature helps you develop a comprehensive understanding of the topic, making you aware of what is known and what questions need to be answered. This can help you to decide exactly what to research and how to go about it.

Familiarity with the body of literature on a topic will help you to identify how your proposed study will fit into the body of literature already available. For example, you might discover that the question you wanted to answer has already been researched using a particular theoretical framework.

Reviewing the literature can also help you to narrow down the topic for your study. In reading the literature, you may see that your topic is too broad and would entail too many areas of investigation. Knowing the literature can help you select a facet of the topic that would be beneficial to study and that can be kept within realistic bounds.

Reviewing the literature can also help you with the design of your study. By exposure to the approach used by previous researchers investigating the area, you can see the nature of the designs chosen, for example, experimental, phenomenological or historical. You would find that homelessness has usually been studied using interview and fieldwork because it is impossible to contact the homeless through survey methods such as postal questionnaires.

Reviewing the literature can also help you with the details of the study's methodology. You will be able to see the specifics of the previous designs, how they related to their theoretical frameworks, how the data were collected and how they were analysed.

You should be aware that in some qualitative approaches, justification is given for not reviewing the literature prior to the study. In some qualitative research approaches, such as grounded theory, it is not appropriate to do more than a superficial reading of the literature in order to identify whether the topic needs to be studied. This will be discussed in Chapter 12.

Identifying relevant literature

The first step in reviewing the literature is to identify possible sources. An enormous amount of information is readily available, and even the identification of information can be time-consuming. It is important to understand the process of identifying relevant literature and to use that process efficiently in order to select only that which bears directly on your topic. This approach will minimise the amount of work involved.

Preparing to search

Before heading off to the library, it is important to organise your search. Being systematic in both searching and record-keeping is the key to an efficient search. Even if you think you have a small topic that requires little organisation, it is important to get into good habits of searching and record-keeping that will become second nature to you. Not only will these habits stand you in good stead in simple projects, they will be useful for non-research projects and for larger research projects, should you progress to them.

EXERCISE

If you are not usually overly systematic in your approach to your work, how can you engender an organised and systematic approach to reviewing literature? In what ways will you need to change to become more diligent in developing systematic research habits?

You need to start by defining your topic in sufficient detail to enable you to find the relevant information. In previous chapters, we looked at how you select, narrow and refine your topic. By now, you should have a good idea of the keywords that define your topic. It is essential to know these so that you can use them as terms under which to search.

Beginning researchers often wonder when to search for material. For quantitative research, you will always search at the beginning of the project. If it is a longer project, say a year, you will search at the end as well in order to make sure that you have included the latest information. If it is a very long project, such as a major thesis, you will need to do a top-up search at least every six months. This is not difficult using electronic media.

For qualitative research, there is a different approach to timing the review of the literature. You may choose not to review the literature before undertaking a study because it can narrow a study too early and too much, causing you to miss important observations.

You may choose to review the literature as the study progresses so that you can see what others are doing, or wait until the end. The problem with the latter approach is that you may spend much time and energy finding what is already known. A middle ground is to read the literature for highlights of major findings and theories only, thus achieving an informed stance but still remaining open to possibilities.

Setting boundaries to the search

Beginning researchers often find it difficult to decide how much to search and frequently under-estimate the amount of time it takes to do a search. How much to search will depend on your experience, searching skills and financial resources. You should normally spend no more than one-quarter of your time reviewing the literature. It is important to search enough to be sure that you have found all of the relevant information but not to search so much that you are in danger of sinking under the weight of information. You should not spend so much time reading that you never carry out the research project. On the other hand, if you do not spend enough time reading you may miss important information. The extent of your reading depends partly on how much information is available on your exact topic. If there is not very much, it may be necessary to read related material. If there is a lot, it may be necessary to narrow the topic. Difficulty in locating sources can also influence the amount of time available for reading.

It is best to begin at the most current references and work your way back until you cannot find any more. If the topic is new, then it may not be necessary to go back very far. For instance, the topic of AIDS was unheard of before 1980. If the topic is in and out of vogue, then beware of stopping the search prematurely as there may be more information in earlier years. As a rule of thumb, 10 years is a reasonable period to search, with those papers leading you to previously published 'classics' which should be included.

Another factor that affects the extent of your search is your reason for doing it. If you are a student undertaking a brief undergraduate project, your lecturer should not expect you to have every reference ever written on the topic; a dozen main papers will normally be sufficient. At the other end of the spectrum, a PhD thesis will normally require an extremely thorough review of the literature. The higher up the academic ladder you climb, the more comprehensive and exacting will be your review of the literature. A world expert on a topic will be thoroughly conversant with the literature on that topic.

EXERCISE

How can you ascertain the scope of a research project? What will you do if you suspect the expectation for the scope of the literature review is beyond the level of the course you are undertaking?

Financial constraints can also have a bearing on how much you search. While sources close to home are reasonably cheap to photocopy, it is expensive to acquire material on interlibrary loan. Often, universities have funds dedicated to interlibrary loan materials for students, so check with your supervisor or lecturer about sources of money for this purpose. Hospital libraries may have financial arrangements to assist you as an employee.

Your own expertise in searching can also be an important factor. Students just beginning to learn about research will not be as skilled at uncovering sources or using other resources.

Sometimes it is necessary to narrow either the scope of the literature review or the topic reviewed. If the topic is producing too much literature, it may be too complex and you should narrow it to make it more manageable. You may be reading non-research material that does not belong in a literature review. If so, you should narrow your search to look only at actual research papers and exclude non-research material or, at most, read it for background information. It is important to identify the boundaries of your search. Sometimes a diagram or flow chart of the topic and design is helpful to identify the limits of the literature review.

Possible resources
Who can help you?

We tend to think of literature resources as paper-based or electronic, but it is important to remember that there are people who can be of great assistance and who are often happy to help students. First, if it is a class project, consult your lecturer. Lecturers have almost invariably done research themselves, or they would not be assigning you a research project. Frequently they will help you to narrow down the topic or point you in the direction of some appropriate resources. Before you consult them, make sure you have thought through the topic somewhat and can talk about it. If it is a thesis or dissertation, you should consult your supervisor frequently, as it is part of their job to assist you in this way.

Second, consult your colleagues. They may have some material on the subject. Also, if they know you are interested in a topic, they may keep their eyes open for information for you. They can also help you to talk through the topic and may give you ideas or a perspective on the topic that you had not thought of. Electronic mail allows researchers to contact colleagues easily and discuss common interests. For example, NURSRES is a list of a large number of nurses interested in research and a message to them will usually result in some useful resources or dialogue. However, be warned that a request that shows that you have not first made an attempt to find the information yourself will not usually be well received. You must first do a thorough search through the indexes (see the section on indexes in Chapter 2).

Library staff will also be helpful. They know how to find information and are usually willing to help, provided you do not expect them to do all your work for you. The staff at the circulation or information desk can help you locate items that you need. Similarly, the staff familiar with the catalogue can help you find out whether an item is in the library. The interlibrary loan staff can help you to obtain items that you need from other libraries. Some libraries have specific reference librarians for particular areas of knowledge and they are familiar with the main materials in that area. The reference librarian can advise you on the type of search that will be most productive. This advice can include which databases to use, and which strategies will be most effective for searching. Most libraries have orientation sessions on how to use the technology, especially CD-ROM or WWW databases. The librarian can also help you find items that are not in the usual databases.

Types of literature sources

There are various types of materials available. One distinction is between primary and secondary sources. **Primary sources** are those written by the author and have the advantage of being the author's own ideas. **Secondary sources** are those to which an author refers. They have the disadvantage of being filtered through the writer's own attitudes and biases, but sometimes you cannot access the source in any other way. A clue to a secondary source is a reference 'cited by . . .' Indeed, the Review of the Literature section of any paper is full of secondary sources.

Another distinction is between scholarly and unscholarly work. Scholarly works are usually the more valuable sources for research purposes. Such works as theoretical papers, reports of research methodologies, procedures or instruments, reports of research results, review papers and books written by authorities are scholarly literature. Refereed journal articles are considered more scholarly than non-refereed articles. A refereed journal article is one that has been sent out for peer review before being accepted for publication. Sources from the lay literature, newspapers and magazines are not scholarly work. Anecdotal or impressionistic reports or opinions on how to carry out health care are not normally scholarly, but certain projects using discourse analysis (see Chapter 14) may read and analyse lay literature. Ordinarily, you should use lay literature for background reading only. Similarly information obtained from the WWW is unlikely to be scholarly unless it is from a refereed journal that is accessible from the web.

Useful sources of literature
Books

Books are not usually in the forefront of research unless they are research books. This is primarily because of the timelag of up to five years between the time a research report project is written up, appears in a journal and is then cited in a book. However, books can be valuable sources of literature and ideas. Their bibliographies can also be useful sources of references. There are now electronic databases of books that are in print. For example, the database WorldCat lists all books in print. It is accessible through a portal called First Search, which lists many databases. These may be available at your library.

Conference proceedings

Conference papers and proceedings are also useful and can be listed as references. Sometimes there will have been a conference on exactly the topic you are researching. These documents are usually harder to access, but they can sometimes be obtained on interlibrary loan. With the growth of electronic media, this type of paper will probably become more accessible.

Reports

Reports from government and institutions are also useful sources of information. These are becoming easier to access now that many institutions are listing their reports on their websites. For example, the Australian Bureau of Statistics has a large number of statistical reports that can be ordered for a nominal sum. Some reports can be difficult to find out about and to access, but reading the bibliographies of journal articles and other reports can lead you to relevant reports, as can searching the indexes.

Theses

A thorough search of the literature will include a search for relevant theses. It is possible to find information about theses on the FirstSearch master database. The specific database is 'Dissertations' and it lists theses, in some cases back as far as 1975. However, the listings are incomplete. Not all universities list their theses this way and not all theses are listed by the universities that do list them. A search by the author for Australian nursing theses listed only 25 theses, which is a gross under-representation of the number of theses that have been written in nursing. The list is of abstracts only, so if you want to read beyond the abstract you must still obtain a copy of the thesis on interlibrary loan. However, the abstracts themselves are useful to get an idea of what has been done in the field. If you need to satisfy the criterion of originality for a doctoral thesis, this can help you to rule out certain topics that have been researched already.

EXERCISE
What are the benefits of searching for thesis abstracts and documents?

Journals

Professional journals are the most valuable resource for researchers. These journals have varying degrees of scope for their various audiences. The scope varies from broad interest journals such as the *Australian Journal of Advanced Nursing*, *International Journal of Nursing Practice* and *Nursing Inquiry* to more specific specialty journals such as the *Australian and New Zealand Journal of Mental Health Nursing*, or concept-specific journals such as the *Australian Journal of Holistic Nursing*. Journals can be discipline-specific to nursing, for example, *Collegian* or *Contemporary Nurse*, or they can be multidisciplinary, like the *Australian Journal of Rural Health*. Some journals are dedicated to research, such as *Clinical Nursing Research*, *Nursing Research* and *Western Journal of Nursing Research*. Some journals have a particular methodological focus, for example, *Qualitative Health Research*. Others include theoretical scholarship and/or clinical scholarship. Frequently, nursing knowledge incorporates knowledge from other disciplines. Journals of medicine, public health, anthropology, sociology and psychology, and paramedical disciplines such as physiotherapy or occupational therapy, for example, may be a useful source of material.

Journals can be international, for example, *Clinical Nursing Research*, which accepts papers from any country, or they can have a national focus, for example, *Collegian* and *Contemporary Nurse*, which deal with Australian research. State-based journals have a more restricted focus, for example, *The Lamp*, which is concerned mainly with events in New South Wales. You can find resources for your topic, depending on how specific it is, in a few journals or in many.

Electronic journals, or journals published only on the Internet, are also being developed. The *Online Journal of Issues in Nursing* emanates from the USA and the *Australian Electronic Journal of Nursing Education* comes from Australia. Electronic journals will undoubtedly proliferate. They are gradually becoming accessible through university information technology services and libraries.

Articles

The bibliography or reference section of useful articles will probably contain references to other useful articles. The text of the article will be a guide to selecting articles from that bibliography to follow up.

Indexes

Each health and health-related discipline has an index of its journal holdings. These indexes are accessed mainly through computers and are described in Chapter 2.

Where do you find the sources?

When you have your list of potential references, the next step is where to find them as easily and economically as possible. It is important to realise that you will be unlikely to find all of them. This problem is more acute now than ever before because electronic media can give you a list of everything written on a topic regardless of how accessible it is. Unless you are doing a PhD thesis it is not necessary to find everything, just the main sources.

The obvious place to start looking is in libraries. There are various types of libraries that may be useful. University libraries carry a large range of resources. Hospital libraries may carry resources that a university library does not have. Members of professional associations will have access to their associations' libraries. Some government departments have specialist libraries, for example, drug and alcohol or family planning libraries. Public libraries may have useful material, depending on your topic. Electronic libraries are also starting to become available. For example, the Virginia Henderson Library is now open. Named after Virginia Henderson, a prominent twentieth-century nurse, it is run by Sigma Theta Tau, the nursing honour society in the USA.

Libraries will have materials available in the reference section, the shelves and the current serials section. Larger libraries may have separate journal and book areas. Some may also have closed stacks from which only the librarian can retrieve items. The National

Library in Canberra operates exclusively on a closed stack basis – the reader submits an order form for each item, then the library staff locate the item for the reader.

If you live in a large city, you may need to visit several libraries. This is cheaper than interlibrary loans unless your institution provides the latter service free of charge. It is helpful to identify which libraries have the journals you are looking for. The librarian will be able to assist you by looking up the information on an index of journal locations. If you locate enough items in another library to justify a trip, it is then worthwhile to visit.

A library's catalogue is the index for information. The catalogue will normally be electronic, stored on a computer that may be linked to a network of library computers. You can search through the catalogue by author, title and subject, with variations on these themes. You select the search mode, for example, key word, and then type in the information. The computer searches its database and prints the items on the screen. Computer searching is fast and can also give you up-to-date information about the status of the item – whether it is checked in or in closed reserve.

Each library item is classified alphabetically, numerically, or by a combination of letters and numbers. One popular system is the Dewey Decimal System, which uses a three-number prefix, a decimal point and a multi-number suffix. Nursing and medical items are listed at 610. The other main system is the Library of Congress system, which uses a combination of letters and numbers. Nursing items are listed at RT.

In the library it is also useful to browse the shelves, particularly if you have identified fairly clearly what you are looking for. Sometimes you will find information in current issues of serials which often have their own section in the library. You may find some items on the re-shelving shelves. Historical research may require a search of the archives.

Don't overlook informal locations such as in-house collections of materials or the personal libraries of your colleagues, and the vast amount of information available on the WWW (see Chapter 2).

If you cannot obtain an item easily by the above methods, then it may be necessary to acquire it using the interlibrary loan service of your institution. Universities and hospitals both have interlibrary loan services, staffed by specialist librarians. The librarian consults the index of locations of books or journals on the Australian Bibliographic Network, and sends for the item. The lending library then either sends the book or a photocopied article to your institution, and your library loans you the book or sells you the photocopy. Usually the item is sent by post, but in cases of extreme urgency a journal article can be faxed or emailed. However, the interlibrary loan option is expensive and the library may pass on the costs to you. It is also relatively slow if items are posted rather than faxed or emailed. It can take a month or longer if the host library is understaffed or has to recall a book from a borrower. If the item is in an overseas library, it can take even longer. It is wise to allow plenty of time to acquire items on interlibrary loan.

Libraries are now increasingly using electronic delivery services to obtain items that they do not hold themselves. Indeed, the increasing availability of journal articles from the Internet will probably eventually make that part of the interlibrary loan service obsolete.

Selecting literature

Before you start reading the literature, you need to select what is appropriate to read. The aim of this exercise is to end up with the most relevant literature – and only literature that is relevant. Suppose you are doing a search for material on a topic such as the effect of circumcision on the infant's ability to breastfeed in the immediate post-operative period. There is a huge body of literature on breastfeeding and a large amount of literature on circumcision. It would be impossible to read all of it and most of it would not directly bear on your topic, although some might be useful background reading. You would want only research articles about the relationship between circumcision and breastfeeding. You would not be interested in articles debating the advantages of circumcision unless they contained observations relevant to breast-feeding. Similarly, you would not want articles on breastfeeding that did not address circumcision. Therefore you would combine the two keywords 'circumcision' and 'breastfeeding' on the computer literature search, which would then extract only articles that dealt with both topics. Figure 4.1 shows you the interaction between the two bodies of literature. By looking only for articles dealing with both topics, you will save yourself a considerable amount of time.

When searching for literature, you can eliminate many items by reading the abstract. It is best to do this at the literature search stage to avoid wasting time and money. However, not all entries in an index have abstracts, and it is then necessary to look at the article itself, just skimming lightly through the introduction and conclusions. By reading these, it is often possible to decide whether the article is relevant. You can also eliminate articles that are in non-research journals since you are interested only in research. When you have eliminated the irrelevant and the unobtainable, you will be left with only a small percentage of your original sources. This is normal and it shows an ability to discriminate between useful and irrelevant literature.

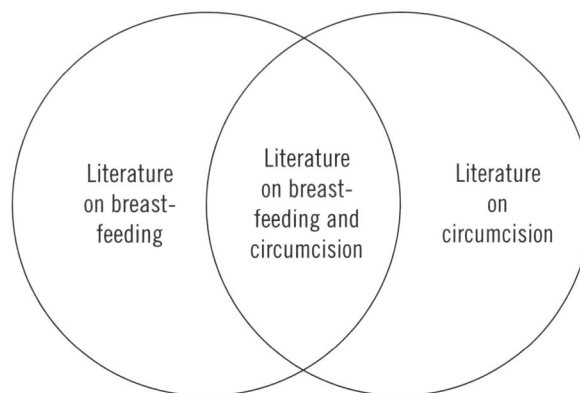

Figure 4.1 Elimination of irrelevant literature

You should also consider whether the article is written by someone who has the authority and credibility to produce a valuable article. Other considerations about the quality of the article are the date when the study was carried out and the type of journal in which it appears.

If it is a refereed journal you can be assured that the article was reviewed by at least two peers of the writer. This system of peer review entails the journal editor sending out the article to two identified reviewers who critique the article using a similar process to the critique method detailed later in this chapter. The editor then sends the critiques to the author, who revises the article. This process continues until the article either meets the standards of the editor and reviewers or the author gives up or decides to send the article to another journal. Thus, the peer-review system helps to maintain a standard of excellence in research scholarship.

The mechanics of searching for and filing literature using a computer are described in Chapter 2.

Acquiring your own collection of information

Having decided that an article or other material is relevant, you now have the problem of how to capture this information for your own future use. You should decide which method to use before you undertake close reading of any material. The pre-technology approach is to take notes of key ideas by hand from the article. This is time-consuming and has a disadvantage in that the notes are your own interpretation of the material and thus subject to bias. Also, if you want to consult the reference later, you will have to look it up again. However, this method is relatively cheap and can be effective provided you do not need much information from the source.

The second method is to capture the article in hard copy. This can be done by photocopying it. This method is more expensive, but more flexible. Photocopying captures the entire article, conference paper or section of a book. You can take the material elsewhere to work on and re-read as many times as you like, which you will need to do when new ideas or insights occur. Be sure that each photocopy has physically written on it information about the volume, year, issue and so forth. The current trend is for journals to print this information at the top or bottom of the page, but not all do. You can either write it on the photocopy or photocopy your reference information onto a blank space on the article when you are photocopying it. When photocopying material, make sure that you do not infringe the copyright laws. It is against the law to copy more than 10 per cent of a book. Most libraries have signs near the photocopy machines informing you of the copyright laws.

You can also capture a hard copy of a document by downloading it from a computer source and printing it. You would be likely to do this from a WWW document or from an electronic source of a journal that has what is called 'full text' capability. More and more libraries are converting journal subscriptions to electronic form. The advantages of this are obvious. The library reduces its need for shelf space for journals, and researchers are able to have virtually instantaneous access to documents, including from a home computer via the library portal if they have the appropriate authorisation and password information.

By using these techniques, you should end up with a collection of all of the material relevant to your topic and be ready to process it.

You will also need to organise the copies of the literature that you have if there are more than a few papers. An expanding file is useful for this purpose, or a portable file, i.e. a box with file hangers. If there is a large amount of material or you are involved in several projects, you may want to invest in a filing cabinet. The articles can then be filed by author or by topic. If you have scanned electronic copies, you can organise them on computer in various files and perhaps even store them on a CD-ROM. The latter method will require a CD-ROM burner and appropriate software. Storing literature in electronic form is described in Chapter 2.

Reading and documenting the information

The next step is to read the relevant material. At this stage you may need to narrow down your topic even further, or you may redirect it slightly as a result of your reading. The first stage is to read all the material superficially once or twice. This will give you a feeling for the important issues in the topic and the methodologies of research previously used on the topic. The next stage is to read the material critically, identifying major points. This may require several readings, but you should at this stage be reading only the most relevant material.

Reading a research report

In order to become familiar with the body of research on your topic, you will have to read research reports. It is helpful to understand the structure of research reports. They usually follow a logical standard order. The title, of course, comes first. Next comes the **abstract**, which summarises the study. The introduction will give the problem being researched, its scope and its significance. The theoretical framework will be identified and its relationship to the study will be discussed. The previous findings will then be summarised and specific research questions given. If it is a quantitative design, specific hypotheses and variables will be identified, either formally or informally. This section usually answers the questions 'what' and 'why'. If it is a qualitative study, hypotheses and variables will not be stated. Rather, the project will be introduced in exploratory terms, and the theory underlying the choice of methods may be described, because qualitative research usually outlines the basis on which knowledge of a particular kind is collected and analysed.

The **methodology** section will outline the design of the study, the subjects used or participants involved and the methodology used to answer the research question, including methods of data collection and analysis. In the **results** section, the findings of the study will be given. The discussion section will discuss the significance of the findings and how they relate to previous findings and the theoretical framework. Conclusions and recommendations for implementing the findings will then be given. At the end of the paper, the references will be given. This section usually answers the questions 'how', 'when', 'where' and 'to whom'.

In reading research reports, beginning researchers often have problems with the scholarly language used, particularly research terminology and statistics. Sometimes it seems as though the writer has difficulty in communicating in plain language, particularly if they are using a formal style of writing. These are conventions that have developed over the years. However, if you want to learn to read research, you have to come to terms with the language. It is really no different from being dropped into the middle of a nursing specialty such as critical care and having to learn the jargon. If you are reading research in a clinical area that is your own specialty, you should be familiar with the clinical terminology. It is usually the research terminology that is difficult. The best way to handle this problem is to read the paper and make notes of the words you do not understand. Look up these words in your research textbook, making particular use of the glossary. Then re-read the paper. Sometimes a paper requires several readings before you will understand it, but it usually gets easier with each reading. It may help to bring together a group of students and do this as a group exercise.

Documenting key ideas from the readings

Since it is impossible to work with a considerable number of whole reports, it is necessary to identify the key passages so that you can refer to them again. There are several ways of doing this. Whichever method you use, you must be able to link the source and the idea so that you can attribute the idea to its rightful source and thus avoid plagiarism.

One system is to indicate key ideas on a photocopy of the article or book chapter. This method works best where there is little material on the topic. You can indicate the key ideas with highlighters, even developing a colour scheme for coding topics. Another way is to make symbols in the margin of the paper. This system can also be adapted for use on an electronic copy of a paper, using keyboard symbols. This method is faster initially but has the disadvantage that you have to go back and use the whole document every time you want to refer to an idea.

Another way is to organise material under topic headings so that you have all of your ideas on one topic together. The keywords that you used for your literature search are a start, but you will probably need subheadings.

One way of organising key ideas is a paper-based method, where you write your ideas on separate cards or pieces of paper with identifying headings at the top. A 12.5 × 20 cm filing card or one-third of an A4 sheet of paper is ideal for this purpose. While the cards are more expensive, they are also more robust and easier to flick through when you are looking for a particular bit of information. They can also be re-used by using the reverse side. At the top of the card, write the author and date of the source on the left-hand side. This will allow you to find the passage again in the original article. Also write the keyword under which the idea fits at the top of the card on the right-hand side. This will allow you to file the idea under keyword headings in a filing box. Then write the key idea on the card. This method forces you to be selective and to think about how the idea fits into the overall picture. Then file the card under the keyword heading in a shoe box or other file. The accumulated cards under the keyword headings will form the beginning of a draft of the paper. All you need to do is sort them into a logical sequence and start writing.

If you have access to a word processor, a much more modern and flexible way to do the above procedure is to type key ideas into the word processor rather than writing on paper, using the same principles of identifying the information. This can be done either as you read or by first taking notes manually and then typing them into the word processor. By doing the former, you avoid double work for yourself. You can then either print out the information and file it mechanically, as above, or file it electronically in the computer by creating a file for each keyword and pasting the information in there. Be sure to keep the author, date and keyword identifiers attached to each piece of information so that you can cite them when you are writing the paper. You can also cut and paste the information into various files that are the electronic equivalent of the sections of the shoebox or flip-top box.

If you have an electronic copy of the whole document, either generated by your scanner or downloaded from a database, you can adapt several of the above techniques to the electronic copy. You can use italics, symbols or bold font to emphasise key passages. You can use the colour facility of the word processor to colour-code key passages. You can copy and paste chunks of the manuscript into your various keyword files. In writing your paper, you could even copy quotations directly from the electronic version. The same principles of identifying the passages by author and date and attributing cited material to the original author also apply to this method.

Critiquing individual reports

A critique is a balanced assessment, developed through a process of critical appraisal, of both the positive and negative qualities of a research report. A good critique offers constructive criticism, with suggestions as to how the researcher could have improved the research report.

People critique research reports for several reasons. One is to promote student learning. Most research training will require students to learn to critique existing research reports in order to teach them to differentiate between good and bad research. Critiquing will teach students to discriminate wisely about what to include in a review of the literature. Learning to critique also helps students to interpret their own research findings in light of previous findings. Another reason for critiquing is for clinicians to evaluate research reports in terms of whether they offer a foundation for change in clinical practice (discussed in Chapter 1). Still another is for researchers to scrutinise research reports for their suitability for a literature review in a research proposal or report. Finally, critiquing can be done by experienced researchers who review journal submissions to make recommendations on the publication of an article.

A good way to learn about what constitutes a critique is to look at some models. Try reading the critiques that frequently accompany journal articles in *Clinical Nursing Research* and *Western Journal of Nursing Research*. However, a journal critique may not be complete because the author may be able to raise only major points in the space available. The reader must rely on the reviewer to evaluate the research on all of the relevant criteria below and raise significant issues in the critique.

If you have to choose an article on which to practise critiquing, you will find that those in refereed journals offer less scope for critique than those in non-refereed journals. Research reports in refereed journals have already been critiqued before publication. They are therefore more likely to be high-quality reports, although the perfect report has not yet been published. Reports in non-refereed journals are more likely to offer scope for finding flaws. To find out whether a journal is refereed, look at the introductory part of the journal where information about it is given, or look in the 'Instructions to authors' section. One of these will usually say whether the journal requires manuscripts to be peer-reviewed.

Critiquing quantitative research reports

Assuming you have selected appropriate material, the process of critiquing is to read through the article quickly for general meaning, then read it in detail several times, asking questions about the article and taking notes. Then you build the material in your notes into a structured, logical argument. You may choose to use the same structure as a research report, looking at the introduction, method, results and discussion in turn. Indeed, it would be wise to read the section in Chapter 18 on research reports before attempting to critique. Right now, we are not going to provide extensive examples to follow. However, you might like to use the examples provided in Chapters 6 and 18 for practice in critiquing.

When critiquing a research report, you should ask general questions about the quality of the research and the document reporting it, and specific questions about parts of the research. We will look at these in turn. In assessing the general quality of the research, we need to ask whether it is significant, that is, do the findings make a difference? For example, there may be studies that give instruction about research design, but which did not get results that could impact on clinical practice. It is also important to ask whether the study is sound science: Does it have a good methodology? Does it have a good design? Does it have a logical progression of links between the purpose of the study, the method, the findings and the conclusions? With regard to the quality of the writing of the report, is it well written with a smooth flow between parts? Is it clear and concise and stated in terms that the reader can understand easily?

In assessing the research report, you need to ask whether it is complete. Most journals require authors to use the IMRAD system, or Introduction, Method, Results and Discussion. The National Standards Institute of the United States of America has adopted this system as the industry standard (Day 1998). Does the report have all of these sections? Are they in a logical order? According to Day (1998), IMRAD is a logical order because it progresses from problem to solution. However, in critiquing, remember that some journals have particular formats that they require authors to follow.

You may not address all of the points below in every critique because they may not all be relevant to the research being critiqued.

Preliminaries

When you start your critique, look at the title first.
- Is it concise, yet informative?
- Does it indicate the research approach?
  The next area for appraisal is the abstract. Most articles these days have abstracts for the convenience of their readers.
- Does the abstract correctly and concisely describe the problem, methods, design, results, conclusions and implications?
- Does it provide a good basis for deciding whether or not the study is worth reading?

Introduction

- Does the introduction explain the purpose of the study, that is, what the study was investigating?
- Does it state the actual problem the researcher investigated or the question the researcher answered?
- Does it give a rationale for doing the study in terms of a theoretical question, unanswered previous research findings, or observations of the researchers or their colleagues?
- Does it set the study in context – does it give the background to the study in terms of some previous work that led to the study question?
- Does it set the scope of the problem, or the limits of the study?
- Does the introduction talk about the potential importance of the study – how this study would advance knowledge on this topic, what significance it might have? In other words, does it answer the question 'so what?'

Literature review

The next part of the introduction in a quantitative study will address the conceptual framework of the study and the literature review or previous findings.

- Does the study have a conceptual framework?
- If so, is it an appropriate framework for the study?
- Is it a nursing framework or a framework from another discipline, for example, sociology?
- Has the author linked the framework to the research question? In what way?
- Are the concepts clearly defined?
- Is the literature relevant to the topic and the concepts being investigated?
- Is it directly related or is it more marginal?
- Is appropriate literature from the conceptual framework included?
- Is the review comprehensive and complete?
- Are classic and current sources included?
- Is there a majority of primary sources?
- Is the literature review just a summary of individual research publications, or is it an integrated review that includes an objective analysis of the strengths and weaknesses of the various studies?
- Does the review develop logically, producing an argument that justifies carrying out the study?
- Does the author summarise the key points of the literature review?

Hypotheses and variables

- If the study design goes beyond description, are there hypotheses? Are they stated or implicit? If stated, are they clearly stated?
- Do the hypotheses flow from the problem statement or arise from the previous findings?
- Do the hypotheses suggest a proposed relationship between two or more variables?
- Are the hypotheses stated as directional or null hypotheses?

- Are they capable of being tested?
- Are they operationally defined (stated in terms that allow the reader to see how they will be measured)?
- Do the hypotheses make it clear what variables are being tested?
- Are the dependent, independent and extraneous variables conceptualised or defined? In operational terms?

Methodology

Generally, the methodology should give enough detail to permit replication of the study. For example, if it is an experiment, the exact procedures for administering the treatment should be given. The methodology section is usually broken down into subsections according to the journal's formula. There may be variations in the organisation of this section depending on the journal. The main subsections are usually the design, participants (subjects), setting, procedures for data collection and analysis, and the instruments and materials.

The methodology section should give the design fairly early so that the readers will know whether they are reading about a descriptive study or an experiment.

- Has the author addressed all sections?
- Is the design the most appropriate one to answer the research question?
- Was the selected design likely to control threats to validity, thereby promoting internal validity?
- If it was an experimental design, was the way of testing the hypotheses valid?
- Has the author included a section about the participants?
- Has the paper stated what the target population was and how the participants were selected, that is, what the sampling procedures were?
- Does the sample appear to be representative of the target population or is it biased in some way?
- What type of sample was it and how could this impact on the findings?
- How many participants were selected, and were there enough to ensure valid findings?
- How did the researcher determine how many participants should be in the sample, for example was a power analysis used?
- What processes were used to recruit the participants?
- After the sample was recruited, what procedures were used to assign them to groups if warranted?
- Were there any losses of participants from the sample during the study and did this affect the findings?
- Did the author report on the ethical aspects of the study?
- Was permission gained from the appropriate human research ethics committee or committees?
- Did the participants volunteer to take part in the study?
- Was informed consent obtained?
- Were participants protected from potential physical, social, psychological and financial harm?

- Were the procedures of the study designed so as to protect the privacy, confidentiality and anonymity of the participants where appropriate?
- Did the author report on what instrument or instruments were used, including their suitability?
- Did the instrument measure accurately with sufficient sensitivity?
- How was it developed, and by whom?
- If the instrument was previously in existence, did the author report the validity and reliability?
- Did the author get permission from the owner of the copyright on the instrument?
- If the instrument was researcher-developed, was the trialling procedure reported, including acceptable validity and reliability tests?
- Who collected the data? Did the data collectors have the appropriate training on the instrument?
- Did the author report the data collection procedures in detail?
- Was a pilot study done?
- Were data processing and management procedures reported? Were they accurate?
- Were data analysis procedures reported in sufficient detail, including statistical tests? Were they adequate?

Results

- Is the results section concise and clearly presented?
- Are the graphics and tables informative and necessary?
- Do the data appear to be sufficient, valid and reliable?
- Did the author describe the participants and their relevant characteristics?
- Did the author give all of the results that were related to the research question or hypotheses?
- Were the findings consistent with the hypotheses?
- Were the findings statistically significant with levels of significance given?
- Were the findings clinically significant?

Discussion

This section should wrap up the report. It should be concise but should bring out the important aspects of the study. A poor discussion section only summarises the findings. A good discussion section discusses their meaning and significance.

- Does the discussion section discuss the contribution made by the study to the development of knowledge?
- Does it point out the strengths and weaknesses of the study and how weaknesses could be addressed in future research?
- Does it relate the findings to the conceptual framework?
- Does it compare the findings with the previous findings identified in the review of the literature?
- Does it say how the findings of this study extend the previous findings?

- Does it say whether the findings could be generalised to other people?
- Do the authors discuss any relevant implications for practice?
- Are any conclusions drawn from the findings; if so, are they appropriate?
- Are any recommendations made for further research, theoretical development or practice?
- Do the recommendations arise appropriately out of the conclusions?

References

- Are the majority of references recent?
- Are they complete and accurate?
- Are all citations listed in the references? Are all of the references cited in the study?

EXERCISE
Locate a quantitative research report and critique it using the above criteria.

Critiquing qualitative research reports

In the preceding section you were given many important questions to ask to assist you in critiquing quantitative research reports, and many of these apply equally well to qualitative reports. Keeping in mind the questions raised previously, this section will emphasise some key questions to ask when critiquing a qualitative research report. The approach taken here will be to use the structure for writing qualitative research reports presented in Chapter 18 of this book as a basis on which to raise questions for research critique.

The points for critiquing a qualitative research report will be listed and some explanation will be given as necessary. You may find that many of the points have been covered elsewhere in this book. There are close and direct connections between critiquing qualitative research and qualitative research processes (Chapter 1), the format of a qualitative research proposal (Chapter 6), presenting the results in qualitative research (Chapter 17) and the elements of a qualitative research report (Chapter 18).

Title, research summary and literature review

Qualitative critiques begin with attention to preliminaries. Look again in the preceding section at what has been written about how to critique the title, the research summary or abstract, and the literature review in quantitative research. All of the questions apply equally well to qualitative research.

It is important to check that the literature review contains all of the elements of a good literature review as described in this chapter. Remember, it is probably more difficult to write a literature review than it is to critique it. Some specific questions that can be asked to assess the completeness of a literature review in a qualitative report are:
- What is the relationship between the literature review and the research area/questions that are considered to be important in the area that has been selected for study? What rationale is given for their selection?

- What do the practitioners, administrators, researchers, governments, community, media, and so on have to say about the area? To what extent are these views represented?
- What key ideas have been raised? What has been seen as problematic? Have solutions and/or actions been proposed and/or evaluated in response to perceived difficulties?
- Has the material been identified clearly as to paradigms of knowledge? Has the material challenged existing knowledge and theory, or does it serve to reinforce current conceptions?
- What research methods have been employed in these studies? Have these methods been appropriate in terms of the research questions that have been investigated? Is there attention to ensuring that the methods are congruent with the underlying theory guiding the research approach (methodology)?
- What are the major findings associated with these studies? Do they reflect an approach that is quantitative, qualitative or a combination of both?
- What debates have there been in the area with respect to both the content of the research and the underlying theory guiding the research approach (methodological) aspects? What have been the main issues involved in these debates?
- What important issues appear to have been overlooked in the area? Are there any gaps, omissions or 'silences' in the literature?
- What 'common threads' emerge in terms of issues, debates, research findings and themes? How can these 'common threads' guide an evaluation of the knowledge that has been gathered to date, and how can they be employed to propose important and potentially fruitful areas for further inquiry?

Research plan, including methodology, methods and processes

The body of a qualitative report contains sections on the methodology, methods and processes. The definitions for each of these sections, as they apply specifically to qualitative research, are given in Chapter 6. Questions follow that you need to keep in mind in order to critique a qualitative project in relation to methodology, methods and processes.

Methodology
- What theoretical assumptions about the way knowledge is generated underlie the methods?
- Have explanations been given of the basic nature and intent of the chosen methodology?
- Is there an explanation of how the methodology relates to this project?
- Are the main references to the methodological literature included?

Ethical requirements
In qualitative research, it is important to critique the ways in which the ethical rights of the participants were safeguarded throughout the project. The report should be checked carefully to see that it includes explanations regarding the ethical requirements. Some questions to ask are:
- Has ethical clearance been obtained?
- From which committees was ethical clearance obtained?

- Are there comprehensive statements about appropriate ethical considerations?
- Are there indications that informed consent, privacy and anonymity were honoured?
- Has any attention been paid to maintaining the integrity of ethical considerations and interpersonal relationships throughout the research?

Methods and processes

Some questions that may guide the critique of methods and processes are:
- Is the sequence of the research methods clearly explained?
- How were participants enlisted into the project?
- Has an explanation been provided of the reasons for the number of participants in the project?
- Are the processes used appropriate for the underlying methodological ideas of the project? That is, does the project demonstrate as appropriate a level of negotiation, collaboration and sharing of power between the researcher and participants as might be reasonably expected?
- Is there a clear account of how the data were collected?

Analysis and interpretation

Some questions that may guide you in critiquing the analysis and interpretation phase of the project are:
- Are the analysis and interpretation phases easily discernible in the report?
- Has a rationale been given for the choice of analysis methods?
- Have the steps in analysis been set out clearly?
- Has the researcher explained who did the analysis, that is, was it done by an individual or by a group?
- Are the processes described clearly as to how the individual/group went about doing the analysis?
- Are there examples of the data organised in their analysed form?
- Are excerpts provided of actual dialogue between researchers/co-researchers/ participants?
- Have sub-themes/collective themes/competing discourses been described clearly?
- Has the researcher explained who made the interpretations?
- Is there a clear account of how the interpretations were made?
- Are the interpretations set out systematically and clearly?
- Is there a clear account of how the interpretations were validated?

Discussion, insights, recommendations, suggestions and conclusions

Some questions to guide the critique of this part of the research report are:
- Does the report document provide a comprehensive discussion of the findings/ insights/examples of changed practice that emerged from the project?
- Does the report offer practical suggestions and/or recommendations for practice?
- Are the final discussion and conclusions congruent with the overall plan, methodology, methods and processes of the research?

In summary, the questions relating to critiquing a quantitative research report's preliminaries apply equally well to qualitative research critiques. Even so, there are some differences to note in critiquing a qualitative research report. It is important to be aware of the differences and to judge the overall integrity of a qualitative project on qualitative research assumptions of what equals a good research report.

It is useful to keep a brief summary of your critique of the articles that you read. As well as the citation, you can record the problem studied, the theoretical framework, the methodology, your own evaluation of the work and how it links into your work. You may not feel that this is necessary if you only have a few articles to deal with, but it is important for keeping order in a larger body of literature. Most of the information, except your evaluation, is already present in the abstract of the article. You can make handwritten evaluations. You can also type this sort of summary straight into a word processor. If you are downloading information from an electronic database you can copy the abstract, which gives you a ready-made summary of the article, written by the author. You can either copy and paste the abstract into your word processor document or you can download it into an electronic reference manager. You can also enter other comments or information into the word processor document or the space provided for notes on the entry in the reference manager.

EXERCISE

Locate a qualitative research report and critique it using the above criteria.

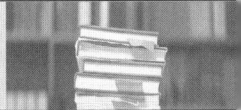

Putting it together

The reasons for reviewing the literature were given at the beginning of the chapter. By the time you have obtained and read the information, you should have a good overview of the literature on the topic. By the time you have read it thoroughly several times and made notes, you should be starting to see patterns and to understand how various parts fit into the whole. You should be able to follow the important themes through the literature. You may even begin to see where you could shape your study further, usually by narrowing it.

If you are interested in exploring literature acquisition and review techniques in more detail, there are books on the subject, such as *Health Sciences Literature Review Made Easy* by Garrard (1999).

The process of reviewing the literature may seem at first to be a chore that is difficult and complex. As you move through the process, however, you will find that the time and energy that you invest will bring rewards in terms of learning new ideas. You will also feel a sense of accomplishment when you have become thoroughly conversant with the literature on a topic. You can discuss the topic intelligently with other researchers. You are now ready to move on to writing a literature review.

Summary

In this chapter, you have learned the meaning of 'review of the literature', and the reasons for reviewing the literature. You have learned ways of identifying possible sources and how to assess the sources for relevance. You have also learned ways of organising this process. Finally, you have learned how to critique individual research reports. You are now ready to move on to considering your conceptual framework (if it is appropriate) and writing a research proposal.

Main points

- The literature is the total body of writing dealing with the topic being researched.
- In preparing to search, be systematic, define your topic, identify key words, set boundaries to the search.
- A search can be limited by availability of time and information, financial constraints and the skills of the searcher.
- Colleagues, experts, librarians and lecturers can be resources.
- Information can be found in books, reports, journal articles, conference papers, electronic indexes, email and the WWW.
- Keep good records of the details of your search using a suitable manual or electronic organising system.
- In selecting material, stick to the topic, exclude non-research material, eliminate non-obtainable material and consider the quality of the source.
- Types of reading can include reading superficially and critically.
- Research reports have a distinct structure including the preliminaries, introduction, methodology, results and discussion.
- Information can be extracted from your readings by photocopying, downloading from the Internet, or a note-taking system.
- Key points can be recorded on cards, in a word processor, or by a highlighting system on hard copy.
- References can be compiled using a manual card system, a word processing system or an electronic reference manager.
- Research reports are critiqued to: promote learning, discriminate what to include in a review of the literature, interpret research findings in light of previous findings, judge whether findings offer a foundation for change in clinical practice, determine suitability for a literature review in a research proposal or report, and to make recommendations on the publication of an article.
- Detailed and systematic questioning processes are required to undertake high-quality critiques of quantitative and qualitative research reports.

CASE STUDY

You may remember Maxwell, who needed your help in Chapter 3. To recap, Maxwell is a 45-year-old physiotherapist, with qualifications in physiotherapy and business administration. He has been accepted into PhD studies through his local regional university, which has professional and academic links with a large city teaching hospital and university. Maxwell is interested in the extent to which complementary therapies have influenced clients' help-seeking behaviours in attending 'orthodox' physiotherapist services. He suspects that the decline in attendance at his physiotherapy clinic may be due to clients preferring to seek naturopathic services and/or to self-medicate with herbal therapies. Maxwell is now at the point of searching for relevant literature in his research area and he asks you for help in how to go about the process. What will you tell Maxwell in relation to:

- locating possible sources of relevant literature
- setting up an efficient system for keeping track of sources
- identifying the literature that is pertinent to the project
- obtaining the identified literature
- effectively reading the literature that has been obtained
- extracting the relevant information from the literature
- critiquing research reports
- setting up an efficient system for dealing with references?

Multiple choice questions

1   A literature review involves:
  a   finding and written and verbal sources on the topic
  b   collating the research findings relevant to the topic
  c   finding, reading and sorting the relevant literature
  d   reading, sorting, analysing and critiquing literature

2   The best literature in academic terms is a:
  a   recent book
  b   refereed journal article
  c   conference proceeding
  d   scientific publication

3   The key to an efficient literature search is:
  a   being systematic in both searching and record-keeping
  b   enlisting the helping services of a knowledgeable librarian
  c   setting up a home computer connected to the WWW
  d   understanding the process of identifying relevant literature

4 The scope of the literature search depends on:
   a   whether there is assistance
   b   all the reasons for doing it
   c   opening hours in the library
   d   the project's methodology

5 Scholarly literature includes:
   a   theoretical interviews, reports of research methodologies, procedures or instruments, reports of research results, review papers and books written by authorities
   b   theoretical interviews, reports of research methodologies, procedures or instruments, reports of research results, review papers and books written by lay people
   c   theoretical papers, reports of research methodologies, procedures or instruments, reports of research results, review papers and books written by authorities
   d   theoretical papers, reports of research discussions, procedures or instruments, reports of research results, review papers and books written by authorities

6 Books are not usually in the forefront of research because:
   a   of limited distribution and relatively high cost
   b   of the timelag in reporting research findings
   c   researchers write articles faster and easier
   d   computer-based information is more fashionable

7 Refereed journal articles are considered more scholarly than non-refereed articles, because:
   a   they are the opinions of people discussing areas of interest in well-set-up chat rooms
   b   only the journal's editor makes the decision on what is considered scholarly
   c   they have been sent out for peer review before being accepted for publication
   d   they focus solely on quantitative research projects with high scientific credibility

8 The specific database for finding theses is:
   a   'Reports'
   b   'Indexes'
   c   'Monologues'
   d   'Dissertations'

9 The logical order for a research report is:
   a   abstract, title, introduction, theoretical framework, methodology, results, discussion
   b   title, abstract, introduction, theoretical framework, methodology, results, discussion
   c   introduction, title, abstract, theoretical framework, methodology, results, discussion
   d   title, abstract, introduction, theoretical framework, methodology, discussion, results

10 A balanced assessment of both the positive and negative qualities of a research report, developed through a process of critical appraisal, is:
   a   an evaluation
   b   a correction
   c   a critique
   d   an examination

Review topics

1 Why is it important to review the literature before commencing a research project?
2 Describe how to narrow the search for literature.
3 Who can help you to undertake an effective literature search?
4 Discuss how you will document the key ideas from the readings.
5 Differentiate between the means of critiquing quantitative and qualitative research reports.

Online reading

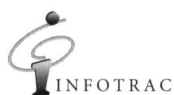

INFOTRAC

INFOTRAC® COLLEGE EDITION

When accessing information use the following keywords to retrieve information relating to refining your literature review knowledge and skills:

➤ literature review
➤ literature search
➤ qualitative research
➤ quantitative research

Then, use specific keywords relating to the research project for which you are searrching, for example:

➤ dietetics
➤ health
➤ medicine
➤ nursing
➤ occupational therapy
➤ physiotherapy
➤ (any other health profession)

References

Day, R. 1998, *How to Write and Publish a Scientific Paper*, 5th edn, Cambridge University Press, Cambridge.
Garrard, J. 1999, *Health Sciences Literature Review Made Easy: The Matrix Method*, Aspen Publishers Inc., Gaithersburg, Maryland.

CHAPTER 5

ETHICS IN NURSING AND HEALTH RESEARCH

CHAPTER OBJECTIVES

The material presented in this chapter will assist you to:

- cite examples of unethical research
- examine a Statement on Human Experimentation
- outline the role, composition and functions of an institutional ethics committee
- discuss the principles of beneficence and non-maleficence in relation to research ethics
- discuss the principle of respect for human dignity, applied in informed consent
- discuss the principle of justice, applied in anonymity, privacy and confidentiality
- discuss ethical aspects in special cases, including reproductive technology, Indigenous participants and multi-site projects
- analyse research issues in clinical practice
- recognise scientific misconduct
- evaluate the ethical aspects of a research paper.

Introduction

Ethics is concerned with moral questions and behaviour. In nursing and other health disciplines, research is usually concerned with investigating the effects of interventions on people. Therefore ethics in nursing and health research concerns moral questions and behaviour in conducting research. Research participants' rights must be respected throughout the research process. Ethical researchers guarantee that no harm was done to any person involved in the research process. They also guarantee the validity of the research findings so that clinicians who apply those findings to client care can have confidence in them.

Sometimes there are problems in reconciling scientific rigour with ethical research practices and there are many examples of researchers acting unethically, with disastrous consequences. This chapter demonstrates the need for ethics surveillance and principles of ethical research conduct. It discusses the obligations of health professionals to conform to high ideals.

Historical examples of unethical research conduct

There have been numerous instances of researchers harming participants in the name of medical research. Indeed, research history abounds with examples of disregard for ethical behaviour, whether from ignorance or indifference to the welfare of others. Many researchers have committed unethical acts in their desire to develop knowledge or their drive to accumulate research papers for their own glory. In the eighteenth century, medical researchers deliberately injected bacteria into people to see if they would cause venereal disease and typhoid fever. In the nineteenth century, doctors tested surgical operations and anaesthetics on slaves (McNeill 1993).

More has been documented about **unethical research** practices in the twentieth century. In the 1920s, the United States Public Health Service carried out what has become known as the Tuskegee Syphilis Study, in which researchers deliberately did not treat 400 African-American men for syphilis even after treatment was available, simply to observe the natural outcomes of the disease. The study was carried over 40 years and terminated only in the 1970s because of moral outrage. A public health nurse, Eunice Rivers, was involved in carrying out that study and it was partly because of her success in recruiting and retaining participants that the study continued for so long (Vessey & Gennaro 1994). The Tuskegee study had disastrous and long-reaching results because many African-Americans believe HIV is an instrument of genocide that has been made by humans (Thomas & Quinn 1991).

The most famous unethical medical experiments were carried out during World War II. Doctors in Nazi concentration camps conducted medical experiments, presumably to improve the efficiency of the camps and to advance their own careers by building up a research profile. They carried out these experiments on camp prisoners, particularly identical twins and persons they considered subhuman on racial grounds. People were subjected to transplants, high-altitude decompression and submersion in ice-water. Doctors tested the efficiency of different methods of killing and the effects of starvation (Caplan 1992). While some of these experiments concerned developing knowledge that could apply to aviation or to exposure of sailors at sea, they nevertheless violated human rights. Participants were selected on racial grounds, were forced to participate, and were harmed by their participation. Most did not survive, but those who did sustained permanent physical and psychological damage.

In the same era, the Japanese conducted germ warfare 'experiments' on the Chinese in mainland China using anthrax, cholera, typhoid, typhus and bubonic plague. They subjected some Chinese to prolonged exposure to X-rays, replacement of human blood with horse blood, and murder by surgical experiments. Again, their motives were to advance the war and their own careers. They may have killed 3000 people in all (McNeill 1993).

During the same war, the Australian Department of Defence subjected many Australian servicemen to high levels of exposure to mustard gas in tropical conditions. These trials were unethical, not only because the government already knew that the outcome would be unfavourable, but also because the servicemen were not informed of the risks and so could not give **informed consent**. Many received burns as a result and although the Department of Defence will not disclose information, it is believed that there has been an out-of-court settlement (McNeill 1993).

In the postwar period, the New Zealand Cancer Study at the National Women's Hospital in Auckland, described by Johnstone (1999), provides a classic example of unethical research. A gynaecologist, Dr Herbert Green, had a theory that pre-cancerous changes in the cervix (carcinoma in situ) would not necessarily progress to carcinoma if untreated. In the study, which had been approved by the hospital ethics committee, he set up an experiment in which 817 women were treated and 131 women (without their knowledge) were in an untreated group. The women in the untreated group had a mortality rate of four times that of the treated group. The study was eventually stopped because of pressure from the hospital colposcopist and pathologist. At the subsequent inquiry, the judge found that the study had been unethical because the women had not given informed consent, the study design was poor, there had been inadequate scientific and ethical review, and there was a known risk that the women would die if untreated. The judge criticised the other doctors and administrators for failing to intercede on the women's behalf. The judge also found that the hospital ethics committee was inadequate because it comprised mainly medical doctors, had a limited understanding of ethical research, did not require informed consent, and did not assess the scientific merit of projects adequately. The New Zealand Medical Council found the chair of the hospital ethics committee guilty of unprofessional conduct for his failure to review the study adequately but as he was retired, he was not subjected to any further action. The Medical Council dropped the charges against the gynaecologist because he was mentally and physically unfit to face them (*Weekend Australian* 11 Oct. 1990).

Lest we think that the record is any better in recent times, in 1992 questions were asked about consent procedures used in the Tamoxifen breast cancer prevention study in the USA and about subject recruitment materials for a women's health initiative clinical trial (Vessey & Gennaro 1994). In the United Kingdom, over a period of 40 years, hospitals removed and stored, without parents' consent, the hearts of more than 10 000 children (Anon. 19 Sep. 1999, *Sunday Age*, p. A20). The hearts were removed during routine post-mortem examinations, for which the parents had given consent; however, the parents were unaware that the hospitals had retained the hearts for research purposes and that the babies had been buried without their hearts.

These examples show that at every period in recent history researchers have exploited participants, who were often people at their mercy. In all of these cases, the researchers' dedication to research or to their own advancement led to disregard for the welfare of the individual participants. The ethical researcher will select means that are consistent with what the research can achieve and will ensure that no harm arises from the study.

Codes of ethics and research ethics guidelines

Several codes of ethics have been developed since the World War II. In the course of judging those accused of the concentration camp atrocities, the Nuremberg Tribunal, in 1949, promulgated the Nuremberg Code of research ethics, which formed the basis for subsequent codes. In 1964, the World Medical Association adopted the Declaration of Helsinki, which distinguished therapeutic research, in which participants receive beneficial treatment, from non-therapeutic research, which does not benefit participants but may benefit future patients. The Declaration of Helsinki stated that researchers should exercise even greater care to protect participants from harm in non-therapeutic research than in therapeutic research and that ethics committees should require strong, independent justification for exposing a healthy volunteer to substantial risk of harm just to gain new scientific information.

In Australia, the National Health and Medical Research Council (NHMRC) developed the Statement on Human Experimentation (NHMRC 2001). This statement has since been updated to become a more general statement applying to all research on humans, not just medical research, which was the focus of the earlier version (Spriggs 1999). The statement exemplifies the principles of ethical research and the rights of participants that are discussed in this chapter. All researchers who carry out projects involving human participants are required by the **human research ethics committee (HREC)** of their institution to read this statement before carrying out the research. The statement is available from your research management unit or on the NHMRC website: http://www.nhmrc.gov.au.

Several codes exist for researchers overseas. For example, the national nursing associations in the USA, Canada and the United Kingdom have developed guidelines for conduct in nursing research. In Australia, the WA Teaching Hospitals Nurse Researchers Network developed a set of Standards for Nursing Research, which stated that 'nurses undertaking research will respect the basic human rights of the individual at all times' (Robertson 1992). The WA group submitted the standards to the Australian Nursing Federation (ANF), which reviewed the standards and incorporated them into its own beginning standards (Robertson 1992). The standards, published by the ANF in 1997, are, along with the NHMRC guidelines, the national standards for ethics in nursing research. In addition, the Royal College of Nursing, Australia has stated in its document *Nursing Targets into the Twenty-first Century: A National Statement* that nursing research will be fostered by 'recognition as a legitimate, professional, ethical and socially relevant area of inquiry' (Royal College of Nursing, Australia 1992).

Thus, there are several codes to guide the researcher and the research consumer. Professionals must be familiar with a relevant code of ethics for their disciplinary research. Researchers will use the code to guide their action, thus ensuring ethical research. Relevant professionals who read research for its applications to practice will be able to judge the ethical aspects of research papers. Nevertheless, it is not sufficient for you as a health professional to be merely familiar with a code of ethics. You must understand the principles behind the code. These are outlined in the following section.

Human research ethics committees

A human research ethics committee (HREC), or its equivalent internationally, is a committee that is constituted to conduct research surveillance in an institution. HREC is the name of the committee in Australia. In Britain an HREC is called a research ethics committee (REC), while in the USA it is an institutional review board (IRB) and an institutional ethics committee (IEC) (Berglund 1998). (HRECs were formerly known as IECs in Australia.) Wherever it is, and whatever its title, an ethics committee is composed of persons inside and outside the institution. In Australia, the HREC should be distinguished from a clinical ethics committee (CEC) whose job it is to oversee ethics pertaining to client care.

Role

The role of the HREC, or any ethics committee otherwise named, is to deal with ethical matters pertaining to research on human participants. For simplicity's sake, this chapter will refer to HRECs. You should ensure that you explore your own country's ethics committee structures and processes and compare these with the statements made in this chapter. All institutions in which research is carried out must have an HREC. The HREC considers the ethical implications of all proposed research projects and decides whether they are ethically sound, monitors ongoing research projects to ensure continued conformity with ethical principles, maintains records of all research proposals, and in Australia communicates with the NHMRC's Medical Research Ethics Committee (NHMRC 2001).

A researcher who wishes to carry out a research project that involves humans or access to confidential records must obtain an ethics clearance from the HREC within their country. The researcher submits a research proposal which will provide information about the design of the project, the participants, and provisions for data handling. Preparation of such a proposal is discussed in Chapter 6.

The HREC will consider the proposal, giving due weight to compliance with ethical principles, institutional procedures, measures to protect the participants from harm, maintenance of cultural safety, and data storage procedures. If the HREC gives approval, the research may proceed. During the life of the project, the researcher submits a report on its status and either seeks renewal of the clearance or informs the HREC that the project has been completed. At the conclusion of the project, the HREC signs it off.

Composition

Compositions of HRECs vary from country to country. For example, in Australia the HREC must comprise at least seven men and women representing different age groups. Members include:

a) a chairperson;

b) at least two members who are lay people; one man and one woman, who have no affiliation with the institution or organisation, are not currently involved in medical, scientific, or legal work, and who are preferably from the community in which the institution or organisation is located;

c) at least one member with knowledge of, and current experience in, the areas of research that are regularly considered by the HREC (eg, health, medical, social, psychological, epidemiological, as appropriate);

d) at least one member with knowledge of, and current experience in, the professional care, counselling or treatment of people (eg, Medical practitioner, clinical psychologist, social worker, nurses, as appropriate);

e) at least one member who is a minister of religion, or a person who performs a similar role in a community such as an Aboriginal elder; and

f) at least one member who is a lawyer (NHMRC 2001, p. 16).

Most members of HRECs have had no training in ethics and are not likely to be as able as an ethicist to judge the ethical aspects of a research proposal. The lay and minister members are not likely to be as influential as the medical doctors and other health professionals.

The composition of the HREC as it is has been constituted usually means that it applies the logical-positivist model of research to all types of research, regardless of its suitability. Some health disciplines such as nursing often need to use a qualitative research design to answer significant questions. The present application forms of many HRECs assume a scientific experimentation model. This makes it awkward for nurses and other health professionals to frame ethics clearance proposals in a naturalistic paradigm. Researchers need to ask who is constructing the ethical standards for their disciplinary research, are these appropriate for their research, and whose interests are really being served by these standards (Johnstone 1999).

EXERCISE

Contact your HREC or equivalent committee chairperson and ask for a list of members on that committee. Compare the list to the NHMRC or national equivalent guidelines for committee composition. Can you see any difficulties, due to the potential power and knowledge differences in the ethics committee, that you may have in getting submissions through the committee?

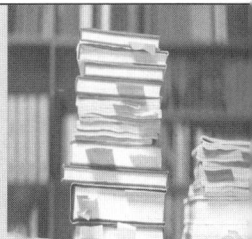

Functions

HRECs or equivalent committees scrutinise and approve the applications that come before them and monitor the progress and conclusion of the projects. They are concerned to uphold ethical principles and protect the public from harm. They must ensure that proposed research conforms to the relevant guidelines (NHMRC 2001). HRECs are concerned to protect the institution's own researchers from inadvertently committing unethical practices. For example, in Australia HRECs are also required to conform with the NHMRC's Statement on Human Experimentation and Supplementary Notes on research in particular fields such as research on human embryos.

At present in Australia, the HREC must review all proposals. Although there is a mechanism for 'fast-tracking' a proposal, it is time for the introduction of a set of guidelines for exemption from HREC review. Studies involving educational research, surveys, existing records or evaluation programs could be exempt from review provided that the principles of provision of **anonymity, confidentiality** and **privacy** are maintained and there is no risk to the participants. A mechanism for expediting review by means of delegation has been recommended.

The HREC has the responsibility of monitoring approved projects to ensure continued compliance with ethical requirements. It also monitors the researchers to ensure that they practise responsible science and thus maintain the good reputation of their institution (NHMRC 2001). The HREC incorporates confidential mechanisms for receiving complaints on the conduct of projects from participants, research workers or others. It requires that the researchers provide a written report to the HREC about the status of the project and compliance with the conditions imposed. In addition, the principal investigators are responsible for notifying the HREC immediately of any factor that might affect the ethical status of the project.

Protecting the rights of human participants
Participants' rights/principles

The Belmont Report in the USA has cited three principles that underpin most research standards: **beneficence, respect for human dignity,** and **justice** (National Commission for the Protection of Human Subjects of Biomedical and Behavioral Research 1978). These principles, plus **integrity,** are cited in the Australian NHMRC Statement (2001). In the Principles of Ethical Conduct the first mentioned value is integrity.

> The guiding value for researchers is integrity, which is expressed in a commitment to the search for knowledge, to recognised principles of research conduct and in the honest and ethical conduct of research and dissemination and communication of results (NHMRC 2001 p. 11).

Principles of beneficence and non-maleficence

Beneficence is 'doing good'. In the health care research context, this means that the researcher's aim should be to produce results that ultimately will benefit individuals or society as a whole through better treatment. In the research context, beneficence can be achieved by producing outcomes that will benefit humankind.

More crucial, however, is the principle of **non-maleficence** or 'doing no harm'. In applying this principle, researchers need to consider the potential for harm to or exploitation of the participants and whether the risks of the research outweigh the benefits. It is important to apply this principle in the planning and implementation stages of the research. HRECs examine applications closely to ensure that they meet this principle.

The right not to be harmed means that human participants should not be harmed as a result of participating in a research study. Obviously, the examples of experiments cited earlier, such as the New Zealand study on cervical cancer, resulted in harm to the participants. In this context, harm means excessive harm beyond slight discomfort involved in such things as blood tests. The researcher should always respect the rights, beliefs and autonomy of the individual participant.

The right not to be harmed includes being protected from harm that may arise through being involved in research studies of dubious scientific merit. The researcher has the ethical responsibility to the scientific community to ensure the integrity of the study throughout the process, from planning to publication. Ethical aspects related to good science include the value of the study in terms of the development of knowledge in nursing or health, and the use of an appropriate and valid theoretical framework and methodology for the question. The HREC is usually the arbiter of what is 'good' science. This assumes that the HREC members have the necessary expertise to decide what is good science, a value judgement that may affect whether they approve qualitative research. For example, in Australia since 2001 the members who can claim to be 'scientists' in their fields are, as quoted earlier:

c) at least one member with knowledge of, and current experience in, the areas of research that are regularly considered by the HREC (eg, health, medical, social, psychological, epidemiological, as appropriate);

d) at least one member with knowledge of, and current experience in, the professional care, counselling or treatment of people (eg, Medical practitioner, clinical psychologist, social worker, nurses, as appropriate) (NHMRC 2001, p. 16).

Thus the authority in the power structure determines the criteria for 'good' or 'valid' science. This means that qualitative projects may be viewed less favourably, because the authority has been socialised into a view that experimental research is the only valid methodology.

Only persons who have the qualifications and facilities to conduct the work properly should conduct or supervise research. If researchers or supervisors fall short in knowledge or experience, they should seek the help of a consultant.

Specific harm to research participants can include physical harm, psychological harm, emotional harm, social harm, financial harm and exploitation. Physical harm can range from minor discomfort to permanent injury or death. The Nazi and Japanese wartime experiments resulted in death for thousands of people. The New Zealand Women's

Hospital experiment was a classic example of extreme physical harm including death from cervical cancer. The experiment on the Australian troops resulted in permanent injury to participants.

Research studies can also cause psychological harm by damage to the participant's mind. A classic example of a study that caused psychological harm is the Milgram obedience experiment in which the researcher encouraged participants to administer electric shocks to other people (Milgram 1963). This experiment was carried out after World War II in an attempt to show that people will obey orders from superiors regardless of the results. An actor played the part of the subject of the experiment and in reality there was no electricity connected. With the encouragement of the researcher, the participants continued to escalate the amount of 'electric current' to lethal levels despite the 'subject's' agonised pleas to stop. We can only speculate on the psychological harm suffered by the real subjects of the experiments, even if they were debriefed later.

Qualitative research can also cause emotional harm, for example, in the interview process when the researcher seeks intimate details of participants' lives. Emotional harm can result from invasion of privacy when a researcher obtains information that the participant would rather have kept secret or perhaps has revealed in an unguarded moment, and later regrets doing so. It can be distressing for participants to recollect memories that they would prefer to avoid. Emotional harm can also result from disclosure of confidential information by the researcher, which could lead to embarrassment to the participants or worse. Unauthorised use of organs from patients has caused anguish for relatives.

Research could also cause social harm if, for example, the research interfered with the participant's kinship and family relationships, or the participant lost employment as a result of participating in the research project. For example, if people participated in a study on AIDS that led to disclosure of their condition to family and/or employers, that could cause irreparable social harm.

Financial harm could result if, say, the researcher or health agency charged the participant for investigative tests associated with the project. This is less likely in Australia where the individual does not pay directly for tests under Medicare. However, there is still financial harm in charging the government for research tests for which the researcher should pay because the taxes that people pay for Medicare will be higher. Another example of financial harm is a nurse carrying out a research project and billing the client for time used for the research. Other potential costs to the participants are the loss of their time and the hidden costs of participating such as baby-sitting or transport costs. People have a right to decide how to use their time effectively. Exploitation occurs if the researcher uses the participants' contribution for profit in any way, such as the selling of names for a mailing list, or expecting the participants to participate in ongoing research projects because they participated in the initial research project.

Tension can arise between the ethical consideration of doing no harm on the one hand and the need for scientific rigour on the other. For example, the accepted test of a new drug or treatment is a classic experiment in which one group of patients receives the new treatment and another group receives a placebo. A placebo is a treatment that looks exactly the same as the active treatment but does not contain the drug. The question then arises whether it is ethical to withhold the treatment from one group. If the treatment turns out to be beneficial, then the placebo group may be harmed by not having the treatment. The issue of fair access to experimental drugs may arise in terminal illness, as happened with AIDS in the 1990s. If, on the other hand, the treatment has unforeseen side effects, the experimental group may be harmed. There is also a question as to whether it is ethical to remove patients from established treatment to test a new drug. There is a risk of complications to the patient who is not even receiving standard treatment but receives a placebo instead.

At all costs, researchers must avoid harming participants. One way of doing this is to test out a new treatment, wherever possible, on animals or tissue cultures. This is not foolproof because, for example, some drugs may be teratogenic for certain species and not others. Testing on animals, at worst, does not consider an animal's right not to be harmed and, at best, judges that the prevention of harm to humans justifies the harm to the research animals. Most universities now have an animal ethics committee that ensures the humane use of animals for research purposes.

Researchers can also avoid harm by making provision in the research protocol to stop the study if there is reason to suspect that harm would result from continuing it. In addition, the researcher must remove individual participants from the study if there is evidence that they are suffering untoward effects. The safety of the participants must in all cases take priority over the research project. The NHMRC requires that an emergency contact number be given to all research participants so that they can contact the researcher if they are having any adverse effects. In addition, studies of new drugs or procedures should have statistical analysis built into them that ensures the study concludes as soon as it is possible to ascertain the potential value of the drug or procedure. This allows the commencement of the new treatment for those receiving a placebo; conventional treatment if the new drug or procedure is clearly superior; or resumption of the participants' previous treatment if that is superior. Thus, there is minimal risk for the participants.

In considering research proposals for their potential to do harm, the researcher and the HREC balance the risks to the participants with the benefits to society or the profession. The benefits should normally outweigh the risks. There are several potential benefits to the participants. There is the possibility of accessing a new nursing intervention or medical treatment that would otherwise not be available. There is the opportunity to acquire knowledge and experience by participating in the research process. There is a possible material reward for participation. Participants may achieve increased awareness of an experience through reliving it. Finally, participants such as the terminally ill may be comforted by the knowledge that they are helping others and advancing scientific knowledge.

If costs outweigh benefits, the researcher should not carry out the project. In an ethical trial, the advantage of the experimental treatment over the conventional treatment should not yet have been established. If an experiment has the potential to result in a valuable new treatment and if the participants know and accept that they have only a limited chance of receiving the real treatment, the benefits outweigh the risks.

Principle of respect for human dignity

This principle affirms the right to self-determination, that is, the rights of humans to determine their own actions. It concerns the right to decide whether to participate in a research project after full disclosure about the project. Participants have the right to self-determination, full disclosure and freedom from harassment. They also have the right to refuse to participate and to withdraw from a study at any time without penalty.

Informed consent

Informed consent is the agreement of the participant to take part in the research project after having been thoroughly briefed about the project and its possible outcomes. Informed consent has two elements: information and consent. Ethical research involves full disclosure of information to the prospective participant. This will include the identity of the researcher; the purpose and nature of the study; the right to refuse to participate; the right to withdraw at any time; the responsibilities of the researcher; possible benefits of the study; possible risks or side effects; any alternative treatments; and measures to be taken to protect privacy and to ensure anonymity and confidentiality. As a researcher, you should give information to the participants in a form and language that they can understand easily. This is usually done in the form of a plain language statement, which is written so that it is comprehensible to a layperson who does not have an advanced education. Figure 5.1 (opposite) shows an example of a plain language statement.

Silva and Sorrell (1984) demonstrated that research participants did not always understand procedures to which they had consented and that the amount, clarity and complexity of information affected participants' comprehension of information they had been given. Age, occupation or gender did not affect comprehension, but illness, passage of time and amount of threatening information did. It is therefore important to be vigilant in ensuring that the participant understands the nature of the study. The full disclosure of information may also be problematic in cross-cultural research, such as that with Indigenous or migrant participants where problems of differences in language, cultural values and beliefs may be present. Written consent may not be feasible and arrangements must be made to record the consent in some other way, for example, by audiotape recording.

Informed consent can also be a problem if, as happens in exploratory ethnographic research or action research, the researcher cannot state the explicit problems and research questions at the outset. The researcher should discuss difficulties openly with the participants

A Plain Language Statement for Registered Nurses about the Research:

Improving the quality of palliative nursing care through reflective practice and action research

You are invited to participate in research about facilitating reflective practice processes with experienced Registered Nurses working in palliative nursing areas. My name is Professor X of Y University and I will be undertaking the project as the principal researcher/facilitator. 'In a nutshell', this research will help you to identify constraints in your nursing practice and to bring about improvements using action research and reflective practice. Action research is a series of cycles of collectively planning, acting, observing and reflecting, in problem-solving practice issues of relevance to you. Reflective practice is a process for thinking back on what has happened at work, so that you can make sense of it and change it for the better, if necessary.

Up to 10 experienced Registered Nurses working in palliative nursing in this hospital will be invited to volunteer to participate. If you need information extra to this description, I will give a verbal and written explanation of the project at a regular meeting of palliative nurses. The nurses who join in the research need to be interested in reflecting on their practice in order to improve it. The focus of the research is on what you will learn as you experience the action research process. If you agree to participate this is what will happen:

Firstly, you will finish reading this Plain Language Statement and listen to the verbal explanation of the project, before you sign the attached Consent Form.

Then, as one of the participating nurses, you will meet weekly for one hour with the group to discuss clinical problems raised through activities such as sharing practice stories, journalling, critical analysis and discussion. I will facilitate the meetings, and explain the project materials including reflective practitioner guidelines and action research aims, processes and strategies, so you will be guided throughout the entire research project.

As a nurse in the research group you will be expected to maintain a journal of your experiences, the non-confidential parts of which you will be expected to share with your peers in the weekly group meeting. The types of questions that could be posed when engaging in practical reflection might include: 'What is happening here?', 'What is the nature of … ?', 'What is the experience of … ?' If you intend to change the constraining nature and effects of political, economic, cultural, social, historical elements in your practice, you may reflect on: 'What is happening here?', 'What factors have made it this way … ?', 'How might this be different …?'

In each action research cycle the findings will be pooled and discussed and the appropriate action will be planned and taken. Successive observation of the effects will follow, before further reflection leads to further action and analysis. If you sign the Consent Form and change your mind later, you can withdraw at any time if you choose and there will be no problem with that at all. If you have any questions to ask or comments to make, please feel free to phone me on (number). If you get my answering service, please leave a message and I will phone you back.

Signed:

Professor X

Figure 5.1   Example of a plain language statement

during the study and obtain their consent. The researcher and the participants make mutual decisions concerning ethical issues throughout the study.

Informed consent can also be a problem when the participants cannot speak English. Special provisions must be made to translate the consent form and plain language statement into the participants' first language. If participants cannot read well, it may be necessary to make arrangements to have the plain language statement read out to them.

Participants must agree to participate in the project and they, or, in the case of those not able to give consent, their agents, are the only ones who can make this decision. The participant must give consent without any coercion or unfair inducement. Coercion is the obtaining of research participants through their fear that harm will befall them if they do not enter the study. Examples of persons vulnerable to coercion are patients who fear inferior treatment or care if they do not take part in a medical research project, or students who are afraid of failing a course if they refuse to participate in a research project for the lecturer. Some groups are especially susceptible to coercion. Patients are especially vulnerable when their clinician is also the researcher, which is at the base of the NHMRC requirement that the clinician and researcher be different people. Unfair inducement is the holding out of undue material gains for the purposes of recruiting research participants. A reasonable monetary payment that merely compensates participants for inconvenience or time spent is not unfair inducement. For example, the payment of participants at a rate equivalent to an hourly wage is a reasonable recompense for time and expenses, but offering more than this, especially to captive participants, is not ethical. An example of unfair inducement is offering prisoners a remission off their sentence if they take part in a research project. The NHMRC guidelines for ethical aspects of qualitative health research point out that the crucial issue is whether the potential participants' belief that there is some gain for taking part affects their freedom to consent (NHMRC 1995).

Participants must also be free to withdraw from the study at any time. In qualitative research, where unforeseen events may occur, the researcher should remind participants periodically of their right to withdraw. Participants must be able to withdraw without a penalty, such as discriminatory treatment from a researcher who has some power over the participants. There is a moral dilemma in the use of participants who are unconscious or otherwise unable to give their own informed consent in that they are unable to withdraw from a study themselves and must rely on their agents.

The researcher must obtain informed consent from participants before collecting data. An agent can act for either the researcher or the participant. The participant usually signs a document that is specific to that study and includes all of the relevant information. The same considerations of language and literacy apply to the consent form. An example of a consent form is seen in Figure 5.2 (opposite).

Obtaining consent can be problematic in some situations, particularly in naturalistic observation. Consent is not necessary for observation in public places such as the street. In large institutions, where there are many people being observed, it may be impractical to obtain written consent from everyone being observed. Consent from the institution, with general information given to the employees about the project, must suffice. Applying the principle of consent can also be difficult in cultures that do not possess the Western idea of individualism and where the family and community make the decisions (Davis 1990). There are also situations in which written consent is unnecessary. The return of a questionnaire implies consent since the prospective respondent is free to refuse to participate by throwing the questionnaire away. Indeed, it is better research practice to have anonymous questionnaires. A signature on a consent form attached to a questionnaire invalidates the anonymity of the respondent and diminishes the validity of the data. However, a plain

Informed Consent Form for Registered Nurses in the Research:

Improving the quality of palliative nursing care through reflective practice and action research

You are invited to participate in research about facilitating reflective practice processes in experienced Registered Nurses working in palliative care. The project is being undertaken by Professor X of Y University. This research will help you to identify constraints in your nursing practice and to bring about improvements using action research and reflective practice. If you decide to participate, I (Professor X) will describe the procedures set out in the Plain Language Statement. Please ensure that you have read this statement and have received the verbal description before you sign this document. If you have any questions, please phone me on (number) and I will be happy to answer them. You will be given a copy of this form to keep.

I _____(name) have read the Plain Language Statement Description of the Project: *Improving the quality of palliative nursing care through reflective practice and action research*. I have also received a verbal explanation of the project by the researcher.

I understand that:

- the research is about facilitating reflective practice processes in experienced Registered Nurses working in palliative care;
- any information that is obtained in connection with this study and that can be identified with me will remain confidential and will be disclosed only with my permission;
- the information will be used to improve palliative nursing care;
- ethical measures will be taken to ensure my anonymity and privacy;
- I am free to withdraw my consent and to discontinue participation at any time without any coercion or penalties;
- I can contact Professor X to discuss the project if I have any questions to ask or comments to make;
- I will be one of possibly 10 nurses working in this hospital who is interested in reflecting on their practice in order to improve it;
- I will meet weekly with the group for one hour to discuss clinical problems raised through various exploratory activities;
- I will be expected to maintain a journal of my experiences, the non-confidential parts of which I will be expected to share with my peers in the weekly group meeting.

I have read the information above and agree to participate in this study. I am over the age of 18 years.

Name of participant...............................   Signature of participant...............................
Date...............................

Name of witness (independent of project)...............................   Signature of witness...................................
Date...............................

Figure 5.2   Example of a consent form (*continued*)

I certify that the terms of the form have been verbally explained to the participant, who appears to understand the terms prior to signing the form, and that proper arrangements have been made for an interpreter where English is not the participant's first language.

Signature of researcher.............................. Date..............................

Professor X
School of Z
Y University
(Town), (State)
Email: XXX@scu.edu.au Phone: (number)

The ethical aspects of this study have been approved by the Y University Human Research Ethics Committee (HREC). The Approval Number is (Insert when approved)

    If you have any complaints or reservations about any ethical aspect of your participation in this research, you may contact the HREC through the Ethics Complaints Officer, Ms X, telephone (number), fax (number), email:XXX@scu.edu.au

Any complaint you make will be treated in confidence and investigated, and you will be informed of the outcome.

Figure 5.2 (*Continued*)

language statement explaining the project is still necessary and should be sent as an attachment to the letter.

EXERCISE

Analyse the plain language statement and the informed consent forms (Figures 5.1 and 5.2) to judge the extent to which they reflect the ethical principles of integrity, beneficence, respect for human dignity and justice.

The main ethical and legal requirements of consent are explained by the NHMRC (2001, p. 12) as having two aspects: 'the provision of information and the capacity to make a voluntary choice'. Therefore, consent should involve:

a) provision to participants, at their level of comprehension, of information about the purpose, methods, demands, risks, inconveniences, discomforts, and possible outcomes of the research (including the likelihood and form of publication of research results); and

b) the exercise of voluntary choice to participate (NHMRC 2001, p. 12).

Special participants

Special participants are persons who have a diminished ability to give informed consent and are therefore at risk of exploitation. Some special participants have an impaired ability to understand information, may or may not have the capacity to give informed consent, depending on their mental state. Such persons include developmentally disabled people, confused elderly, and mentally ill persons. Persons in a dependent relationship are also special participants because they are unable to give their own consent. These include children, elderly persons who cannot give free consent, wards of state and unconscious patients.

These groups should be treated with the same ethical standards as all others and require even greater protection because of their inability to give informed consent. Special participants should not be used as research fodder because of their vulnerability to exploitation. They should be used only for therapeutic research from which they have some hope of deriving a benefit, or in situations in which other populations are not suitable to answer the questions posed by the study (NHMRC 2001).

The principle of obtaining informed consent from special participants is that informed consent should be obtained from an agent, that is, a person who has the intelligence or capability to give it on behalf of the other dependent person. The person giving informed consent should be in a legal capacity to the proposed participant, such as a parent or guardian. Children are considered to be below the age of legal consent, and consent should be obtained from the parents or legal guardian. Consent should also be obtained from the child where the child is of sufficient maturity and intelligence to make this feasible.

However, obtaining informed consent from such groups as the elderly is not always straightforward. Elderly people frequently have visual and hearing impairments that can make the use of written consent forms inappropriate, or they may be reluctant to sign without a family member present.

An interesting issue has arisen with regard to obtaining consent for the use in research studies of tissues and body parts that were obtained for clinical purposes. For example, slides may be taken for diagnostic purposes and a research project planned for later, in which it is intended to use those slides. Should consent be obtained? In many cases it is difficult to track down the clients to get their permission. It is possible to avoid this situation by obtaining consent to use the slides or tissues for later research purposes at the time of collection of the material. Of course, if a research project is planned before the tissues are collected, consent should be obtained. It should not just be assumed that if the tissues are there, they can be used freely for research purposes.

Deception

Sometimes a researcher seeks to deceive participants to facilitate data collection or because giving full information can lead to invalidation of the study. This is most likely to occur in methods involving participant observation (NHMRC 2001). Participants might not behave naturally if they know they are being observed, especially in cases where illicit activity is concerned. Participants might also censor information at interview if they know the real purpose of the study.

Deception can be passive, where the researcher omits to give information to participants, or active, where the researcher actually tells lies to the participants. Passive deception usually involves covert data collection or obtaining data by false pretences without actually lying. Techniques for covert data collection include observing participants who do not know they are being observed, interviewing participants who do not know that what they say will become research data, or participating in activities with a group who do not know they are participants. For example, a researcher might wish to study the conversation of professionals at tea breaks. Believing that if the clinicians knew they were being observed their behaviour might change, the researcher might elect to collect data on them without their knowledge. Covert research can also take place through the study of confidential documents (NHMRC 2001). More sinister techniques involve the use of devices such as one-way mirrors or hidden video cameras and microphones.

Apologists for covert data collection justify it by saying that it is sometimes the only way to obtain valid data. However, studies may be unethical if the design involves covert observation of subjects behaving in ways that they would not wish a researcher to observe or record, or that they might later regret. It can be argued that workers ought to be able to carry out work without unknowingly being observed by a researcher and that researchers who use covert observation fail to take into consideration the feelings of the subjects when they find out that they were observed without their knowledge. In ethnographic studies it is sufficient to get permission from the community. Individual consent is necessary only if specific data, for example, interviews, are sought.

Active deception consists of deliberately withholding some information or giving false information about the study to secure people's participation. The researcher may resort to this when knowledge of the true purpose of the study would invalidate the findings. The Milgram obedience experiment cited earlier in this chapter is a classic case of deception. Another less harmful instance of deception occurred in England. A researcher asked nurses to evaluate the same research paper that had two false names and qualifications on them: one paper was purported to have been written by a doctor and one by a nurse; both were female (Hicks 1992). The participants thought they were critiquing the papers, but the true purpose of the study was to see whether nurses ascribed greater research expertise to doctors than to nurses. There was no difference in the perceptions of the quality of the paper overall, but the participants ascribed superior research methodology and statistical analysis to the paper supposedly written by the doctor. The other classic method of active deception is the use of placebos in experiments. The researcher should inform participants that they have an equal chance of getting a placebo or the treatment.

Is it ever justifiable to deceive research participants, for example, if the benefits of the research to society outweigh the risks to the individual? The NHMRC (2001, p. 51) guidelines say that:

> as a general principle, deception of, concealment of the purposes of a study from, or covert observation of, identifiable participants are not considered ethical because they are contrary to the principle of respect for persons in that free and fully informed consent cannot be given.

The guidelines go on to acknowledge that there may be 'exceptional circumstances where studies cannot be conducted without deception …' (p. 51), so certain requirements must be satisfied before a HREC can grant ethical approval for such a project.

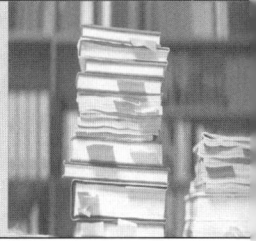

Principle of justice

The principle of justice is that all participants have the right to be treated fairly and with respect and courtesy at every stage of the research process, from the design of the project to the reporting of findings. At the design stage, it is necessary to build fair selection and treatment of participants into the process. Participants should be selected on criteria related to relevance to the topic rather than availability or on inability to refuse. The Australian Army study of mustard gas calls into question whether the soldiers were truly volunteers. Once the group has been selected, each participant should have an equal chance of receiving the active treatment, both for reasons of fairness and for reasons of scientific validity. The researcher should assign participants to the group randomly, not on the basis of favouritism. If the researcher is in a position of authority over participants, participants who decline to participate or who withdraw from a study should not be penalised in any way, regardless of the effect of their withdrawal on the research project. The informed consent document, or another written agreement that outlines the commitment of the participant and the researcher in terms of time, procedures and benefits, should be adhered to by the researcher. The participants should be provided with access by telephone or in person to the researcher in case of problems, and the researcher should provide any necessary assistance if inadvertent side effects occur. At the end of the study, any promised benefits or reports should be provided.

Anonymity

Anonymity means the concealment or obscuring of the identity of the participants. Total anonymity occurs when even the researcher cannot identify the research participants, for example, when a questionnaire is returned anonymously. Partial anonymity occurs when the researcher knows the identity of the participants but conceals it from any outsiders. If anyone beyond the team knows the identity of the participants, or can link findings to any participant, then the participants do not have anonymity.

The researcher should act at all times in such a manner as to protect the anonymity of the participants and should build appropriate procedures into the study design to separate the identity of the participants from the data. For example, if the design of the study requires that a written consent form is attached to the data, this is separated from the data as soon as possible and the data are entered into the computer using a code number or pseudonym. If the design of the study requires the linking of two sets of data, a list is created that records the participants' names and pseudonyms or code numbers, and this is stored in a different place. An alternative to this is a code number or combination of numbers and letters such as the participant's mother's maiden initials, number of siblings and so forth. This code, which may be used according to a formula generated by the researcher but which will be unique to each participant, will be attached to all protocols. If the researcher must know the identity of the participants, as happens in qualitative research, the full name of the person should not be used in the primary data, including tape-recordings. A pseudonym or code number should be used in the transcribed or processed data. Also, with this type of data a list linking the code numbers or pseudonyms should be kept separately and securely.

Several years ago, an issue arose with respect to anonymity and research on the Internet. Some researchers had posted questionnaires to all members of a list of subscribers to the Internet, using the facility that allows them to post one message through the central list-server to all members of the list. If respondents unwittingly used the 'reply to all' option, rather than the 'reply' option, which returns only to the individual initiating the response, the answered questionnaire went back to all of the members of the list. This obviously destroyed the anonymity of the respondents. The correct procedure is for the researcher to warn respondents to send the answered questionnaire back to the address of the researcher. This procedure keeps the data in the hands of the researcher who can then institute procedures to separate the data from the names and thus protect the anonymity of the participants.

Privacy

Privacy in the research context refers to the right of participants to decide which information they wish to disclose. Participants have a right to privacy, particularly concerning their attitudes, beliefs, behaviours, opinions, and records such as diaries and other private papers. Researchers do not have any automatic right to information by virtue of the fact that they are doing a research project and they must not invade the privacy of the participant beyond what is reasonable and what is approved by the HREC for the purposes of the study. Even then, researchers must be sensitive to the private nature of some information and guard its confidentiality. Invasion of privacy can also occur in covert data collection, which was discussed under the topic, informed consent. Watching people in non-public places for data collection when they are not aware of it is an invasion of privacy.

A special problem concerning privacy of records has occurred since the rise in popularity of epidemiological research, where it has become increasingly commonplace for nurses and other health professionals to carry out research utilising records which identify the individual. Often access is sought by researchers for records of births and deaths, which are open to inspection for the purposes of research at the discretion of the appropriate state or territory registrar. In addition, records of living persons are often needed for research purposes. The principle laid down by the NHMRC is that medical records should be made available for legitimate research purposes; in practice, this means HREC-approved research projects. This principle also has legal force since several states, including New South Wales, Victoria, Queensland and South Australia, have statutes providing access to hospital medical records for research purposes. The issue which then arises is whether the individual needs to give consent to their use. However, the task of tracking down all persons whose records one might wish to access to obtain written consent would be impossible. Even if it were possible, it might alarm some participants, as could happen if one wished to do a study on the link between previous miscarriages and probability of abortion. With regard to the use of medical records, there is a distinction between information obtained for further experimentation and the study of records. In the former case, informed consent must be obtained for any research which adds further risk to the participants. In the case of a pure study of records, consent from the individuals is not necessary. However, it is possible to build in consent for future examination of records into an initial consent form.

Procedures can be put in place to safeguard the privacy of records. Where two types of records are linked together, once the linkage has been made, the names must be removed from the file and replaced with a code number. The list linking the names and code number or pseudonym must be kept in a secure place. It is recommended that standard measures be taken to ensure anonymity and confidentiality, as discussed in the previous sections.

Anonymity may be violated if the identity of the participants is not concealed in the reporting or publication stage. This can happen if the researcher reveals a cluster of characteristics that would identify a person, for example 'a female professor at University X' where there is only one.

Privacy legislation issues

The Privacy Act 1988 requires HRECs 'to conform to the Information Privacy Principles (IPPs) in dealing with personal information' (NHMRC 2001, p. 52). There are guidelines for 11 privacy principles for dealing with personal information including its: manner and purpose of collection; solicitation from the individual concerned; solicitation generally; storage and security; records kept by the record-keeper; access to records; alterations of records; accuracy; its use for relevant purposes; limits on use; and limits on disclosure. For the specific guidelines read the NHMRC (2001) document.

A principle of interest and concern to health researchers is Principle 10, which sets out the limits on use of personal information. The principle makes clear and distinct links between researchers' ethical and legal requirements. For example, a 'record-keeper' (researcher) who keeps and controls data for research 'shall not use the personal information for any other purpose unless:

a) the individual concerned has consented to use of that information for that other purpose;

b) the record-keeper believes on reasonable grounds that use of the information for that other purpose is necessary to prevent or lessen a serious or imminent threat to the life or health of the individual concerned or another person;

c) use of the information for that other purpose is required or authorised by or under law;

d) use of the information for that other purpose is reasonably necessary for enforcement of the criminal law or of a law imposing a pecuniary penalty, or for the protection of the public revenue; or

e) the purpose for which the information is used is directly related to the purpose for which the information was obtained (NHMRC 2001, pp. 60-1).

Reading just one principle, such as Principle 10 above, shows the degree of researcher knowledge and diligence necessary to use personal information ethically and legally. Research projects in nursing and health can be of a risky nature in relation to personal information, because projects may focus on human experiences of illness and the personal circumstances around diagnoses and treatments. Therefore, researchers need to become acquainted with the privacy legislation in their own country and ensure that projects they undertake conform fully to the ethical and legal requirements implicit in principles relating to accessing, analysing, storing and disseminating private information.

EXERCISE

If you are an Australian researcher, locate a copy of the Information Privacy Principles (IPPs) in dealing with personal information (NHMRC 2001). Alternatively, locate your own country's national ethics statement.

Use the document to ascertain the complexity in ensuring privacy in human research and the extent to which health professionals are responsible for ensuring privacy.

Right to confidentiality

The researcher has the responsibility to keep data confidential so that individuals are not compromised. This means that you do not allow anyone access to the data unless they are authorised to have it, and you do not tell anyone information given to you in confidence.

Maintaining confidentiality includes protecting data from unauthorised access. You can prevent inadvertent unauthorised data access by storing it in a secure place such as a locked filing cabinet. This is especially important for data that are not anonymous. Researchers must refuse any requests for data access from unauthorised persons. You can also prevent identification of participants by concealing their names and identities in a report. Even geographical locations should be concealed if they are easily identifiable.

During the course of a research project, the participants may tell the researcher confidential information. The researcher has an obligation to respect the participants' wishes concerning the confidentiality of information as far as possible. Confidentiality is especially important for sensitive data such as that concerning sexual matters or use of illicit drugs, or while the participants' names are linked to the data. Confidentiality is broken if you disclose information to persons outside the project, either by careless gossip or by allowing unauthorised persons to access the data.

The unpredictable nature of qualitative research means that new information may arise during the course of the study, and participants should periodically be reminded of their right to withhold information. Confidentiality in qualitative research can be difficult to maintain in small settings where everyone knows everyone else. However, in some qualitative projects, participants may choose to be named.

In the case of medical records, the researcher must exercise care concerning confidentiality and ensure that the information is restricted to those who need it.

Sometimes, persons in authority may pressure the researcher for access to data; for example, in a study of health in an industrial setting, the participants' supervisor may ask to see data on workers. This should not be granted. The only persons in authority who can legitimately demand access to confidential research data are police if they have a search warrant.

The NHMRC guidelines on ethics point out that researchers need to be aware that they cannot guarantee participants absolute confidentiality because they may be legally compelled to testify in court (NHMRC 2001). If, for example, a participant confessed to a crime, in some states or territories the researcher could be called to testify in court and would not be able to claim client–professional privilege.

A moral dilemma concerning confidentiality may arise if one discovers irregularities in practice during the course of a research project. This places the researcher in a difficult position – whether to break confidentiality and report irregularities to the authorities, or to keep quiet about them and condone patient abuse. Reporting to the authorities will likely jeopardise the continuation of the research, whereas keeping silent will allow the researcher to retain the trust of the participants.

Broken confidentiality destroys trust and may have consequences for present and later research. If confidentiality is broken during the project, the researchers may be asked to leave before the project is completed, with disastrous consequences for the outcome of the research project. If participants feel that they have been betrayed, they are not likely to consent to further research by that researcher. Furthermore, they are unlikely to grant access to future researchers. The ethical dilemma is whether to give priority to the research or to patient safety. The resolution of such a dilemma is not easy. The researcher may wish to start with a discussion with the participants about the problem and try to raise their awareness of the problem and attempt to solve it that way. If the problem cannot be resolved 'in-house', the researcher must make a decision based on the moral issue. The safety of clients must take priority over research aims. The NHMRC guidelines on ethics state that the researcher is not legally protected against mandatory reporting if abuse is seen during a study (NHMRC 2001).

Ethical aspects of research in special cases
Research involving assisted reproductive technology

Since the development of *in vitro* fertilisation (IVF), research on the human embryo or foetus has become more controversial. The embryo is the product of the union of the sperm and ova at fertilisation and before implantation. The foetus/foetal tissue is the continuation of the embryo from the time of implantation to the time of complete gestation, regardless of its status at birth. The foetal membranes, placenta, umbilical cord and amniotic fluid are considered to be part of the foetus before separation. There is concern about experimentation on embryos, either spare embryos left over from IVF treatment or embryos specifically created for research purposes. The central issue is whether embryos have human status and therefore should be protected from harm. To decide whether embryos have human status requires a determination of when life begins. These issues are under debate in legal, moral, religious and research areas. In recent times, several states (South Australia, Victoria and Western Australia) enacted legislation that restricts experimentation on human embryos and that overrides guidelines of government agencies. Embryos, which are of concern in IVF, are treated differently from the foetus and foetal tissue, which are considered to exist when implantation occurs. The sperm and ova produced for IVF should be treated as belonging to the donors rather than the institution or researcher and the donors' wishes concerning the usage of these must be respected. Embryos belong to the donors or a single surviving donor. It is considered unethical to store frozen embryos for more than 10 years, grow them beyond the stage at which implantation would normally occur or conduct cloning experiments designed to lead to the production of multiple genetically identical humans. However, the law does permit stem cell research which could lead to cures for genetic diseases.

According to the NHMRC guidelines, it may be ethical to carry out experiments on the foetus *in utero* where such experiments may promote life or health of the foetus or where the research provides the mother with information about the health or normality of the foetus, thereby giving her choices concerning the future treatment and disposition of the foetus. It is unethical to administer drugs to or carry out any procedure on the mother to find out any harmful effects on the foetus, even if abortion is anticipated. Once abortion is inevitable, some research procedures may be permissible. Consent should be obtained from the mother and, where practicable, the father before the research commences and permission should be obtained for use of foetal tissues, including cells, membranes, placenta, umbilical cord and amniotic fluid to be stored or propagated in tissue culture. Permission to transplant cells into a human recipient should also be specifically obtained. The decision to approach the mother for consent to such research must be made by the clinician rather than the researcher.

There are also issues concerning research on a separated pre-viable foetus or foetal tissue. A pre-viable foetus is one that has not reached an age of 20 weeks gestational age and that weighs 400 g or less. The foetus should have separated by natural processes or lawful means, should not be dissected while there is any obvious sign of life, and should be removed from the nearby clinical area before research is carried out. Again, there should be separation of clinical and research decision-making to avoid a conflict of interest. The main Australian publication to be consulted in these matters is the *NHMRC Ethical Guidelines on Assisted Reproductive Technology* (NHMRC 1996). Researchers in other countries should consult their guidelines through relevant medical research authorities.

Indigenous participants

Indigenous participants are not special participants under the previous definition; nevertheless their situation requires special consideration. The history of relationships between Indigenous people and non-Indigenous researchers has produced a suspicion of the motives of non-Indigenous researchers. Research involving Australian Aboriginal and Torres Strait Islander communities must take account of sensitive ethical issues, particularly with regard to culture. The Special Purposes Committee of the NHMRC convened a national conference in 1986 in Alice Springs from which it emerged that a high priority was ethics in relation to Aboriginal and Torres Strait Islander health. A national workshop of ethics in Indigenous health was then held in New South Wales in 1987, attended by 30 Indigenous representatives from all around Australia. From this workshop, a set of advisory notes, later converted to comprehensive guidelines, was developed. At the time of the workshop, the Medical Research Ethics Committee believed that the issue of Aboriginal and Torres Strait Islander communities deserved special consideration because they had an obvious level of poor health that past research had failed to address. It cited reasons for this failure as a priority of interest in scientific research or research interests of white Australians and an insensitivity among researchers to the 'values, needs and customs' of Aboriginal and Torres Strait Islander peoples. Specific concerns were: lack of understanding of cultural values concerning gender issues, inappropriate treatment of organs post-mortem, inappropriate requests for and handling of blood and other biological specimens, and publication of inappropriate pictures, such as of dead people (NHMRC 1992).

Prior to the guidelines, the lack of appreciation of ethical issues in research on Aboriginal and Torres Strait Islanders had led to deficient practices including approval being sought from individuals instead of from the appropriate community authority, lower standards being applied for obtaining consent among disadvantaged Aboriginal and Torres Strait Islander communities, a failure to appreciate that access to sensitive areas would be dependent upon the researcher's social status, conflict between the mores of scientific research and Aboriginal and Torres Strait Islander cultural and social values, and the increased vulnerability of Aboriginal and Torres Strait Islander groups to exploitation by researchers. The highest standards of ethical conduct in research should apply to research concerning the Aboriginal and Torres Strait Islander people, who must set their own research priorities rather than merely responding to those set by non-Indigenous people (Johnstone 1991). Indigenous people have the power to set their own ethics guidelines and insist that these be enforced because they now control access by researchers to their communities.

In some Australian states, organisations controlled by Aboriginal and Torres Strait Islander people have established their own HRECs. In addition, some ethics committees have an Indigenous subcommittee, for example, the Top End Ethics Committee in the Northern Territory. These committees and subcommittees can decide or recommend on research proposals that relate to research on Aboriginal and Torres Strait Islander people, whether internally or externally developed. It is now very difficult, if not impossible, to obtain access to Indigenous participants without an Indigenous co-researcher.

The NHMRC (1991) recommends that a HREC should satisfy itself that a proposal concerning research on Aboriginal and Torres Strait Islander communities should demonstrate that:

- the researcher has sought advice from Aboriginal and Torres Strait Islander health agencies and local community controlled Aboriginal and Torres Strait Islander health services and agencies
- the Aboriginal and Torres Strait Islander community, or the agency representing the community, has indicated that the research will be potentially useful to the community or the people in general

- the research will be conducted in such a way that it is sensitive to the cultural and political situation of the community
- the researcher has written consent from the community concerned or has documented the reasons why this is not possible.

In the process of obtaining informed consent from Indigenous communities, the researcher should provide information concerning collection and analysis of data, the drafting and publication of reports in a format understandable by the community, and the potential costs and benefits of the research. The researcher should have face-to-face discussions with the people concerned, where possible, or document reasons for lack of success. Sufficient time for the community to absorb and reply to the information should be allowed. There should be a demonstrated process for obtaining free consent from individuals, as well as written evidence of consent from the whole community. There should be provision for informing participants of their right to withdraw consent at any time (NHMRC 1991).

Aboriginal and Torres Strait Islander communities must have involvement in research on their own people. They must be given decision-making power at every stage of the research project and receive appropriate financial recompense (NHMRC 1991). This approach will help to compensate for past injustices and enhance Indigenous control and participation in research. However, the guidelines unquestionably make it difficult to do research in Indigenous health, which may lead to less research and consequently militate against improving Indigenous health.

Multi-centre and multi-site research

Multidisciplinary health team collaboration in research projects and competition for large funds from funding bodies often result in multi-centre and multi-site research. This means that researchers from different departments within and across health care institutions and universities generate team projects reaching across many centres and sites. Because the projects are significant for health outcomes and research funds must be expended within a given time, the guidelines expedite the multi-site ethical approval processes. For example, the NHMRC (2001) suggests that HRECs ascertain whether the submission has been reviewed by another HREC. For example, for 'prompt and efficient consideration of multi-centre research protocols an individual HREC may:

a) communicate with, and give advice to or receive advice from, any other HREC;

b) accept a scientific/technical assessment of the research by another institution or organisation;

c) review, and where the same research project is conducted at two or more institutions or organisations, adopt the reasons for ethical approval or disapproval of another HREC in reaching its own decision; or

d) adopt other administrative procedure to accelerate timely consideration and avoid unnecessary duplication (NHMRC 2001, p. 23).

If your project is not as large or as highly funded as the projects inferred above, but it nevertheless occurs across two or more sites, you must ensure that you have ethical approval from the relevant HRECs associated with those sites. For example, a nursing research project in three different hospitals must secure ethical approval from the relevant committees within the specific health regions. This means that you will need to allow time for the project to be reviewed by several committees, who most probably meet at different times of the year. Sometimes the multi-site approval may be facilitated by an expedited review, where approval at one site helps approval at the other sites. It is of great importance that you check the requirements for multi-site review before you make a final decision on research settings and participants, lest you find yourself very much behind time in your project timelines while awaiting ethical approvals.

Research ethics in health practices

With the research explosion of recent years, clinicians are more likely than ever to be involved in nursing, health or medical research in various ways. They may collect or transport specimens for research, for example, foetal tissue. They may be responsible for administering experimental medications in research protocols in the course of their client care. Or they may be involved as members of a research team. If you are involved in a research project, whatever your role, you have certain rights and responsibilities.

As a participant in research, you have the rights of voluntary and informed participation, and of withdrawal without penalty. You should also be able to withdraw from a project without being put at a disadvantage.

If you participate in a research project as a part of the research team, you must assure yourself about the ethical aspects of the project. You have the responsibility for being aware of relevant research guidelines and codes of conduct and for ensuring that you are not taking part in illegal or unapproved research. You must ensure that the researchers protect the clients' rights. You need to understand the aims and design of the project, including whether it has ethics clearance. You should also assure yourself about the credentials of the investigator to conduct the research.

As a clinician with clients involved as participants in research projects, you also have certain responsibilities towards those clients. If you give clients experimental drugs the effects of which are not completely known, you should know the action, possible side effects and expected clinical outcomes of the drug and should observe the client for reactions to it. You will need to be competent in assessment of clients undergoing clinical trials so you can recommend that the clients be removed from the trial if they are being adversely affected in any way.

You also have certain rights as a clinician requested to be a data collector for others' research projects. You have the same rights as clients to refuse to participate without fear of reprisal. One situation that may arise is a conscientious or religious objection to a particular type of research such as that on foeti. No-one should be required to participate in a project against their will or suffer reprisals because of their objection.

Scientific misconduct

Scientific misconduct is an act of deception or misrepresentation of one's own work. It can take the form of fraud, such as fabrication of data to report non-existent research, or falsification of data, such as changing records. It also includes irresponsible authorship, such as plagiarism, and false attribution of authorship. Furthermore, it includes publishing the same article in more than one journal and fragmenting a study unnecessarily to increase the number of publications (Australian Vice-Chancellors' Committee n.d.). Scientific fraud usually occurs when a researcher desires a shortcut to rewards such as promotion, or is convinced that the desired outcome justifies altering the results to achieve the 'correct' findings.

Scientific fraud comprises both unintentional fraud, in which the researcher makes an honest mistake, and intentional fraud, in which there is a deliberate deception. Unintentional fraud can involve failure to recognise the important factors that affect the observed evidence or can involve misinterpretation of data. Intentional fraud, however, is a more serious matter. It usually involves the data management phase of the research process. The three most common ways of faking data are smoothing out irregularities, discarding results that don't fit the theory, and inventing the data. The publishing process is supposed to detect fraud through the process of peer review. However, peer review is inadequate as a control mechanism because reviewers generally assume that other researchers are honest and even if they do suspect fraud, they may be reluctant to report it because of considerable risk to their own careers.

In Australia, there have been two documented cases of scientific fraud in the area of medical research, one on birth control pills and one on hyoscine. Both took place in the early 1980s. The first was the case of Dr Michael Briggs, a Professor of Human Biology at Deakin University, who had faked research on the effects of contraceptive pills on blood metabolism in women using the pill for longer than 18 months and in a study on progesterone and breast tumours in beagle bitches (Kohn 1986). Briggs resigned from the university and went to Spain where he died a short time later.

The second case concerned Dr William McBride, who was lionised for discovering that the drug thalidomide could produce phocomelia, a congenital malformation or absence of limbs. McBride is alleged to have made a habit of duplicity in research, including the use of unauthorised data in his MD thesis, taking more than his share of the credit for the thalidomide discovery, stealing the neural crest theory of thalidomide action, giving false witness at a trial of a drug company in the USA, and fabricating data on a study of the effects of hyoscine on birth deformities (Nicol 1989). A medical tribunal that lasted four years found McBride guilty of 24 charges of medical research fraud and he was struck off the medical register as being not of good character in the context of fitness to practise medicine (Humphrey 1994). An appeal was later dismissed.

A researcher or clinician may discover a case of scientific misconduct or unethical research processes and must decide whether to become a 'whistle-blower', or one who reports suspected misconduct to the authorities. Or you may be the first to observe the deleterious effects of a drug in a clinical trial. Should you report it, and, if so, to whom? On one hand, you have a duty of care to the client. On the other hand, repercussions may result if a nurse reports the incident. Nevertheless, your moral duty to put the protection of the patient above other considerations is clear. However, anyone in such an invidious position would do well to read the literature on whistle-blowing and take account of protective mechanisms before 'blowing the whistle'.

How can scientific fraud be prevented? The Australian Vice-Chancellors' Committee states in its guidelines that a principle of research is the validity and accuracy in the collection and reporting of data (NHMRC 2001). Institutions should have policies in place to deal with prevention of scientific fraud, including maintenance of records and retention of data. Researchers should be familiar with those policies. Institutions should cultivate an ethos that discourages scientific fraud. Established researchers should serve as role models and/or mentors to less experienced researchers. Finally, institutions should reward quality rather than quantity of publications, although this is not likely to happen while university funding gives precedence to quantity, as is often currently the case.

Reading a research report: ethical considerations

You will probably need to read research reports in the course of your professional practice and you should be familiar with the ethical aspects of evaluating these reports. Research papers frequently do not address ethical aspects very well, but an informed reader is able to critique the implied ethical aspects. Most journals have a policy of publishing only research that conforms to ethical standards. As a reader, you will ask questions about the appropriateness of topic or participants, research design, approval by a HREC, treatment of participants and ethical procedures. The advanced reader may examine the results for evidence of propriety: results that are too good to be true may not be!

EXERCISE
Locate a research report in a refereed journal in your health discipline. Read the report to ascertain the extent to which ethical safeguards are discussed. Criteria for critique of ethical aspects of research reports can be found in Chapter 3.

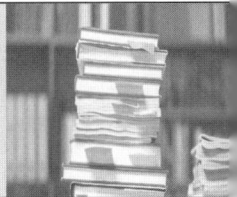

Summary

This chapter presented the ethical issues that nurses and other health carers need to know to be effective researchers, consumers of research and participants in research projects. Historical instances of unethical medical research have set the scene for understanding ethical issues and the need for codes of ethical conduct in research. The rights of participants and the responsibilities of researchers have been discussed and ways in which researchers can protect the rights of participants have been outlined. The role, composition and function of HRECs has been discussed. The issues of ethics affecting clinicians have been presented.

Scientific misconduct has been outlined and the reader has been given a set of guidelines for evaluating the ethical aspects of research.

Main points

- Ethics is concerned with moral questions and behaviour; it asks what ought to be done and is a guide for research procedures.
- All research should be carried out with the highest moral standards.
- There are examples of unethical research conduct in all times including the present.
- Codes of ethics and research ethics guidelines are based on the Nuremberg Code and the Helsinki Declaration, as is the NHMRC Statement on Human Experimentation, which forms the ethical standard for human research in Australia.
- Ethical principles on which the codes are based comprise integrity, beneficence, non-maleficence, respect for human dignity and justice.
- Human research ethics committees (HRECs) are charged with scrutinising and approving applications and monitoring progress and conclusion of projects involving research on humans.
- Participants have the right to informed consent, anonymity, privacy, confidentiality, to not participate or to withdraw at any time, and to not suffer harm.
- Special cases such as embryos, foetal tissue, vulnerable subjects/participants and Indigenous participants have extra protection under the guidelines.
- Scientific misconduct is an act of deception or misrepresentation of one's own work and includes fraud, fabrication or falsification of data, plagiarism, irresponsible authorship, and false attribution of authorship.
- Whether conducting or assisting with research, clinicians ought to uphold the highest ethical standards.

CASE STUDY

Our case study continues with Maxwell, who you met in Chapter 3. To recap, Maxwell is a 45-year-old physiotherapist who has been accepted into PhD studies. Maxwell is interested in the extent to which complementary therapies have influenced clients' help-seeking behaviours in attending 'orthodox' physiotherapist services. He suspects that the decline in attendance at his physiotherapy clinic may be due to clients seeking naturopathic services and/or to self-medicate with herbal therapies. So far, you have helped Maxwell formulate a research question and prepare to review the literature. He is now at the point of considering the ethical implications of his research. To gather research data, Maxwell intends to send a postal survey to all previous clients who are no longer attending his clinic, to ascertain, what, if any, health care they are now seeking. He also intends to follow up with an in-depth interview with 20 previous clients to explore their help-seeking behaviours in greater depth. Maxwell is appreciative of the help you have given him so far and he requests a discussion with you about the ethical implications of his proposed research. What will you tell Maxwell in relation to:

- the need for integrity in conducting research
- the importance of non-maleficence and justice and how to apply these ethical principles in his research
- special considerations if he is intending to include Indigenous participants?

Multiple choice questions

1   Human research ethics committees:
    a   decide on funding for institutional projects
    b   conduct research surveillance in institutions
    c   ensure research institutions operate legally
    d   arrange multi-site institutional research
2   The application of the ethical principle that ensures no harm is done to research participants is:
    a   non-maleficence
    b   confidentiality
    c   justice
    d   integrity
3   The agreement of the participant to take part in the research project after having been thoroughly briefed about the project and its possible outcomes is:
    a   human dignity
    b   full disclosure
    c   self-determination
    d   informed consent
4   Giving information about a project to the participants in a written form they can understand easily is a:
    a   list of keywords
    b   guide to experimentation
    c   plain language statement
    d   research consent form
5   Special participants with diminished ability to give informed consent and in dependent relationships:
    a   do not know what is happening so they do not need to give their consent to participate
    b   do not require the researcher to be ethical because they do not understand the project's intentions
    c   should be given a chance to explain why they are unable to participate before being excluded
    d   should be treated with the same ethical standards as all others and even greater protection

6 The ethical principle that all participants have the right to be treated fairly and with respect and courtesy at every stage of the research process, from the design of the project to the reporting of findings, is an example of the application of:

a privacy

b confidentiality

c anonymity

d justice

7 Protecting data from unauthorised access is an example of:

a confidentiality

b privacy

c anonymity

d justice

8 If your project is not large or highly funded, but it occurs across two or more sites, you:

a only need to gain ethical approval from the HREC from which the project originates

b must gain ethical approval from all relevant HRECs associated with those sites

c only need to take an official copy of the original ethical approval to the other sites

d must gain ethical approval from the national HREC overseeing all research sites

9 An act of deception or misrepresentation of one's own research and scholarly work is considered to be:

a scientific misconduct

b highly unreasonable

c acting competitively

d ethically irresponsible

10 If you participate in a research project as a part of the research team, you:

a have the responsibility for being aware of relevant research guidelines and codes of conduct

b do not have to concern yourself with ethical implications unless you are the Principal Investigator

c can defer to other team senior members if questioned about the ethical integrity of the research

d have the ethical responsibility for being aware only of your role and functions in the project

Review topics

1 Why are ethics important in conducting and disseminating research?

2 Discuss how your country oversees ethical safeguards in research.

3 Describe your country's privacy legislation and how it is applied in health research.

4 What are the ethical implications of conducting research in multiple sites?

5 Describe the process for critiquing the ethical components of research reports.

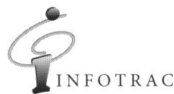

References

Anon. 19 September 1999, 'Doctors store child cardiac victims' hearts without parents' consent', *Sunday Age*, as cited in *Monash Bioethics Review,* 1999, vol. 18, no. 4, 7.

Australian Vice-Chancellors' Committee n.d., 'Guidelines for Responsible Practice in Research and Dealing with Problems of Research Misconduct', AVCC, Canberra.

Berglund, C. 1998, *Ethics for Health Care*, Oxford University Press, Melbourne.

Caplan, A. 1992, 'How did medicine go so wrong?', in A. Caplan (ed.), *When Medicine Went Mad*, Humana Press, Totowa, New Jersey.

Davis, A. 1990, 'Ethical issues in nursing research', *Western Journal of Nursing Research*, vol. 12, no. 3, 413–16.

Hicks, C. 1992, 'Of sex and status: a study of the effects of gender and occupation on nurses' evaluations of nursing research', *Journal of Advanced Nursing*, vol. 17, 1343–9.

Humphrey, G. 1994, 'Scientific fraud: the K McBride case – judgment', *Medicine, Science and the Law*, vol. 34, no. 4, 299–306.

Johnstone, M.-J. 1991, 'Improving the ethics and cultural suitability of Aboriginal health research', *Aboriginal and Islander Health Worker Journal*, vol. 15, no. 2, 10–13.

Johnstone, M.-J. 1999, *Bioethics: A Nursing Perspective*, 3rd edn, Harcourt, Sydney.

Kohn, A. 1986, *False Prophets: Fraud and Error in Science and Medicine*, Basil Blackwell Ltd, Oxford, UK.

McNeill, P. 1993, *The Ethics and Politics of Human Experimentation*, Cambridge University Press, Cambridge, UK.

Milgram, S. 1963, 'Behavioral study of obedience', *Journal of Abnormal and Social Psychology*, vol. 67, no. 4, 371–8.

National Commission for the Protection of Human Subjects of Biomedical and Behavioral Research 1978, *The Belmont Report: Ethical principles and guidelines for research involving human subjects*, US Government Printing Office, Washington, DC.

NHMRC 1991, *Guidelines on Ethical Matters in Aboriginal and Torres Strait Islander Health Research*, Australian Government Publishing Service, Canberra.

NHMRC (ed.) 1992, 'NHMRC Statement on Human Experimentation', in *NHMRC Statement on Human Experimentation and Supplementary Notes,* NHMRC, Canberra, 2–4.

NHMRC 1995, Ethical Aspects of Qualitative Methods in Health Research – an Information Paper for Institutional Ethics Committees, Australian Government Publishing Service, Canberra.

NHMRC 1996, *NHMRC Ethical Guidelines on Assisted Reproductive Technology*, Australian Government Publishing Service, Canberra.

NHMRC 2001, *National Statement on Ethical Conduct in Research Involving Humans*, Australian Government Publishing Service, Canberra.

Nicol, B. 1989, *McBride: Behind the Myth*, Australian Broadcasting Commission, Crows Nest.

Robertson, J. 1992, 'Standards for nursing research: a WA initiative', *Australian Nurses Journal*, vol. 21, no. 9, 14–15.

Royal College of Nursing, Australia 1992, 'Nursing Research Targets into the Twenty-first Century: A National Statement', RCNA, Melbourne.

Silva, M. & Sorrell, J. 1984, 'Factors influencing comprehension of information for informed consent: ethical implications for nursing research', *International Journal of Nursing Studies*, vol. 21, no. 4, 233–40.

Spriggs, M. 1999, 'Human subjects research: review of the NH&MRC National Statement on Ethical Conduct in Research Involving Humans', *Monash Bioethics Review*, vol. 18, no. 4, Ethics Committee Supplement, 5–13.

Thomas, S. & Quinn, S. 1991, 'The Tuskegee syphilis study, 1932 to 1972: implications for HIV education and AIDS risk education programs in the Black community', *American Journal of Public Health*, vol. 81, no. 11, 1498–505.

Vessey, J. & Gennaro, S. 1994, 'The ghost of Tuskegee', *Nursing Research*, vol. 43, no. 2, 67.

Weekend Australian 1990, 'Guilty medic?', 11 Oct., 27–8.

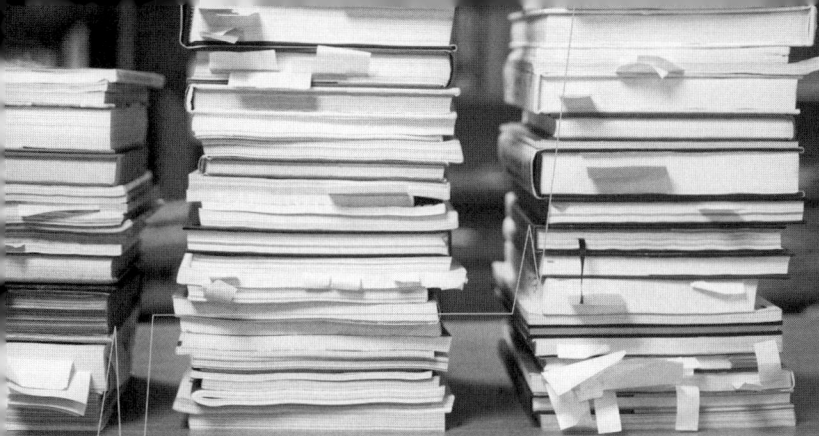

CHAPTER 6

OBTAINING APPROVAL AND SUPPORT FOR YOUR PROJECT

CHAPTER OBJECTIVES

The material presented in this chapter will assist you to:

- understand the reasons for preparing a research proposal
- identify the intended recipients of the research proposal
- develop a research proposal
- write a research proposal
- submit a research proposal
- evaluate a research proposal
- understand some funding mechanisms and processes
- gain entry to data collection sites
- gain access to research participants.

Introduction

In this chapter, we will discuss writing a research proposal. When research is undertaken with human participants, formal approvals, including ethics clearance, must be gained from the university, health service or other agency responsible for oversight of the project. If clinical research is involved, approval must be gained from the appropriate authorities in the clinical field. Informal support is also needed from key people in these areas. Financial support may also be gained from funding bodies to support the project. This process of applying for approval and support is initiated by writing a research proposal and forwarding it to the necessary committees, boards and organisations for approval and support.

The research proposal

A research proposal is a written account of the plan for the research project. It presents an argument as to why a particular problem should be investigated and what the appropriate research design is to investigate it. It sets out what the researcher intends to do – how, why, where, when and at what cost. For quantitative research, the research proposal is like a pattern for a garment or a blueprint for a building in that it assists the researcher to follow a process that has been laid down. For qualitative research, the research proposal is much more flexible because the method tends to evolve with the research.

You may ask yourself why it is necessary to have a plan for the research as long as you know what you are doing. Just as a dressmaker would not start to cut into fabric without a pattern, or a builder to lay bricks without knowing where the walls were going, a plan helps you, the researcher, to design and organise the project. A plan allows you to see and think through the relationships between different parts of the proposal, for example, the purpose, research design and expected outcomes. It helps you to foresee potential problems, and to solve them at the planning stage rather than the implementation stage. It also allows you to consult other researchers before the study is carried out so that they can comment and make constructive suggestions for improvement – they may be able to view your proposed research more objectively than you and be more able to see the pitfalls of your project. A **research plan** is the best way to ensure that you avoid mistakes when carrying out the actual project.

Once you have formulated a rough plan, the next step is to write a formal **research proposal**. The purpose of writing a formal proposal is to communicate to readers in a clear and concise style exactly what you propose to do in your research project. The process of writing down your ideas helps you to clarify them. It is almost always necessary to write a proposal for any intended research project because approval to carry out the research must be gained from the appropriate authorities such as a university research committee, a human research ethics committee (HREC) or a funding body. This mechanism protects the researcher because if there are any repercussions from the research, such as a lawsuit, the researcher has had the appropriate approvals. The committees giving the approvals would have to take some of the responsibility in the form of legal liability. This mechanism also protects participants, as they are assured of anonymity, confidentiality and privacy. It is therefore essential for the beginning researcher to learn how to write a satisfactory research proposal.

Preliminary steps in preparing the proposal

Before you write the proposal, you must have identified what your research problem is, regardless of what type of proposal you are making. You will usually have read and reviewed the literature, unless you are working using a qualitative approach such as grounded theory in which this may not be appropriate. You will have identified your research design. These processes have all been discussed in previous chapters. Unless you have identified these aspects, you will not be able to complete a satisfactory research proposal.

Another step that you must take before commencing is to identify the audiences at which the proposal is aimed; these are usually individuals or committees that have the power to approve your proposal. It is important to direct the proposal to their concerns. Naturally, all committees will be concerned with the quality of the proposal. However, different committees have specific concerns. HRECs will be most concerned with protection of the people from whom you intend to collect data, the risk/benefit ratio, and scientific rigour. Research committees will be especially concerned with the adequacy of the research design and with budgetary aspects. Clinical research committees or gatekeepers will be concerned with the impact on the institution, such as how your proposed project will impact on other projects and if it will interfere with the agency's routine. Funding bodies will be concerned that the proposal is consistent with their identified objectives and priorities, and whether the proposed budget is appropriate. Indeed, where there is a competitive process, for example, for scholarships or funding, committees often will have developed a points system for scoring proposals. If you are submitting a proposal under those conditions, it is wise to direct the bulk of your energies to where the most points can be scored.

The formal approval mechanisms may be simple or complex, depending on your situation. Undergraduate students in a beginning research unit may have to submit a proposal only for assessment, with an indication of the approvals that they would have to acquire should the project be carried out. All projects undertaken under the auspices of the university in which data collection is involved will require the approval of university committees. In addition, all projects carried out in the clinical field must have the approval of the relevant committees in the clinical facility. Furthermore, an approval will have to be given from each clinical facility involved, unless there are joint committees operating. Table 6.1 shows the committees required for approval and under what conditions you must seek their

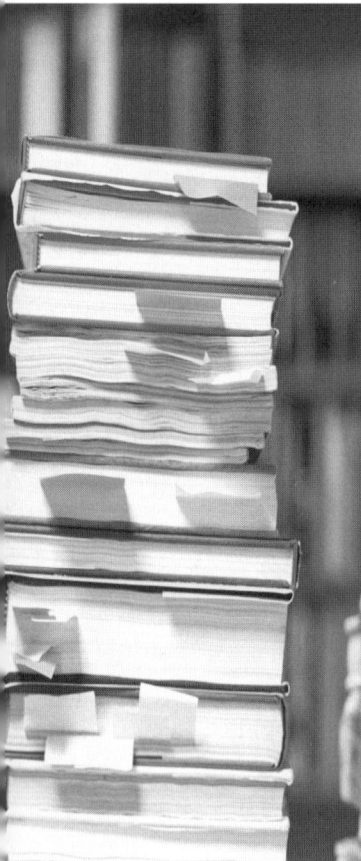

Table 6.1 Necessary approvals for different types of projects

	Student in course unit: full project		Honours/postgraduate student		Clinical researcher
	Laboratory	Clinical field	Laboratory	Clinical field	
Lecturer/supervisor	✓	✓	✓	✓	
University research committee			✓	✓	
University research ethics committee	✓	✓	✓	✓	
Clinical site human research ethics committee		✓		✓	✓
Clinical field research committee		✓		✓	✓

approval. Remember that a proposal is a contract and cannot be altered substantially without agreement from the persons or agencies giving the initial approval.

As Table 6.1 shows, clinical field projects require the most approvals. Most funding bodies will require a letter of approval from all of the relevant committees listed here, plus an application for funding.

Many organisations and committees provide application forms and guidelines which you are required to use. Guidelines have been developed by an organisation to expedite the process and to help the reviewers make decisions about the proposal. The guidelines will be consistent with the aims and priorities of the organisation. They are there to help the readers make decisions about the proposal, so it is important to follow them to facilitate a positive outcome. Before you start to write your proposal, obtain a copy of its guidelines from every committee or agency that has to give approval. This is usually a matter of a telephone call or an email to the secretary of the committee. Although this can seem like a lot of forms to fill in, you will find that most forms follow the NHMRC model, so it is often a matter of a judicious cut and paste from the word processor. Some committees make their guidelines and application forms available on electronic media as a word processor file that can then be transferred straight into your word processor. Some of the application forms are quite brief, but some committees will require a full scientific protocol, or detailed research proposal, as well.

Generally, you will acquire the necessary university approvals first, so any errors are addressed 'in-house' before the proposal goes out to external committees. The proposal should first be assessed and approved by your supervisor and then be sent through the appropriate university committees, followed by external committees. Figure 6.1 (overleaf) shows the approval process.

Allow plenty of time to prepare your proposal: it can take up to six months to develop a proposal and get all of the necessary approvals. It is wise to find out each committee's approval process, meeting schedule and deadlines for submission of proposals.

Meetings can be four to six weeks apart, or even longer over the summer holidays or midyear break. Most committees require submission at least 10 days before the meeting to allow time to circulate the papers to members. Make sure that you get your application in on time or even early – committee managers like to send the papers out all together and will not take kindly to sending your proposal out individually because it is late. If you cannot meet the deadline, it is better to wait for the next meeting than to put in incomplete papers that waste the committee's time. If you put in incomplete papers, the committee will send your application back to you for revision, so you are no further ahead.

Content of a research proposal

The overall structure of a research proposal is fairly standard. The proposal begins with the title, then an abstract or summary, an introduction section, and a methods and procedures section. At the end, there are references and appendices. The proposal should develop a logical flow of ideas from problem to budget and should be laid out in the correct order. This may be set by guidelines of the committee or agency reviewing the proposal. Figure 6.2 shows a sample of a format for a standard research proposal.

Elements of a quantitative research proposal

In this section, we use as an illustration a research proposal for a survey of the health-related quality of life of retirement village residents.

Preliminaries

The first part of the proposal is the 'preliminaries' – the pages that precede the body of the proposal. The preliminaries comprise a title page, an abstract and the details of the research team.

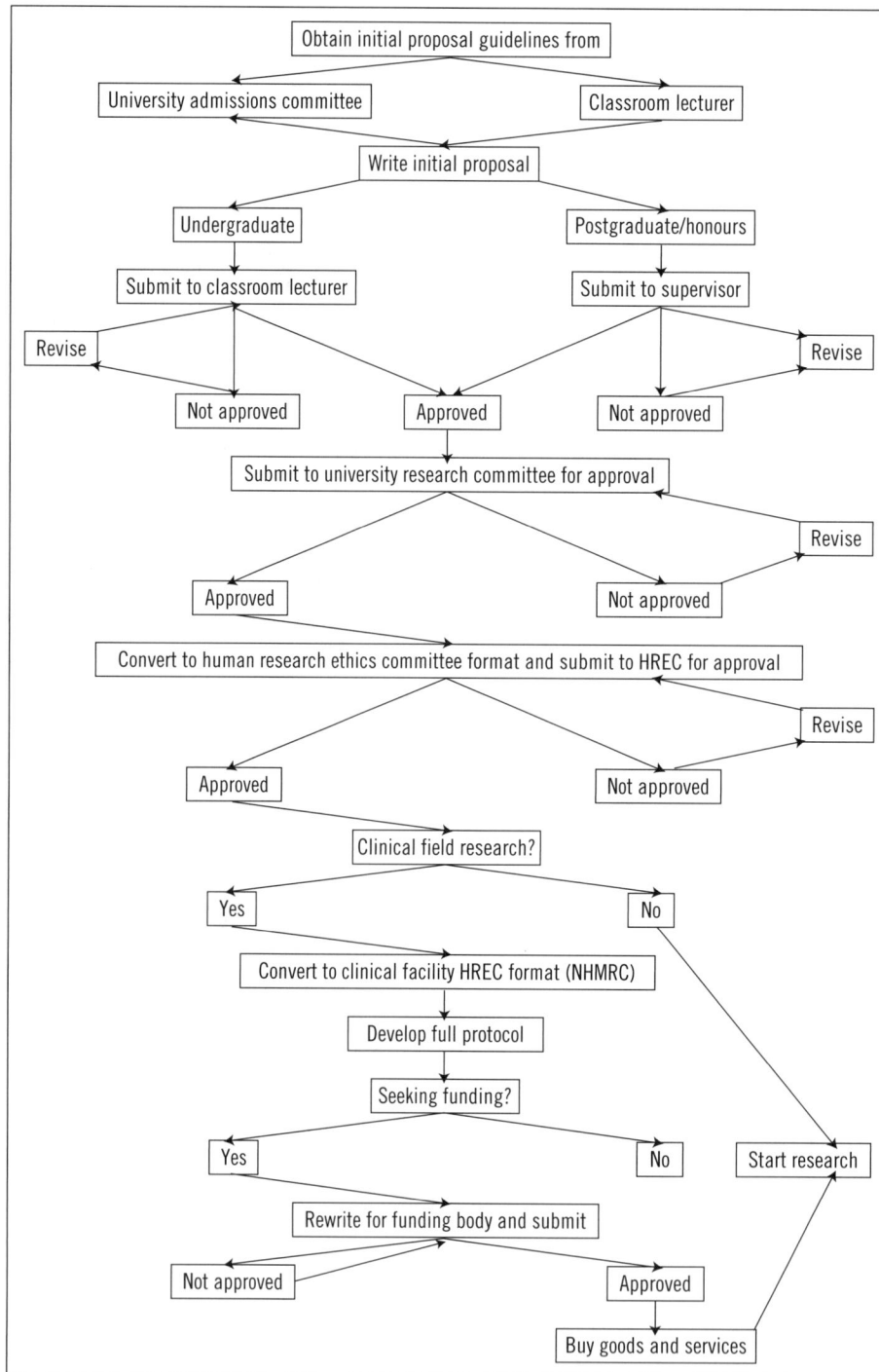

Figure 6.1 The approval process

```
Preliminaries
 •  Title page
 •  Abstract
 •  Details of researchers
Body of proposal
 •  Introduction
      •  Purpose statement
      •  Background, significance and review of literature
 •  Research design
      •  Design for the study
      •  Setting
      •  Participants
      •  Methods and procedures
 •  Ethical implications
 •  Dissemination of results
 •  Work plan
 •  Budget
 •  References
 •  Appendices
```

Figure 6.2 Sample format of a research proposal

The title

The title of the proposal should convey the intention of the proposal. This can be achieved by using keywords. The title should be no longer than 20 words. Some agencies require both long and short titles. An example of a title for a quantitative proposal is: *A survey of the health-related quality of life of retirement village residents.*

As well as the title of the proposal, the title page gives the author's name, position and qualifications. If the proposal is being submitted for ethics, funding, or other outside approvals, the author's postal and email addresses should be given, as well as telephone and fax contact numbers. The date should be placed somewhere on the page, and this can be done easily as a footer if you are using a word processor.

The abstract

The abstract is a brief summary of the proposal. It gives the reader an overview of the project, and should include the major themes or threads of the project. Primarily, it should focus on the objectives and design of the project. It should be concise, with a word limit of 250 to 300 words. Some application forms specify a limit of seven lines. An example of an abstract is as follows:

> This study will use a survey design to assess the quality of life (QOL) of retirement village
> residents in one metropolitan setting, using the WHOQOL instrument developed by the

World Health Organisation (WHO). It will produce data to provide baseline comparisons across demographic variables and major International Classification of Diseases (ICD) diagnostic categories.

Details of researchers

This section usually requires a statement of the names, positions and qualifications of the researchers. It requires that one person be named as the person responsible and contact person for the project.

For proposals other than classroom projects, you should include in the appendix the curricula vitae (CVs) of the researchers involved in the project. The CV is included so that the person evaluating the proposal can judge whether the applicant has the necessary relevant experience to carry out the project successfully. The CV should include qualifications, relevant experience, a list of publications, if any, and any other research projects you have done. It is also advantageous in some applications to include any previous research grants awarded to members of the research team.

Body of the proposal

The introduction

The body of the proposal begins with the introduction. The purpose of the introduction is to state clearly what the project is trying to do and present evidence as to why it is a worthwhile and/or interesting study. The introduction should convince the reader that the study should be carried out.

The purposes or objectives section of the introduction should clearly state what the study is attempting to find out. It should state the problem that the study is investigating. Specific aims should be stated in terms of the objectives and the research question and, if it is an experimental or quasi-experimental study, should lead to the hypotheses. An example of a purpose statement is:

> The purpose of this study is to identify the QOL needs of sub-groups of retirement village residents in order to improve service provision to these groups. It intends to quantify well-established QOL variables and compare these for a range of sub-groups of residents categorised according to ICD categories.

The background to the study is a brief section that establishes the rationale for doing the study. It answers the question 'why?' This rationale should be developed logically. The rationale may be that previous research has left questions unanswered; that you may be able to devise an improved way to answer a question; that a theory suggests such line of inquiry; or that it is a new line of inquiry that may be justified by logical argument. The rationale should show why your study will provide a solution to the problem.

The background to the study begins by orienting the reader to some previous key research in the area or key theoretical issues. It should show how the problem was identified, mentioning any key theoretical issues. It should show how the proposed research builds on what has already been done in the area.

The statement of significance of the study should follow the discussion of background and rationale. It should show why this study is worth doing. It should answer the question 'so what?' A good research proposal will contain a significant research problem. It should show how the results of this study could advance knowledge or practice in your field. If there are possible applications of the results of this study, state them. You should have reflected on these points already, when you were selecting your problem to study. You may also incorporate relevant statistics about the incidence, prevalence, distribution, relevance to health, and impact on morbidity or mortality related to the problem.

A good quantitative research proposal will contain an adequate review of the literature. This literature is what provides your arguments regarding background, rational and significance. Generally, it comprises two sections: a review of the theoretical literature that constitutes the theoretical framework for the study, and a review of the empirical literature, or research findings, that are relevant to the study. The literature review demonstrates that the researcher has a command of the current empirical and theoretical knowledge concerning the proposed problem. The theoretical basis for the study includes statements about the major ideas on which the study is based and it establishes a conceptual framework for the major variables being addressed in the study.

The literature review should summarise the previous relevant findings and it should also critique them. The research studies chosen should relate to the research question or hypotheses that you are trying to answer.

The depth of the review varies according to the purpose of the proposal. For an undergraduate research proposal, half-a-dozen decent papers will suffice, and you may need to include only the most recent research on the topic. For a doctoral degree, the complete literature on the topic must be reviewed. For proposals for ethics committees, a few recent relevant papers will usually suffice.

The breadth of the review varies according to the topic itself and the amount of literature acquired. If the topic is a complex one, much literature will be needed to cover the area properly. If it is a narrow one, much less will be required. The breadth of the review also relates to the amount of literature available. If you have found a lot of literature on your topic, you will have to be selective, but not biased. Your literature review should include only research findings, and only findings that are pertinent to your topic.

Original references should be used where possible rather than citations. If there is very little or no literature on the subject, you may need to bring in peripheral literature that is related to the topic. For example, if you want to study the effects of negative ion therapy on cancer patients, but the only research has been on children with asthma, you may use this. At the end of this section you should summarise the main findings of the literature. You should show how your proposed study will extend the previous research, if any.

Writing a literature review is not easy. The review is meant to integrate the research findings on the topic and critique any weaknesses in the previous studies so that they can be taken into account in the design of your study. The process of critiquing individual studies was detailed in Chapter 4. However, developing a literature review requires more than just piecing together separate studies. A literature review is a logically constructed argument. An effective way to organise the review, particularly if you have several independent variables, is according to the independent variables or questions being asked, and to then write about all of the findings on each variable, with a summary at the end. At the end of the literature review, you should lead into and express your specific research question. An example of this process follows:

Quality of Life (QOL) has become a major concern in health care with the growing importance of patient-centred health outcome measures. WHO defined quality of life as 'an individual's perception of their position in life in the context of the culture and value systems in which they live and in relation to their goals, expectations, standards and concerns' (WHOQOL Group 1993).

Quality of life in elderly populations has a special significance in relation to the impacts of chronic and degenerative illness as well as the changes associated with post-work lifestyles. Kermode and MacLean (2001) found that QOL is actually higher in older persons than in younger persons and that having good relationships with their partner and with their children were important components of this.

Clarke and Black (2005) found that quality of life can be seriously diminished following stroke, but that many persons find ways to adapt and still report a high quality of life. Masoudi et al. (2004) also found that functional limitations do not necessarily result in diminished QOL in older patients with heart failure, but that they are at risk for worsening Health Related Quality of Life (HRQL) if functional status declines too far. Functional status and mood do not necessarily impact on QOL in the same way, however. In aged care residents with dementia, it has been found that among those with a higher level of cognitive functioning, apathetic behaviour was associated with low QOL, and vice versa for those with low levels of apathy (Gerritsen et al. 2005). Hoe et al. (2005) also found that QOL does not decrease as cognition worsens.

Bryant et al. (2004), in a national study of Canadian elders, found that health care concerns and socioeconomic concerns were major factors affecting their quality of life, while Blieszner (2004) argues that factors such as a focus on wisdom, a sense of acceptance of life outcomes, satisfying close relationships, meaningful use of time, and spiritual beliefs and values are the major factors affecting quality of life for older women. He further argues that these factors need to be incorporated into the delivery of health care services.

There is little doubt that QOL has specific dimensions among elderly populations, whether those populations are well or sick, and it is likely that these dimensions may vary according to the presence or absence of illness or disability. Previous studies have linked QOL to specific pathologies. Indeed, some studies have found QOL to be predictive of health outcomes such as mortality, hospitalisation, and outpatient utilisation (Sprenkle et al. 2004). Other studies have found QOL to differ between those with and without health problems, with factors such as psychological health, social relationships, and level of independence impacting on overall QOL (Schok & de Vries 2005).

The rationale for this proposed study comes from a body of research which suggests first, that QOL among the elderly seems to have different dimensions to QOL among the young, and second, that there is a relationship between QOL in the elderly and the presence of specific pathologies. It is hoped that this study will facilitate further exploration of this latter finding in order to facilitate the development and implementation of appropriate services for at-risk elderly residents.

Accordingly, the research question for this study is: 'Are there differences in QOL profiles between different sub-groups of elderly residents living in a metropolitan retirement village?'

The research design

The research design section describes in detail the framework for the study. This includes the design of the study, the setting, participants, instruments and procedures proposed for the study. This section should answer the questions: 'on whom?', 'how?', 'when?' and 'where?' Each choice should be justified. A good research proposal will have a design that is suitable to answer the research question.

The design that you will choose depends entirely on the question you are trying to answer. It is impossible to overemphasise the importance of this point. Quantitative approaches are used when data are collected as numbers. In health, the question of cause and effect is crucial, for example, whether certain exposures cause certain health problems, or whether certain treatments cause certain health outcomes. Different quantitative designs answer these cause and effect questions in different ways, and with different levels of veracity.

In writing the research design section, you begin by stating the design, framework or overall approach of the study, for example, experimental, correlational, descriptive or comparative. Quantitative designs are discussed in detail in later chapters. You should explain why you have chosen the particular approach, that is, why it is appropriate to the research question. If it is a complex design, a diagram or flow chart may assist the reader to understand it. In deciding how much detail to give in the design of the study section, consider the level of the question. If it is a descriptive design, less detail will be required than for an experimental design. You should give enough detail to enable a reader to understand how you intend to answer the research question.

A statement of study design is as follows:

> This study will use a comparative design. Data will be collected using a well-validated and reliable survey questionnaire instrument. In 1993, the World Health Organisation (WHO) established a working party to develop a QOL assessment instrument, and this resulted in the WHOQOL. There are two versions of the WHOQOL – the full 100-item version, and the revised 26-item version. The 26-item version (WHOQOL-BREF) will be used in this study.
>
> The WHOQOL-BREF measures four domains – physical health, psychological health, social relationships and environment. It has high internal consistency, test–retest reliability, construct validity and content validity (Frank-Stromborg & Olsen 2004).
>
> It is not disease-specific, but it has been used to assess quality of life across a number of conditions such as schizophrenia (Hasanah & Razali 2002), HIV (Fang, Hsing & Yu 2002; Starace, Cafaro & Albrescia 2002), chronic pain (Skevington, Carse & Williams 2001) and liver transplantation (O'Carroll, Smith & Couston 2000), as well as natural disasters (Wang, Gao & Zhang 2000). It is available from WHO in 29 different languages.

If the design is experimental or quasi-experimental, there should also be a statement of the hypotheses. The hypotheses should be stated as a description of the anticipated outcomes. They should be well-defined, logical, clear, and necessary to answer the research question. They should show the relationships between the variables, and be stated in measurable terms. The independent and dependent variables should also be identified and where possible, stated in measurable terms.

The setting for the research should be given. In a proposal, it is quite appropriate to give the names of agencies in which you will carry out the research. You should show that the agency is capable of supplying sufficient participants for the study by giving the numbers of potential participants that the agency has.

The participants should be described next. State the characteristics of the group from which they will be selected and where they are to be found. State your rationale for selecting this particular group of participants. You should give the size of sample you wanted to end up with and say how you arrived at this figure. If it is a design that has the potential for participant mortality, you should address participant attrition and build in extra participants, usually about 10 per cent, so that you will end up with enough participants. A good research proposal will include plans to acquire sufficient participants to make the results meaningful.

It is customary to state the type of sample that you intend to use, for example, a random sample, convenience sample, stratified random sample, and so on. Types of samples will be discussed in later chapters. If it is a convenience sample there will not be much to say except the basis of the convenience, for example they were the first 50 patients treated in a clinic. If it is a random sample or a stratified random sample, say how the sample was drawn from the population. You should describe the criteria for participant selection and give the rationale for the criteria. You should give the details of how they were recruited, for example, by letter, telephone or personal contact.

Once you have described your sampling procedures, you should state the number of groups, the number of participants in each group, and whether and how they were allocated to the groups. Any special procedures, such as matching participants on criteria, should also be described.

You should also describe the instruments or materials that you will use. An instrument is any tool, including questionnaires, that you use to collect the data. The instrument should be the best possible one to assist you to answer the research question. It is not necessary to explain any standard tests, but you should explain any unconventional techniques, tests or instruments. You should state or describe any questionnaires that you propose to use, and refer the reader to an appendix, where you will include a full copy of the questionnaire. If the questionnaire is subject to copyright, you should obtain permission from the author to use it. If you propose to use a physical instrument, it should be named if it is well known, for example, a sphygmomanometer, or described if it is unusual or new. You should say how the instrument is scored or measured, for example, on a Likert scale or in millimetres of mercury. You can use diagrams or photographs of an instrument to avoid a long description. You should include a brief discussion of how the instrument has been used previously, according to the literature. You should justify your choice of the instrument in terms of its appropriateness to the research question or design. You should discuss the strengths and weaknesses of each instrument in terms of its reliability and validity. These concepts are discussed in later chapters.

It is always wise to use an instrument that has been developed already, but if you are developing your own instrument, you will need to show why no existing instrument meets your needs.

You will also need to describe the procedures for the study. If it is an experiment, you describe how an experimental treatment will be applied. You state how, when and where you will collect the data. This information should be given in enough detail to allow someone to replicate your procedures. You will give your procedures for collecting the data in terms of what you intend to do to the participants. This will include procedures such as observing subjects or participants, administering a questionnaire, applying an instrument or administering an experimental treatment. Any lengthy instructions to the participants may be included in the appendix, but summarised here. Describe any calibration of the instruments or training to be given to the data collectors.

You should say when you will carry out your procedures and how long they will take so that each participant's time commitment is clear. If there is a particular time of day, week, month or year involved, this should be made clear. If the timing is complex, a diagram or flow chart may be helpful. In this section, you should also state how you will record your data. If it is quantitative data, you can include a sample data roster as an appendix, or you can state that one is being devised.

Next, you should state your procedures for managing the data. These include coordination of data management if a multiple site is involved; data entry into the computer; and storage of original data, including how, where and for how long it will be stored. You should also consider the ethical aspects of data management, including confidentiality of the data (addressed in Chapter 5). You should address the aspects of data coding: who will do it and how will it be done? Provision should be made for checking the data for errors in data entry.

A good research proposal will show a strong, clear, rigorous program for analysing the data. The methods of data analysis should follow from the research question, research design and hypotheses. In the proposal, you should state how you intend to analyse the data. You should say whether you intend to analyse the data by hand or computer, and if the latter, you should name the data analysis package that you intend to use. You should justify your data analysis by showing which tests you intend to do to describe the variables and to check the validity of each hypothesis, including a restatement of the hypothesis. This allows the reader to assess the appropriateness of the data analysis in terms of the hypotheses and research questions. If the data analysis is complex, a flow chart may help. An example of a data analysis statement is: 'data will be subjected to a range of analysis techniques including descriptive statistics, Chi Square, t-Tests and Multivariate Analysis of Variance (MANOVA)'.

If you are planning to do a pilot study, which you should, if at all possible, give the details here. If you have done a pilot study already, you should also give an outline of the methods and results here; it gives the reader confidence in your expertise and provides an indication of the feasibility of your study. An example of a research design section follows:

Design
This will be a comparative design using a well-validated and reliable survey questionnaire instrument developed by WHO (WHOQOL 1993).

Setting
This study will be conducted at the Riverside Retirement Village in the suburb of Billington North. It is a managed retirement village with a nursing home on-site. Residents occupy individual units as couples or as individuals.

Participants

The current population of Riverside Retirement Village is 320, of which 198 are female and 122 are male. This study will invite all residents of the village to participate. The sample size will be determined by the response rate, and it is estimated that the response rate will be in excess of 75%.

Methods and procedures

Copies of the WHOQOL-BREF questionnaire will be distributed to all residents via the mail distribution system in the village. A covering letter will explain the purpose of the study, and residents will be invited to participate by completing the questionnaire and returning it to a central collection box in the foyer of the village administration office.

The standard WHOQOL-BREF form will be used with data collected for demographic variables and current ICD diagnoses. Data from the completed questionnaires will be entered into a database and analysed using the SPSS statistics package. Scales and sub-scales scores will be compared for a range of sub-groups of the participants using t-Tests, ANOVA and other procedures as appropriate. ICD classifications and demographics represent the independent variables and the WHOQOL scores represent the dependent variables. In the first instance, it is anticipated that comparisons by gender, age group and diagnosis will be undertaken.

Ethical implications

Now that the reader knows how your study is going to be carried out, it is appropriate to discuss the ethical implications inherent in the study procedures. For a general research proposal that goes to a university research committee, this section can be brief. You will need to state your proposed procedures to obtain ethics clearance from university ethics and/or clinical ethics committees.

A proposal for an ethics committee is somewhat different. An ethics committee asks about the general design of the study, not only to assess its scientific merit but also to determine the ethical implications of the study. Therefore, you should outline any ethical implications and how you propose to deal with them. These include prevention of harm to participants, and protection of the participants' rights to confidentiality, anonymity and privacy. These issues were covered in Chapter 5. You should state whether a written consent is to be obtained from the participants, and justify the reasons if it is not to be obtained. For a discussion of when consent is necessary, see Chapter 5. If informed consent is being sought, you should satisfy the reader that you have made provision for the participants to be informed as to what will be required of them and the risks and benefits of participating in the study. You should include with your application a copy of your proposed plain language statement and consent form. On the consent form, make sure that you say that the participants will not be pressured into being in the study, will not be discriminated against if they do not take part in the study, and that they have the option of withdrawing from the study at any time without any penalty.

There are some special considerations that may have to be dealt with in some studies. If you are using vulnerable participants, you must justify the choice of these, describe the procedures you intend to put in place to protect their rights, and state who will give consent on their behalf. If you are seeking to observe participants without their express individual consent, you must justify why you have selected this method and show that the costs in terms of potential invasion of privacy are less than the potential benefits of such a study.

At the end of the research design section, it is customary to acknowledge any weaknesses of the approach that you have chosen. Remember that the reader may be an experienced and distinguished scientist who will spot flaws in your design. It is better to acknowledge the flaws in your design, that is, the threats to validity, and explain how you will deal with them than to try to gloss over them and hope no-one will notice. Remember that no-one expects your study to have a perfect design and what counts is that you are aware of the limitations and can deal with them. An example of an ethics statement is as follows:

> All participants in this study will be adults. The population of the village is a homogenous, English-speaking, Caucasian one. There are no Indigenous residents or non-English speaking residents. Participation will be voluntary, informed and completely confidential. No written consent will be used, so as to ensure that participant and non-participant identities are protected. Agreement to participate will be taken as consent. Participants will be able to withdraw at any time. There are no perceived risks to participants.

Dissemination of results

The proposal should include a plan for the dissemination of results and the implementation of the findings. For example, it could state that you will be giving a presentation on the results of the study and/or a written report to the institution, you will be presenting a paper at a conference or you intend to submit the results for publication in a journal. You could also state any plans for implementing your findings to change ward practice. Such a statement may look as follows:

> A report of the study will be produced for the Care Manager of the village, including recommendations regarding any specific sub-groups. A formal research report will be submitted for publication to the journal *Age and Ageing*. A brief summary of findings will also be circulated to all residents of the village.

Work plan or timeframe

A work plan may be included in a proposal for university or funding committees. This is an overall description of the sequence and duration of tasks that must be carried out. It indicates to the reader how realistic the research plan is, and how thorough the researcher has been in considering all that needs to be done to carry out the research project. The work plan incorporates the tasks, personnel requirements, estimate of time required to carry out each part of the project, and date by which each part should be done. It is often shown as a schedule or as a flow chart. For an example of a work plan, see the section later in this chapter on qualitative research proposals.

Resources and budget

A good research proposal will show that the physical and human resources available are sufficient to carry out the project satisfactorily. A section on the background of the researcher, the physical resources and the budget required to run the project will be required by granting agencies and universities. In the budget section, you will give the costs for all of the materials, personnel and equipment that you will require to carry out the project to a successful completion. The major cost components are direct costs, that is, costs that are specific to the project, and indirect costs, that is, infrastructure costs that are incurred by the institution as a result of supporting your project.

Direct costs are usually broken down into salary costs and costs for equipment, materials and procedures. Salary costs would include salaries of secretaries, research assistants and the researcher. They should also include salary costs of clinicians who may be acting as data collectors. Salary costs also include a component for on-costs such as annual leave, payroll tax and the like. Your financial services personnel can advise you as to the appropriate costs to charge. There may also be costs for work carried out by non-salaried personnel such as typing, consulting, data entry and data transcription services. Costs for equipment would include any instruments, computer software, equipment such as video cameras or tape recorders, and purchase or rental of computers. Materials would include stationery, videocassettes, audiocassettes, postage, report preparation and dissemination. Procedure costs would include printing, photocopying and laboratory analysis of data. There may also be other incidental costs, such as travel and accommodation, if you are collecting data out of town.

Indirect costs are usually referred to as 'infrastructure costs'. These include use of the telephone, fax, office, computing time, etc. Students carrying out projects for a qualification will not usually have to include infrastructure costs in a proposal because it is taken for granted that the university supplies these as a part of the student's educational package. However, proposals for grants from outside the institution will normally be required to include an infrastructure component in the budget. Infrastructure costs are usually calculated by a formula devised by the institution and you should use this formula to calculate any such costs. For an example of a budget statement, see the qualitative proposal section later in this chapter.

EXERCISE

Think of a research project you are interested in doing, which involves collecting data in number form. Answer the following questions related to this project:

- What would be your research question?
- Why is this a worthwhile question to ask?
- Where would you go to gather data?
- From whom would you gather data?
- How could you gather the data you needed?
- Who would you need to get support and/or approval from to do this project?

Elements of a qualitative research proposal

To some extent, there are similarities in quantitative and qualitative research proposals. For example, the preliminary pages are much the same and within the body of the report the introduction has a similar structure. However, the rest of the body of the proposal may be substantially different from a quantitative proposal. Indeed, qualitative proposals may also differ from one another depending on the kind of approach they intend to take.

Qualitative proposals have to be scrutinised by academic departments, health agency organisations, funding bodies and ethics committees that are often composed of people with backgrounds in quantitative research. Therefore, qualitative proposals must conform to some extent with these people's expectations of what constitutes a 'proper' research proposal. Too much creativity at this stage of the research may result in obstruction to the research at the outset. Therefore, it is important that qualitative proposals are written carefully, clearly and with a sound rationale for all of the proposed steps in the project.

To demonstrate how to prepare a qualitative proposal, we will work through an example of a proposal, pointing out how other qualitative proposals may differ. The example given is of a proposal that was submitted to an institutional ethics committee, in which there was only one nurse member with qualitative expertise deciding on the merits of the proposal. Other members were representative of roles required for an ethics committee, but they did not necessarily have expertise in qualitative research. Therefore, it was important to be clear about the focus and methodology of the project, as it would have to 'stand alone' against predominantly quantitative interests at the meeting.

The title

Be clear about what it is you want to know and why you want to know it, so that you will be able to give the research a title. The title should clarify the research approach, what the research is about and the people and setting involved. For example, it might read: 'Improving the quality of palliative nursing care through reflective practice and action research.'

Research summary

Sometimes called an abstract, the research summary provides an overall picture of what the project hopes to achieve, as well as when and how. It is important to be concise. For example:

> This project involves experienced Registered Nurses (RNs) practising palliative nursing. The research will use reflective processes in an action research approach, to achieve the research objectives. The research aims to raise critical awareness of practice problems RNs face every day; work systematically through problem-solving processes, to uncover constraints against effective nursing care; and improve the quality of care given by palliative nurses in light of the identified constraints and possibilities.

Research significance, aims and objectives

At this point, a statement may be made about the significance of the project. The statements of significance inform readers why this research is worthwhile. Aims are overall intentions and objectives are specific subsets of the intentions. For example:

Significance
The significance of the project is in improving palliative nursing care and in educating nurses in a process, which they can use for any clinical problems that emerge in their practice well after the completion of this project. Palliative nurses need to think quickly and carefully in the course of their everyday work to make accurate and effective clinical decisions to ameliorate patients' distress. Reflective processes will allow them to reflect effectively in and on action. Also, nurses work under complex historical, economic, cultural, social and political constraints, which they need to identify and work towards changing. Using action research in this project will give the nurses the 'research tools' they require for collaborative research in the future. Therefore, the project will not only serve as a medium for immediate improved practice, but also as a lifelong educating process for nurses for future practice improvements.

Aim
This project aims to facilitate reflective practice processes in experienced Registered Nurses.

Objectives
in order to raise critical awareness of practice problems RNs face every day, to work systematically through problem-solving processes to uncover constraints against effective nursing care, and to improve the quality of care given by hospital nurses in light of the identified constraints and possibilities.

EXERCISE

How do research aims differ from objectives? Why is it important to state the research aims and objectives 'up front'? What are some possible reasons for a research project not achieving its stated aims and objectives?

Research questions

Specific questions related to the research objectives may be posed at this point. These questions will indicate the problem focus you are taking in the research. Questions of this nature may not be appropriate to all qualitative proposals, as some critical approaches may intend to use participatory processes in which the participants work collaboratively to raise questions as the research moves through cycles and group processes. However, if a proposal chooses to pose questions they may resemble the following examples:

- What practice problems do palliative nurses face every day?
- What constraints weigh against effective palliative nursing care?

- How can the quality of nursing care given by hospital nurses be improved, in light of the identified constraints and possibilities?

Background and literature review

Sometimes a background statement precedes the literature review, to set the context for how the ideas for the research came into being. For example:

> The research will be the fourth project with nurses at (this) hospital (Taylor 2001; Taylor et al. 2001; Taylor et al. 2002). This project comes from a direct request by palliative nurses for the researcher to facilitate another action research and reflection project.

The reasons for the literature review are similar to those already outlined in this chapter under 'Elements of a quantitative research proposal'. You may choose to refer to these comments to refresh your memory of them. However, there are some areas that need to be highlighted in a general approach to writing a literature review for qualitative proposals.

First, the suggestion to base the project in a nursing model is a good one, but it is not one all researchers may choose to take up. If the model fits well, use it. If not, do not. Also, it will be important to choose a model that fits with the particular methodological approach you are taking. For example, the model put forward by Parse (1987) may suit some but not all phenomenological projects.

Second, there may not be much empirical literature in a highly unusual area of interest as is the case with many qualitative projects that try to push the boundaries of what can be known about phenomena. In this case, the literature may need to be linked indirectly to the main ideas in the research. Allied, non-specific information may be shown through the proposed methods and processes to be related to and informative for the research interest.

Lastly, some approaches such as grounded theory may claim that their inductive style suggests that literature should not be amassed at this stage. This is a good enough stance if it can be substantiated. However, be aware that some people reading the proposal may assume that the failure to present a literature review is a 'cop out' and that the prospective researchers may not even be aware of literature in the area.

With these disclaimers in mind, the rules of a thorough literature review still apply just as much to qualitative proposals as they do to quantitative proposals. Continuing the proposal in this section, an example of a literature review may be:

> Palliative nurses work in clinical settings, which have a direct bearing on the quality of the care they can provide. Reflective practice and action research are the methodological approaches for the proposed project. Therefore, the literature reviewed included areas relating to the nature of palliative nursing practice, reflective practice and action research in nursing.
>
> **The nature of palliative nursing practice**
> Palliative nursing care is complex, because nurses are involved with the care of dying people and their grieving families. Taylor et al. (2001) explored the degree of congruency in patients',

families' and nurses' perceptions of the nature and effects of palliative nursing care. In the three research phases, transcripts of the audiotaped interviews were analysed by a method of collaborative thematic analysis, to find specific themes within stories.

The research team compared the results of the three phases and found that the three groups agreed about the work involved in palliative nursing care, and that the information revealed two main categories in relation to palliative nursing care. The stories conveyed the essentials of the experience for various groups of people involved in giving and receiving palliative nursing care.

The major difference in the stories was the relative emphasis on the personal qualities palliative nurses bring to their work and the activities in which they engage. Nurses emphasised their work activities, whereas patients and relatives emphasised equally nurses' qualities and activities. In a focus group meeting at the end of the third phase, nurses discussed their reactions to caring for dying people, including their grief and work dilemmas associated with giving effective care.

Bolmsjo and Hermeren (1998) described situations in palliative care where nurses were faced with more than one alternative action. They pointed out that clinical decision-making can lead to psychological and ethical problems for nurses, as they attempt to make correct decisions for action. Further sources of conflict and stress result from an inability to relieve distressing symptoms in patients. This contradicts the nurse's care values, such as personal beliefs in caregiving, altruism, accountability, integrity, trust, freedom, safety, knowledge and ongoing self-evaluation (Weis & Schank 2000). Perfectionism, idealism, competence and nursing values are closely related concepts.

Shared values and beliefs, assumptions and norms are also central to organisational culture and determine the characteristics of specific organisations. Values determine what people think ought to be done and are closely associated with moral and ethical principles. Fitzgerald and van Hooft (2000) maintain that Western-style health care systems restrict nurses in the degree to which they can express their values in care, ethical decision-making and love expression. In fact, professional codes and organisational culture, which prescribe professional boundaries, may inhibit individual nurse development, lateral thinking and holistic care (Lillibridge, Axford & Rowley 2000). Part of the organisational culture is reflected in rules and routines, which are often the source of practice issues in palliative nursing. Action research with an emphasis on reflection is an effective research approach for identifying work issues and improving nursing practice (Taylor 2001a&b; Taylor et al. 2002).

Research involving reflection and action research

Reflection and action research combine well to create an effective collaborative qualitative research approach for identifying and transforming clinical issues, because reflection is part of the action research method. Action research involves a four-stage phase of collectively planning, acting, observing and reflecting (Dick 1995; Stringer 1996). Each phase leads to another cycle of action, in which the plan is revised, and further acting, observing and reflecting is undertaken systematically, to work towards solutions to problems of a technical, practical or emancipatory nature (Kemmis & McTaggart 1988; Taylor 2000). The planning and acting phases may include any appropriate methods of gathering and analysing data, such as participant observation, reflective journalling, surveys, focus groups and interviews. Cycles of action research lead to further foci and co-researchers can keep an action research approach to their work for as long as they choose, to find solutions to their practice problems.

Nurses have been using action research successfully in a variety of settings with differing thematic concerns (for example, Chenoweth & Kilstoff 1998; Keatinge et al. 2000; Koch, Kralik & Kelly 2000). Taylor (2001a&b) and Taylor et al. (2002) used action research and reflection to work on thematic concerns common to the nurses' research group. Both projects gave nurses a regular forum in which to discuss their reflections on practice and to generate an action plan to bring about change. The benefits of action research and reflection are that there are immediate, practical outcomes for participants, because they can share their experiences with peers, work together on thematic concerns, and bring about local changes in their practice. Thus, co-researchers experience participatory research, while developing their reflective skills, and in this sense the research offers them personal and professional gains in lifelong appreciation for their participation.

Taylor (2001b) facilitated reflective practice processes with 12 experienced female Registered Nurses, working in a large Australian rural hospital. Participants shared their experiences of nursing during three action research cycles. A thematic concern of dysfunctional nurse–nurse relationships was identified, as evidenced by bullying and horizontal violence. The negotiated action plan was put into place and co-researchers reported varying degrees of success in attempting to improve nurse–nurse relationships. This project confirmed the necessity for reflective practice and continued collaborative research processes in the workplace to bring about cultural change within nursing.

Taylor et al. (2002) used a combination of action research and reflective practice processes to explore idealism in palliative nursing care. Six experienced Registered Nurses identified their tendency towards idealism in their palliative nursing practice, which they defined as the tendency to expect to be 100% effective all of the time in their work. Participants collaborated in generating and evaluating an action plan to recognise and manage the negative effects of idealism in their work expectations and behaviours. Participants expressed positive changes in their practice, based on adjusting their responses to their idealistic tendencies towards perfectionism.

The references may be included immediately after the literature review, or may appear in an appendix attached to the proposal. You will find the references for this literature review at the end of this chapter.

Research plan, including methodology, methods and processes

A research plan is roughly equivalent to the methodology section of a quantitative proposal, in that it includes information about the study setting, participants and methods to be used. However, there are differences which relate mainly to the use of specific language. For example, generally speaking, when qualitative researchers refer to methodology, they are referring to the theoretical assumptions underlying the choice of methods. This means that in the proposal under the word 'methodology' there will appear a short description of the theoretical tradition informing the project. For example:

Methodology

In the context of qualitative research, methodology means the theoretical assumptions of how knowledge is generated and validated, which underlie the choice of methods. This project is informed by reflective practitioner concepts and the technical, practical and emancipatory intentions of action research, as described in the literature review.

Methods and processes

Qualitative research often differentiates between the ways of organising the research and collecting and analysing the information (methods) and the interpersonal processes that are used in accessing, informing, maintaining and closing relationships with participants throughout the research (processes). With these differences between methods and processes in mind, it is still important to give a full account of all your intentions in doing the research. For example:

Accessing participants

Full ethical clearance processes from (the) university and (the) Hospital Ethics and Research Committee will precede the commencement of the project. The researcher will send copies of the Plain Language Statement to the RN manager in the palliative care unit and she will distribute them to nurses. Some nurses who collaborated on previous projects may choose to be involved again; others may become involved for the first time by a 'snowballing' effect. It is anticipated that there will be a quick response to the invitation to be involved in the research because the request for the project has come from the nurses themselves. If recruitment is slow or delayed, the researcher will go to the hospital and speak to nurses at a clinical meeting, to explain the project and the benefits and risks (minimal, as explained in this application) of their involvement.

The research will be for approximately three months. Up to 10 experienced RNs working in palliative care will be invited by the researcher to participate in the group processes within the project, but three or more will be sufficient for effective group reflection and discussion.

EXERCISE

In qualitative research, what are the differences between methods and processes? Why is it important to propose particular methods and processes, rather than to simply let them evolve during the project?

It may be necessary to provide a rationale for the number of participants, especially if the proposal is likely to be judged against empirico-analytical criteria. Committee members may not be aware of the assumptions of the nature of knowledge generated and validated through qualitative research. The extent to which you produce a strongly referenced rationale will depend on the likelihood of its being needed. It may be worthwhile checking on the composition of certain committees judging research proposals to see if they are open to and aware of the assumptions of qualitative research. For instance, you might decide that it is advisable to write a few (non-patronising, non-jargonistic) sentences about the relative and context-dependent nature of knowledge.

You may also decide that it is wise to give a sound set of reasons for what may be construed by some commentators as a 'small sample size'. You might also need to justify your 'sampling' methods, that is, how you will go about accessing the participants. Be clear about what you write. For instance, you might consider statements such as: *'This research approach is interested in accessing participants who have experience in the research interest. They have been sought intentionally for their ability to inform the research from their personal perspectives'*. In the case of the example in this section, I wrote:

> Convenience sampling will be used to intentionally target those research participants, who are interested in reflecting on their practice in order to improve it. The number of participants is appropriate for this qualitative project, because of the potential of the research to generate rich data sufficient to bring about changes in work practices. The number of participants is also congruent with the assumptions of qualitative research, which emphasise the context-dependent quality of process, experience, and language (Roberts & Taylor 2002). Therefore, this project does not seek high numbers to generalise results or use them for predictive purposes. Also, in collaborative research of this nature, the process becomes as important as the potential outcomes, because the focus is on what people learn as they experience the research itself.

You will need to decide whether it is advisable to compare and contrast quantitative and qualitative methods of accessing participants. If you choose this option, be careful not to overdo the teaching angle. Intelligent people do not necessarily like to feel they are 'being hit over the head' with details that make them feel ignorant. However, they may respond to a clear and succinct synopsis which justifies qualitative research activities that differ from those to which they are most accustomed.

Data collection

Be sure to include all of the points about what data you will collect and how you will collect it. Provide examples of the questions you intend to ask. Even if they are open-ended to facilitate a spontaneous conversation, they need to be included. For a collaborative project it may not be possible to predict questions that may arise from group processes. Nevertheless, this should be explained at this point of the proposal, so that people who are uninformed about the methodology you are using will be able to understand why the questions are not given in this instance.

If the methodology you are using allows for questions to be posed, be sure that you intend to ask questions that will give you the information you need. For example:

Data collection and analysis
Over the three-month period, the RNs will meet weekly with the researcher/facilitator for one hour, to discuss clinical problems raised by them in their journal writing and group discussion. The sequence of research activities will be based on previous projects (Taylor 2001a&b). The data collection activities are embedded in the group processes and they are that:

- RNs will be given opportunities to write journal reflections of practice experiences, by using participant observation during the normal course of their work in ward areas. As with all nursing care, the details of patients' care will be completely confidential
- the reflections will be shared in the group meetings
- the individuals and the group will critically analyse the content of all the shared practice stories and identify common themes and issues in palliative nursing practice
- a theme common to all of the reflections will be identified as the thematic concern (issue) as a focus for the group
- action cycles of planning, assessing, observing and reflecting will generate an action plan for addressing and amending the identified thematic concern
- the action plan will be instituted in nursing practice and the results of the changed approach to the thematic concern will be noted through continued planning, acting, observing and reflecting
- the action plan will undergo revision until it achieves positive changes in successfully managing the identified thematic concern.

As reflective practice may be undertaken in many ways, the kind of reflection may be determined to some extent by the kind of knowledge nurses are seeking to generate in and through their practice (Taylor 2000). If nurses intend to increase their understanding of procedures and experiences, they might lean towards technical and practical reflective strategies respectively. The types of questions they could pose when engaging in interpretive reflection might include: 'What is happening here?', 'What is the nature of . . . ?', 'What is the experience of . . . ?' If nurses intend to change the constraining nature and effects of political, economic, cultural, social, historical elements in their practice, they will require emancipatory reflective strategies. The types of questions that they could pose when engaging in critical reflection might include: 'What is happening here?', 'What factors have made it this way . . . ?', 'How might this be different . . . ?'

Ethical requirements

It is necessary to provide a full account of ethical considerations to be given to participants, including informed consent to ensure their privacy and anonymity, and the assurance that they can choose to withdraw from the research at any time, without penalty. Full ethical clearance will need to be sought from participating institutions. It is usual to submit a full research plan, including ethical statements, a plain language statement and a consent form for each category of participants. Ethical considerations may include these sorts of statements:

> Research participants have the right to consent freely and without coercion. They will be offered the right to refuse to participate, or to withdraw at any time with no explanation, and without penalty or coercion of any kind. Measures taken to ensure that research participants have the capacity to understand the research project will be to ascertain that each participant can comprehend English, and to provide the services of an interpreter should this be necessary.

The forms given to participants will be relative to their comprehension. Participants will receive detailed explanations, verbally and in writing, of what the research involves, the aims and the processes of the research, and participants' commitments in it.

Nurses are the participants in this research, so the Plain Language Statement and the Consent Form will be written relative to their comprehension, bearing in mind that nurses are professionals conversant with language used in higher education institutions and health care settings. Even so, any words and sentences which may cause confusion, will be paraphrased into simple English so that the meaning is clear and unambiguous. The project will also be explained in plain language verbally by the researcher. Participants will have opportunities to ask questions, make comments and voice any concerns that they may have concerning the project at the outset and throughout the duration of the project.

As this research encourages nurses to share their practice stories, likely minimal risks are that the privacy and confidentiality of patients may be breached and that nurses may feel vulnerable in sharing their experiences, leading to embarrassment or possible emotional catharsis, such as tearfulness or anger. Trusting group processes will be discussed and agreed to in the first two meetings and the facilitator will carefully monitor the emotional status of meetings and raise any concerns about participants' emotional integrity, as they arise.

Nurses are educated in the need for patient confidentiality and they practise it daily in their work, thus minimising risks to patients. Even so, the researcher will ensure that privacy and confidentiality measures are instituted and maintained. Stories written in journals and shared in group meetings will be devoid of information that could identify institutions, patients, relatives and/or staff. Pseudonyms will be used and identifying material will be omitted or renamed to protect the identities of people within the written transcripts of the stories. Reflective journals will remain the personal property of participants and they will not be read or sighted by the researcher, unless it is a participant's expressed wish that this occurs. Reports and published material will describe the participants' stories and interpretations according to the issues they raised and the practice improvements they caused, rather than to identify specific people, places and situations.

All data collected in the course of the research will be secured in a locked storage compartment for five years and the responsibility for the safety and security of it will reside with the researchers.

With respect to risks associated with emotional catharsis, the group will offer support to its members and the researcher/facilitator is an experienced nurse with 30 years of group management and support. Should any member become emotionally upset beyond the ability of the group to support them, he or she will be offered professional counselling (See 'Free Counselling Services' attached with this proposal).

Analysis and interpretation

The proposal must clearly set out the methods for sorting (analysing) and making sense of (interpreting) the data. This is the main way the project will be judged as trustworthy when completed. Therefore, the proposal should be very clear about how you intend to analyse and interpret the data, so the people judging the merits of the proposal can consider whether your plans for this phase are reasonable in relation to the rest of the project.

Continuing the example in this section, the analysis and interpretation part of the proposal may include statements such as:

> The data analysis methods will depend on the types of data collection used. Analysis of journal experiences will be managed by individual and group critical reflection and problem-solving strategies. Group discussion will also be used to identify the specific nature and determinants of problems, as well as the most appropriate methods to investigate problems further and the most practical and useful plan of action. Descriptions of participant observation will be analysed by manual thematic analysis techniques (Roberts & Taylor 2002).
>
> As mentioned previously, in each action research cycle the findings will be pooled and discussed and the appropriate action will be planned and taken. Successive observation of the effects will follow, before further reflection leads to further action and analysis.

Dissemination of findings

The proposal should contain a plan for the dissemination of findings. This will show that you are aware the research will be rendered meaningless if the results are not shared with the people who may benefit from them. For example:

> The researcher will teach RNs how to plan for verbal presentations to peers, and to write for publication in refereed professional journals. A potential target for national presentation is the annual clinical practice conference. Local venues for speaking about the research may also include nurses' seminars at local hospitals and various nurse interest groups in the region. National refereed journals, which could be targeted for publication, include *Contemporary Nurse* and the *Australian Journal of Advanced Nursing Practice*. International refereed journals for which the project is suitable include *The International Journal of Nursing Practice* and *The International Journal of Palliative Nursing*. Articles will be written by a combination of group members, depending on who is interested and willing to expend time and energy in getting quality articles ready for publication. In all presentations and articles each member of the group will receive acknowledgement, although they may not necessarily be listed as contributors if they have not taken a share of the workload for the verbal presentation or written article.

Of course, participants' first point of dissemination may be in thesis form to the tertiary organisation in which they are enrolled. The organisation will deposit the thesis in the library for access by borrowers. It is also a good idea for students to make plans to disseminate the research findings at professional conferences, and in journals and monographs. These avenues for dissemination will be discussed later in this book.

The project timeframe

The proposal needs to show that you are organised as far as time is concerned and that you have allowed enough time to complete the project within the prescribed period. The funding body and/or your organisation will want to know what you are going to do, and when, so that they can be assured that the project will be completed on time. An example of a timeframe might be:

Proposed timing

(Year)

August	Finalise ethics approval
September	Recruit participants
	Begin reflective and action research methods and processes
October	Continue and document action cycles of planning, acting, observing and reflecting
November	Facilitate tuition and practice in preparing for professional presentations and publications
December	Submit the journal article(s).

Budget

If you are applying for a research grant to assist you in completing your research award, you will need to give careful consideration to the costs involved. Most grant bodies require a detailed budget, outlining costs for the research personnel (research assistants, desktop publishers, clerical assistance and so on); equipment (computer data analysis system, audiotapes and so on); travel at × cents per kilometre; and other costs, such as photocopying, mailing and so on. The grant application form will make it clear what the funding body will or will not fund, so be sure to read the information carefully.

The example in Table 6.2 (overleaf) was not part of the example given in this section, but was part of a different project funded internally by a university. However, it may give you some idea of what is expected in an itemised budget where justification is required for funds.

Funding bodies want to know about each item of research expenditure in your budget, to know that the money is justified and that you will use it prudently. You need to be as clear as possible in writing this section. For example:

Justification of the budget

Although I will be responsible for the conduct and evaluation of the project, I will need the help of an experienced Research Assistant (RA), who is also a Registered Nurse with an honours degree. My role as an academic has many research, teaching and community liaison facets; therefore, I need to delegate some of the practical aspects of research projects to an RA. Duties will include assistance in arranging access and consent, and helping in the conduct and evaluation of cycles. Specific duties will include the preparation and sequential data collection of surveys and interviews in the clinical area. Some 240 hours of work are needed to assist me in these duties over a nine-month action research period (seven hours per week for 34 weeks). The HEW Level 5/1 reflects the level of qualification and experience of an RA with established clinical competence and a high degree of confidentiality, capable of working with minimal supervision in a sensitive area of research.

The transcription assistant costs reflect the lengthy and tedious process of transcribing audiotapes. It takes three hours to transcribe a one-hour tape, and it must be done by a

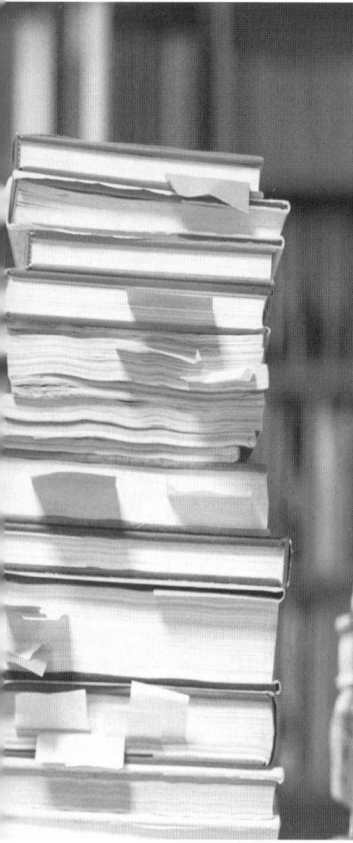

Table 6.2 Example of a budget

Detailed budget items	Priority	Amount requested		
		2005	2006	2007
Research assistant				
Paid at HEW Level 5/1, at a base rate of $22.01/hour (includes 16.5% on-costs) for 240 hours, to assist CI in arranging access, consent, and conduct and evaluation of cycles, including sequential data collection, analysis, and interpretation over a nine-month action research period	A	5282.00	Nil	Nil
Transcription assistant costs				
40 half-hour tapes x 1.5 hours/tape, equals 60hrs @ $18.76/hr (includes 16.5% on-costs)	A	1125.60		
Maintenance				
40 TDK audiotapes ($32 4 boxes of 10)	B	$ 128.00		
Total	**(n/a)**	**6536.00**		

proficient and reliable person to maintain the integrity of the data. The number of tapes is an estimate for a nine-month data-gathering period in a wide variety of nursing settings with a range of people, including patients, relatives and health care workers.

High-quality audiotapes are required for safe recording and storing of interview data for analysis.

EXERCISE

Why is it important to predict a timeline for a project? Why are plans proposed for the dissemination of the results?

Summary

There are similarities in quantitative and qualitative research proposals; however, there are also differences. The similarities are in the structure of the format of a proposal. The differences relate to the use of words in the body of the report to describe the chosen research methodology, methods and processes. Qualitative researchers also need to be discerning in presenting their proposals to committees who may come from an empirico-analytical background, as criteria from that background may be used as a frame of reference for judging the merits of a qualitative proposal.

Common final elements

The final pages of any research proposal contain supporting materials – information that relates back to the material in the body of the proposal. Principally these materials are a full reference list and any appendixes containing additional material not central to the proposal but providing additional information and examples.

References

The list of references should come at the end of the proposal but before the appendixes. You should follow the referencing system recommended by your institution. Usually it is only the university that will have requirements for a particular referencing system. If you have a choice, you should use a user-friendly referencing system such as the author–date system (Harvard) unless your guidelines stipulate a different one. The Harvard system is economical in terms of time and is very flexible, as entries can be added, deleted or changed with a minimum of disruption to the rest of the document. In addition, the reader is able to tell immediately who the author is and when the reference was published. Other systems, such as the endnote system or the footnote (Oxford) system, require an adjustment of all following reference numbers whenever a reference is inserted or removed.

   The Harvard system has been used in this book, so for details on how to apply it, consult the references in this book. References for the two proposals in this chapter can be found in the reference list at the end of this chapter. For further details, consult the Australian Government Printing Service *Style Manual for Authors, Editors and Printers*, 6th edn (Snooks & Co. 2002). The Harvard system puts the author(s) and date of the work being referred to at the appropriate point in the text, rather than using a number. This is called a 'citation'. All of the works cited are then listed at the end of the paper in alphabetical order according to author. The reader can then refer from the text to the reference. It is not necessary to reference well-known facts.

   Textual references should be given in a consistent manner throughout the document. Each citation in the text should refer to a reference in the reference list and each reference in the list should be cited in the text; that is, they should match. The list of references is alphabetical, by author's surname. It contains only works cited in the text; others are listed as a bibliography, if used. The reference list must contain all of the works cited in the text.

Appendixes

Appendixes are included if it is necessary to provide material that is too cumbersome for the main text, for example, questionnaires and so forth. Use appendixes judiciously to avoid filling the proposal with unnecessary detail and interrupting the flow of the main text. Include only material that supports or expands on the information in the body of the text.

Examples of things that are best put in an appendix are questionnaires, instruments, or tests, diagrams of instruments, consent forms and letters of support. Start each appendix on a new page and name them alphabetically, i.e. Appendix A, Appendix B and so on. You should be aware that it is common committee practice for the committee secretary not to copy appendixes to the committee but to have them available on the day. However, if you supply enough copies for the committee members you can ensure that they receive the appendixes.

Writing the proposal

Style

The style of a research proposal is fairly prescribed. It is not like an essay, and creativity is inappropriate in writing a research proposal (Barnard 1986). In writing the research proposal, aim for clarity, coherence, conciseness and completeness. Remember that the reviewers are busy people who want a succinct proposal because they have to read a lot of them. You should use the formal scientific style in a quantitative paper, but in a qualitative paper, the personal style is appropriate. Construct the proposal in a logical order, such as the one given in this chapter. Avoid preaching or adopting a value-laden stance since you are supposed to be an objective researcher and bias is considered to be poor science.

Aim to use good English, with short, crisp sentences. It is important to use language that can be understood by lay strangers and/or members of other disciplines. The reason for this is that some of the people on an ethics committee will fall into that category. You should avoid jargon, especially that of your specialty, but where you must use specific terminology, clearly define the terms that you use. Use terms consistently and do not attempt to change terms to make your proposal read more like a novel.

It is important to avoid sexist language: never use the pronoun 'he' to refer to everyone. It is possible to avoid sexist language by using the plural rather than the singular, for example 'participants will have their blood pressure taken before and after the treatment'. However, be specific about the gender of the participants where it is relevant. For example, if your study is going to be done with females only, say so.

Using the correct tense can be difficult. Use the future tense for the parts of the proposal that state what you intend to do. Use the past tense for the literature review and the section on the pilot study if it has already been completed. Write statements of everyday knowledge in the present tense.

There are specific books on writing research proposals and reports, for example, *Assignment and Thesis Writing* (Anderson & Poole 1998). Pro formas from ethics committees or funding agencies may set out sections for your guidance. If you are writing a full scientific protocol, use the format suggested above.

Use of headings

Headings assist the reader to understand the structure of the proposal and to prepare the reader for what is to come. While the use of headings is inappropriate in creative writing or an essay, it is mandatory in a research proposal. Whatever system you decide on, you should use headings and subheadings generously to guide the reader. However, use your commonsense. If you find that every paragraph has a heading, you are probably using too many headings.

There are two major systems of headings. One uses differences in the physical appearance of the heading and the other uses a numbering system, with or without differences in physical appearance. For longer reports such as theses, the numbering system is better because it makes it easier to see the structure of the proposal. However, for shorter proposals, such as student classroom projects, the other system is quite adequate. In a thesis, a combination of the two systems can be used, but the heading system should be consistent. Modern word processors include a function that allows you to build in a heading style.

The physical appearance system

This system relies upon differences in the appearance of the letters. It uses a combination of lower- and upper-case letters in the headings, position of the headings, and underlining or boldness (heaviness) of the font. This system is suitable for only about three or four levels of headings in addition to the title. Variations can be made by using italics, or different colours if you have a colour printer. A simple example of a heading format using physical appearance of lettering is seen in Figure 6.3.

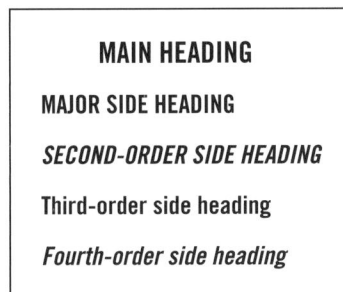

MAIN HEADING

MAJOR SIDE HEADING

SECOND-ORDER SIDE HEADING

Third-order side heading

Fourth-order side heading

Figure 6.3 Physical appearance system of headings

Note that the centred heading, and the major and second-order side heading are all upper-case/capital letters. The second-order side heading is italic. The third- and fourth-order side headings have only the first word capitalised and the fourth-order side heading is also italic. This system can be varied by using normal-face as well as bold-face (heavy black) and italic fonts.

The numbering system

This system relies on numbered sections. As stated earlier, it is usually used for larger proposals and in theses. Each section is given a number, and the number is used as the beginning of each heading in the section. The second-order headings begin with the number 1, and go up from there, and the third-order headings begin with 1, and so on. An example is shown in Figure 6.4 (overleaf).

Notice that this system may also use physical characteristics. The numbers at the same level are indented the same amount. The disadvantage of this system is that an alteration to the text may require changing subsequent numbers within the section.

```
SECTION 2

METHODOLOGY

2.1     Setting

2.2     Participants

2.3     Instruments and Procedures

            2.3.1 Instruments

                    2.3.1.1 The questionnaire

                    2.3.1.2 The physical instrument

            2.3.2 Procedures for data collection

2.4     Data Analysis
```

Figure 6.4   Numbering system of headings

The process of writing a proposal

Before starting to write your proposal, see if you can acquire both a good proposal and a weak one and compare them. This allows you to see the differences and implement the good points while avoiding the bad ones. When you are ready to begin writing, tackle what you see as the easiest part first. You do not need to write the proposal in the order in which it finally appears. The abstract is usually written last.

After you are satisfied with the structure and content of your draft, you should polish it. Check the spelling. Use the spellchecker on your word processor by all means, but don't rely on it. Check the grammar, punctuation and style using a book such as *The Elements of Style* (Strunk & White 2000) or the AGPS *Style Manual*. You can also use the grammar checker on your word processor, but remember that you cannot exclusively rely on it. You must proofread all your documents, but especially your final copy, to eliminate grammatical errors; the spellchecker is unable to pick up some errors such as 'their' when you mean 'there'.

When you are satisfied with the first draft of the proposal, leave it for a fortnight or longer. Then read it critically and analytically, and from the point of view of the lecturer, supervisor or committee member who will be reading it. Then revise it. At this point, if possible, you should get an objective colleague, friend or relative to critique it, then revise it again. Finally, proofread it again and ask someone else to proofread it as well.

Your next task is to transfer the final draft of your proposal onto the application form, or pro forma specified by the organisation. It should be typed or word processed. This is worth an investment of your time and effort in learning to type yourself, or paying someone else to do it. You may have an electronic copy of the application form on your word processor, in which case make a duplicate and use that, retaining the blank original for future use. If you do not have an electronic copy, you may type the forms into the word processor yourself: most organisations will accept facsimiles without the fancy boxes as long you respect the page limit and keep the format and the font size the same. You may have to type the material onto a paper copy, in which case use a photocopy of the form and save one clean copy in case you have to make revisions.

The document itself should be double-spaced (unless on a pro forma with limited space) and printed in black. Use A4 bond of at least 80 gsm weight. Print the document on white paper since coloured paper doesn't provide enough contrast for photocopying. Ideally the font should be 12 point if you are typing on blank paper. However, the size on the pro forma should be matched if you are using a pro forma. Use a legible font such as Palatino, Times New Roman or Bembo. Make sure that the pages are numbered. At the very end, check that the submission is complete, that is, it contains all pages including appendixes and references.

Submitting the proposal

Having completed the proposal, your next step is to submit it to the committee or agency. Make sure you provide the exact number of photocopies required – you may be required to provide one copy for each member of the committee. Or you may be able to submit the application electronically. In any event, make sure that you retain a copy of the document, in case of loss. In the case of a word-processed document, make sure that you have a backup copy. Better yet, keep two backup copies in different places in case of fire or theft.

It is possible, but by no means usual, that you may be asked to appear before a committee, most likely an institutional ethics committee, to explain or defend your proposal. If so, you will be notified that you are required to attend. You may bring your supervisor. In preparation for the meeting, you should rehearse a concise overview of your study because you will probably be asked to describe it. You should know the proposal thoroughly. You must be able to justify the value of your study and its impact on practice. You should also be aware of any ethical aspects that you think the committee could raise. Make sure your supervisor is well briefed. On the day, make sure you have a copy of your application with you and provide one for your supervisor too. Remember to dress appropriately and present a cool and confident manner. You can expect about 10 people to be there. During the meeting, ask for a question to be repeated if you don't understand it. You can refer to your supervisor if you get out of your depth.

You can expect that you will receive a written response from the committee, usually at least a fortnight after its meeting. Only if you are under pressure of time should you telephone the committee chair or secretary. An informal approval over the telephone would permit you to start making arrangements for carrying out your study. However, under no circumstances should you ever commence data collection without a written approval from the appropriate committees.

If your proposal is not successful, you can use any feedback provided by the assessors of your application to improve the proposal. Often the committee may require only minor modifications, or may stipulate that approval is granted subject to certain conditions. It is then your job to respond in writing to the committee, stating how you will fulfil the conditions. If the response from the committee is very discouraging, you may need to rethink the entire proposal from an objective point of view. If it is appropriate, you may consult with members of the committee to clarify their points of concern.

Funding

Frequently, the cost of a project makes it imperative to acquire funding from a source other than the researcher. For student projects, you, the researcher, will have to bear the costs in excess of any funds granted by your institution. For graduate students, the university may give a stipend or you may be able to get a grant from an outside body. In addition, the university provides the infrastructure described earlier. Some graduate students may do work that is funded by their supervisor's research grant.

For clinicians, the sources of funding are from their own institution's research fund or from collaborative projects with university staff, who may be able to get a grant from the university. Alternatively, the other source of funding is from independent organisations, government or corporate bodies. The NHMRC controls government funds for clinical research, while the Australian Research Council controls funding for non-clinical research such as disciplinary systems or education. The amount given by various bodies may vary from a few hundred dollars to many thousands of dollars. Often grants are advertised in prominent newspapers such as the *Sydney Morning Herald* and the *Australian*. If your institution has a research management unit, it will probably have the details of funding sources and may be able to advise you of them.

It is important when identifying a possible source of funds for your grant to match the aims of your research project with those of the granting body, and to make sure that the amount of funding given by the body is in line with the amount you are seeking (Hamilton 1994).

Obtaining informal approvals

The formal approval for the research project given by the ethics and research committees will gain you entry to the institution for the purposes of your research project. However, you will also need to secure informal approvals from other parties in the clinical field in order to gain access to participants. If you plan to do a research project in a hospital, for example, you will need to see the director of nursing and the appropriate administration staff to brief them and get their approval. If you are going to use the patients of medical practitioners, it is courteous to acquire their approval. These people function as gatekeepers and it is as well to get them on side. Similarly, you will need the approval of the staff concerned, for example, the staff on the hospital ward. A wise researcher gets this approval and arranges to brief the staff on the project and get their cooperation. All this may seem like a lot of work, but it pays dividends in staff cooperation. Staff who feel resentful at your presence or who feel that they have not been consulted can sabotage your research project.

You can improve your access to participants by gaining credibility within the institution, and attending to the social amenities. You can enhance your credibility by promoting the benefits of your study to the staff, being visible in the clinical area during the course of the study, and by minimising the intrusions and demands that the project makes on the daily operations of the site. Social amenities include keeping key people informed of the progress of the study, acknowledging staff participation and behaving with professional courtesy at all times.

If the study is carried on over a period of time, it is essential to implement strategies to ensure continued access to participants. If staff turnover is a problem, you may need to do more than one briefing session. Continuing to carry out the above strategies will help to ensure continued access. In addition, at the end of the project, you should thank the staff formally with a letter. You may also wish to thank them with a small gift, such as a box of chocolates or an afternoon tea, depending on your budget. This helps to keep the channels open for further research. Above all, don't forget to send the ward staff, as well as any other key persons, a written summary of your findings. It is also appropriate to present your findings at an inservice session as well.

If your research is being carried out at the university, you will need to brief the key people there, such as the head of the nursing or physiotherapy department, and the academic staff. If you are using a laboratory you will need to organise this with whoever handles the bookings for using the laboratory. You will also need to liaise with the laboratory technician, who may be able to help you with setting up and returning the laboratory to its previous state. The above principles with regard to social amenities and feedback apply in the university setting as well as the clinical field.

Summary

In this chapter we have discussed the mechanisms for gaining approval for your research project, including from your supervisor, the university, and the clinical field. We have shown you the process for constructing a research proposal and the content of the proposal. In addition, securing funding for the project and gaining the necessary approvals from the clinical field have been discussed briefly. Now that you have the necessary approval, you are at last ready to move to the next exciting part of the process: collecting your data!

Main points

- A research proposal is a written account of a plan for a project that argues why a particular problem should be investigated and what the appropriate methodology is to investigate it; and it sets out what the researcher intends to do – how, why, where, when and at what cost.
- A plan helps to design and organise a project, allows you to see and ponder relationships between different parts of the proposal, helps to foresee potential problems and solve them at the planning stage, permits consultation with other researchers before the study is carried out, and is the best way to prevent mistakes occurring when you are carrying out the project.
- Proposals are written to gain approval of funding bodies, university research committees, ethics committees and other bodies giving approval.

- The preliminary steps in writing a proposal are to: identify the research problem, read and review the literature, identify a research design, identify the proposal's audience, acquire protocols and guidelines from institutions and identify pathways for approvals.
- All proposals consist of preliminary pages, the body of the proposal and supporting materials.
- The body of a quantitative research proposal has a particular structure: introduction (including a literature review that elucidates the theoretical framework for the study), methodology (including participant recruitment, and data processing and analysis), ethical requirements, dissemination plan, work plan and budget.
- Qualitative research proposals have a title page and a research summary or abstract but in the body of the proposal the use of words is specific to describe the chosen research methodology, methods and processes.
- Qualitative research proposals contain clear and concise statements about the research summary; the significance, aims and objectives of the study; the research questions; background and literature review; the research plan, including methodology, methods and processes of participant recruitment; data collection, analysis and interpretation; ethical requirements; dissemination of findings; the project time frame; and the budget.
- The writing style of the proposal should aim for clarity, coherence, conciseness and completeness with the proposal constructed in a logical order. The language should be understandable by all people, avoiding jargon but defining specific terms.
- The proposal should be submitted according to the guidelines of the scrutinising body and a response can be expected to take at least a fortnight after that body's meeting.
- Seek informal approvals from gatekeepers of the institutions in which you will be collecting data and develop strategies for recruiting and retaining participants.

CASE STUDY

In this case study we return to Wendy, to whom you were introduced in Chapter 1. Wendy is an experienced Registered Nurse with a Masters qualification, who works as a diabetes educator in a large rural hospital. So far, Wendy has enlisted the help of the members of the multidisciplinary team to offer their clinical expertise in formulating a research interest. The team decided that they were all interested in how diabetics manage their everyday activities of living after initial adjustment to lower limb amputation.

Wendy now needs to write a research proposal. Although she realises that this project could be done with a mixed methodology using quantitative and qualitative approaches, she has decided to use a qualitative approach. She intends to interview 20 people, over the age of 18 years, who have accessed the local diabetic services and who are at least one year post amputation. Although there are many other details to consider, she is at the point of being able to write the first draft of her research proposal. She requests a discussion with you to help her clarify the proposal writing process. What will you tell Wendy about:

1   how to decide on what to write for the title, significance, aims and objectives of the research
2   the literature that could be included
3   how she can choose a particular methodological approach, e.g. grounded theory etc
4   how she can justify interviewing 20 people only in a qualitative project?

Multiple choice questions

1   A written account of the plan for the research project that presents an argument as to why a particular problem should be investigated is a research:
    a   proposal
    b   methodology
    c   design
    d   matrix

2   All projects undertaken under the auspices of the university and/or clinical facility in which data collection is involved will require the approval of the:
    a   executive managers
    b   ethics committees
    c   participants involved
    d   department head

3   Which of the following would be found in the body section of a research proposal:
    a   data analysis procedures
    b   title page
    c   abstract
    d   researcher details

4   In which section of a research proposal would you most likely find the ethical implications? In the:
    a   preliminaries
    b   budget
    c   abstract
    d   body

5   The statement of significance of the study should show:
    a   the intentions for the study
    b   the researchers' details
    c   why the study is worth doing
    d   the summary of the project

6 The section of the proposal which describes in detail the framework for the study, including the justification for choices about the setting, participants, instruments and procedures is the research:

    a design

    b abstract

    c summary

    d context

7 Generally, when qualitative researchers refer to methodology in a proposal, they are referring to the:

    a choices about the setting, participants, instruments and procedures

    b estimation of time to undertake the research activities including publication

    c theoretical assumptions underlying the choice of methods

    d risks involved in undertaking research with human participants

8 Examples of documents that are best put in an appendix are:

    a the detailed background of the research project, including a well-referenced literature review

    b the abstract, title, significance, aims, objectives, and data collection and analysis methods

    c complete copies of the documents submitted for university and health facility ethics approval

    d questionnaires, instruments, or tests, diagrams of instruments, consent forms and letters of support

9 Justification for items in a research budget is necessary because funding bodies:

    a are composed of mistrustful people

    b give the money to the cheapest proposal

    c need to be sure that the money is used wisely

    d know that some projects have no costs

10 Obtaining informal approvals relates to:

    a gaining permission to access participants in the research settings

    b lobbying members of the ethics committees for their support

    c checking to see that participants will be willing to be involved

    d ensuring that staff in clinical settings know you are a researcher

Review topics

1 Discuss the reasons why research proposals are necessary.

2 What basic information do you need before you can hope to write a research proposal?

3 Why is it necessary to ensure that every part of the proposal demonstrates that all of the ideas are linked?

4 Describe the differences between quantitative and qualitative research proposals.

5 Why are research proposals and ethics submissions linked in human research?

Online reading

INFOTRAC® COLLEGE EDITION
When accessing information about research proposals use the following keywords:

INFOTRAC

➤ aims
➤ background
➤ data analysis
➤ data collection
➤ design
➤ dissemination of results
➤ literature review
➤ methodology
➤ methods
➤ objectives
➤ plan
➤ processes
➤ qualitative
➤ quantitative
➤ significance

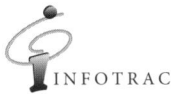

References

Anderson, D. & Poole, M. 1998, *Assignment and Thesis Writing*, 3rd edn, John Wiley & Sons, Brisbane.

Barnard, K. 1986, 'Writing a research proposal', *MCN: Maternal Child Nursing*, vol. 11, January–February, 76.

Blieszner, R. 2004, 'Supporting health-related quality of life for old women', *Journal of the American Medical Women's Association*, vol. 59, no. 4, 244–7.

Bolmsjo, I. & Hermeren, G. 1998, 'Challenging assumptions in end-of-life situations', *Palliative Medical* vol. 12, no. 6, 451–6.

Bryant, T., Brown, I., Cogan, T., Dallaire, C., Laforest, S., McGowan, P., Raphael, D., Richard, L., Thompson, L. & Young, J. 2004, 'What do Canadian seniors say supports their quality of life?: Findings from a national participatory research study', *Canadian Journal of Public Health*, vol. 95, no. 4, 299–303.

Chenoweth, L. & Kilstoff, K. 1998, 'Facilitating positive changes in community dementia management through participatory action research', *International Journal of Nursing Practice*, vol. 4, 175–88.

Clarke, P. & Black, S. 2005, 'Quality of life following stroke: negotiating disability, identity, and resources', *Journal of Applied Gerontology*, vol. 24, no. 4, 319–36.

Dick, R.A. 1995, 'A beginner's guide to action research', *ARCS Newsletter*, vol. 1, no. 1, 5–9.

Fang, C., Hsing, P. & Yu, C. 2002, 'Validation of the WHO quality of life instrument in patients with HIV infection', *Quality of Life Research*, vol. 11, no. 8, 753–62.

Fitzgerald, L. & van Hooft, S. 2000, 'A Socratic dialogue on the question "What is love in nursing?"' *Nursing Ethics: International Journal of Health Care Professionals*, vol. 7, no. 6, 481–91.

Frank-Stromborg, M. & Olsen, S. 2004, *Instruments for Clinical Health Care Research*, 3rd edn, Jones & Bartlett, Boston.

Gerritsen, D., Jongenelis, K., Steverink, N., Ooms, M. & Ribbe, M. 2005, 'Down and drowsy? Do apathetic nursing home residents experience low quality of life?', *Aging & Mental Health*, vol. 9, no. 2, 135–41.

Hamilton, H. 1994, 'Winning finance for your project', in J. Robertson (ed.), *Handbook of Clinical Nursing Research*, Churchill Livingstone, Melbourne.

Hasanah, C. & Razali, M. 2002, 'Quality of life: an assessment of the state of psychological rehabilitation of patients with schizophrenia in the community', *Journal of Research in Social Health*, vol. 122, no. 4, 251–5.

Hoe, J., Katona, C., Roch, B. & Livingston, G. 2005, 'Use of the QOL-AD for measuring quality of life in people with severe dementia – the LASER-AD study', *Age and Ageing*, vol. 34, no. 2, 130–5.

Keatinge, D., Scarfe, C., Bellchambers, H., McGee, J., Oakham, R., Probert, C., Stewart, L. & Stokes, J. 2000, 'The manifestation and nursing management of agitation in institutionalised residents with dementia', *International Journal of Nursing Practice*, vol. 6, 16–25.

Kemmis, S. & McTaggart, R. (eds) 1988, *The Action Research Planner*, 3rd edn, Deakin University Press, Geelong, Victoria.

Kermode, S. & MacLean, D. 2001, 'A study of the relationship between quality of life, self-esteem and health', *Australian Journal of Advanced Nursing*, vol. 19, no. 2, 33–40.

Koch, T., Kralik, D. & Kelly, S. 2000, 'We just don't talk about it: men living with urinary incontinence and multiple sclerosis', *International Journal of Nursing Practice*, vol. 6, 253–60.

Lillibridge, J., Axford, R. & Rowley, G. 2000, 'The contribution of nurses' perceptions and actions in defining scope and stabilising professional boundaries of nursing practice', *Collegian*, vol. 7, no. 4, 35–9.

Masoudi, F., Rumsfeld, J., Havranek, E., House, J., Peterson, E., Krumholz, J. & Spertus, J. 2004, 'Age, functional capacity, and health-related quality of life in patients with heart failure', *Journal of Cardiac Failure*, vol. 10, no. 5, 368–73.

O'Carroll, R., Smith, K. & Couston, M. 2000, 'A comparison of the WHOQOL-100 and the WHOQOL-BREF in detecting change in quality of life following liver transplantation', *Quality of Life Research*, vol. 9, no. 1, 121–4.

O'Connor, R. 2004, *Measuring Quality of Life in Health Care*, Churchill Livingstone, Edinburgh.

Parse, R. 1987, *Nursing Science: Major Paradigm Theories and Critiques*, WB Saunders, Philadelphia.

Roberts, K. & Taylor, B. 2002, *Nursing Research Processes: an Australian Perspective*, 2nd edn, Nelson ITP, Melbourne.

Schok, M. & de Vries, J. 2005, 'Predicting overall quality of life and general health of veterans with and without health problems', *Military Psychology*, vol. 17, no. 2, 89–100.

Skevington, S., Carse, M. & Williams, A. 2001, 'Pain management improves quality of life for chronic pain patients', *Clinical Journal of Pain*, vol. 17, no. 3, 264–75.

Snooks & Co. 2002, *Style Manual for Authors, Editors and Printers*, 6th edn, John Wiley & Sons Australia, Canberra.

Sprenkle, M., Niewoehner, D., Nelson, D. & Nichol, K. 2004, 'The Veterans Short Form 36 Questionnaire is predictive of mortality and health-care utilization in a population of veterans with a self-reported diagnosis of asthma or COPD', *Chest*, vol. 126, no. 1, 81–9.

Starace, F., Cafaro, L. & Albrescia, N. 2002, 'Quality of life assessment in HIV-positive persons: Application and validation of the WHOQOL-HIV, Italian version', *AIDS Care*, vol. 14, no. 3, 405–15.

Stringer, E.T. 1996, *Action research: A Handbook for Practitioners*, California, Sage Publications, Thousand Oaks.

Strunk, W. & White, E. 2000, *The Elements of Style*, 4th edn, Allyn and Bacon, Boston.

Taylor, B. 2000, *Reflective Practice: A Guide for Nurses and Midwives*, Allen and Unwin, Melbourne.

Taylor, B., Glass, N., McFarlane, J. & Stirling, K. 2001, 'Views of nurses, patients and patients' families regarding palliative nursing care', *International Journal of Palliative Nursing*, vol. 7, no. 4, 186–91.

Taylor, B.J. 2001a, 'Overcoming obstacles in becoming a reflective nurse and person', *Contemporary Nurse*, vol. 11, no. 2–3, 187–94.

Taylor, B.J. 2001b, 'Identifying and transforming dysfunctional nurse-nurse relationships through reflective practice and action research', *International Journal of Nursing Practice*, vol. 7, no. 6, 406–13.

Taylor, B.J., Bulmer, B., Hill, L., Luxford, C., McFarlane, J. & Stirling, K. 2002, 'Exploring idealism in palliative nursing care through reflective practice and action research', *International Journal; of Palliative Nursing*, vol. 8, no. 7, 324–30.

Wang, X., Gao, L. & Zhang, H. 2000, 'Post-earthquake quality of life and psychosocial well-being: longitudinal evaluation in a rural community sample in northern China', *Psychiatry and Clinical Neuroscience*, vol. 55, no. 4, 427–33.

Weis, D. & Schank, M.J. 2000, 'An instrument to measure professional nursing values', *Journal of Nursing Scholarship*, vol. 32, no. 2, 201–4.

WHOQOL Group 1993, 'Study Protocol for the World Health Organisation project to develop a quality of life assessment instrument (WHOQOL)', *Quality of Life Research*, vol. 2, no. 2, 153–9.

CHAPTER 7

QUANTITATIVE RESEARCH DESIGNS

CHAPTER OBJECTIVES

The material presented in this chapter will assist you to:

- describe the different types of quantitative research designs
- compare the strength of various types of quantitative research designs
- discuss the advantages and disadvantages of the different types of quantitative research designs
- choose an appropriate quantitative design for a research project.

Introduction

A **research design** provides the framework by which a project will answer a particular research question. It guides the researcher in carrying out the study, much as a recipe guides the cook in preparing a dish, or as a blueprint guides the engineer in constructing a bridge. A research design also provides the researcher with signposts to guide them through the research process. Well-established research designs have well-known signposts.

In this chapter, we will be concerned with quantitative **descriptive designs, comparative designs, correlational designs** and **experimental designs**. These designs answer specific types of research questions, and produce different levels of 'evidence'. A descriptive design only describes a phenomenon, a comparative design allows descriptive data from two or more groups to be compared, a correlational design looks for relationships between different variables, while an experiment attempts to show whether one thing causes another. In this chapter, we will describe these designs as pure types, although a study may combine elements of more than one of these. It could, for example, be both descriptive and correlational.

There is no one answer to the question: 'What is the best research design?' The best research design is the one that is most likely to help you answer your particular research question. It is a matter of selecting the design with the best 'fit' to your question.

Major types of research design

There are various types of research design ranging from the simple descriptive design, through designs that compare groups, to experimental designs. Table 7.1 (overleaf) shows the major types of research designs and their features.

Descriptive designs

Descriptive designs are designs that describe phenomena in order to answer a research question. These designs may vary in complexity. They are also found in qualitative research where the purpose is to describe or draw a picture of a phenomenon using words, art, music or other media. Many of these designs focus on 'experience' of a phenomenon, rather than objective analysis of a phenomenon. That type of research will be described in Chapter 12. In this chapter, we will be concerned only with quantitative descriptive research. This is research that uses numbers to describe phenomena. Quantitative descriptive research may also allow simple comparison of the incidence of the phenomenon in different groups of people, but does not set out to confirm differences between them.

Quantitative descriptive designs produce very weak 'evidence' in comparison to experiments, but nevertheless they have a place, particularly when little is known about the topic being investigated. They are a way to start building up knowledge about a topic and are used to conduct an initial exploration on a research question.

Table 7.1 Comparison of major research designs

	Simple descriptive	Comparative descriptive	Correlational	Pre-experimental	Quasi-experimental	Experimental
Describes participants	Yes	Yes	Yes	Yes	Yes	Yes
Compares groups	No	Yes	Yes	Yes	Yes	Yes
Investigates cause-and-effect relationships	No	No	No	No	Yes	Yes
Manipulates independent variable	No	No	No	No	Yes	Yes
Has control group	No	No	No	No	Yes	Yes
Random assignment to groups	No	No	No	No	No	Yes

Simple descriptive designs

Simple descriptive designs measure known variables in a population. For example, suppose that you wanted to measure self-care capabilities in adults with arthritis. You could take a questionnaire that measured self-care abilities and administer it to a group of people with arthritis and come up with a measure of self-care ability for that group. The Australian census, which is undertaken every five years, draws a statistical 'description' of the Australian population. Various methods can be used to collect descriptive data but the most common are surveys using questionnaires or interviews and observation by people or monitoring equipment. These methods will be discussed in Chapter 8.

In designing a descriptive study, it is necessary first to decide what you want to investigate. Once you decide on your research question, you need to select the group or population that you want to study. You then identify the aspects of the group that you want to study. These must be defined clearly and in sufficient detail that they can be measured. These characteristics may be identified through existing theory, through the literature and through your own knowledge. These are your variables. Once you identify them, you can measure them in the sample or population you have chosen.

An example of a simple descriptive design can be found in Peden et al. (2004), who studied the characteristics of negative thinking and the mental health of low-income single mothers. They surveyed a sample of 205 women using a number of psychometric questionnaires. They found that more than 75 per cent of the participants were at least mildly depressed and that negative thinking was an important factor in this depression.

The simple descriptive design produces weak evidence because it cannot determine degrees of difference between groups, relationships between variables or whether one variable causes another. It has the advantages of being quick, relatively inexpensive and useful for preliminary research that may lead to further research questions.

Comparative descriptive design

A comparative descriptive design is one in which two or more groups are being compared on particular variables. For example, if you wanted to measure the relative self-care abilities of male and female arthritis sufferers, you would administer your self-care instrument to one group of males and one group of females and see if they got different scores on their self-care abilities. Of course, you would want to compare males and females of equal ages, stages of the disease, and any other characteristic that might affect the results.

An example of a comparative descriptive design is a study by Bostrom et al. (2003), in which comparison of pain and health-related quality of life was made between two groups of cancer patients with differing average levels of pain. Both groups were assessed using a number of instruments, and it was found that pain has a negative impact on quality of life, especially on physical health, and that pain increases towards the final stages of life. Even if patients have to endure symptoms such as fatigue and anxiety during their short survival time, dealing with pain is an unnecessary burden which can be prevented.

This type of design generally has the same advantages and disadvantages as simple descriptive design, but has the added advantage of allowing comparison of groups. The evidence produced by such a design therefore is a little stronger than a simple descriptive design.

Correlational designs

A correlational design examines the relationship between two or more variables within one group without aiming to determine cause and effect. It examines the direction of the relationship (positive or negative) and also the strength of the relationship. It does not have an independent variable that can be manipulated by the researcher, that is, there is no intervention by the researcher, just observation. The researcher identifies the variables of interest and chooses the most appropriate way to measure them. Where pools of data already exist (such as nursing charts) such a design can be implemented very quickly. Then the researcher carries out a statistical analysis to determine whether there is a relationship between the variables, and if so, how strong, and in what direction.

An example of a study with a correlational design is one that examined the relationships between the symptoms of insomnia and fatigue and the psychological factors of anxiety and depression, and the relationships between these psychological and symptom variables and quality of life in cancer patients who were receiving chemotherapy (Redeker, Lev & Ruggiero 2000). The researchers found that insomnia and fatigue are related to depression and that depression is more closely associated with quality of life than are insomnia and fatigue.

The advantage of a correlational design is that it is a relatively easy, fast, and inexpensive way to acquire and process a lot of data that can be used to investigate relationships among variables. A correlational design has the advantage that it is useful in exploratory research to determine relationships that can later be tested out more explicitly by more exacting methodologies. In comparison to an experiment, a correlational design is more straightforward and easier to implement, and the data are collected more quickly, usually by a survey, or chart audit. A correlational study is also less intrusive than an experiment.

Experimental designs

The classical experimental design is one in which one group of subjects are exposed to a treatment, while another group is exposed to something inert. The responses of the two groups are then examined to see if there was any difference between them. Experiments can occur naturally by the intervention of nature (e.g. acts of 'God'), or artificially by the intervention of an experimenter. An experiment may be carried on in the laboratory or in the clinical setting. If a new type of drug or treatment is tested in the clinical setting, it is called a clinical trial.

Experimental designs are considered to be the quantitative research designs that produce the best evidence for cause and effect relationships between variables. This is the prime purpose of an experiment – to conclusively determine whether one variable has an effect on another variable. The researcher sets up a situation in which one variable can be manipulated. This variable is called the independent variable, treatment variable or causal variable. It is expected that the manipulation of the independent variable will have an effect on another variable, called the dependent variable, outcome variable or effect variable. This variable is called the dependent variable because any changes in it are dependent on changes in the independent variable.

The experimental design is characterised by the use of a control group to which an experimental group is compared. The control group does not get the treatment that the experimental group gets. A design without a control group is called a pre-experimental design. A design that has a control group but does not allocate the subjects to the control and treatment groups randomly is called a quasi-experimental design.

In nursing and health research, independent variables are usually such things as nursing interventions, nurse-prescribed drugs, educational programs, types of staffing or systems of patient care. The independent variable may be varied by giving it to one group, called the experimental group and not giving it to another group, called the control group. For example, one group may receive pre-operative teaching while another group does not. Or the researcher may give different amounts or types of the independent variable to two or more different groups. For example, suppose that you wanted to test out a new dressing technique on the rate of infection in clients. The use of the dressing technique would be the independent variable while the rate of infection would be the dependent variable because it is dependent on the dressing technique.

Although the experimental design is considered to be the classic research design, most nursing research is not experimental, for a number of reasons. First, experimental research assumes that the relevant variables have been identified so that they can be controlled. Not all of the important variables associated with nursing care have been clearly identified. Second, there are many social variables of importance to health and nursing outcomes that cannot be manipulated. Third, it is difficult to carry out experimental research in the clinical setting where random assignment to groups and standardisation of research procedures may be impossible to achieve. And finally, the ethical questions concerning the best care of the patient cannot be ignored. For those reasons, the application of experimental designs to nursing research has been limited.

EXERCISE

If your research question is: 'Is the prevalence of decubitus ulcers greater in patients who are overweight for their height than in patients who are normal weight for height?', which of the following research designs is appropriate:
- simple descriptive design
- descriptive comparative design
- correlational design
- experimental design?

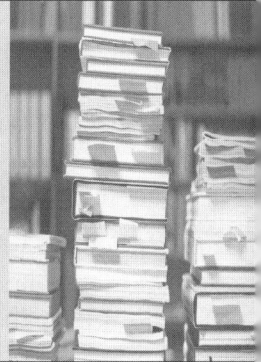

Validity in scientific research

Before we can understand why the different types of experimental research design have developed, we need to understand certain concepts related to validity. A study is said to be valid if it measures what it claims to measure. Validity in research is usually of two kinds: external validity and internal validity.

External validity

The findings of a study have external validity to the extent that they can be generalised, or applied, to the population. In order to achieve external validity, the subjects should be selected at random from the population so that they are as representative as possible. This allows the researcher to be confident that the results found from the sample would be the same as those that would be obtained if a different part of the population, or the whole population, were tested. Random sampling is often used in social science research. However, it is frequently not possible to select randomly from a whole population in health science research. If participants are not sampled randomly from the population, the results cannot be applied to the whole population, but only to that portion of the population from which the sample was taken. For example, suppose that you had done a study using 40-year-old females in a country hospital. Your findings could then only be generalised to 40-year-old females in that country hospital, and not to the entire population of 40-year-old women in the state or the country.

Internal validity

An experiment is said to have internal validity if it measures what it is supposed to be measuring and the effects measured are therefore attributable to the manipulation of the independent variable. For example, if you wanted to measure the effects of a new method of mouth care on the state of the oral mucosa, you would want to be sure that it was the effects of the mouth care that you were measuring and not some other factor that came into effect during the study, for example the introduction of vitamin therapy.

Threats to validity

There are various problems that can arise to threaten the internal validity of a study. In their classic treatise on experimental design, Campbell and Stanley (1966) discussed various threats to validity, some of which are outlined here.

Changes related to subjects

Experimental mortality

Experimental mortality does not refer to death of the subjects during the study! It refers to the loss of subjects from the study. Subjects may drop out from the experimental and control groups at different rates, leaving an imbalance in the number of subjects in the two groups. Different kinds of subjects may drop out from the groups, leaving an imbalance in the composition of the groups. If this happens, comparisons between the groups may be invalid.

History

History refers to events that happen during the course of the study, specifically between the introduction of the independent variable and the measurement of the dependent variable, that were not a part of the study design and that may affect the study results. For example, if you were studying the effects of an educational program on attitudes to use of contraceptives and during the course of the study there was a major television campaign about contraception, this may affect the attitudes of the subjects. Therefore, the results of the study could be attributed to the television campaign and not the educational campaign.

Maturation

During the course of the study the subjects change in such a way as to affect the results. This can be important in longitudinal studies because of the length of time that the study runs. It can also be important in studies in which children take part because of their physical, mental and social growth. Even in short studies, effects such as fatigue and hunger can affect certain results. However, the effect of maturation can be countered by using shorter intervals between observations.

Testing effect

Taking an initial test can affect the results of a second test. The testing effect can result from learning from a test and may be a problem when testing learning or skills. Suppose that you wished to test whether an educational program in diabetes management had any effect on control of blood sugar. You decide to measure the subjects' pre-program levels of knowledge and so you test their knowledge before you give them the education program. This then stimulates them to learn about diabetes, which interferes with your measurement of the effects of the educational program.

Selection effects

The selection effect is found after non-random selection of subjects from the comparison groups. For example, if subjects are allowed to choose the group they enter, the groups may be unequal which may make comparison invalid. This effect can be avoided by random allocation of subjects to control and treatment groups.

Placebo effect

The placebo effect is the effect on a person's mind or body from a belief that a treatment works. If the participant believes that the treatment works, this can result in artificially high ratings of the effectiveness of the treatment. This can be a problem for a researcher testing out a treatment that has not yet been shown to work. The placebo effect can be controlled for by administering to a control group a placebo or inert substance that looks exactly like the active drug. Any change in this group will demonstrate the effect of belief and can be subtracted from the ratings of the group that receives the active treatment. The recipients must be 'blind' to whether or not they are receiving a placebo or the active treatment.

Changes related to measurement

Changing procedures and instrumentation

If the measurement procedures change during the course of the study, then the readings will change and the comparison will be invalid. This can be controlled by ensuring that the exact procedures to be followed are written down and all data collectors are trained to follow them precisely every time measurements are taken. The major method of dealing with this problem is by running a rigorous trial on a small group, that is, a 'pilot study' to iron out the problems and develop an adequate procedure before embarking on the full experiment.

Differences in instruments

If several instruments are used, they may measure differently and this can affect the results. This can be avoided by calibrating the instruments so that they measure a standard unit in the same way, and to the same degree of accuracy. For example, if you wished to measure body temperature during a study, you should calibrate all thermometers to be used in a liquid that was a known temperature to check the accuracy and similarity of the thermometers' measurements. Any defective thermometers could then be eliminated and you could have confidence in your equipment.

Differences in measurement

If several data collectors are used, they may make measurements differently. This can be controlled by training the data collectors to take the measurements in the same way and testing them until they can achieve inter-rater reliability to a set standard. Conditions must be kept the same during the study. For example, if temperature is an important condition, it must be kept controlled. Laboratory conditions may be preferable to the clinical setting because more control can be exerted over the conditions during the study.

Changes related to observation

Hawthorne effect

The Hawthorne effect (Robbins 1994) was named for a study that was done in the Hawthorne Electric plant many years ago. Researchers were attempting to measure the effects of light levels on worker productivity. They found, to their surprise, that whether they raised or lowered the light, the productivity levels increased. The workers produced more, perhaps because they were being watched, or because they perceived that the management cared about them. This suggests that people behave differently when they know they are being observed. It is difficult to control for this variable without violating ethical principles. The researcher is in a dilemma: it is unethical to watch people without their knowing it, but if they know they are being watched they may behave differently, thus producing invalid data. The only way to surmount this problem, aside from deception, is to use unobtrusive observation.

Experimenter effect

The experimenter may consciously or unconsciously affect the results of the experiment. For example, a researcher who is convinced of the value of a treatment may consciously or unconsciously 'sell' the treatment to the recipient and cause artificially high ratings of the new treatment, augmenting the placebo effect. For this reason, in placebo trials of new drugs, the person prescribing or giving out the drug should also be 'blind' to whether the client is receiving the placebo or the active treatment.

Confounding variables

Some variables are known or suspected to cause the outcome under study, or are statistically associated with it, but are not actually being measured in the research study. For example, there may be an association between coffee-drinking during pregnancy and low birth-weight babies. However, women who drink lots of coffee might also be more likely to smoke cigarettes, and cigarette smoking might be the real cause. Matching of subjects in your design can help to eliminate confounding effects. It may also be identified and adjusted statistically to give a true picture if cause and effect are to be established. Sophisticated statistical procedures such as multivariate analysis of variance (MANOVA) and multiple regression can do this.

Effect modifiers

When the magnitude of an association between two variables is affected by the level of a third variable, this is the result of 'effect modification'. For example, obesity increases the risk of breast cancer in post-menopausal but not pre-menopausal women. Menopausal status is therefore a modifier of the effect of obesity on breast cancer. Likewise, asbestos is a modifier of the effect of smoking on lung cancer.

Bias

If the measured value of a variable varies from the true value of that variable, this is due to some kind of bias in the design. Bias has a number of typical sources. It can be due to sloppy measurement, interviewer bias where interviewers unintentionally favour a particular view of an issue, participant recall bias due to the effects of memory on reporting events, reporting bias where participants deliberately report the aspects of a phenomenon which are of most importance to them, or poor selection of participants resulting in a sample that has a biased concentration of some variable.

EXERCISE

You undertake a study of surgical patients in your hospital to see whether the incidence of post-operative wound infections is higher among males than among females. List three of the variables which might modify, confound or bias your findings in some way.

1 _____

2 _____

3 _____

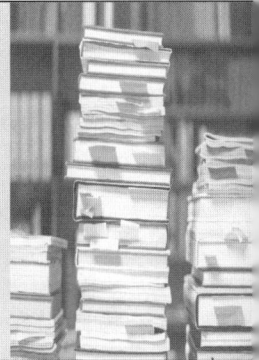

Reliability in scientific research

Reliability refers to the 'reproducibility' of the results of a measurement technique. This means that, given the same circumstances, the technique will 'reliably' produce the same measurements. If multiple measurements of the same thing agree, then reliability is good. There are some useful measures of reliability that can be reported by researchers to demonstrate that their research is reliable.

Test–retest reliability

If you take two sets of measurements of the same thing some time apart, and compare the measurements to see how similar they are, it will be an indication of test–retest reliability. A correlation coefficient is calculated to demonstrate the strength of the reliability. This type of reliability is sometimes called 'stability'. It is a particularly useful approach when evaluating whether the phenomena measured by questionnaires are 'stable' over time. You might, for instance, use a mental health assessment tool to determine the presence of depression, but need to know whether it is subject to fluctuation due to everyday events.

Inter-observer reliability

If two sets of measurements taken by different observers are compared to see how similar they are, it is possible to determine inter-observer reliability. A correlation coefficient is calculated to demonstrate the strength of the reliability. This type of reliability is sometimes called 'inter-rater reliability'. It is a particularly useful approach when using observational data collection techniques to make sure that all observers are actually measuring the same thing with the same degree of precision. You might be observing the activity levels of school children in the playground at recess using a scoring system. It would be important to know that each of the observers is 'reliably' scoring the activity.

Types of experimental design

Experimental design is shown diagrammatically, using symbols. This method was developed by Campbell and Stanley (1966), who developed the typology of designs explored here.

R = random allocation to groups
O = observation or measurement
E = experimental group
C = control group
X = exposure of the group to the experimental variable
The **X**s and **O**s in any line apply to the same specific participants
Left to right indicates time sequence
Xs and **O**s directly above each other indicate events taking place at the same time.

Pre-experimental designs

A pre-experimental design is one that does not use a control group. The evidence it produces is therefore considered relatively weak. However, pre-experimental designs can still be useful, particularly in exploratory research or where there are limitations on the numbers of subjects that preclude the use of a control group. These include one-shot case studies, pre-test/post-test design and static group comparisons.

One-shot case study

In a one-shot case study design, the effect of an event or phenomenon, or the administration of a substance, or other treatment is tested on a group after it has occurred. The conclusions are based on the general expectations of what the findings would have been if the experimental event had not occurred. Usually, this design is used for events that have happened without warning, or a situation in which it is not possible to design a scientific experiment. In this design, subjects are selected because they have been exposed to some experience or substance; frequently they are self-selected. They are then measured on a selected variable to see if it is different from normal. This design is diagrammed as follows:

$$X \quad O1$$

An example of a one-shot case study is a study carried out by Armstrong and Barrack (1995), in which a convenience sample of 30 subjects was given an educational program in taking blood pressure at home. After the educational program the subjects were tested for their ability to meet a criterion of accuracy as measured against an instructor. Subjects were recruited into the study only after the educational program was given so that a pre-test was not used, and the researchers did not use a control group from whom the educational program was withheld. The researchers claimed that patients 'can be taught to accurately and confidently measure their blood pressure'. This claim rests on the assumptions that the subjects did not know initially how to take a blood pressure and that their ability to do so after the educational program was a direct result of it.

The advantage of this design is that it does permit investigation of phenomena to explore whether or not a phenomenon may have had an effect on some characteristic of the participants. This type of design can point the way to more sophisticated designs to measure the same effects. However, it is considered a very weak design because the researcher has no control over the intervention and there is no control group.

One group – pre-test post-test design

In this design, a pre-test and post-test are both done but the measurements are only made on one group. This design is used where it is not possible to use a control group, for example where there are too few subjects available. This design can be diagrammed as:

O1   X   O2

This type of design was used in a study by Roberts, Brittin and deClifford, who measured the effects on respiratory capacity of frail, elderly women lying on boomerang pillows for 10 minutes (Roberts, Brittin & deClifford 1995). This design was chosen because there was a shortage of subjects and a previous study had shown that there was no difference between respiratory capacity in well women on boomerang and ordinary pillows. The subjects were first made comfortable on ordinary pillows, and given a trial on the instrument to accustom them to it, then their pre-test breathing capacity was done. The subjects were then placed on boomerang pillows for 10 minutes and the post-test was carried out. The pre- and post-test respiratory capacities were compared and it was found that there was a decrease between the two readings.

The advantage of the pre-test post-test design over the one-shot case study design is that it allows comparison of the measurement of the dependent variable after the experimental treatment with the results before the treatment. This then allows you to draw some conclusions about the size of the effect of the treatment.

However, there are several threats to the validity of the findings in such a design. For example, suppose you wanted to test the effect of hyperbaric pressure on the size of pressure sores. You do a pre-test measurement of the size of the sores, and then apply the hyperbaric pressure treatments, and then measure the size of the pressure sores again. If the average size of pressure sores at the end of the program was lower, you might conclude that the hyperbaric pressure treatment had reduced the rate of pressure sores. However, the validity of the findings of your study may be challenged on the grounds of history, for example if other events occur during the course of the study, such as increased mobility of the patients. The findings can also be challenged by the problem of maturation, or changes in the subjects that occur spontaneously during the course of the experiment, for example, spontaneous remission of the pressure sores. This challenge could have been easily avoided by comparing the results to another group who had not been exposed to hyperbaric pressure but had shared all of the other experiences of the experimental group: in other words, a control group.

This type of design can be weakened by a testing effect where learning or skills are involved. It is known that people being tested for a second time tend to do better on the test. Furthermore, just taking the test may serve to stimulate the effect you are looking for. For example, suppose you want to test the effect of an anti-smoking campaign on people's rates of smoking. You decide to do a pre-test on your group of smokers selected for this campaign so you ask them to keep track of the number of cigarettes they smoke during the week before you start the intervention. You then find that after your campaign many of the smokers decide to quit and you conclude that your campaign is successful. However, it may have been that it was not your campaign that led your participants to the decision to quit smoking but the realisation of the number of cigarettes they smoked. Again, this challenge to validity could have been avoided by the use of an equal group who did measure their cigarette usage but was not exposed to your intervention.

There can also be a problem of instrument decay in which changes in the assessing instrument can affect the results. This is more of a problem where physical instruments are used over a longer period of time. This can be avoided by recalibrating the instruments against a known stable reference.

The static group comparison

The static group comparison is a design in which, in order to determine the effect of an event, a group that has experienced the event is compared with a group that has not. In the previous two examples, only one group was used. In this design, two groups are used but they are groups that occur naturally. There is no pre-test. This design can be diagrammed as follows, with the broken line indicating that the groups are not equivalent:

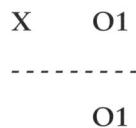

$$X \qquad O1$$

$$\text{- - - - - - - - -}$$

$$O1$$

The advantage of the static group comparison design is that two groups are being compared so that different practices can be compared and conclusions can be drawn. However, the problem with this design is that there is no way to establish whether the groups were initially equivalent and so you do not know whether the differences in the two groups are caused by the event, X. Or, put another way, you have no way of knowing if the groups would have measured the same if not for X. This is especially worrisome if the subjects have been allowed to select whether they are going to have X or not. You might, for instance, want to measure body mass of vegetarians compared to non-vegetarians. You have no idea what their body mass might have been had they all been vegetarians, or all been non-vegetarians. It makes forming conclusions about your findings a little risky.

An example of this type of design can be seen in the study by Bennett, Ohrmundt and Maloni (1996). This study examined the preventing intravasation in women undergoing hysteroscopic procedures. An experimental group, in which intra-uterine pressure was controlled, was compared to a control group. It found a reduction in complications in the experimental group.

True experimental research designs

A true experimental design enables a researcher to draw valid conclusions from their research. It has three major features: use of an equivalent control group to control for extraneous variables, random assignment to experimental and control groups, and the ability to control and manipulate the independent variable.

Use of control group

A control group is one that is equivalent in every way to the experimental group except for the experimental variable. The group controls for extraneous variables and thus allows significant comparisons. The use of a control group allows the researcher to control for extraneous variables because anything that is going to happen to the experimental group that might affect the results will happen to both groups and this can be accounted for in the interpretation of the results. For example, the problem of history is removed since both groups have exactly the same experiences and a comparison of their results on the variable X will represent a true effect of X. In the same way, maturational differences will be accounted for because both groups will grow or become tired at the same rate.

A placebo, or substance that has no physical effect but mimics the experimental treatment, will usually be included for trials of new drugs. This ensures that the control group receives the same psychological effects of the treatment that the experimental group receives, without actually being treated. Any differences in the post-treatment outcomes of the two groups can then be explained by the treatment alone. The reason for a placebo trial is that with new drugs it is imperative to be absolutely sure that any treatment effects are caused by the new drug and not by the placebo effect.

Subjects are 'blind' to the treatment if they do not know which drug they are receiving. If the person who prescribes and/or administers the drug also does not know which drug is being given, the design is said to be 'double blind'.

The use of an untreated control group in clinical therapeutics allows the researcher to see what would happen without the treatment. For example, if you wished to test out the effect of treatment X on outcome Y, if you only applied treatment X and measured the outcome Y before and after the treatment, you would not know at the end whether any effect was from the treatment or from other factors such as attention or spontaneous remission. If a control group is used that does not receive any treatment at all, you can eliminate spontaneous remission as a problem because it could occur in both groups, but you still might be measuring the psychological effects of treatment. However, you can avoid these problems in most studies if you use an equivalent control group that receives a placebo, with both participants and those administering the treatment being 'blind' to which group gets the active treatment and which gets the placebo. If the groups are treated the same, and are measured at the same time and in the same way, any differences between the two groups could be attributed to treatment **X** and not other factors. However, in some studies it is difficult to find a placebo, for example, aromatherapy studies, so another design must be used to overcome this difficulty.

The use of a control group does not preclude unforeseen events happening to one group and not the other. It is important in the design and implementation of the study to ensure that the groups have the same experiences. For this reason, it is recommended that both groups are studied at the same time.

Random assignment to groups

The subjects must be randomly assigned to the treatment and control groups, that is, they must have an equal probability of being in either group. This eliminates any systematic bias in the groups that may affect the variable being studied. It therefore allows the researcher to be confident that any other variables would be evenly distributed between the groups so that they should be alike except for the independent variable. An example of the need for random allocation to groups is as follows: suppose the researcher allowed the mothers to choose which group they went into in a comparison of the effect on duration of breastfeeding of early discharge from hospital or normal discharge. The mothers that were going to breastfeed longer might have been more confident and therefore more likely to choose the early discharge. If this group then had a longer duration of breastfeeding, it might have reflected the initial attitude of the mother rather than the time of discharge. If the subjects are not randomly assigned to groups, the design becomes quasi-experimental.

There has been more emphasis on randomisation with the recent development of evidence-based practice, which is discussed more fully in Chapter 19. Randomised controlled trials are considered by advocates of evidence-based practice to be the epitome of research evidence on which to base practice.

An example of a randomised controlled trial is a study done by Rickard et al. (2004), which examined the prevention of hypothermia during continuous haemodialysis. The study was a prospective randomised controlled trial carried out in the intensive care unit of a metropolitan, tertiary-referral, teaching hospital. It found that intravenous fluid warmers do not prevent hypothermia during continuous veno-venous haemodiafiltration and that female patients, and those with a low-normal baseline temperature, are most likely to become hypothermic during this form of dialysis.

Manipulation of the independent variable

In a true experiment, the researcher must be able to manipulate the independent variable or variables. The manipulation of the independent variable by giving the intervention to only one group ensures that, providing all other things are equal, any change in the group receiving the independent variable is then attributable to the effects of that variable.

This manipulation should ensure that the levels of the independent variable are sufficient to produce different findings between the groups. For example, if an experimental group is subjected to relaxation therapy as the independent variable, it should be sufficiently long to actually produce a significantly relaxed state in the participants.

The experimental design has the advantage that it is the only one that can truly demonstrate a causal relationship between variables because of its tight control over the experimental conditions. On the other hand, this very degree of control can create an unrealistic situation.

An example of an experimental study can be seen in Chen and Chen (2004), in which the effects of acupressure on primary dysmenorrhoea were studied. An experimental group received acupressure, while a control group received relaxation. A range of questionnaires and a visual analogue scale were used to assess pain. The findings suggested that acupressure can be an effective, cost-free intervention for reducing pain and anxiety during dysmenorrhoea.

Types of experimental design
Equivalent control group pre-test post-test design
This design features random allocation of subjects to the control and experimental groups, pre-testing of both groups on the dependent variable, administration of treatment to the experimental group but not the control group, and measurement of the dependent variable on a post-test.

$$RE \quad O1 \quad X \quad O2$$
$$RC \quad O1 \qquad O2$$

The results of the experiment are established by a set of comparisons. The pre-test measurements of both groups (O1) are compared to establish whether the groups were in fact initially equivalent. Pre-test measurements will also establish a baseline measurement. The post-test measurements for both groups (O2) are compared with the pre-test measurements to establish if there has been a change and if so in what direction. If the treatment has been successful, the experimental group should achieve a significantly different post-test measurement from its pre-test measurement. It should also achieve a significantly different post-test measurement from the control group not receiving the treatment. The control group may also demonstrate a slight change in the same direction because of the placebo effect.

An example of this type of design is one in which a cabbage extract ointment was tested for its effectiveness in treating breast engorgement (Roberts, Reiter & Schuster 1998). The active ointment was compared to a placebo, an inert cream that could not be distinguished from the active cream. The clients were randomly assigned to the control and treatment groups. The midwives and the clients were blind to the type of cream. The subjects were pre-tested for chest circumference, pain perceptions and hardness of breast tissue. The cream was then applied and subjects were tested after it had been on for two hours. Then the measurements were repeated. The pre-test readings of the two groups were compared to establish if they were in fact equivalent. Post-test readings were compared with the pre-test readings to see if there was any change. The post-test readings of the two groups were then compared to see if there was any difference in them. This design enabled the researchers to have confidence in the validity of the findings.

This design is considered to be the best because it controls for any changes during the course of the experiment.

Post-test only control group design

This design is often used when a pre-test is not possible or desirable. There are still two groups, a control group and an experimental group. A post-test is given to both groups. A control group is used and subjects are allocated randomly to the two groups. The advantage of this design is that it eliminates any testing effect so may be used where the measurement is a test of learning or skill. This design can be diagrammed as follows:

RE X O1

RC   O1

An example of this type of design can be seen in Lin et al. (2003). This study examined the efficacy of swallowing training for patients following stroke. The experimental group was given swallowing training, and the control group was not. The experimental group had improved outcomes for body weight gained and frequency of choking episodes.

A potential problem with this design is using it where the pre-test post-test design should be used instead. As we have seen above, sometimes it is not possible to do a pre-test. However, if you use a control group with randomisation to groups, you can reasonably assume that the groups were the same to start with and that the results were due to the treatment. If the treatment was effective, there should be a significant difference between the two groups' readings. On the other hand, if you do not do a pre-test when you should, you are not really sure whether the groups were in fact equal before the treatment so you do not know how much change might have occurred and in what direction.

Solomon four-groups design

This is a special type of experimental design that is used when the experimenter is worried that the use of a pre-test would affect the post-test readings, but is concerned to achieve equality of the groups. In this design, there are two control groups and two experimental groups. One control and experimental set is given the pre-test and the other is not. This design could be diagrammed as follows:

RE1 O1 X O2

RC1 O1   O2

RE2   X O2

RC2   O2

The results of an experiment with this design would be interpreted as follows. If the pre-test did not have any effect, the two experimental groups should have the same result on the post-test. If the pre-test did sensitise the subjects, the two experimental groups would have different results on the post-test. The comparison of the control with the experimental groups should be interpreted in the same way as for other experiments.

This design is a powerful design to control for testing effect and intervening variables. However, its disadvantage is that it requires many more subjects.

Factorial designs

Factorial designs involve the measuring of two or more independent variables on a dependent variable. For example, if you wanted to measure the effects of both type and timing of back care on the development of pressure sores, either you would have to do two different studies or you could develop a design that had two different independent variables, or factors. Type of back care – e.g. re-positioning versus back cream – would be one factor, while frequency of back care – e.g. four-hourly versus two-hourly – would be the second factor. This design would have four cells, to which subjects would be assigned randomly. More complex designs with more factors and levels are possible.

	Four-hourly care	Two-hourly care
Re-positioning	Group 1	Group 2
Back cream	Group 3	Group 4

Thus, one group would have two-hourly back care using only re-positioning, one would have two-hourly back care with back cream, and so on. This would be called a two by two factorial design because there are two factors and two levels of treatment.

An example of this type of design can be seen in Dowding (2001). This study examined the effects that manipulating information given in the change of shift report has on nurses' care planning ability. It found that the type of report had a significant effect on an individual's ability to plan patient care, and type of information content affected their ability to accurately record and recall the information they heard.

Quasi-experimental designs

The word 'quasi' means 'almost' in Latin. Quasi-experimental designs are so called because they do not quite meet the requirements of classic experimental design. Quasi-experimental designs fall short of the standards set for experimental designs because there is no random allocation to control and experimental groups. Much nursing research is of this type, because random allocation in the clinical setting is often impossible. Often a control group uses a conventional treatment and the experimental group uses a new treatment. This design is susceptible to the placebo effect.

Campbell and Stanley (1966) point out that an inability to conceive and execute the perfect experimental design should not cause a sense of hopelessness in the researcher. They state that it is important to do the research but to be aware of which specific variables your design fails to control so that you interpret the findings accurately.

An example of a quasi-experimental design can be seen in a study by Smith et al. (2002), which examined outcomes of therapeutic massage for hospitalised cancer patients. Twenty participants received therapeutic massage and 21 received the control therapy, nurse interaction. The outcome variables were measured on admission and at the end of one week using a range of instruments. The findings supported the potential for massage as a nursing therapeutic for cancer patients receiving chemotherapy or radiation therapy.

Non-equivalent control group designs

The most common design of the quasi-experimental type is the non-equivalent control group design. While this design does use a control group, it varies from the classic experimental design by using groups that either have been established already or are going to be established but not randomly. The subjects are self-selected into the groups or selected on some criterion. Therefore, the non-equivalent control group design does not meet the criterion for random allocation to groups. The biggest problem with a non-equivalent control group design is that you cannot be absolutely sure that the groups were equal to begin with because subjects were not randomly assigned to the groups. Collection of data about possible extraneous variables such as gender, age and educational levels will help to establish whether or not the groups were equivalent on these variables. A pre-test will help to establish whether or not the groups were initially equivalent on the dependent variable.

For example, suppose that you wanted to test out the effect of a new dressing technique on wound healing compared with a traditional technique. If subjects were randomly allocated to control and experimental groups, each group must always have the same type of dressing technique. This would mean that the nurses would probably have to do dressings using the two different techniques because of changing patient allocations, which would be confusing and difficult to manage. By the same token, randomly allocating the nurses to two different techniques on one ward would not work because of shifting patient allocations – patients would mostly end up in both groups because you couldn't guarantee the continuity of nurse-patient allocation. For these reasons, you would probably have to settle for using two wards, an experimental and a control ward, and introduce the new technique into the experimental ward. This then becomes a non-equivalent control group design.

Sometimes where random allocation to groups is not feasible and the groups are therefore not equivalent, subjects in the experimental group are matched with subjects in the control group on critical variables and their results are compared. This is not considered as tight a design as random allocation.

Within the non-equivalent control group design, there are two types, the pre-test post-test type and the post-test only type. The pre-test post-test design can be diagrammed as follows:

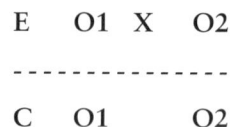

$$E \quad O1 \quad X \quad O2$$
$$\text{---------------}$$
$$C \quad O1 \quad\quad O2$$

This design has the advantage of establishing whether or not the groups were equivalent on the experimental variable before the treatment.

Another quasi-experimental design is the post-test only non-equivalent control group design. This design is similar to the pre-test post-test non-equivalent control group design except that it has only a post-test. This design can be diagrammed as follows:

```
E       X       O2
- - - - - - - - - - - - - -
C               O2
```

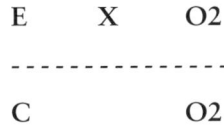

Without the pre-test, normally you have no way of knowing whether the groups were initially equal on the experimental variable. However, as noted earlier, not all studies are suited to a pre-test.

An example of a non-equivalent group post-test only design can be found in a study in which the rate of Caesarean section was compared in women presenting to a birth centre and a conventional labour ward (Homer et al. 2000). The researchers found no significant difference in rate of Caesareans but that the women in the birth centre were less likely to use analgesia in labour.

Cross-sectional designs

Cross-sectional designs are 'snapshots' or cross-sections of a population studied at a single point in time. They are sometimes called 'one-shot' designs because they aim to study a population in one go. Many quantitative designs fall under the heading of 'cross-sectional'. Virtually all descriptive designs are cross-sectional, including simple descriptive, comparative and correlational. Many experimental designs are also cross-sectional. The defining characteristic of a cross-sectional design is that there is only one snapshot of data taken.

EXERCISE

There are three essential features of a true experiment. What are they?

1 _____

2 _____

3 _____

Why are placebos used in clinical trials?

A. _____

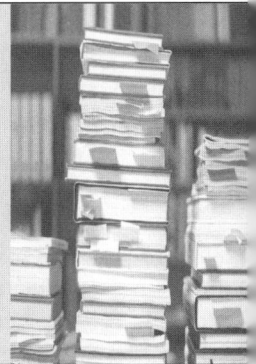

Longitudinal designs

Longitudinal studies set out to study a group at various points in time. In longitudinal designs, the primary objective is to see whether a phenomenon changes over time by identifying time-dependent patterns in data. Longitudinal designs can be used with correlational, experimental and quasi-experimental designs. The time period in a longitudinal design may be several years, or even a lifetime. Many experimental designs in health research (such as clinical trials) are longitudinal because there is a need to follow people through a full course of treatment, repeatedly gathering data, to determine whether any changes in their condition are occurring.

Cohort studies

A cohort is a defined group of people, all of whom will be studied over a period of time. Cohorts occur naturally, such as birth cohorts. Typically, a cohort is studied repeatedly at points of time over a number of years. One birth cohort that has been the subject of much research are the 'baby-boomers' – those people in Australia born after the World War II up till about 1960. A simple cohort study might be diagrammed as:

EX   O1   O2   O3   O4   O5   O6   O7   O8

Another type of cohort is a 'one-off' cohort. This is a unique group of people, all of whom were exposed to something unusual which may have affected their health. In Australia, there have been studies done on military servicemen who were exposed to the atomic bomb tests at Maralinga, and the servicemen exposed to Agent Orange in the Vietnam War.

Some cohort studies are 'concurrent', meaning that the exposure occurs now, and researchers commence collecting data now and move forward, collecting it into the future. Other cohort studies are non-concurrent, meaning that the exposure occurred a long time ago, and researchers need to look back in time at data which may have been collected, as well as collecting new data.

Time series design

A time series design differs from a cohort study in that the participants are selected by the researcher, and are not a naturally occurring group. In a time series design the experimenter makes several measurements, both before and after the treatment. This helps to measure any variations in the data that are dependent on time. A simple pre-experimental time series design is diagrammed as follows:

E   O1   O2   O3   X   O4   O5   O6   X   O7   O8

Time series designs can help show that any changes that occur just after the institution of the treatment are related to the treatment. Nevertheless, without the use of a control group, it is a weak design because it does not control for other events that happen during the course of the study. With the use of a non-equivalent control group, this design can become quasi-experimental, or with the use of random assignment to control and experimental groups it can become experimental.

An example of a prospective time series design can be seen in a study done by Cimiotti et al. (2003), which examined the adverse reactions associated with an alcohol-based hand antiseptic among nurses in a neonatal intensive care unit. It found that nurses who had adverse reactions had been employed on the study unit and in the nursing profession for significantly less time than those with no reactions and were significantly more likely to report a history of itchy, sore skin.

Counterbalanced designs

This is a group of designs that attempt to achieve control by entering all subjects into all treatments. It is usually used where pre-tests are not advisable and control groups are not available. As noted earlier, counterbalanced designs can be used in true experiments as well. This design can be diagrammed as:

$$X1 \quad O \quad X2 \quad O$$

An example of a counterbalanced design is a study in which electrocardiographic tracings were compared on the same subjects using both tap water and electroconductive gel (Birks et al. 1993). In all subjects, the first tracing was done using water and the second using the gel. No significant difference was found.

This group of designs includes crossover designs. This can be diagrammed as:

$$\text{Group A} \quad X1 \quad O \quad X2 \quad O$$

$$\text{Group B} \quad X1 \quad O \quad X2 \quad O$$

An example of this type of design can be seen in Ducharme (2003). This study set out to find what was the best topical anaesthetic for nasogastric insertion, by comparing lidocaine gel, lidocaine spray and atomised cocaine. This study used a triple crossover design with each participant having three nasogastric tubes inserted and acting as his or her own control for the three study medications. It found that 2 per cent lidocaine gel appeared to provide the best option for a topical anaesthetic during nasogastric tube insertion.

Sometimes in clinical trials using placebos, there is a refinement called a 'crossover' effect built into the design. This means that at a certain point in the experiment, persons on the experimental drug are switched over to the placebo and vice versa. If the outcome data vary with the crossover, then this is additional evidence that the drug is effective. This design could be diagrammed as follows:

$$\text{RE O1 X – active O2} \quad \backslash \text{Crossover} / \quad \text{RC O3 X – placebo O4}$$

$$\text{RC O1 X – placebo O2} \quad / \text{Crossover} \backslash \quad \text{RE O3 X – active O4}$$

The advantage of counterbalanced designs is that in the absence of an equivalent control group of different subjects, some degree of control is achieved because the same subjects essentially serve as their own equivalent control group. This design, however, has the weakness of possible testing effects.

Single patient trials (n=1 design)

It is possible to construct a counterbalanced design using a single participant. This is called a single patient trial or n=1 design. The patient is their own control. If, for instance, you wanted to know which aromatherapy oil had the most beneficial effect on a patient's sleep patterns, you could measure their sleep as a baseline, then introduce an oil for a week or so, measure their sleep, remove the oil, measure their sleep, introduce a new oil, measure their sleep and so on. Diagramatically it would be represented as:

$$C \quad O \quad X1 \quad O \quad C \quad O \quad X2 \quad O$$

The advantage of this kind of design is that as well as being a useful guide to individual care for patients, it can also be carried out using single patients in multiple settings at different times on an ongoing basis, and the data can then be aggregated.

Summary

In this chapter, we have discussed the four major types of quantitative design: descriptive, comparative, correlational and experimental. We have examined the advantages and disadvantages of each type, with references to examples from the Australian nursing literature. You should now be able to carry out one of the most interesting parts of the research process: choosing a research design that will give you the best possible opportunity of answering the research question that you set out to ask.

Main points

- A research design guides you in carrying out your study, tells you exactly what must be done, and answers the questions 'how?' 'when?' and 'where?'
- Types of designs include descriptive designs, which only describe phenomena; comparative designs which look for differences between groups; correlational designs, which look for relationships between variables; and experimental designs, which attempt to demonstrate cause and effect between variables.
- The best research design is the one that is most likely to help you answer your research question.
- Simple descriptive designs measure known variables in a population, often by questionnaire surveys, interviews and observation. They are inexpensive and relatively quick to administer. They are useful for preliminary research but they can't determine the amount of difference between groups, relationships of characteristics or causality.
- Comparative descriptive designs compare two or more groups on particular variables. They have the same advantages and disadvantages as simple descriptive design but allow comparison of groups.
- Correlational designs examine the relationship of variables within one group without aiming to determine cause and effect. They can examine the direction and the strength of the relationship but they do not have an independent variable that can be manipulated.
- The researcher identifies the target variables and chooses the best way to measure them, usually by observation, interviews or surveys. The researcher then carries out a statistical analysis to determine if there are relationships between the variables, and if so, how strong, and in what direction they are.
- A correlational design is relatively easy, fast and inexpensive to use, and it is useful in exploratory research to determine relationships for later, more rigorous testing. However, it too does not show causality.
- In an experimental design, the subjects are exposed to the event or treatment, and the response is measured. A control group can receive a standard treatment or be untreated. An experimental design can show whether changes in one variable cause effects in the other and has the potential to show the strength of an association between variables. However, it is usually unnatural and not always suitable for answering important nursing questions.

- Broadly, experimental designs can include many types of design, including pre-experimental and quasi-experimental designs. A true experimental design is characterised by the use of an equivalent control group, with subjects allocated to the two groups by random methods, and the manipulation of an independent variable.
- Internal validity in scientific research is that the research measures what it claims to measure. External validity refers to generalisability to the population.
- Threats to validity can include changes to the participants, changing procedures and measurements, changes in observation and extraneous variables.
- Other types of design include cross-sectional design, which uses only one instance of data collection for a cross-section of the population; longitudinal design, which repeatedly collects data at various points in time over a prolonged period; cohort study, which follows a specific group of people (cohort) over a prolonged period of time, and repeatedly collects data about them; and time series design, which is a repeated measures design using a sample of participants, rather than a cohort.

Case study

At the monthly meeting of the Nursing Practice Committee of the residential aged-care facility in which you work, one staff member raised the issue of constipation among residents. As the chair of the committee, you suggest a research project to see if a daily glass of prune juice for each patient will help the problem.

Discussion questions:

1   If you want to establish a cause and effect relationship between prune juice and bowel activity, what kind of research design would be best?
2   What would be the independent variable?
3   What would be the dependent variable?
4   What other factors might modify, confound or bias your findings?
5   What would you need to do if you wanted to be able to generalise the results of your findings to all nursing homes in Australia?
6   How would you deal with the problem of inter-observer reliability in the data collection for this study?

Multiple choice questions

1   The purpose of a comparative design is:
   a   to look for differences in one variable between two groups
   b   to establish a causal relationship between two variables
   c   to measure the extent that one variable makes changes in another variable
   d   none of the above

2 An experimental design is used primarily to:
   a provide an overview of the range, size and characteristics of a group of variables
   b find which variables have the strongest influence on another variable
   c establish cause and effect relationships between variables
   d provide an explanation for existing health problems in a particular group

3 The 'maturation' effect refers to:
   a natural changes in research participants over the course of a research project
   b changes in behaviour of participants because they know they are being observed
   c improvements in performance due simply to the expectations of participants
   d scores becoming closer to the average when measurements are repeated

4 A researcher intends to study staff working in the hospitality industry. Participants in both smoke-free settings and smoking-allowed settings will be counted into two groups – those who have a regular cough and those who don't. The design to be used would probably be:
   a experimental
   b case-control study
   c randomised controlled trial
   d correlational

5 A researcher wants to find out whether tobacco and alcohol use have an effect on the length of hospital stay of orthopaedic surgical patients. The most appropriate type of design would be:
   a ethnographic
   b correlational
   c experimental
   d comparative descriptive

6 A researcher wants to study the effect of a video teaching program on weight loss. The most appropriate design for this would be:
   a equivalent groups pre- and post-test design
   b equivalent groups post-test only design
   c correlational design
   d comparative descriptive design

7 A researcher wants to determine which of two treatments is more effective in reducing local haematoma following femoral angiography. The most effective design would be:
   a correlational
   b comparative descriptive
   c one-shot case study
   d experimental

8 When an association between two variables is accentuated by a third variable, this is an example of:
   a a confounder
   b an effect modifier
   c the Hawthorne effect
   d the placebo effect

9 Establishing that your research design is reliable will:

   a mean that your study is reproducible

   b ensure that there will be no placebo effect

   c remove the need for sampling

   d allow you to generalise your findings to the population of interest

10 A longitudinal design differs from a cross-sectional design in that:

   a a longitudinal design is done as a single, one-shot measurement

   b a cross-sectional design is done as repeated measurements over a long period of time

   c longitudinal designs are always experimental

   d none of the above

Review topics

1 Distinguish between a descriptive, a comparative, a correlational and an experimental design.

2 What is the reason for using a control group?

3 What is an independent variable? What is a dependent variable?

4 What is internal validity? What is external validity?

5 What is reliability?

Online reading

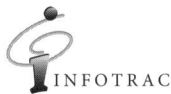

INFOTRAC® COLLEGE EDITION

Access information using the following keywords to retrieve information relating to quantitative research designs:

➤ **causality**

➤ **comparative descriptive design**

➤ **correlational**

➤ **cross-sectional design**

➤ **dependent variable**

➤ **descriptive design**

➤ **experimental**

➤ **external validity**

➤ **independent variable**

➤ **internal validity**

➤ **longitudinal design**

➤ **reliability**

INFOTRAC

References

Armstrong, R. & Barrack, D. 1995, 'Patients achieve accurate home blood pressure measurement following instruction', *Australian Journal of Advanced Nursing*, vol. 12, no. 4, 15–21.

Bennett, K., Ohrmundt, C. & Maloni, J. 1996, 'Preventing intravasation in women undergoing hysteroscopic procedures', *AORN Journal*, vol. 64, no. 5, 792–9.

Birks, M., Santamaria, N., Thompson, S. & Amerena, J. 1993, 'A clinical trial of the effectiveness of water as a conductive medium in electrocardiography', *Australian Journal of Advanced Nursing*, vol. 10, no. 2, 10–3.

Bostrom, B., Sandh, M., Lundberg, D. & Fridlund, B. 2003, 'A comparison of pain and health-related quality of life between two groups of cancer patients with differing average levels of pain', *Journal of Clinical Nursing*, vol. 12, no. 5, 726–35.

Campbell, D.T. & Stanley, J.C. 1966, 'Experimental and quasi-experimental designs for research on teaching', in N.L. Gage (ed.), *Handbook of Research on Teaching*, Rand McNally, Chicago.

Chen, H.M. & Chen, C.H. 2004, 'Effects of acupressure at the Sanyinjiao point on primary dysmenorrhoea', *Journal of Advanced Nursing*, vol. 48, no. 4, 380–7.

Cimiotti, J.P., Marmur, E.S., Nesin, M., Hamlin-Cook, P. & Larson, E.L. 2003, 'Adverse reactions associated with an alcohol-based hand antiseptic among nurses in a neonatal intensive care unit', *AJIC: American Journal of Infection Control*, vol. 31, no. 1, 43–8.

Dowding, D. 2001, 'Examining the effects that manipulating information given in the change of shift report has on nurses' care planning ability', *Journal of Advanced Nursing*, vol. 33, no. 6, 836–46.

Ducharme, J. 2003, 'What is the best topical anesthetic for nasogastric insertion? A comparison of lidocaine gel, lidocaine spray, and atomized cocaine', *Journal of Emergency Nursing*, vol. 29, no. 5, 427–30.

Homer, C., Davis, G., Petocz, P. & Barclay, L. 2000, 'Birth centre or labour ward? A comparison of the clinical outcomes of low-risk women in a NSW hospital', *Australian Journal of Advanced Nursing*, vol. 18, no. 1, 8–12.

Lin, L.C., Wang, S.C., Chen, S.H., Wang, T.G., Chen, M.Y. & Wu, S.C. 2003, 'Efficacy of swallowing training for residents following stroke', *Journal of Advanced Nursing*, vol. 44, no. 5, 469–78.

Peden, A.R., Rayens, M.K., Hall, L.A. & Grant, E. 2004, 'Negative thinking and the mental health of low-income single mothers', *Journal of Nursing Scholarship*, vol. 36, no. 4, 337–44.

Redeker, N.S., Lev, E.L. & Ruggiero, J. 2000, 'Insomnia, fatigue, anxiety, depression, and quality of life of cancer patients undergoing chemotherapy', *Scholarly Inquiry for Nursing Practice*, vol. 14, no. 4, 275–98.

Rickard, C.M., Couchman, B.A., Hughes, M. & McGrail, M.R. 2004, 'Preventing hypothermia during continuous veno-venous haemodiafiltration: a randomized controlled trial', *Journal of Advanced Nursing*, vol. 47, no. 4, 393–400.

Robbins, P.R. 1994, *Management*, 4th edn, Prentice-Hall International Inc., USA.

Roberts, K., Brittin, M. & deClifford, J. 1995, 'Boomerang pillows and respiratory capacity in frail elderly women', *Clinical Nursing Research*, vol. 4, no. 4, 465–71.

Roberts, K., Reiter, M. & Schuster, D. 1998, 'Effects of cabbage leaf extract on breast engorgement', *Journal of Human Lactation*, vol. 14, no. 3, 231–6.

Smith, M.C., Kemp, J., Hemphill, L. & Vojir, C.P. 2002, 'Outcomes of therapeutic massage for hospitalized cancer patients', *Journal of Nursing Scholarship*, vol. 34, no. 3, 257–62.

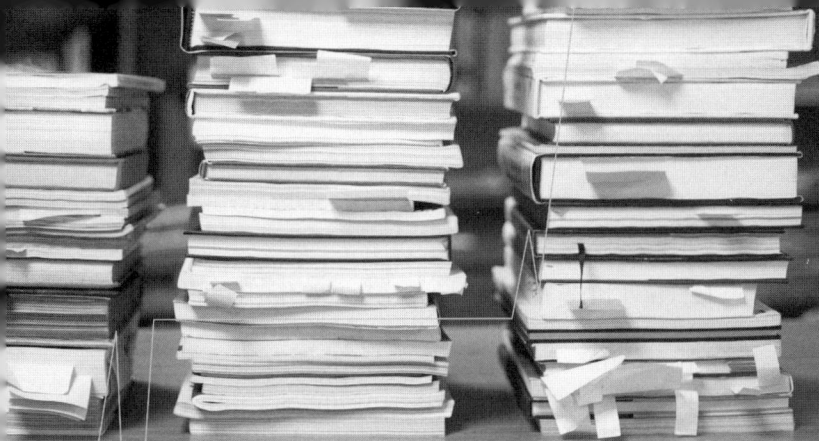

CHAPTER 8

QUANTITATIVE METHODS

CHAPTER OBJECTIVES

The material presented in this chapter will assist you to:

- identify a suitable setting in which to collect data

- choose an appropriate sampling method

- choose a data collection method that is suited to the design of the study

- outline the advantages and disadvantages of triangulation.

Introduction

In this chapter, we are going to talk about the types of methods that can be used in carrying out quantitative studies. In previous chapters, you learned how to select a problem that you want to investigate, review the literature on the problem and choose a design that suits the problem. This chapter will narrow down the focus into the data collection methods that need to be considered in order to implement the study. We will consider the appropriate setting, and types of sample. We will also explore types of **measurement** and **instrumentation**, observation and information collection. Finally, we will examine the concept of **triangulation**.

Choosing a setting

The setting for the study is the place in which you, the researcher, carry it out and in which you can observe the phenomenon in which you are interested. There are a range of places in which research can be done, varying from a naturalistic setting to a laboratory.

A **naturalistic setting** is a place in which people carry out the activities of daily life, such as working, playing, or whatever phenomenon is under investigation. For example, in nursing research, a naturalistic setting might be a clinical field setting such as a hospital ward, a clinic or a nursing home. You would choose a naturalistic setting if you wanted to observe events as they occur naturally.

Data acquired from a natural setting have the advantage of increased ecological validity since the phenomenon was observed in its real situation. Other researchers will be able to compare your setting with theirs and make judgements about whether they think your findings would be valid in their setting. The disadvantage of natural settings is that they are difficult for the researcher to control. For example, there are many things in a hospital ward that you cannot control, such as routines for care, intervention of staff, presence of visitors, noise levels and so forth. Furthermore, in the natural setting it may be more difficult to make observations and to use the equipment that you need. Since the environmental factors in the clinical field cannot always be controlled it is often advisable to measure any of the factors that you think may have an effect on the study and then see if they affect the findings.

An example of a study carried out in a naturalistic setting was one which examined the influence of animal-assisted therapy, specifically fish aquariums, on nutritional intake in individuals with Alzheimer's disease in an aged care facility (Edwards & Beck 2002). It found that residents' weight increased significantly over the 16-week period of the study, and in addition, that participants required less nutritional supplementation, resulting in health care cost savings.

A **laboratory setting** may be used instead of a natural setting. A laboratory is a place that is specially constructed for the purposes of practice or research. A laboratory setting is used when the researcher needs to have a great deal of control over the research situation, which often gives greater internal validity to the study. The advantage of using a laboratory is that you can control such environmental factors as temperature and procedures. You can also control who has access to the laboratory and can often prevent unforeseen events from affecting your investigation. Because experimental designs require manipulation of the independent variable they are often done under the more controlled conditions in a laboratory. Another advantage of a laboratory setting is that the equipment may be easier to use and observation methods may be easier. The disadvantage is that while the study may have greater internal validity, it may have less ecological validity because the conditions are artificial. That is, you cannot guarantee that the findings would be the same if the study were carried out in the actual clinical setting.

An example of a study carried out in a laboratory is a study in which the researchers examined wound secretions to help understand the trajectory of wound healing (Wysocki et al. 1999). Another laboratory-based study involved examining the effects of dietary supplementation with linoleic acid for mice with cancer. It found that the supplementation helped to preserve muscle mass (Graves et al. 2005).

It is important to decide which setting to use while planning your study. You need to go back to your research question and ask yourself what setting will best help you answer the question. You should also ask yourself whether it is more important to observe the phenomenon in its natural setting or to be able to control the variables. Despite the advantages of a laboratory setting, most nursing studies are carried out in the clinical setting. This may be because it is more realistic or because it is cheaper to use readily available facilities than it is to set up a laboratory.

Defining the population

A **population** is a group whose members have specific common characteristics that you wish to investigate in your research study. It is important to select the population that will enable you to answer your question. A single unit of the population under study is an element. The elements do not have to be people, although often they are. The elements of the population can also be places, such as hospitals; objects, for example, syringes; or events, such as immunisations. You identify your population by reviewing the literature, the conceptual framework for your study and the definition of the problem that you wish to investigate.

The population that you wish to study or to which you would like to generalise your findings is called the target population. For example, the target population in a study investigating remedies for breast engorgement would be 'all lactating women with breast engorgement'. The target population is sometimes called a 'universe'. However, one is not usually able to include the whole target population because of limited money and time. Furthermore, the members of the population may be geographically dispersed or unwilling to participate. The part of the target population that you are able to access is the accessible population. For example, the accessible population might be only those women with breast engorgement who live in a particular geographical area.

EXERCISE

If your research question is: 'What is the incidence of patient falls in hospitalised surgical patients?', what would be the population of interest for this study?

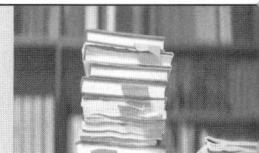

Sampling

For various reasons, one cannot usually collect data on all of the target population of a particular study. First, it is unlikely that the whole population would agree to be in the study. Second, there are also usually limitations of time and budget. It is better to use limited resources to acquire a smaller amount of accurate data rather than a lot of thin data. It is therefore customary to study only a part of the target population. This part of the population is called a sample. Using a sample often allows you to carry out all of the data collection yourself, thereby increasing your control and avoiding the complication of differences among data collectors. The part of the population used for sample selection is a sampling unit, for example, a hospital, a person, or a patient's chart. Figure 8.1 shows the process of **sampling**.

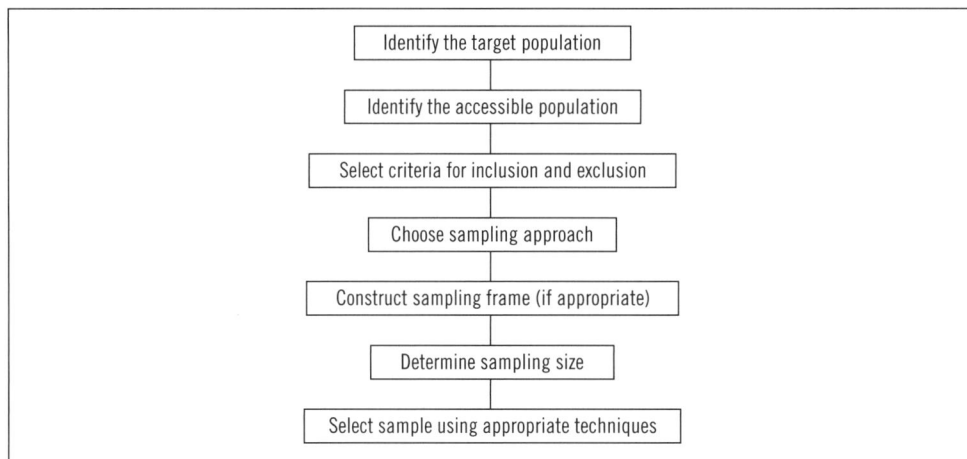

```
┌─────────────────────────────────────────────────────────────┐
│                  Identify the target population               │
│                                                               │
│                 Identify the accessible population            │
│                                                               │
│              Select criteria for inclusion and exclusion      │
│                                                               │
│                    Choose sampling approach                   │
│                                                               │
│              Construct sampling frame (if appropriate)        │
│                                                               │
│                    Determine sampling size                    │
│                                                               │
│              Select sample using appropriate techniques       │
└─────────────────────────────────────────────────────────────┘
```

Figure 8.1   Process of sampling

Before actually drawing a sample, it is important that you make a sampling plan, which you devise in relation to the question that you want to answer and the variables of interest in your study. This allows you to be methodical about the sample and consider the various choices that you can make. By devising a plan, you will be able to see how feasible your desired method is in terms of money and resources, and you will be able to get the most precise sample possible under your particular constraints. The sampling plan will help you to justify your choice of a particular sampling technique in the research proposal and in the research report. It will include the type of sample, the size of sample and the process for choosing the elements of the population that take part in the sample.

Types of samples

The main types of samples and their advantages and disadvantages have been described by Henry (1990) and will be outlined briefly here. The two major types of samples are probability samples and non-probability samples. A **probability sample** is one that resembles the population as closely as possible and is usually selected randomly from the population. It is used to calculate the probability that the results can be generalised to the population. A **non-probability sample** is one that does not attempt to portray the population in miniature and the results cannot be generalised to the population. You will have to make a judgement about which approach will fulfil the objectives of your research.

Probability sampling

A probability sample is one that attempts to portray the target population in miniature. The distinguishing characteristics of a probability sample are, first, that each element in the population has a possibility of being chosen to take part and, second, the probability of its being included in the sample is known. An equal probability sample is one in which every element of the population has an equal chance of being chosen. If some elements of the population have a greater chance of being chosen than others, it is an unequal probability sample.

The probability sample is chosen by objective techniques rather than by the subjective judgement of the researcher in order to prevent sampling bias. Sampling bias occurs when the researcher, either consciously or unconsciously, selects some participants in preference to others. Only if the sample is without bias can findings be generalised to the entire population. The sample is never actually identical to the population and there is always a sampling error, which is the difference between the sample and the population. Statistical analysis can show to what extent the sample is actually representative of the population by calculating the standard error. Larger-sized samples have less sampling error.

Probability samples include the simple random sample, the systematic random sample, cluster sampling and multi-stage sampling. For a probability sample, all members of the population are physically present or listed in a sampling frame. Each element appears once and only once in the sampling frame. If all of the elements of the population are not known, the sample cannot be a probability sample. For example, you could not use the telephone book to draw a probability sample from a city population since not all people have telephones. An example of a study using a sampling frame is one in which the total population of nursing staff in the Western Sydney Health Area were in the frame and a random sample was drawn from the population (Lam, Ross & Cass 1999).

Random samples

A random sample is a sample drawn at random from the target population. Each element in the sampling frame can be selected independently of any other element. A technique for selecting elements randomly must be used in order to prevent any bias in the selection of the sample. This can be done in several ways, for example, by lottery, by random number table or by a computer program. In the lottery method, names or numbers can be drawn out of a container after thorough mixing. If the numbers are not well mixed at the end, the last ones in have a greater probability of being drawn. A random number table can also be used. Random numbers can be generated by a computer spreadsheet program. In this method, each element in the population is assigned a number. The researcher, with eyes closed, then points to any number in the random number table and moves in any systematic fashion selecting every *n*th number until the correct number of potential participants has been reached. The third method is to use a computer program that will generate a random list of units from the list of elements.

The simple random sample is, as its name suggests, the least complicated type of sample. For a simple random sample, you choose elements at random according to the selected method until you attain the previously determined number of elements. Once selected, an element is not replaced in the sample. The best-known example of selection of a simple random sample is a lottery. Throughout Australia we have lotteries where the draw is conducted on television. The 50 numbers are placed in a bowl and a given number of balls, usually six, are selected at random. Each number has an equal chance of being selected. A computer-generated random sample was used by Grindlay, Santamaria and Kitt (2000) in their study of nurse safety in the 'hospital in the home' program.

The systematic sample is a variation on the simple random sample. You take the population list and randomly select the starting point. Then you select every *n*th element. For example, if you wanted a 10 per cent sample, you would select every 10th element. This is called a sampling interval. To find the sampling interval, you divide the population by the number in the sample. For example, if you want a sample of 75 in a population of 3000, you would divide 3000 by 75 and take every 40th person. This method is easier to apply than a simple random sample, but the start must be random in order for every element to have a chance of selection. In addition, it is important to avoid any situation that could interfere with the randomness of the selection process.

Stratified samples

Stratified sampling is the selection of elements from a target population that has previously been divided into groups called strata. For example, a group of university students could be divided into undergraduate and postgraduate strata. Each element is placed into one stratum only. Then you select elements randomly from each stratum in the same way as for a simple or systematic random sample. If you take the same proportion from each stratum, the sample will have elements of each stratum in the same proportion as in the population. If you want to increase the numbers of a particular group in the sample, you can select proportionally more of them. This is then called a disproportionate stratified sample. The analysis of data from a disproportionate sample requires the weighting of elements to compensate for the disproportion of the sample. An example of a study using a stratified sample was done by Thapar et al. (2004). They used a stratified random sample of 30 public buildings to determine functional access to these buildings and their facilities for persons with impairments. They found that wheelchair users reported a lower task performance in comparison to the control group and persons with mobility and visual impairments.

Cluster Sample

In cluster sampling, groups of elements in a cluster rather than individual elements are sampled. The population is divided prior to sampling into unique, non-overlapping groups, or clusters. These can be naturally occurring groups of elements such as schools, hospitals or health areas. Then the clusters are chosen randomly and each member of the cluster is studied. For example, if you wished to study the attitudes of nurses working in hospitals in a particular state but were not able to take a random sample of all of these nurses, you could divide the population into hospitals, which would be your clusters. Then you could randomly select a percentage of the hospitals. You would then survey every nurse working in the selected hospitals. The cluster is the unit of sampling. Cluster sampling is useful where you cannot get lists of the whole population. It can reduce transportation and training costs.

Multi-stage sample

Multi-stage sampling is an extension of cluster sampling. In multi-stage sampling, you first select clusters randomly according to the above method. Then you randomly select units to sample within those clusters. Sometimes there are two stages of cluster sampling before the random sampling. For example, suppose in the above example of wanting to study the attitudes of all nurses in the state hospital system, it was a very large state with hundreds of hospitals. You might, as a first stage, take the health service areas and randomly select a percentage of those. Then you might take the clusters of hospitals within the selected health service areas and randomly select a percentage of those hospitals. Then you could randomly select a proportion of the nurses on the payroll of those selected hospitals. That would be a three-stage sampling process. In addition, it is possible to add stratification to the process to make sure that you include representatives of different-sized hospitals, or nurses working different shifts, or other variables of interest.

An example of a multi-stage sampling procedure can be seen in a study done by Fajemilehin (2000), in which the experiences of care-giving in a population of older Nigerians was studied. It found the pressures of social change were impacting significantly on the care-giving roles of elders.

Non-probability sampling

Non-probability sampling is sampling in which subjective judgements contribute to the selection of the sample. It is carried out where it is not possible or advisable to use probability sampling. You may have limited resources, you may be unable to identify the members of the population, or you may just need to do exploratory research that will establish whether or not the problem exists. In all of these cases, non-probability sampling is acceptable. However, the disadvantage of non-probability sampling is that, because the sample is not known to be typical of the population, you cannot generalise the results or make conclusions concerning the population from your findings about the sample.

The types of non-probability sampling are convenience sample, typical case sample, critical case sample, snowball sample and quota sample.

Convenience sample

A convenience sample is one that uses any available elements of the population that meet the criteria to enter the study. Convenience samples are very common in clinical nursing research where there may not be enough people to form a probability sample. An example of the use of a convenience sample is a study by Wichowski et al. (2003) which examined patients' and nurses' perceptions of quality nursing activities. They found there was a significant difference in the perceived importance of nursing activities by nurses and patients in the psychosocial and safety categories.

Case-Based samples

Some samples are case-based. Typical case and critical case samples contain elements that are chosen specifically by the researcher. That is, the researcher selects cases that are thought to best represent the phenomenon under study in the population. These are also called purposive samples. A typical case sample is one in which the researchers choose a few cases that they judge to be normal or typical. The validity of this type of sample rests on the ability of the researcher to select typical cases. A critical case sample is one that has previously been found to be, or can be argued to be likely to be, generalisable to the population. For example, certain electorates in an election are thought to be indicative of the overall election result. This type of selection is also seen in the Delphi technique (see later in this chapter).

Snowball sample

A snowball sample is one in which the initial members of the group identify other possible members, and those members in turn identify other members. Thus the sample grows like a snowball. This type of sampling is used when the researcher is unable to identify the elements of the population in advance, for example, with homeless people or illegal aliens. A snowball technique was used by Pelletier et al. (2000) in a study of cardiac educators and clinicians. The cardiac educator panel was determined first, and then each educator was asked to identify two suitable clinicians. Other examples of the use of snowball samples in Australian nursing research are in studies on the work of nurse-practitioners (Offredy 2000) and a study on the perceptions of Thai women of prenatal testing (Rice & Naksook 1999).

Quota sample

A quota sample is one in which elements that meet the criteria are chosen until the subsections of the sample are full. Quota sampling is used in research in which it is desirable to access different sub-groups of the population. For example, you might decide that it was necessary to interview a certain percentage of people from different ethnic groups. The interviewer would keep selecting people who fit the criteria until the quota was filled. The problem with quota sampling is that the researcher selects the participant and may unconsciously select certain types of people. Thus quota samples are considered to be biased.

It is important to determine the characteristics of the sample before you select it. You need to ensure that the characteristics of the sample are linked to the variables that you want to measure. A simplistic example is that if you want to measure gender, it is not appropriate to confine your sample to only men or women.

Sample size and power calculations

It is important to determine the size of the sample before you collect your data. There are scientific and ethical considerations concerning the size of the sample. It must be sufficiently large to yield valid data or the study will lack internal validity. However, where there is the possibility of harmful effects from participating in the study, the size of the sample should be the minimum sufficient to answer the research question. There are formulas available to assist with calculating the size of the sample to give sufficient power to the results.

'Power' refers to the likelihood that a study will find a significant result if such a result actually exists. It means that the sample was large enough to reasonably assume that the result was not an accident. The statistical power of a study is the probability that you have found a true result. Large studies have greater power than small studies, if all other factors are equal. Undertaking sample size and power calculations at the beginning of a study helps to make sure that you have enough participants in your study to find a significant result if one actually exists. It also prevents you from inadvertently having unnecessarily large samples which may waste your time and money.

Sample size and power calculations are appropriate mechanisms for determining sample size only where all data in the study are collected on the same **scale of measurement**. Where a study collects multiple types of data, such as a survey questionnaire involving a range of different types of questions, these calculations are not possible. In such cases a researcher would need to calculate a power analysis for every single item on the questionnaire.

In order to undertake sample size calculations and power calculations the following conditions must be able to be met in your study:

- Because these calculations rely on estimating the likely variation in a single measurement between the sample and the population, the design must facilitate all data being collected on, or reduced to a single scale of measurement.
- It must be possible to estimate the actual proportion of a condition in the population of interest, or the standard deviation of the mean of the parameter of interest in the population. Sometimes the 'smallest practical difference' is used as an estimation of this.

If both these conditions are satisfied, sample size and power calculations can be done. There are a range of sources available to help you make sample size decisions including tables, computer and compute applications, some of which can be downloaded from Internet sites. A useful discussion of power analysis can be found in Dawson-Saunders and Trapp (2001).

The size of the population for a potential survey also needs to be taken into consideration. For large groups, for example where there are thousands of potential respondents to a questionnaire, often a 10 per cent sample will be enough. Another consideration concerning the size of the sample is the number of variables. The more sub-groups you want to compare, the greater the size of the sample must be. For example, if you merely wanted to compare males and females, you would need only a minimum of data. However, if you wanted to compare males and females of three ethnic groups, considerably more data would be required for you to be able to draw meaningful conclusions.

The most common mistake of beginning researchers is to attempt a study that is too comprehensive and tries to answer too many questions. The process of determining the sample size is very effective in bringing home the idea that it is better to have a manageable sample size and answer one significant question than it is to assemble masses of data on a great many things and thus learn very little about anything.

EXERCISE

A researcher wants to find the demographic characteristics of new mothers-to-be in their health region. They develop a questionnaire to give to all participants attending antenatal classes in their hospital and collect them each day till they have 100 completed questionnaires.

- Is this a probability sample?
- What type of sample is this?

Quantitative methods of obtaining data

Data are obtained in quantitative research by a variety of methods that fit in with the variety of research designs. In this chapter, I have placed them into three major groups: instrumentation, observation and information. In addition, triangulation involves the combination of methods. There is some overlap with qualitative research methods, particularly in the areas of observation and information. However, before we discuss these methods, we are going to talk about measurement because it is a concept that can apply to all three areas.

Measurement

Measurement is the determination of the size or range of an object, characteristic or phenomenon. Measurements are carried out using instruments. Nurses are very familiar with instruments and measurements as they use them in their daily practice, but they tend to think of them as equipment and procedures. For example, as a nurse you would know how to measure body temperature using a thermometer, blood pressure using a sphygmomanometer, and blood glucose using a glucometer. When these procedures and pieces of equipment are used in research they are called measurement and instruments.

Measurement is important in quantitative research. By measuring the phenomenon of interest, we can produce data that describe phenomena and show the relationship of variables to each other. We can evaluate nursing actions to see how they affect client outcomes. We can obtain data that are reliable and valid. By having common procedures of measurement and common units of measurement, we can compare our findings with those of other researchers. For example, a thermometer is an instrument that always measures in degrees, which are standard units. Thus, the meaning of a degree in one study is the same as that in another study. Even if different temperature scales, such as Celsius and Fahrenheit are used, data can be converted to the other scale for purposes of comparison of findings. Measurement also allows us to get an accurate determination of an effect. As a nurse, you will be familiar with the concept of accuracy in measurement. For example, when giving medications it is important to measure the dose accurately, and when taking a urinalysis, blood pressure or blood glucose, it is important to carry out the procedure properly to get an accurate reading. In both clinical practice and research, the conclusions reached are only as good as the accuracy of the data on which they are based.

Before deciding on a method of measurement, it is essential to identify what is to be measured. What is the characteristic or measurement in which you are interested? This is determined by the research question, the hypothesis that has been drawn and the variables that have been identified and operationally defined. You may need to measure the independent variable and/or the dependent variable. Measurements may be used in various designs such as experimental, quasi-experimental, correlational or comparative descriptive designs.

Measurement is usually carried out by instruments. The word 'instrument' is used in research terminology to describe any tool that measures, whether a sophisticated piece of machinery, a questionnaire or a simple checklist on a piece of paper. Even the researcher can be considered an instrument, for example, where observation is the method of choice. The advantage of using instruments is that they can increase the accuracy of the measurement and can allow measurement in more detail. In addition, they facilitate recording of data and analysing it by numerical methods such as statistical analysis on computers. The disadvantages are that they may be expensive, mechanical and prescriptive. Furthermore, the person using the instrument may require special skills to operate it and/or the researcher may require special skills to interpret the data that come out of it.

Direct and indirect measurements

A direct measurement measures an actual characteristic directly, without having to make an inference. The measurement of height by a ruler, temperature of the mouth by a thermometer, weight by a scale, and tidal volume of the lung by a spirometer are all examples of direct measurement using instrumentation. An example of a study where direct measurement was used was the influence of animal-assisted therapy, specifically fish aquariums, on nutritional intake in individuals with Alzheimer's disease (Edwards & Beck 2002). In this study, direct measurement of weight was the dependent variable. It found that residents' weight increased significantly over the 16-week period of the study, and in addition, that participants required less nutritional supplementation, resulting in health care cost savings. Other aspects of the client such as gender, race, religion and marital status can also be measured directly without using instrumentation.

Where direct measurements are not possible, an indirect measurement of one characteristic or phenomenon is taken and the value of another is inferred. These may be done where it is not possible or feasible to take direct measurements. Pain is a phenomenon that cannot be measured directly. It is therefore necessary to use indirect measurements such as a visual analogue scale in which the research participants indicate the level on the scale that corresponds to the amount of pain that they are suffering. Indirect measurements may also be done where the concept is abstract rather than concrete. For example, cardiac status is an abstract concept that has to be inferred from other measurements such as an electrocardiogram. Questionnaires which measure attitudes, beliefs and behaviours are also forms of indirect measurement.

An example of an indirect measurement from use of a questionnaire can be seen in a study done by Ammenwerth et al. (2003), where nurses were surveyed regarding their acceptance of computer-based nursing documentation. The study found that computer experience and acceptance of the nursing process were the key factors in achieving acceptance.

There is considerable scope for error in indirect measurement. For example, only part of the characteristic may be measured, or irrelevant measurements may be made unintentionally. Often it is necessary to extensively pilot indirect measurement tools to develop validity and reliability. Questionnaires, observation checklists and other such tools tend to become modified over time to meet these challenges.

Some phenomena or characteristics may be measured either directly or indirectly. For example, suppose you wanted to measure blood pressure. You could measure it either indirectly by a sphygmomanometer, or directly by an arterial line.

In vitro *and* in vivo *measurements*

Biophysiological measurements may also be classified as *in vitro* or *in vivo*. In Latin, *vitro* means glass (i.e. a test tube), while *vivo* means living person. Thus, *in vitro* means a measurement that is done on a sample taken from the participant, but analysed after it has been removed from the participant. *In vitro* tests usually measure chemical components carried out as hormone assays or blood components such as cholesterol; microbiological components such as infection carried out in microbiological cultures; and tissue or cell components carried out in pathology or cytology tests. *In vitro* tests may be done at the patient's bedside, for example, a glucometer reading. However, many *in vitro* tests are sent to the laboratory for analysis. If you are involved in collecting *in vitro* specimens involving body fluids you should be aware of the dangers of infection. As a researcher handling *in vitro* specimens, you should ensure that appropriate procedures are carried out for labelling specimens, sending them to the laboratory and storing them.

An example of *in vitro* measurements can be seen in a study by Senner, Johnston and McLachlan (2005), which compared peripheral and centrally collected cyclosporine A (CSA) blood levels in paediatric patients undergoing stem cell transplant. The blood samples were analysed in a laboratory setting. They found no significant differences in CSA blood concentrations between the different collection sites.

In vivo measurements are those taken directly on the participant and the value is obtained at the time of measurements. *In vivo* measurements are usually physiological characteristics of participants. Examples of *in vivo* measurements are blood pressure recordings, and temperature, pulse and respiration recordings. An example of *in vivo* measurements can be seen in a study by Smolen, Topp and Singer (2002) in which the effect of self-selected music during colonoscopy on anxiety, heart rate and blood pressure was studied. *In vivo* measurements of these vital signs were taken to determine the effect of the music. It found that heart rate and systolic and diastolic blood pressure significantly decreased among the music intervention group.

Scales of measurement

A scale is a 'measuring stick' or standard reference for comparison of measurements between cases. Measurement is the assignment of numbers or codes to observations of phenomena. Different types of data are measured on different scales. It is important to know exactly what type of data you are collecting and the scale on which you are measuring your variable because this will determine what type of data analysis you can carry out.

Data occur in two broad groups – qualitative and quantitative. Within these two groups there are a number of sub-groups of data types.

Qualitative (unstructured) types of data includes data, such as interview transcripts or tapes, works of art or bodies of text. There is no real scale of measurement applied to collection of these type of data. They are collected in a measurement-free way.

Categorical/**nominal** (structured) qualitative data includes all qualitative data which have been summarised into categories, as well as qualitative data which exists naturally in categories, such as gender (male/female) or yes/no responses to simple questions. The scale of measurement used in the collection of these type of data is categorical, which means that it lends itself to primitive numerical analysis, such as counting the number of cases in each category.

Quantitative data is far more precise when it comes to issues of measurement, because it is gathered in numerical form to begin with. There are, however, varying levels of precision attached to different scales of measurement. There are three broad types of quantitative or numerical data:

1   *Ranked (ordinal) data* – these are data that can be ranked in order from 'first' to 'last' in some way. It usually refers to variables that are not able to be measured precisely, but are able to be compared to one another in order to rank them. In the absence of a ruler, for instance, you might line children up from tallest to shortest, and give each one the label 'first', 'second', 'third' etc. Much international public health data makes cross-national comparisons on the basis of **ordinal data**. 'Highest' rates of youth suicide or Indigenous mortality are two such examples used when describing Australia. Absolute numbers are not the issue with these data, only the relative position of this case to other cases. The scale of measurement used in the collection of these type of data is an ordinal one – it lends itself to ranking data in some kind of order for a variable.

2   *Discrete data* – such data are often obtained in response to 'how many?' questions. They are naturally distinct units or whole numbers. Examples might be the number of cigarettes smoked per day, the number of admissions to hospital, the number of clients treated etc. Each datum is a whole number, and cannot be broken down into fractions of a whole number as they are being counted. In social or behavioural research, rating scales are assumed to represent **interval level data** because they require making a response which is translated into a whole number, which in turn represents a measurement of the strength of the variable. The scale of measurement used in the collection of these type of data is a discrete one – it lends itself to collection of whole number data for a variable.

3   *Ratio (continuous) data* – these are data that can be measured on a scale from zero to infinity, with every possible graduation in between, with a potentially unlimited number of decimal places. Measurements of weight, length, time and blood chemistry are all examples of continuous/**ratio data**. Each datum may be represented in decimal

form or fractions of whole numbers. The scale of measurement used in the collection of these type of data is a continuous one – it lends itself to collection of very accurate data for a variable.

Often, a high level of precision, or a large number of decimal places, is not required for the purposes of a research study and would only confuse the picture and make computation laborious. Consequently, potentially continuous data are often 'reduced' to discrete data, even if the intervals between measurements are very small.

As we move from purely qualitative and categorical 'measures' through interval to ratio scales there is an increasing amount of 'definiteness' about the relationship between any datum and another. This gives rise to the concept of 'levels of measurement', with categorical 'measures' as the lowest and ratio scales as the highest.

The mathematical basis of statistical procedures depends upon assumptions about the relationship between variable values. More precise or powerful statistical procedures are appropriate for data collected using higher levels of measurement.

The type of data analysis procedures you use depend on the type of measurement procedures you use. Data analysis procedures become more powerful as measurement procedures become more precise.

The term **parametric** means that the data involved have come from variables which are based on measurable population characteristics or variables that have a distribution in the given population of interest, and which were measured at least on an interval scale. A parameter is a 'measurement across' a population. Height, weight, blood pressure, intelligence and attitudes are all things which have a range of possible observations and are therefore distributed throughout the population. The distribution has some arithmetically meaningful characteristics. It would be possible to plot each of these things on some kind of curve. This curve would represent the distribution.

Some things are considered to be measurable only in non-parametric forms. In other words, they have no distribution. Something like gender, where there are only two possible classifications, is a good example of non-parametric data. However, if a sample of data are selected from a population of parametric data (like height, for instance), but the sample was selected in such a way that it cannot be assumed to adequately represent the population, it should also be considered suitable only for non-parametric analysis techniques.

Generally, data must be at least at the interval level of measurement (or assumed to represent interval level data) and have some sort of distribution before it can be subjected to parametric analysis techniques.

Measurement-related error

Whenever measurements are carried out, there is the potential for error. As a researcher, you will need to be aware of possible errors in order to prevent, control or take account of them in the design and conduct of the research. This will diminish the threat to the validity of your findings. We have considered already error in the design of a study (see Chapter 7). Errors can also result from the sampling and measurement phases of the study. Typically, sources of measurement error may come from:

- poor sampling (sampling error)
- lack of precision (sloppy measurement)
- lack of validity (using an instrument to measure something which it really does not measure very well)
- lack of reliability (not getting consistent, accurate measurements from the same measuring instrument).

One of the major errors in the measurement phase can result from mistakes made by the researcher in carrying out the measurements. The researcher may make mistakes in administering the instrument in such a way as to cause a false reading. Usually this results from sloppy measurement.

Errors can also result from variations in the participants, the environment and the procedures. The participants may be tired, hungry or emotionally affected, which could affect their response to an instrument. The environment may vary, for example noise, temperature or electric current could cause an error in measurement. The procedures may vary from one participant to another. There could be mistakes in processing specimens – for example, laboratory specimens can be improperly collected or labelled. In the laboratory, some measurements can be made inaccurately. Sloppiness and lack of reliability are the culprits here.

Error in measurement terms means 'how accurate is a particular measurement?' It has to do with the resolution and repeatability of the measurement and this concerns both the instrument and the object being measured. Errors can be classified as random or systematic.

A group of researchers could use a micrometer to measure the thickness of a piece of steel and everyone would probably get the same answer within ± 0.01 mm. But if the same researchers tried to measure the thickness of a piece of skin with the same micrometer the tolerance might well be ± 0.1 mm. Such errors are random and can be readily determined as the standard deviation of the observations.

There may also be systematic error in an experiment. Systematic error refers to errors within the system that generate bias. It is an error that occurs whenever a procedure is carried out or at regular intervals. Systematic error may result from faulty equipment, for example a thermometer that always reads one-half of a degree too high. Pulling too hard on a tape measure around someone's chest results systematically in a measurement that is too low. Systematic error can also result from the use of multiple instruments that have not been calibrated and are thus not measuring the same. Finally, there may be a regular effect of a stimulus that changes the reading of the instrument, for example, an electric current that interferes with an electronic reading. Systematic error can be avoided by taking multiple measurements and comparing the results.

Instrumentation
Selecting an appropriate instrument

In choosing an instrument, whether biophysiological or not, it is necessary to consider several factors. You should consider primarily whether the proposed instrument is the most appropriate one to help you answer the research question. The primary consideration is the validity of the instrument, or the extent to which it measures the characteristic that you are trying to measure. If the instrument is not the right one, other considerations are not important. This is easy with known factors; for example, everyone knows that the correct instrument for measuring temperature is a thermometer. However, it is less easy with instruments such as questionnaires, which measure more abstract concepts. When you are choosing an instrument, it is useful to consult previous studies to see how they have evaluated the validity of an instrument.

You should also consider the sensitivity of the instrument or how precisely it measures. It must be sensitive enough to pick up the amount of change that you want to measure. For example, if you wanted to measure temperature change in tenths of a degree, a thermometer that measured only fifths of a degree would not be sensitive enough. For a known instrument, you can check the manufacturer's specifications to see how sensitive it is.

You should also consider how accurate you need the measurement to be. Invasive instruments may be more accurate but they have a greater potential for injury. The accuracy of an instrument may be affected by the quality control in the manufacturing process, by wear and tear and by environmental factors such as temperature or humidity. Before they are used, many instruments will need to be calibrated against a known measurement so that their accuracy is established. The manufacturer's specifications will usually give the accuracy, or tolerance of the instrument.

You need to consider also the reliability of the instrument. It should measure consistently over time, that is, measurements should not vary very much with subsequent recordings or an error may creep in and the data will not be very accurate. Reliability can be checked by calibrating the instrument periodically.

You need to consider the cost of the instrument and the extent to which specialised training will be required. Although research budgets are limited, the validity and accuracy of the instrument should be a primary consideration. It is worth approaching the manufacturer of the instrument; sometimes a manufacturer will be willing to donate an instrument for research purposes.

Availability and suitability for the participants may be considerations too. You will need to check that the instrument is available when you want it. You should also ascertain that the instrument will be suitable for your proposed participants.

If a suitable instrument is not available, you may have to develop one, although this is not to be undertaken lightly by the beginning researcher. In developing an instrument, it is important to ensure that it is valid. This can be done by exposing it to a proven developmental process. The instrument is scrutinised by experts in the field for face validity in terms of the effectiveness of the structure, and its validity. Then it is put through a trial to see if it measures what it is supposed to be measuring. It should also be checked for reliability to see if it consistently measures the same on repeated measurements. Finally, it is revised. If there have been a lot of revisions, it would be wise to trial it a second time.

An excellent, comprehensive book on instruments for clinical health care research is by Frank-Stromborg and Olsen (2004). If you are seeking a particular type of instrument, you should look it up in such a book.

Biophysiological instrumentation

In recent times, there has been an increase in clinical nursing studies which tend to use biophysiological instrumentation to measure biophysiological variables such as body temperature, blood pressure, biochemical values, blood gases and types of infection. However, not all data in clinical research are obtained by biophysiological instrumentation. Observation, questionnaires, chart audits and direct questioning of the patient are also used. An example of biophysiological instrumentation can be seen in George et al. (2002). In this study, measurements of oxygenation, ventilation and bloodflow were measured in single lung transplant patients for a range of positions. The study found that no single position maximises oxygenation in the immediate postoperative period in single-lung transplant recipients; and that transplant recipients can be safely turned in the immediate post-operative period without compromising oxygenation or hemodynamic status.

There are many biophysiological research instruments that have been developed and tested. In addition, there are many biophysiological instruments already used in clinical management of the patient that can also be used for research purposes, such as cardiac monitors, spirometers, pulse oximeters and so forth. Ethics approval must be gained for the use of instruments in research, even if they are already in place for treatment purposes.

Biophysiological measurements as a means of data collection have various advantages. They are objective because they are not normally sensitive to errors on the part of the person who measures: if the instrument is properly calibrated any two readers should get the same reading on it. Biophysiological instruments are usually sensitive; they can record relatively small changes. They are also accurate and they have the advantage that they give quantitative, numerical data that are comparatively easy to analyse.

Biophysiological instruments also have disadvantages. They are usually expensive to purchase, and the data collector has to have the appropriate training in the use of the instrument. Biophysiological instruments may be adversely affected by changes in the environment such as the temperature. They may also be affected by the Hawthorne effect since the participant usually knows that a test is being made. In addition, biophysiological instruments may be invasive so there is a potential for harm to the participant in the study.

Observation

Observation by the human eye is a way of obtaining data about people's behaviour when and where it actually happens. We can observe how often behaviours occur, how long they last or how long it takes to carry out an action or achieve an objective. Observation can be used in both qualitative and quantitative research. It can be used as a method of obtaining data in various research designs. It is carried out by observers who are objective, reliable and trained in the skills and techniques of observation. Observation is not useful if the intention is to study people's thoughts, values, attitudes, beliefs or feelings.

Observation may be objective or subjective. In quantitative research, the observer is aiming for objectivity. However, total objectivity is unattainable; for example, observers tend to rate behaviour more positively if the person observed is someone who is attractive or whom they like. However, you aim to be as impartial as possible by putting aside your own values, attitudes and emotions. Objectivity can be enhanced by being a total observer rather than a participant observer.

Observation may be covert or overt, depending on whether the participants are aware they are taking part in a study. Overt observation entails the observed being aware of the observation, while covert observation conceals the act of observation from the observed. A discussion of the ethics of covert observation can be found in Chapter 5.

Observation may be obtrusive or unobtrusive depending on whether the observer is visible to the observed. Obtrusive observation is observation in which the participant cannot help but be aware of the observer. Unobtrusive observation is observation in which the observer is either not visible or keeps a low profile. It is less likely to result in the effect of the participants changing their behaviour because they know they are being observed. Obviously covert observation must be unobtrusive in order to remain covert. However, overt observation may be either obtrusive or unobtrusive. If you are trying to be unobtrusive, it is helpful to observe in a busy area in which you will be less noticeable. It can also be helpful to keep out of the line of sight of the observed.

There are various dimensions of observation depending on the amount of involvement of the researcher, the degree of structure, the extent to which the observation is known to the observed and the extent to which the observer is visible to the observed.

There may be varying degrees of involvement of the researcher in what is being observed. The researcher may be a complete non-participant, engaged only in observing the scene. An example of a study using non-participant observation was one which assisted in the development of competency standards for specialist critical care nurses. More than 800 hours of specialist critical care nursing practice were observed and classified into domains of practice (Dunn et al. 2000). Proctor (2000), on the other hand, used participant observation to study the impact of the Balkan conflict on the culture and emotional health of a community of Serbian Australians.

Observation may range from the unstructured, in which the observer is attempting to observe the scene without imposing any structure on the observations, to the highly structured, in which the observer categorises observations using a tool such as a checklist with predetermined categories. In quantitative research, the observation will be highly structured because the observations are used to generate measurement rather than to describe situations or generate meaning as in qualitative research. However, structured observation has the disadvantage of not accommodating unexpected behaviours.

Observation as a research tool has several advantages. It allows us to see what people actually do in a situation. It allows us to see the finer nuances of behaviour, for example, body language. Observation can be used with participants who cannot give verbal data, such as unconscious patients and infants. For the purpose of studying behaviour, observation is considered better than relying on participants' verbal accounts of their behaviour, which they may edit or distort, consciously or subconsciously, to give a positive picture.

Observation also has disadvantages. If it occurs in a laboratory setting, it may be somewhat artificial. However, if you want to observe naturalistic behaviour it is necessary to go to the natural setting and wait for the behaviour to happen, which may involve extra time and expense. Access may be a problem if the activity under observation is not something that people want to be observed doing, for example, sexual behaviour. Furthermore, it is not possible for the observer to see everything in a situation or to record everything that is seen. The data are therefore limited by the amount that can be seen and recorded. Nor is it possible for the observer to be completely objective since the observer's frame of reference is superimposed on what is seen. Two observers may see the same thing differently. The data are therefore limited by the accuracy or framework of the observer.

Structured observation

Structured observation is the predominant observational method in quantitative research. It is characterised by systematic planning, and recording the data according to a framework. Imposing such a structure is intended to improve the accuracy of the observations. This framework is predetermined by the researcher and will reflect the research question, the conceptual framework, the hypotheses and the operational definitions of the variables. The researcher needs to know what will be observed and how it should be recorded. To design this framework, the researcher needs to know what behaviours to expect. This can be determined from the literature on the subject, and/or a preliminary pilot observational study in the setting to observe and categorise the behaviour.

Structured observation normally involves an instrument. One type of instrument used in structured observation is a 'paper and pencil' instrument. A simple example is a checklist in which the observer simply indicates whether or not an explicit behaviour, for example, crying, happens. Another such instrument is a set of mutually exclusive categories in which to sort the observations.

Automated methods may be used in place of or in addition to paper and pencil instruments. These include such instruments as stopwatches, audiorecordings and videorecordings. Stopwatches can be used to determine how long a behaviour lasts. Audiorecordings are not, strictly speaking, observation, but they can be used to analyse verbal behaviour or augment visual observation. Videorecordings are becoming popular because they offer a visual record of behaviour. An example of this technique can be seen in a study by Andersen and Adamsen (2001), in which 142 hours of continuous video recording of patient–nurse interactions were examined. It found that nurses were with patients for approximately one-quarter of the available time and the majority of any communication with patients centred around physical care.

Automated methods such as audiorecordings and videorecordings are used when the action is too rapid or too complex to analyse in situ. They are also convenient because they allow researchers to capture the data at the time of the behaviour but analyse it at their convenience. They also improve accuracy of data analysis as they allow the data to be played over and over until a decision is reached. However, these methods also have some drawbacks. Good-quality equipment and consumables are expensive. Editing videotapes is time-consuming. Furthermore, the videorecording process requires special skills of filming and editing, which may not be in the researcher's repertoire.

The process of observation

Before undertaking observation, it is necessary to decide exactly what is going to be observed and when. Do you want to observe according to time, for example, a set amount of time per hour? Do you want to observe a whole event, for example, the changing of a dressing? You will also need to consider questions of whether the observation is structured or unstructured, covert or overt, obtrusive or unobtrusive, and the degree of involvement that you will have in the activity being observed.

You will also need to decide how many observers are needed to collect the data. If you do it all yourself, you will not have the problem of differing observations of different data collectors. However, the use of more than one observer may improve the validity of the data if they both agree on the observations. If more than one data collector is being used, their measurements can be compared. Multiple data collectors must practise until they achieve the same or similar measurements, thus ensuring inter-rater reliability.

Before observing, you will also have to train yourself and/or other data collectors in order to ensure accurate observations. This can be done by familiarisation of the observer with the instrument and practice to ensure skilled handling of the equipment or recording of the observations.

You should carry out a pilot study in the real research situation so that you or your data collectors will be able to practise the procedure using the equipment to ensure that they develop the skills. A full pilot study can also serve as a rehearsal for the main study, thus increasing the confidence of the observers. If the same participants are being used it can also help them become accustomed to being observed.

Information

When using information as data you, as the researcher, can use either data that have been collected by someone else or data that you collect yourself in the form of information from media, or information given by the participants.

Secondary analysis

Existing data are data that have been collected by you or another researcher but have not yet been analysed for your present purpose. Such data may include any data that have been collected either for research or clinical purposes by another researcher or an organisation. Other researchers may have data that they will make available. Organisations such as the Australian Bureau of Statistics, state and territory health services or individual hospitals often have data that they will make available for research purposes, possibly at a cost. Previously collected data might be raw data or data already entered into a database. You might use these data for exploring new hypotheses and relationships, analysing a sub-group of the data to draw inferences about that group or using a new unit of analysis or a different method of analysis.

Such an approach is sometimes called 'secondary analysis'. An example can be seen in a study by Jette, Warren and Wirtalla (2004), which explored the relationship of patients' outcomes with nursing staff levels and therapy intensity within skilled nursing facilities. The authors examined an administrative dataset of 6897 patients from 68 skilled nursing facilities providing rehabilitation. They found that higher nursing staff levels and therapy intensity are related to improved length-of-stay efficiency and increase the likelihood of patients being discharged to the community.

The major advantage of working with previously accumulated data is that it saves you considerable time in collecting and entering data yourself. It also allows the examination of data for longitudinal trends without waiting years for data to be generated. Another major advantage is that it is less expensive than collecting and entering it yourself, even if you have to pay a fee. Previously accumulated data may also provide a greater amount and range of data than you could otherwise hope to acquire on a limited budget.

However, working with someone else's data has several disadvantages. Since the data have not been collected for the purpose of your present study there are very likely to be areas in which the fit with your purposes is less than ideal. For example, hospital medical records will be unlikely to be complete. Methodological problems may arise such as a deficiency in the sample used, or poor matching of your definition of the variable with the definition in the existing database. The tool that you might consider superior might not be the one that the original investigator used. The data themselves may not be of adequate quality; you are dependent upon the accuracy and completeness of the original data collection and entry process. Data may not be consistent over time; for example, a classification system such as nursing diagnosis may have changed in the middle of the period that you want to examine.

It is important to weigh up the costs and benefits before making a decision on whether or not to use available data. If the discrepancies between the structure and methods of the original data and your ideal data are too great, you may decide that it is preferable to collect your own data.

Content analysis

Content analysis in quantitative research means a numerical description of the appearance of specific ideas or expressions in a body of communications that use language. Content analysis was first developed during World War II to analyse the content of propaganda. It can be applied to oral/aural media, such as radio and television broadcasts, and written media, such as newspapers, books, articles and letters. Since content analysis is not a common technique, it will not be explored in depth here. However, the method depends on formulating rules and categories for the analysis. The unit of analysis may be a word, phrase or theme. Content analysis is often used in mixed method research projects where qualitative data are collected alongside quantitative data. An example of such an approach can be seen in a study done by Badger and Mullan (2004), where they studied staff experiences of violence and aggression in a head injury unit. The qualitative component of their survey was subjected to content analysis. They found that staff needed to identify their own training needs in order for training programs to be effective regarding workplace violence and aggression.

Meta-analysis

Meta-analysis is the analysis of multiple research reports to integrate and synthesise the findings on a particular topic. This is an ever-increasing necessity in these days of expanding volumes of research. Meta-analysis has potential to integrate findings on a clinical research topic and to be useful in evidence-based nursing, particularly the development of clinical guidelines; this will be explored in more detail in Chapter 19. Special statistical approaches, which convert statistical findings to a comparable measurement called an effect size, are used to determine which findings are most powerful. Since meta-analysis relies on published findings it may have a bias in its results. However, it is considered superior to a conventional literature review. An example of meta-analysis can be seen in a study done by Griffiths et al. (2005). They studied all published studies on post-acute intermediate care in nursing-led units (NLUs) in order to determine whether such care in such units is effective in preparing patients for discharge from hospital. The study completed a systematic review of nine random or quasi-random controlled trials involving 1669 patients. They found that the NLU successfully functions as a form of intermediate care, and that, so far, there is no evidence of adverse outcome from the lower level of routine medical care.

Courtney (2005) provides a useful overview of the process of systematic reviews for the purposes of developing a sound evidence base for nursing practice. The Joanna Briggs Institute in Australia was developed for the explicit purpose of developing such evidence bases, and its database is available online to subscribers at http://www.joannabriggs.edu.au/about/home.php#.

Self-report

Self-report is a method of obtaining data directly from the participants in the study, using them as informants. Basically, self-report consists of answers that the participant gives to specific questions asked by the researcher in order to answer the research question. This is particularly effective where you are not investigating something that can be measured by instruments, or observed. It is ideal for things such as values, attitudes, feelings or problems. Self-report methods may be written, for example questionnaires and scales, or oral, for example, structured interviews. Interviews and questionnaires may be used in conjunction with other types of approaches either to generate questions or to augment them. Interview and questionnaire questions can be the same, but the methods of delivery and response are different. The instrument chosen should reflect the purpose of the study, the research question and the variables being measured.

Questionnaires

A questionnaire is the most commonly used instrument for obtaining information by self-report. It is a document containing questions to which the person responds. Questionnaires can be used to obtain a variety of information. Through a questionnaire, you, the researcher, can seek such demographic details as age, gender, income or postcode. In addition, you can ask a series of questions related to a concept, for the purpose of investigating people's attitudes, values, beliefs and stated behaviours. The answers on a questionnaire may also be used to explore relationships between variables, for example, between gender and attitudes. Questionnaires are used frequently in correlational designs.

Questionnaires have several advantages over other types of instruments. They are quick to administer and to receive. Although they may incur postal costs, they are inexpensive compared to more labour-intensive data collection methods such as interviewing and observation. In addition, they have the advantage of enabling you to acquire large amounts of information from the target sample. Because questionnaires can be mailed and distributed electronically, you can distribute them over a wide geographic area, much wider than you could access easily if you had to travel to do interviews. Furthermore, since most questionnaires ask for anonymous replies, the respondents are more likely to answer candidly than they are in interviews where they may give you the answers they think you expect or that they perceive as socially acceptable. Finally, the development of statistical tests has made questionnaire data relatively easy to test for reliability and validity.

On the other hand, questionnaires have several disadvantages. They are suitable for use only with people who can understand them. You cannot use them with people whose judgement may not be valid, for example, the very young, the confused elderly, the illiterate or the developmentally challenged. Even with those capable of filling in a questionnaire there may be misunderstandings and misinterpretations that cannot be clarified, resulting in incomplete or invalid data. The cost of distribution, although relatively inexpensive, may still be high. For 150 three-page questionnaires with covering letters, you would need to pay for two reams of paper, 300 envelopes, photocopying or printing, and 300 stamps. Each round of questionnaires could therefore cost between $200 and $250.

The structure that is frequently needed on questionnaires imposes constraints over the content. The need to confine the length of a questionnaire so that the respondent does not get tired or bored also means that it may be necessary to leave out information that could be relevant. Finally, one of the major problems with questionnaires is that they tend to have a low return rate unless they deal with a burning issue or have been distributed by personal contact. A low return rate raises questions about how well the sample represents the population. This can be overcome partially by including demographic data, which allows you to compare some characteristics of the sample with known values in the population. If the sample is demographically like the population, responses to other questions are more likely to be typical of the population than if it is unlike the population.

Selecting an appropriate questionnaire

Selection of a questionnaire raises the question of whether it is better to use a questionnaire that someone else has prepared or to develop one yourself. Using an existing questionnaire has many advantages, for example, you can compare your results with those of the previous studies that used it. On the other hand, using your own questionnaire allows you to tailor it to your own requirements. We shall discuss the advantages and disadvantages of each approach as well as other aspects.

You will find it much easier to use an existing questionnaire than to develop your own. In using a questionnaire developed by someone else, you will be saving time and energy by capitalising on someone else's work. Those researcher(s) will have done all of the hard thinking work in developing the questions. They will also have piloted their questionnaire and established its reliability and validity.

It is not difficult to find existing questionnaires. There are resource books with schedules of instruments in just about every discipline that uses questionnaires. You can also locate questionnaires by doing a literature search that focuses on instruments in the area in which you are interested. Other researchers in your area of interest or nurse-researchers on the Internet will probably know of relevant questionnaires, perhaps even ones that have been developed and validated but not yet published. If you are using a questionnaire that someone else has developed, you need to check that its reliability and validity have been established. If there is an existing questionnaire that is close to what you require, it may be possible to modify it to meet your needs. However, if you do, you need to recheck its reliability and validity and trial it in your situation before using it in your main study.

In using an existing questionnaire, you should ask yourself if it is suitable for the situation in which you intend to use it. A questionnaire that has been developed for university students may not be suitable for poorly educated people, for example. You need to look at the suitability of the questionnaire in terms of the instructions, language, method of scoring and so forth. Looking at the characteristics of other groups on which it has been used should give you an idea of its suitability for your proposed group. As a matter of etiquette, you should seek permission from the author to use or adapt a questionnaire.

An increasingly popular option among researchers is to develop and use web-based questionnaires, or SMS-based questionnaires on mobile phones. An Internet search on these topics will return a large number of providers who can undertake such activities on a fee-for-service basis. One distinct advantage in using web-based questionnaires is that all responses are automatically loaded into a database, which eliminates any costs associated with data entry.

Developing your own questionnaire

You may decide to develop your own questionnaire. There are really only two valid reasons for doing so. The first is that no existing questionnaire will serve your purpose, even with adaptation. The second is that you want or need to learn how to do it to develop your skills as a researcher. Developing a questionnaire is regarded as a very difficult task, even for seasoned researchers (Street 1995). Street (1995, p. 105) entitled the section of her book that deals with questionnaire development 'How to develop a headache without really trying'. She quoted one of her participants as saying 'If anyone ever thinks, "Aha, we will do a questionnaire", forget it' (p. 105). Reasons given were difficulties constructing questions and limiting the number of questions, and group decision-making problems.

A lengthy discourse on the process of developing a questionnaire is beyond the scope of a book for beginning researchers; however, some guidance and instruction will be given. If you do decide to develop your own questionnaire, you are advised to consult a book that deals specifically with questionnaire development. A useful account of development of a questionnaire and a discussion of the methodological issues involved can be found in Frazer and Lawley (2000).

Your questionnaire can be as short as one page or as long as you wish. However, be warned that the length of a questionnaire affects the return rate. Indeed, the length and the response rate tend to be inversely proportional! Few people are prepared to spend hours doing a questionnaire. The length of the questionnaire should be consistent with the attention span of the respondents. A reasonable length is one that takes less than half an hour to complete.

The response rate can also be affected by the content of the questionnaire. If the respondents judge it to be unbearably intrusive (for example, asking questions about their income) or too sensitive (for example, asking questions about their sex life), they may choose to discard it. Fear that they can be identified can lead respondents to discard the questionnaire.

The process of questionnaire development entails many steps. These are outlined as follows:

- Decide on your primary research questions. These may be at various levels, as outlined in Chapter 2. All of the content items should be congruent with and designed to answer these questions.

- Identify your hypotheses and variables. Again, all of the content of your questionnaire should be designed to test the hypotheses and explore the interactions of the variables.

- Identify relevant concepts. These can come from your own knowledge and ideas on the topic or from your reading of the literature on the topic, including previous research; this may be qualitative research that has identified themes that you now wish to explore in a questionnaire survey. The concepts will normally be abstract, and thus not directly measurable, for example, pain.

- Concepts must then be translated into items on the questionnaire. You will probably find that there are several sub-concepts that might require separate items. For example, if you are measuring stress, it might be broken down into types of stress, such as physical, emotional, social and financial stress. You may wish to focus on only one of these or on all of them. You could ask a person how much stress they perceive they are under, or ask them if they suffer from some of the indicators of stress, such as headache, skin rashes and so forth.

- Ensure that each item is necessary to your study. Every item should relate to a concept, hypothesis or variable. Questionnaires often include unnecessary items such as demographic variables. If age is not one of your variables, do not include it in the questionnaire just because it might be interesting. Eliminating unnecessary items helps to keep the length of the questionnaire under control.

- Ensure that the items are neither biased nor contain an assumption. For example, 'How often do you cheat on your income taxes?' assumes that you do. It should be rephrased to 'Do you cheat on your income taxes?', which could be answered by a range of responses from 'never' to 'always'. Similarly, 'Do you think that nurses should be paid more?' invites the answer 'yes'. It should be rephrased to include options for the pay staying the same or even decreasing. Items should be framed in as neutral a way as possible if you want unbiased answers.

- Ensure that there is only one question per item. Items that contain two actual questions cannot allow for the possibility that the respondent would like to answer the two questions differently.
- Ensure that all items are worded clearly and correctly and are easy to understand in order to eliminate incomplete item response. This is likely to occur if the respondent perceives the item to be unclear or the choice of responses to be irrelevant, unsuitable or lacking. The respondent may leave that item blank and go on to the next one.
- Choose the demographic items, if any, that you need to include and what categories you will break them down into: for example, do you want age in years or to the nearest decade? Some questionnaires ask the demographic information at the beginning to get the person answering easy questions, while others leave it till later so the person will do it, having come that far.
- Pitch the language at the correct level for the respondents. The questionnaire should not contain any jargon or ambiguous language that they may not understand because this will decrease the validity of the responses.
- Cluster related items so that the respondents do not have to jump around in their thoughts. You may wish to put headings at the tops of the sections and use a relevant numbering system.
- Put the most important items at the beginning of the questionnaire so the answers will not be subject to respondent fatigue.
- Ensure correct spelling and grammar.
- Consider the data analysis. Questions that are 'closed', that is, tick-a-box type, permit only those responses supplied by the researcher. The responses are usually numerical or capable of being transformed into numbers. The advantage of these is that their specificity makes analysis easier – the respondent has in effect classified your data for you. However, answers to closed questions are narrow and shallow. Open questions just give the question and allow the respondent to compose the response. Open questions are more qualitative and require a lot more work in data analysis – they need to be classified and coded, and may need to be transcribed into the computer. However, the data are richer and deeper.

Developing questionnaire scales

A scale is a method that asks a respondent to rate an item on a basis that is either a number or can be converted into numbers. There are various types of scales that can be used, but the idea is to locate the respondent on a continuum with a mathematical basis. This makes for ease of analysis of data. Some common types of scales are:

The Likert scale: On the Likert scale, the respondents rank their attitudes or opinions on a continuum of response from 'strongly agree' to 'strongly disagree' (see Figure 8.2, opposite). There is usually an odd number of possible responses, normally five or seven. The continuum is usually phrased as 'strongly agree', 'agree', 'mildly agree', 'neutral', 'mildly disagree', 'disagree' and 'strongly disagree'. These responses are given a numerical score from 1 to 7 (or sometimes 1 to 5). This allows you to calculate a numerical value for the purposes of descriptive and inferential statistical analysis.

| Nurses should be paid more |

SA	A	N	D	SD

Figure 8.2   A five-point Likert scale

The semantic differential scale: The semantic differential scale is a scale that asks the respondents to rate their response to an item using a pair of adjectives at opposite ends of a continuum. For example, one might be asked where one would rate euthanasia on the beautiful/ugly axis (see Figure 8.3).

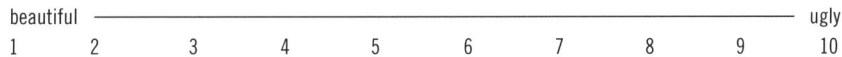

beautiful									ugly
1	2	3	4	5	6	7	8	9	10

Figure 8.3   An example of a semantic differential scale

Rating scales: On rating scales, respondents are asked to rate how often they carry out a behaviour. Responses range from 'never' to 'always', with intermediate steps such as 'sometimes' and 'often' (see Figure 8.4).

How often do you do daily exercise?	Always	Often	Sometimes	Seldom	Never

Figure 8.4   An example of a rating scale

Visual analogue scales: On a visual analogue scale (VAS), respondents are asked to indicate the quality of an experience on a representation of the phenomenon (see Figure 8.5, overleaf). One type of VAS is a linear, ruler-like scale that appears somewhat like a thermometer. The scale has numbers, with extreme ranks at the ends. Visual analogue scales are useful for measuring stimuli such as pain. An example is the Bourbonnais pain ruler, which ranks pain on a scale from 0 to 10, with 0 representing no pain and 10 representing excruciating pain (Bourbonnais 1981).

Pictorial representations of the phenomenon under investigation can be used for participants who cannot use a numerical scale, for example, faces that express varying degrees of pain (see Figure 8.6, overleaf).

Formatting the questionnaire

Composing the questionnaire items is the first stage. The questionnaire as a whole must be formatted and attention should be paid to its presentation. In general, you should make sure that it looks professional and appealing so that the recipient will have confidence in your research ability. The following points can assist you in formatting and presenting the questionnaire:

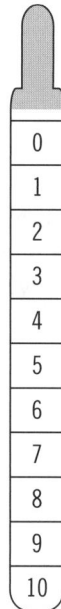

Figure 8.5 An example of a visual analogue scale

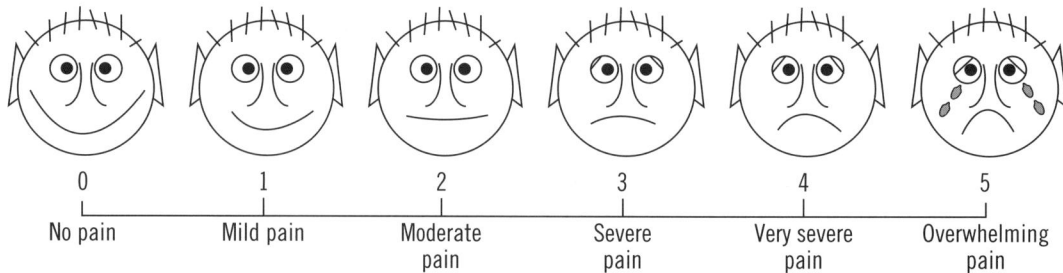

0	1	2	3	4	5
No pain	Mild pain	Moderate pain	Severe pain	Very severe pain	Overwhelming pain

Figure 8.6 An example of a faces scale

- Put a title at the top of the questionnaire that reflects the overall topic. You do not need to include the word 'questionnaire' as that is self-evident.
- Make sure the pages are numbered.
- Put instructions for completing the questionnaire at the beginning. If they are brief enough, put them at the top of every page.
- Do not overcrowd the page – dense print is even less appealing than more pages and it does not conceal excessive length of a questionnaire.
- Use a readable font (12 point is best).
- Consider whether to use one side of the page or both. One side is more expensive but looks more elegant and is easier to use during data entry.

- Make sure every question is numbered to facilitate data entry.
- Put the answers near the questions, but close to the edge of the page on one margin or the other to facilitate data entry.
- Make sure the pages are stapled together securely.

The draft questionnaire

When you are satisfied that the draft is as good as you can make it, the next step is to refine it and then pilot it. Have the items reviewed by several experts for content validity, structure and bias. Send your draft out for comment to at least three experts in the content area of the questionnaire and take account of their suggestions for revising it. You should also ask your supervisor to vet it. Ask any colleague who has developed a questionnaire for their feedback. You will be surprised at the obvious flaws that have escaped your notice.

Once you have refined the questionnaire according to the feedback from the experts on content and structure, you are ready to trial the questionnaire with a pilot sample. The following points can help you:

- The pilot sample should be large enough to give you a realistic trial without compromising your main sample.
- Develop a covering letter (including a plain language statement) asking for participation in the study.
- You should trial all phases of the questionnaire, *including data analysis*. This will enable you to assess realistically the quality of the questionnaire and data, the time it will take and the appropriateness of the methods you have chosen for distribution, data entry and data analysis.
- You should do a statistical procedure on the questionnaire to establish reliability, for example, the Kuder-Richardson test.
- Revise your questionnaire again in light of the findings of the pilot study. If there are major revisions, you will need to pilot it again.

The covering letter

Your questionnaire will need a covering letter, which can incorporate the plain language statement, as described in Chapter 6. You will not need a consent form as return of the questionnaire is implied consent. The letter should inform your potential respondents about the study. You should tell the recipients how you got their names and how they were selected, for example, by random computer allocation. You should tell them what the study is about, why it is being done and who, in general, is participating. State how you plan to use the data and how your procedures will ensure confidentiality of the data. You should give them instructions for maintaining their anonymity and for returning the questionnaire. Finally, you should give a contact number for more information and thank them for considering participating in your survey.

The covering letter should be composed so that it motivates your potential respondents to return the questionnaire. You can appeal to their altruism. If possible, stress the rewards that the respondent will get for helping you. If you personalise the letters by addressing them to 'Dear Ms/Mr (Name)' instead of the impersonal 'Dear Colleague' you will improve your return rate. However, that is a lot of work, particularly if you have a large number of questionnaires to distribute. If you have secretarial resources and a word processor with a mail merge facility, it is achievable. The letter should carry your personal signature or a facsimile, which can be done by signing the original letter before photocopying. If you are using institutional stationery, you can print a letter on plain stationery, sign it, then photocopy it onto the letterhead stationery.

Building in incentives to respond

Low questionnaire return rates are one of the problems facing researchers. Not only is it disheartening after all of the work you put in; it also reduces the external validity of your findings.

In order to encourage people to return the questionnaires, you should enclose a stamped envelope with your return address on it. You might think that a stamp and an envelope are but a small cost to each participant or institution and if you could defray these costs your expenses would be significantly reduced; however, it is not the cost of the stamp and the envelope but the convenience. Even if someone fills in the questionnaire, it may take several days before they get around to buying envelopes and/or stamps or they might decide it is just too much trouble and end up not posting the letter at all. Furthermore, it is not ethical to expect institutions to unknowingly bear the cost of the postage for your research project. One way of reducing costs of postage is to arrange for a 'reply paid' billing at your end rather than putting a stamp on each envelope. This means that the envelope indicates to the participant that postage will be paid by you. Under this system you pay the post office only for the questionnaires that are returned. However, you need to make it clear in your letter that the reply paid envelope precludes the need for a postage stamp. You can consult the appropriate people to see if your institution will provide this service as part of your student stipend, if you have one.

Giving an incentive such as a small monetary reward, e.g. a lottery ticket, might seem like a good inducement. However, this can be expensive and it is difficult to administer unless you can arrange to give it out when the questionnaires are returned. In the case of postal questionnaires, postage for just this purpose is also expensive and unworkable unless the respondents can identify themselves, in which case their anonymity is not safeguarded. I recently heard of one researcher who included a tea bag in the questionnaire packet and suggested that the respondent sit down and have a cup of tea while doing the questionnaire. Perhaps you can think of something equally creative, but beware of giving out a reward unless the questionnaire is returned.

Follow-up rounds

Unless you get your target return rate (which should be at least 66 per cent) on the first round, you will need to plan for a follow-up round of questionnaires. Basically, there are three methods you can use to determine who will receive your follow-up questionnaires and they all have advantages and disadvantages in terms of anonymity. Before choosing one of these methods, you need to ask yourself if you really need to know the identities of the respondents for any reason other than following up the non-responders.

One follow-up method is to send a new questionnaire to everyone on your original list with instructions to discard it if they have already replied. This has the disadvantage of potential double returns if some respondents forget they have already done it and do it again. You will not be able to tell if a person has sent it in twice unless the person is identified by a code number. The time involved may also be a consideration. However, the major disadvantage of sending a full second round of questionnaires is the expense of stationery, printing and postage. You will need to pay for a full set of postage to send out this round but return postage costs can be minimised by using the reply paid method.

The second follow-up method is to sacrifice anonymity and give every potential respondent a code number that you put on both your primary list of names and the questionnaire or envelope. This allows you to identify respondents and eliminate them from the follow-up round. This is much cheaper than the first method but it will almost certainly reduce the return rate, perhaps even to catastrophic levels of less than 20 per cent. This occurs because people are suspicious of strangers and will probably be afraid that you will identify their data, despite your assurances that the numbers will be used only for the stated purpose. This suspicious attitude is even more likely to be prevalent if the content of the questionnaire is sensitive or intrusive.

Sometimes the design of a study requires linking two or more sets of data from each individual, for example pre-tests and post-tests. You therefore need to put a linking system in place. A code number can do this. However, data-linking can be achieved more readily by asking respondents to generate their own unique code and put it on all responses. The recipient can choose the numbers, for example, their mother's day, month and year of birth. The advantage of this method is that you do not know who the respondent is so the response is anonymous, but if they use a unique number that can be reliably generated each time, the data can be linked. People are used to generating pin numbers so will be familiar with this concept and likely to comply, provided you give them a clear explanation in the letter of the procedure and the reasons for it.

The third method is the use of a system that allows you to determine who responded without putting any code number or identifying mark on the questionnaire or envelope. In the author's opinion this is the best method, unless you need to link sets of data, as above. When you are having the questionnaires and reply paid envelopes printed, have postcards printed that have your address on one side and on the other a message that Ms/Mr X has sent back the questionnaire by separate post. If you use this method, make sure that you include the person's name on the card when you send it so that you are not dependent on the respondent putting it on, which they will not always realise they are meant to do. You can do this easily by generating a second set of sticky labels with the respondents' names and addresses on them and sticking them on the postcards. However, be careful to have 'To' and 'From' printed clearly in the appropriate place to avoid confusion in the post office. When you receive the postcard you can cross off the respondent's name from your list and you are left with the non-responders, to whom you send the follow-up round minus the postcard. This is clearly cheaper than the first method, but more expensive than the second as you pay for printing the postcards and for their return postage. However, the increased return rate compensates for the extra cost involved. An illustration of the postcard is shown in Figure 8.7, overleaf.

Front of postcard

```
┌──────────────────────────────────────────────┐
│                                                │
│   ┌─────────┐            ┌──────────────┐     │
│   │         │            │ Stamp if not │     │
│   │   To    │            │ postage paid │     │
│   │         │            └──────────────┘     │
│   └─────────┘                                  │
│                                                │
│       ┌────────────────────────────────┐     │
│       │                                  │     │
│       │  Name and address of researcher │     │
│       │                                  │     │
│       └────────────────────────────────┘     │
│                                                │
└──────────────────────────────────────────────┘
```

Back of postcard

```
┌──────────────────────────────────────────────┐
│   ┌─────────┐                                  │
│   │  From   │                                  │
│   └─────────┘                                  │
│       ┌────────────────────────────────────┐  │
│       │ Dear (your name)                    │  │
│       │ This is to inform you that I have    │  │
│       │ posted back your questionnaire       │  │
│       │ separately.                          │  │
│       │        Yours faithfully,            │  │
│       └────────────────────────────────────┘  │
│          ┌─────────────────────────────────┐  │
│          │ Name of respondent               │  │
│          │ Address of respondent            │  │
│          └─────────────────────────────────┘  │
└──────────────────────────────────────────────┘
```

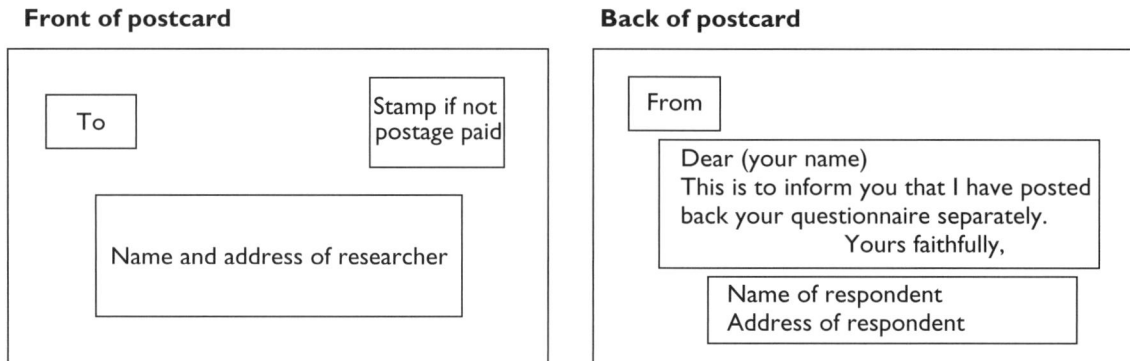

Figure 8.7 An example of a postcard used to increase questionnaire returns

Whatever method you use to follow up non-respondents, you will need to distinguish between the first- and second-round respondents so that you can compare them and see if they are any different. You can do this by making some distinction between the two questionnaires such as a slight change in format, for example, underlining the title of one or the other, or a slight difference in colour of paper that will be obvious to you but not to the respondents.

Distribution of questionnaires

Before you can distribute the questionnaires you must determine the sample that you will use through the sampling procedures discussed earlier in this chapter. Unless you are using a convenience sample, in which you distribute questionnaires until you reach your quota of responses, you will need to identify the potential recipients of the questionnaire.

The actual process of distributing questionnaires will be discussed in Chapter 9, on data collection.

You can now see that the art and science of questionnaires is a very comprehensive topic and requires a lot of attention to detail to be used successfully. If you wish to explore questionnaire development in more depth, read Chapter 14 in Minichiello et al. (2004) or Frazer and Lawley (2000).

The Delphi survey technique

The Delphi technique is a special survey method of obtaining and analysing a range of expert opinions on a topic or issue without having a face-to-face meeting of the group. It is named after the famous Greek oracle at Delphi, who was thought to transmit answers from the gods. A panel of experts is repeatedly surveyed by mail or electronic means, with feedback on each round of results, until a consensus is obtained. The principle is that with each round, the experts will move closer to the prevailing view on the issue. The Delphi technique is used where the objective might be to get a consensus on policy issues, priority of goals, or forecast trends.

A classic Delphi study should meet four criteria: anonymity of panel members, iteration through presentation of a questionnaire over a number of rounds, controlled feedback of information to group members, and statistical group response at the end of the procedure (Crisp et al. 1999). However, Crisp and colleagues argue that researchers have modified the classic Delphi technique over the years to the extent that sometimes little of the technique is recognisable in the method of the study. If you are interested in this technique, the article by Crisp et al. will provide a full discussion of the topic.

The Delphi technique has the advantage of reaching experts over a wide geographic area. In a country as large as Australia this allows people from remote areas to participate. It saves the participants the time and expense of a formal meeting. It also allows a panel of experts to achieve consensus without face-to-face interaction, which can influence the results (Pelletier et al. 2000). The anonymity of the responses allows more candid responses. However, the Delphi technique relies upon a fast turnaround time and it can be time-consuming and expensive for the researcher. The anonymity can reduce the accountability of the respondents for their responses, and responder attrition can be a problem. However, used in the appropriate situation, the advantages can outweigh the disadvantages.

An example of a Delphi survey can be seen in Hardy et al. (2004). This study developed mental health nursing clinical indicators using a three-round reactive Delphi survey. Equal proportions of Maori and non-Maori nurses and consumers rated the importance of 91 clinical indicator statements for the achievement of professional practice standards in New Zealand. The Delphi technique is an ideal method for achieving consensus among participants on matters of policy.

In constructing a Delphi survey, one first identifies an appropriate panel of experts in the area under discussion. They should represent a range of opinion, as well as be representative in other parameters such as geography and gender, otherwise the exercise will not work. After obtaining agreement from the experts for their participation in the survey, you administer the first round of questionnaires, instructing the experts not to communicate with each other about the topic. You then receive the anonymous questionnaires, analyse the data and revise the questionnaire as necessary. The tabulated results and the revised questionnaire are fed back to the experts who are asked to reanalyse the questionnaire in light of the group results. This process is repeated, usually about three times, until the desired amount of consensus is obtained. When the final results are obtained, they become the results of the study.

Q-sort

Q-sort methods use a procedure in which the researcher gives a participant a deck of 60 to 100 cards containing individual items that are developed from the literature of a particular field or discipline (Tetting 1988). The researcher asks the participant to sort the cards according to predetermined criteria such as importance or amount of time spent on an activity. It is useful to describe and compare participants' opinions about such things as the importance of various types of nursing care or nursing behaviours, or self-perceptions, for example of personality and personal characteristics. Q-sort can also be used to sort items for inclusion in a questionnaire scale. The cards contain words, phrases, definitions or other statements about the topic being researched. Pictures could be used for special groups where language is a problem. The researcher specifies how many cards are to go in each pile, to avoid all of the cards being put into the middle or at the ends. Usually the distribution of the cards mimics a normal curve. Each statement is judged in relation to the other statements, which preserves the relationship of the statements, unlike a questionnaire where the statements are independent of each other. The participant sorts the cards into a set number of piles, usually about nine, according to some dimension such as desirable/undesirable, agreement/ disagreement, and like me/unlike me. This technique is reliable, although time-consuming to administer, particularly if there are numerous participants.

An example of the use of Q-sort methods can be seen in a study that used the technique to compare the perceptions of patients and nurses about important nursing behaviour (Gardner et al. 2001). The researchers used the 'Care Q' instrument that measures the concept of caring, using 50 cards containing statements of nursing behaviours ranked from most to least important. They found that patients ranked technological competence first while nurses ranked listening to the patient and patient participation in care first. Another study using Q-sort methods is one by Ryan and Zerwic (2004), who investigated the knowledge of symptom clusters among adults at risk for acute myocardial infarction. They found that people with known coronary artery disease and their significant others had varied expectations of acute myocardial infarction symptoms. The study indicated that new and various strategies need to be developed to help patients accurately identify acute myocardial infarction symptoms.

Interviews

A research interview is a method in which the researcher asks the participant purposeful questions with the intention of investigating a research problem. Interviews differ from questionnaires in that the main response medium is speech rather than writing. The questions may be written down for the guidance of the researcher. There are several types of interviews, on a continuum of structure ranging from the highly structured interview, which uses an undeviating format to an unstructured interview in which only a few introductory questions may be predetermined. In between is the semi-structured interview, which uses written questions as a guide, in order to achieve some consistency of data, but allows unscheduled exploration of topics that arise in the course of the interview. Unstructured and semi-structured interviews are used in qualitative research where the lack of structure is important in grounded theory research. However, in quantitative methods the structured interview is more usual and it will be explored in more depth here.

The structured interview is appropriate when you want factual information and consistency of data across respondents. The aim of structured interviews is to get information objectively, without the interviewer influencing the process. In a sense, the interviewer tries to become as objective as a questionnaire. The structured interview is the form of interviewing that gives maximum control to the interviewer. Structured interviews allow more quantification of responses than semi-structured or unstructured interviews. The disadvantage of the structured interview is that the structure can constrain the data and you can miss things that you might pick up in a less structured format.

If you are developing a set of questions for a structured interview, it is important to undertake the same processes as when developing a questionnaire (see, for example, Minichiello 2004).

To implement the structured interview process, you, the researcher, develop a set script to give the initial information and instructions to the interviewee, and set questions to elicit the information. You train the interviewer to follow the set structure, asking the same questions, in the same order, and with the same tone of voice in order to promote consistency of data across participants. If there is more than one interviewer, it is essential to train them to perform the interview exactly alike, to ensure consistency across interviewers. It is important for the interviewer(s) to practise interviewing under full research conditions in order to develop their skills of interviewing and to check for consistency. Some researchers even videotape the practice interviews for critiquing.

The considerations for the actual interview process of structured interviews are similar to that of unstructured and semi-structured interviews, which will be discussed in Chapter 14.

Interviews can be carried out in different ways. The traditional way is the face-to-face interview. The most satisfactory method of conducting an interview is in person, in privacy. However, this can involve travel and accommodation expenses and can be very expensive if major distances are involved.

Interviews can also be carried out by telephone. The telephone interview is cheaper if great distances are involved but has the disadvantage of lacking visual contact between the interviewer and interviewee. This is not as important in highly structured interviews. Telephone interviews can be captured on audiotape if you arrange it with the telephone company.

The videoconference is also a possibility for a face-to-face interview. It is still relatively expensive, but could be cheaper than travel. It is relatively difficult to arrange since both parties must go to a videoconferencing centre, which may require considerable travel. Videoconferencing has the advantage of visual contact although it is not as intimate as a personal meeting. An added advantage is that it can capture the interview on videotape for future analysis of visual cues, thereby freeing part of the interviewer's attention for other matters. Researchers are also conducting 'interviews' via email on the Internet and via real-time dialogue in chat rooms. At the present time Internet technology restricts the interview to written responses, but it has the element of informality and immediate response that is associated with speech, particularly if it is done in 'real' time through a chat room. Some computers come equipped with a camera on top that could capture interviewees' responses in both video and audio.

Interviews can be carried out with participants either individually or in groups. A method of group interview is a focus group, in which the group meets face to face and is facilitated by an interviewer. This has the advantage of several people discussing an issue, thus allowing for group consensus. However, it is possible that the participants may be less candid in a group than in a one-to-one situation. O'Brien et al. (2004) used focus groups as a means of generating bi-cultural clinical indicators for subsequent use in a Delphi study. Focus groups are often used as part of larger research projects, particularly as a means of using relevant participants to help identify which variables might need to be included at the beginning of a project.

Whatever method of interviewing you use, you will need to decide how to capture the interview data. If the interview is conducted in person, audiotape is the usual method. Some researchers feel that this interferes with the process, but today's sensitive microphones allow an unobtrusive recording process. If this is a concern, written notes can be made, although these interrupt the flow of the dialogue. Videotaping is also a possibility, but involves the presence of another person, which reduces the privacy of the process. Telephone companies offer a recording service with a teleconference call. Obviously if the Internet is used, a written record of the responses is available.

Choosing between questionnaire and interview

Sometimes, as a researcher, you will have to choose between the methods of questionnaire and interview. The advantage of interviews over questionnaires is that the data will be richer and deeper. You can access participants to whom you cannot send questionnaires, such as the homeless, or those who do not have the ability or strength to fill in questionnaires, such as the illiterate or the very ill. You will also get a better response rate since people find it harder to say 'no' in person to an interview than to throw a questionnaire in the waste bin. A questionnaire relies on the correct interpretation by the respondent, but in an interview the interviewer is present and can clarify instructions where needed and observe the interviewee's response to the questions.

The disadvantage of interviews as compared with questionnaires is that they are more expensive in terms of training, administration and travel to access the participants. You may have to pay the interviewees a small fee to compensate them for travel, child care and so on. Interviews can be difficult to arrange and are subject to cancellation if your interviewee has more pressing matters to attend to at the time. They also require more time and expense to collect and analyse the data than questionnaires do. Since it is never possible for people to be completely objective, the interviewer can inject bias into the process by tone of voice or body language, which a questionnaire cannot – unless the items are biased. Interviews require a lot of skill to carry out because you have to both conduct the interview and monitor the process at the same time. Interviewees may find it difficult to answer your questions, particularly if they have never reflected on the matter before or if the questions are on a sensitive topic. Interviewees may also give socially acceptable answers in person, whereas they may give more candid responses to an anonymous questionnaire.

EXERCISE

A researcher wants to study the effects of cigarette smoking on the recovery of post-surgical orthopaedic patients. They are looking for ways to measure various aspects of smoking behaviour. Which of the following measurements represents the highest scale of measurement?

1   Asking patients the average number of cigarettes they smoke per day.

2   Asking patients the reasons why they smoke.

3   Asking patients to list the ways in which smoking affects them.

4   Asking patients to use a peak flow meter to determine their lung function.

5   Asking patients to rank in order of importance all of the health concerns they have, including cigarette smoking.

Triangulation

Triangulation is the use of more than one method in studying the same phenomenon, in order to validate the phenomenon. The concept of triangulation originally comes from the field of surveying where surveyors fixed one data point by taking measurements from different angles. There can be various types of triangulation, from mixing quantitative and qualitative approaches in one study design to using more than one investigator examining the same phenomenon and using several different measurement devices to measure the same variable (Sohier 1988). The goals of triangulation are to confirm data and ensure their completeness (Begley 1996). The principle is that if you collect data based on more than one observation or measurement, the data are more likely to be valid because there will be less investigator bias. There are various different typologies for classifying triangulation.

One of the most well known is the typology developed by Denzin, who identified data triangulation, investigator triangulation, theoretical triangulation and methodological triangulation (Denzin 1989). Data triangulation refers to the use of multiple data sources. These can be collected at different times (time triangulation), from different places (space triangulation) or from people at different levels (person triangulation). In person triangulation, the method entails collecting data from any pair of the three levels of individuals, groups and collectives (Begley 1996). Investigator triangulation refers to triangulation occurring when two or more skilled researchers with different expertise examine the data. Theoretical triangulation refers to the use of different theories in the conceptual framework for a study. Methodological triangulation is the use of more than one research method in the one study (Begley 1996).

Within methodological triangulation, between-method triangulation entails combining methods from two or more research traditions, for example, quantitative and qualitative, in one study. Within-method triangulation involves combining two or more similar data collection methods within one study to measure the same variable (Begley 1996). According to Begley (1996), Kimichi, Polivka and Stevenson (1991) have added 'unit of analysis' triangulation, in which two or more approaches to analysing the same set of data are used.

Triangulation was used by Merkouris, Papathanassoglou and Lemonidou (2004) in their study of patient satisfaction with nursing care. They found that a combination of qualitative and quantitative methods contributed to the completeness of description and understanding of the phenomenon under investigation.

Redfern and Norman (1994, pp. 51–2, cited by Begley 1996) have discussed the advantages and disadvantages of triangulation. The advantages are that triangulation:

* overcomes the bias of 'single-method, single-observer, single-theory studies'
* increases confidence in the results
* allows development and validation of instruments and methods (confirmation)
* provides an understanding of the domain (completeness)
* is ideal for complex issues
* overcomes the elite bias of naturalistic research
* overcomes the holistic fallacy of naturalistic research
* allows divergent results to enrich explanation.

Redfern and Norman (1994, pp. 51–2, cited by Begley 1996) cite the disadvantages of triangulation as:

- no guarantee of internal and external validity
- may compound the sources of error
- methods selected may not be the right ones
- unit of analysis might not apply to all methods
- cannot compensate for researcher bias
- expensive
- no use with the 'wrong' question
- replication is difficult.

As Begley points out, some of these disadvantages are applicable to any method and are not a feature of triangulation as such.

The whole concept of triangulation is based on a positivist view of the world, that it is somehow necessary to augment qualitative findings and that combining various methods will lead to finding the truth (Begley 1996). While triangulation can be useful, it is important to avoid the assumption that qualitative findings are useful only if they are supported by quantitative findings. Further debate on these issues can be found in Shih (1998).

Summary

In this chapter we have discussed the methods you can use in carrying out quantitative studies. We looked at different types of settings and sampling methods. We considered ways of collecting data by measurement and instrumentation, different types of observation, and information-collecting strategies. Finally, we examined the various ways in which multiple methods, or triangulation, can be used. After choosing the appropriate methods to match your aims, question, broad methodological approach and study design, you are now ready to move on to applying for the necessary approvals for your project. This was discussed in Chapter 6.

Main points

- A setting is the place in which the study is carried out, where the phenomenon of interest can be observed. It can be a naturalistic setting, or a laboratory setting.
- The population is a group whose members have specific common characteristics that you wish to investigate in your research study. The 'population' can be people, places, objects or events.
- An element is a single unit of the population studied.
- The sample is the part of the population that you study. The sample can be selected by a variety of methods, but the two major groups are probability and non-probability samples.
- In non-probability sampling, subjective judgements contribute to the selection of the sample and findings will lack external validity.

- In probability sampling, each element has the same possibility of being chosen to take part and the probability of each element being included in the sample is known. This precludes the likelihood of bias, and therefore is representative of the population.
- A random sample can be selected by a lottery, random number table or computer program.
- Stratified samples represent certain 'strata' in a population, most commonly gender or age groups.
- Cluster samples represent groups of elements rather than individual elements.
- Multi-stage samples use clusters and then select elements from clusters.
- Convenience samples use whatever elements are available which fit the design.
- Case-based samples are purposefully chosen by the researcher to fit the aim of the study.
- Snowball samples grow as one participant refers the researcher to the next participant.
- Quota samples keep including elements in certain categories till the quotas for these categories are full.
- Sample size and power calculations can be done to estimate the required sample size for a study.
- Measurement is the determination of the size, range or frequency of an object, characteristic or phenomenon. Carried out using instruments, measurement gives the advantages of standardisation of data, accuracy, and the ability to compare findings with those of other researchers.
- Measurement can be direct or indirect and *in vivo* or *in vitro*.
- Scales of measurement represent the level of precision of any measurement technique.
- An instrument is any tool that measures. An instrument has the advantages of increasing accuracy, allowing measurement in more detail, and facilitating recording and analysing data. It has the disadvantages of being mechanical, prescriptive and relatively expensive and possibly requiring special skills to operate.
- Considerations for choice of instrument include: validity, sensitivity, accuracy, reliability, cost and requirements for specialised training.
- Error in measurement can be random or one-off errors or systematic errors that occur whenever the procedure is carried out or at regular intervals.
- Biophysiological instruments measure biological or physiological events such as pulse or blood pressure.
- Observation is done by the human eye and comprises obtaining data about people's behaviour when and where it actually happens. It can be used in lieu of interview, can see what people actually do as opposed to what they say, allows us to see the finer nuances of behaviour (such as body language) and prevents distortion of data by the person being observed. However, observation can be artificial if done in a laboratory, must await the behaviour, and entails problems of access. Observations can be inaccurate and biased.
- Observation can be unstructured or structured, as participant or observer, covert or overt, and obtrusive or unobtrusive.

- Information can be gained from existing data, secondary analysis, content analysis, meta-analysis or self-report (by questionnaires or interviews).
- A questionnaire is a document containing questions to which a person responds. Questionnaires are relatively quick to administer and receive, are cheaper than interviewing or observation, can yield large amounts of information, can be distributed over a wide area and can yield candid responses if anonymous. The data are relatively easy to analyse.
- Questionnaire data can be limited by the respondents' lack of literacy, language, or misunderstandings and misinterpretations. Questionnaires can be expensive and tend to have a low return rate.
- Questionnaire design is complex and requires attention to content and format, with trials and procedures to ensure content validity and reliability.
- A scale is a tool that asks the respondents to rate their responses on a numerical basis. Common types are Likert Scale, semantic differential scale, rating scales and visual analogue scales.
- Delphi studies attempt to achieve consensus between a group of experts, usually on a matter of policy.
- Q-sort studies ask participants to sort cards with items on each one related to the phenomenon under investigation.
- In an interview, the researcher asks the participant purposeful questions with the intention of investigating a research problem. Interviews can be conducted by a variety of face-to-face or technological methods. Interview data are richer and deeper, the interviewer can access difficult participants, the response rate is usually good and the interviewer can clarify instructions and observe the interviewee's response to the questions.
- Interviews involve training, administration, travel, and possibly a fee to the interviewees, can be difficult to arrange and are subject to cancellation. Data collection and analysis are time-consuming. Interviews can be difficult to carry out; the interviewer can inject bias by tone of voice or body language, interviewees may find it difficult to answer questions and they can give socially acceptable rather than candid answers.
- Triangulation is the process of taking multiple measurements or observations of the same phenomenon in order to increase the validity and depth of understanding of that phenomenon.

CASE STUDY

The North Eastern Rural County Council is concerned about recent outbreaks of giardia infections in the community. It suspects that some domestic water tanks might be infested with the organism. As the public health officer for the council, you decide to carry out a project to see whether domestic water tanks are contaminated with giardia.

Discussion questions:

1 Is this project most appropriately addressed in a laboratory or in a naturalistic setting?
2 How would you define the population of interest for the study?
3 What kind of sampling strategy would be most effective in answering your research question?
4 What kinds of measurements might be made to produce the data needed in this study?
5 What kind of instrumentation would be needed to produce these data?
6 How could you triangulate the data collection in this study?

Multiple choice questions

1 Laboratory research has the advantage(s) of:
   a it can easily be compared with other similar studies
   b it generally has high internal validity
   c it allows for controlled observations
   d all of the above

2 Probability sampling has the advantage of:
   a being representative of the population
   b allowing generalisation of findings
   c contributing to external validity
   d all of the above

3 The most appropriate method of studying the characteristics of wound healing would be:
   a questionnaire
   b participant observation
   c pure observation
   d content analysis

4 The advantage of a stratified random sample is that:
   a it has the same proportion of important characteristics which exist in the population
   b it is easier to recruit participants
   c it is a non-probability sample
   d none of the above

5 The purpose of sample size calculation prior to commencing a research study is to:
   a ensure that a sample is at least twice the size required
   b make sure your study finds an effect if one is there to be found
   c avoid having to use a random sample
   d none of the above

6   The most precise level of measurement is found in:
     a   categorical data
     b   ordinal data
     c   discrete data
     d   continuous analysis
7   Which of the following is a source of measurement error:
     a   lack of precision in the instrument
     b   poor sampling
     c   lack of reliability in an instrument
     d   content analysis
8   Questionnaire scales are used to:
     a   quantify variables which might otherwise not be measurable
     b   produce continuous level data
     c   both a and b
     d   neither a nor b
9   The purpose of triangulation is:
     a   to repeat the same measurement three times in order to demonstrate reliability
     b   to confirm data and ensure their completeness
     c   to ensure that all data are the same for all participants
     d   all of the above
10   In order to maximise the precision of measurements in a research study, the researcher should:
     a   only use observational methods
     b   choose the highest scale of measurement possible
     c   use the smallest possible sample size
     d   avoid non-probability sampling

Review topics

1   Discuss the advantages and disadvantages of laboratory and clinical settings.
2   Compare and contrast probability and non-probability sampling.
3   Describe the different levels of measurement.
4   Compare structured and unstructured interviews.
5   Describe triangulation and state its advantages.

Online reading

INFOTRAC® COLLEGE EDITION

Access information using the following keywords to retrieve information relating to quantitative methods:

➤ data collection

➤ design

➤ instrumentation

➤ interviews

➤ measurement

➤ observation

➤ questionnaire

➤ sampling method

➤ survey

➤ triangulation

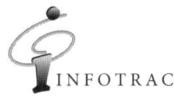

Answers to exercise questions

Exercise on p. 208 (no; quota sample)
Exercise on p. 234 (4)

References

Ammenwerth, E., Mansmann, U., Iller, C. & Eichstadter, R. 2003, 'Factors affecting and affected by user acceptance of computer-based nursing documentation: results of a two-year study', *Journal of the American Medical Informatics Association*, vol. 10, no. 1, 69–84.

Andersen, C. & Adamsen, L. 2001, 'Continuous video recording: a new clinical research tool for studying the nursing care of cancer patients', *Journal of Advanced Nursing*, vol. 35, no. 2, 257–67.

Badger, F. & Mullan, B. 2004, 'Aggressive and violent incidents: perceptions of training and support among staff caring for older people and people with head injury', *Journal of Clinical Nursing*, vol. 13, no. 4, 526–33.

Begley, C. 1996, 'Using triangulation in nursing research', *Journal of Advanced Nursing*, vol. 24, no. 1, 122–8.

Bourbonnais, F. 1981, 'Pain assessment: development of a tool for the nurse and the patient', *Journal of Advanced Nursing*, vol. 6, 277–82.

Courtney, M. 2005, *Evidence for Nursing Practice*, Elsevier, Marrickville.

Crisp, J., Pelletier, D., Duffield, C., Nagy, S. & Adams, A. 1999, 'It's all in a name: when is a Delphi study not a Delphi study?' *Australian Journal of Advanced Nursing*, vol. 16, no. 3, 32–7.

Dawson-Saunders, B. & Trapp, R. 2001, *Basic and Clinical Biostatistics*, 3rd edn, Lange Medical Books-McGraw-Hill, New York.

Denzin, R. 1989, *The Research Act: A Theoretical Introduction to Sociological Methods*, 3rd edn, McGraw-Hill, New York.

Dunn, S., Lawson, D., Robertson, S., Underwood, M., Clark, R., Valentine, T., Walker, N., Wilson-Row, C., Crowder, K. & Herewane, D. 2000, 'The development of competency standards for specialist critical care nurses', *Journal of Advanced Nursing*, vol. 31, no. 2, 339–46.

Edwards, N. & Beck, A. 2002, 'Animal-assisted therapy and nutrition in Alzheimer's disease', *Western Journal of Nursing Research*, vol. 24, no. 6, 697–712.

Fajemilehin, B. 2000, 'Old age in a changing society: elderly experiences of caregiving in Osun Sate, Nigeria', *Africa Journal of Nursing and Midwifery*, vol. 2, no. 1, 23–7.

Frank-Stromborg, M. & Olsen, S. 2004, *Instruments for Clinical Health-care Research*, 3rd edn, Jones and Bartlett, Boston.

Frazer, L. & Lawley, M. 2000, *Questionnaire Design and Administration: A Practical Approach*, John Wiley and Sons, Brisbane.

Gardner, A., Goodsell, J., Duggan, T., Murtha, B., Peck, C. & Williams, J. 2001, 'Don't call me Sweetie', *Collegian*, vol. 8, no. 3, 32–8.

George, L., Hoffman, L., Boujoukos, A. & Zullo, T. 2002, 'Effect of positioning on oxygenation in single-lung transplant recipients', *American Journal of Critical Care*, vol. 11, no. 1, 66–75.

Graves, E., Hitt, A., Pariza, M., Cook, M. & McCarthy, D. 2005, 'Conjugated linoleic acid preserves muscle mass in mice bearing the colon-26 adenocarcinoma', *Research in Nursing and Health*, vol. 28, no. 1, 48–55.

Griffiths, P., Edwards, M., Forbes, A. & Harris, R. 2005, 'Post-acute intermediate care in nursing-led units: a systematic review of effectiveness', *International Journal of Nursing Studies*, vol. 42, no. 1, 107–16.

Grindlay, A., Santamaria, N. & Kitt, S. 2000, 'Hospital in the home: nurse safety – exposure to risk and evaluation of organisational policy', *Australian Journal of Advanced Nursing*, vol. 17, no. 3, 6–12.

Hardy, D.J., O'Brien, A.P., Gaskin, C.J., O'Brien, A.J., Morrison-Ngatai, E., Skews, G., Ryan, T. & McNulty, N. 2004, 'Practical application of the Delphi technique in a bicultural mental health nursing study in New Zealand', *Journal of Advanced Nursing*, vol. 46, no. 1, 95–109.

Henry, G. 1990, *Practical Sampling*, Sage, Newbury Park, California.

Jette, D., Warren, R. & Wirtalla, C. 2004, 'Rehabilitation in skilled nursing facilities: effect of nursing staff level and therapy intensity on outcomes', *American Journal of Physical Medicine & Rehabilitation*, vol. 83, no. 9, 704–12.

Kimichi, J., Polivka, B. & Stevenson, J. 1991, 'Triangulation: operational definitions', *Nursing Research*, vol. 40, no. 6, 364–6.

Lam, L., Ross, F. & Cass, D. 1999, 'The impact of work-related trauma on the psychological health of nursing staff: a cross-sectional study', *Australian Journal of Advanced Nursing*, vol. 16, no. 3, 14–17.

Merkouris, A., Papathanassoglou, E. & Lemonidou, C. 2004, 'Evaluation of patient satisfaction with nursing care: quantitative or qualitative approach?', *International Journal of Nursing Studies*, vol. 41, no. 4, 355–67.

Minichiello, V., Sullivan, G., Greenwood, K. & Axford, R. 2004, *Handbook for Research Methods for Nursing and Health Science*, 2nd edn, Pearson, Frenchs Forest.

O'Brien, A.P., Boddy, J.M., Hardy, D.J. & O'Brien, A.J. 2004, 'Clinical indicators as measures of mental health nursing standards of practice in New Zealand', *International Journal of Mental Health Nursing*, vol. 13, no. 2, 78–88.

Offredy, N. 2000, 'Advanced nursing practice: the case of nurse-practitioners in three Australian states', *Journal of Advanced Nursing*, vol. 31, no. 2, 274–81.

Pelletier, D., Duffield, C., Adams, A., Mitten-Lewis, S., Crisp, J. & Nagy, S. 2000, 'Australian clinicians and educators identify gaps in specialist cardiac nursing practice', *Australian Journal of Advanced Nursing*, vol. 17, no. 3, 24–30.

Proctor, N. 2000, 'Cultural affirmation and the protection of emotional well-being', *Holistic Nursing Practice*, vol. 15, no. 1, 5–11.

Redfern, S.J. & Norman, I.J. 1994, 'Validity through triangulation', *Nurse Researcher*, vol. 2, no. 2, 41–56.

Rice, P. & Naksook, C. 1999, 'Pregnancy and technology: Thai women's perceptions and experience of prenatal testing', *Health Care for Women International*, vol. 20, no. 3, 259–78.

Ryan, C.J. & Zerwic, J.J. 2004, 'Knowledge of symptom clusters among adults at risk for acute myocardial infarction', *Nursing Research*, vol. 53, no. 6, 363–9.

Senner, A., Johnston, K. & McLachlan, A. 2005, 'A comparison of peripheral and centrally collected cyclosporine A blood levels in pediatric patients undergoing stem cell transplant', *Oncology Nursing Forum*, vol. 32, no. 1, 73–7.

Shih, F. 1998, 'Triangulation in nursing research: issues of conceptual clarity and purpose', *Journal of Advanced Nursing*, vol. 28, no. 3, 631–41.

Smolen, D., Topp, R. & Singer, L. 2002, 'The effect of self-selected music during colonoscopy on anxiety, heart rate, and blood pressure', *Applied Nursing Research*, vol. 15, no. 3, 126–36.

Sohier, R. 1988, 'Multiple triangulation and contemporary nursing research', *Western Journal of Nursing Research*, vol. 6, no. 6, 732–42.

Street, A. 1995, *Nursing Replay: Researching Nursing Culture Together*, Churchill Livingstone, Melbourne.

Tetting, D. 1988, 'Q-sort update', *Western Journal of Nursing Research*, vol. 10, no. 6, 757–65.

Thapar, N., Warner, G., Drainoni, M., Williams, S., Ditchfield, H., Wierbicky, J. & Nesathurai, S. 2004, 'A pilot study of functional access to public buildings and facilities for persons with impairments', *Disability and Rehabilitation*, vol. 26, no. 5, 280–9.

Wichowski, H., Kubsch, S., Ladwig, J. & Torres, C. 2003, 'Patients' and nurses' perceptions of quality nursing activities', *British Journal of Nursing*, vol. 12, no. 19, 1122–9.

Wysocki, A., Kusakabe, A., Change, S. & Tuan, T. 1999, 'Temporal expression of urokinase plasminogen activator, plasminogen activator inhibitor and gelatinase-B in chronic wound fluid switches from a chronic to acute wound with progression to healing', *Wound Repair and Regeneration*, vol. 7, no. 3, 154–65.

CHAPTER 9

QUANTITATIVE DATA COLLECTION AND MANAGEMENT

CHAPTER OBJECTIVES

The material presented in this chapter will assist you to:

- prepare for data collection
- collect data
- process data for analysis
- manage the data and products of analysis
- carry out a pilot study.

Introduction

For most researchers, **data** collection is the time when they feel as though they have finally got down to the nitty gritty of the research process. It seems as though you have spent an inordinate amount of time planning the process, but at last you are going out to collect your data! Even if all of your planning has promoted a smooth data collection process, there are pitfalls in this phase of the process and things can still go wrong. You can help to prevent problems from arising, and minimise any damage by anticipating potential traps and managing the data collection phase effectively.

It is not easy to generalise about the data collection phase of the process because so much of the approach to it depends on the design and methods chosen for your study. What might be appropriate for one method could be inappropriate for another. In this chapter, therefore, we will try to confine our discussion to broad principles which you can apply to most quantitative data collection and management.

Preparing for data collection and management

Preparing for the data collection phase in your research project involves selecting and obtaining the equipment and materials, deciding on the participants and how to access them, and determining the location for the research.

In preparing to collect data, it is a good idea to construct a data collection plan using a flow chart or some other method of laying it out and tracking the process. You can do this on paper, but recording it in a computer program is probably more effective and it can then be imported into subsequent documents. You then have a 'road map' of the project against which you can check your progress.

Acquisition and preparation of equipment and materials

Your first task is to select and acquire any necessary equipment, such as biophysical instruments, computers, modems, telephones, recording equipment, statistical packages and so forth. This may involve buying, renting or borrowing pieces of equipment. You have more security if you hire or buy equipment because you are not subject to the lender's needs. If you are borrowing equipment, you need to make sure that it will be available when you need it and for as long as you need it.

It is essential to order any equipment and materials well before you expect to need them. This process inevitably takes longer than you think it will, particularly if you have to order things from overseas. If you are ordering through a university or hospital bureaucracy, you may have to wait for the purchase order to be approved, which can entail waiting for the institution's preferred suppliers to supply goods, or for expensive items of equipment to go out to tender. Furthermore, you do not want to find out at the last moment that the equipment you ordered is no longer being made, is out of stock or is sitting on a wharf due to industrial action. Nor do you want to find out at the last minute that the printery that promised to do your questionnaires by a certain date is unable to meet your deadline. Photocopiers have a way of breaking down at inopportune times. It is also a good idea to get the promised dates of delivery in writing so that there can be no misunderstandings later. For equipment or material that is not too expensive, order a few extra copies or a few spare consumables as insurance against loss or breakage.

If you are buying a statistical package, buy it in advance and learn how to use it so that you can be sure that the data you are proposing to collect will be compatible with the package and with your skills. Ask experienced researchers what package they use and why they find it useful. You can also consult a database such as CINAHL, Medline or a journal such as *Computers in Nursing* for reviews of software. The Statistical Package for the Social Sciences (SPSS) is commonly used by nurse-researchers. It is relatively expensive to buy for a personal computer, but most universities have it available on the network. You would probably need to buy the manual (SPSS 1999). If you are buying a data analysis package for your own personal computer, there are reasonably priced, user-friendly data analysis packages available. The data analysis functions of Excel or Lotus are also useful for simple tasks. Whatever you buy, it is wise to consult the manual to learn how to operate the program. Some universities may have classes in running particular statistical packages.

You will need to order, in plenty of time, any necessary consumables such as consent forms, receipts, information sheets, sticky labels, logbooks and so on. You will need to prepare your informed consent document and your plain language statement. You will need to prepare any protocols for the ward staff: that is, instructions for taking part in data collection for your study.

It is important to check your equipment after you acquire it to make sure it is complete and in running order. Do this in plenty of time to get it repaired if necessary. If you are using any equipment that has been around for some time, you would be well advised to get it serviced before you are going to use it, for example, to make sure that the rubber belts that drive the spindles of the tape recorder have not perished. Do a final check of your equipment immediately before you take it to the site. Check materials such as batteries, audiotapes and videotapes to make sure they are not defective. This is especially important if you have bought materials of lower quality. Check materials when they arrive to ensure there are sufficient copies and that all of the pages in such items as questionnaires are there.

Finally, ensure that you have a secure place to store your equipment and materials so that no-one else can borrow them, leaving your stock empty just when you need it.

Preparing questionnaire materials

You will need to get your questionnaires printed. You can use different coloured paper to identify different sites, or to differentiate the original from follow-up questionnaires, but coloured paper is more expensive than white paper. Be sure that you have proofread the questionnaire carefully before it goes to the printery. If your questionnaire is web-based or SMS-based, you will need to have the questionnaires formatted and loaded and a database of respondents set up and ready to go. This may be either an emailing list or a list of telephone numbers.

If you are doing a questionnaire survey you will need the names of the population so that you can access them. In some circumstances, you may need to construct your own mailing list, although this is time-consuming. Sometimes you can acquire a mailing list that has been already developed. Some organisations keep mailing lists of their memberships and may be willing to give you access to that membership for research purposes. If you need to request a mailing list do so in plenty of time to make other arrangements if your request is not granted. Many organisations will not give you a list of their members' names and addresses because they need to protect the privacy of their members, and prevent them from receiving too many mail requests. However, some of these will distribute your questionnaire packet to their members at your expense. There are also agencies with mailing lists for sale.

If you are selecting a random sample from your population, you will need to do so according to the principles outlined in Chapter 8. It is possible to arrange for a computer to select names randomly from the database, or to follow a set of instructions to select a strati-fied random sample. If you need to do this, you should make the appropriate arrangements with the institution involved. Be warned that there may be a charge for computer program-ming time for specialised requests. However, using a computer to randomise the sample has the advantages of being fast, eliminating investigator bias, and being able to generate multi-ple random samples from the same list without using the same name twice. There is a ran-dom number generating feature in Excel which can do this relatively easily.

The best way to address your questionnaire materials is by using sticky mailing labels generated by computer, especially if you need more than one set. There are computer pro-grams that will create a file that can be printed out on sticky mailing labels. These are worth the money if you have some computer expertise and if you have to do your own mailing list. If you are doing a set of labels, remember to do as many sets as you will need for the round. For example, you may need one set for envelopes and one set for postcards if you are using that system. If you are doing a follow-up round you will need another set of labels.

You will also need self-addressed envelopes for respondents to return the question-naires. You can either get them printed at a printery or use sticky labels, depending on the number. The most cost-effective way is to use reply paid post because you pay only for the actual returns.

Access to the site and participants

In most sites, it is mandatory to secure permission to collect data. The exception is a public place such as a street, where it is not strictly necessary to get permission. However, it is a good idea to let the police know what you are doing. This can save you trouble if somebody reports you as a person behaving strangely. Also, it is a good idea to let the police know if your study involves any approach to members of the public or impedance in the flow of pedestrians.

If you are doing research in a semi-public area, such as a shopping centre, a health clinic lobby, or a hospital waiting room, you must secure permission.

If you are doing research that involves access to a library beyond that to which you may be entitled, you will need to seek permission. Also remember that even in a library in which you are entitled to use the open collections there may be restrictions on access to rare books, theses and other valuable collections. Access to these may require advance negotiation.

Special conditions may apply to data collection in these areas; for example, some rare book rooms allow only pencils to be used for note-taking and the books must not be removed from the room.

You will need to write all necessary letters (or emails) concerning access to the site well before you are ready to carry out data collection. You will need the letters of permission before the time of data collection.

It is wise to make sure beforehand that the site is still there, still available and in a fit state to be used for your research. It would be disastrous for the data collectors to arrive on the appointed day only to find that the venue has vanished or been totally reorganised. If you are using a laboratory, you will need to book it well in advance and confirm the booking a week or two before your projected use.

Before you go to the site, and as part of preparation for your study, make sure that there are sufficient participants available for your project, including extras to provide for participant mortality. If you are in doubt, you may need to acquire access to a second setting that is similar to the first one.

Ensure that the clinicians in charge of your potential participants are going to allow you access. Before the time of data collection, you can write letters requesting access or go and see the clinicians if it is convenient. Involving clinicians in the study will improve access, particularly if they are influential. Often they will be happy to assist you, particularly if you reward them in some way, for example, with a box of chocolates, morning tea, or an inservice. However, sometimes clinical staff such as medical practitioners, nursing unit managers and clinicians caring for the client, may deny you access to their clients. They do so because they do not understand your project, they do not approve of it personally, or they are trying to protect 'their' clients from taking part in a research project.

Just before you are due to go into the site, check and make sure that the gatekeepers are still on side. You can follow up your initial letter with another letter, email or fax asking them to acknowledge that they know you are coming, or you can make a telephone call reminding the relevant people that you will be coming and when. A personal visit close to the time is ideal if you are near the site. You should also confirm that the person who arranged for your access is still in that position and is expecting you to come. If it is another person, you will have to brief them, send them copies of the earlier approvals, and hope that they will be cooperative. It is very important to do this in order to avoid the situation in which you arrive for your data collection, only to find, say, that the very helpful nursing unit manager has been replaced by an uncooperative one who thinks research is a waste of time.

Immediate preparation of the site

You will need to get into the laboratory or clinical field well in advance to check that your equipment can be placed where you want it. Set up your equipment and check that it actually works on site. You will also need to make sure that any special conditions that you require will be fulfilled, such as a specific temperature of the room.

If you are doing interviews, you will need to set up some mechanism to ensure privacy during the interviews. Strategies could include arranging to use a vacant office, making a sign for your office door, and arranging for someone else to answer the telephone if possible. You can also warn anyone who is likely to interrupt that you will not tolerate interruptions during this period. Check again that the tape recorder is working and that you have all the needed equipment such as extension cords, batteries, audiotapes and so forth.

Preparation of people

When preparing for data collection, it is also necessary to prepare the people involved including the gatekeepers, the staff in the clinical area or laboratory, the participants, and yourself, the researcher.

Staff

If you are using busy employees in any setting, remember to brief them in person, if possible – you could do one or more inservice sessions to explain your study and how it will affect the staff. In order to promote cooperation it is useful to prepare a resource folder about the study to leave in each participating area. This folder could contain any procedures, protocols, patient materials (such as informed consent document and plain language statement), and any relevant previous literature. Ensuring the cooperation of the staff is crucial to the success of a study.

Recruitment and preparation of participants

When you get to the site, in either a clinical or non-clinical situation, it is necessary to recruit participants to take part in the study. Depending on the design of your study, you may recruit clients, members of the public or colleagues. Each of these groups has inbuilt problems. Members of the public are often suspicious of strangers. Colleagues require special consideration if they are in a junior position to you to ensure that they do not feel compelled to take part in the study. Special care is needed with participants from another culture, and participants who do not understand English. Care is also needed with vulnerable people such as the elderly, and any special types of participants who cannot give informed consent on their own behalf. Procedures with these participants were discussed more fully in Chapter 5.

You may need to recruit all the participants at the beginning of the study or as you go along, depending on the design of the study. Recruitment is done either by you, the researcher, or by your colleagues on site. Recruitment is best done by someone involved in the study personally so that you can be sure that all possible potential participants are approached.

Personal contact, either by you or by colleagues assisting you with the research, is the best method of recruitment, especially when it is done one-on-one, because people find it harder to say no to you in person than they do to less personal methods. If personal contact is not possible because of distance, you can use a telephone call, fax, letter or email. It helps to use a personal touch if possible. When approaching clients, introduce yourself and give your credentials so that they understand with whom they are dealing. Remember that the system of identification of staff that is so clear to you as a nurse may be incomprehensible to the participants.

Remember that it always takes longer than you expect to get the required sample size. If recruitment is a problem, for example, where you do not have a captive pool of possible participants, you can advertise in suitable sites, such as the newspaper or, in the clinical setting, fliers. Another strategy is to offer some small reward for participation in the study; remember, this should be sufficient to recompense them for their time.

You may be unable to recruit enough participants. This can occur when your criteria are too restrictive – if so, you may need to re-examine them. Another problem of recruitment is occurring increasingly with general trends like shorter hospital stays for surgical operations and childbirth. This can both limit access to participants and decrease the number of potential data collection days for each participant. These influences have also resulted in fewer nursing staff, which means there is not enough time for them to assist with data collection.

One recruitment problem that can occur is that potential participants decline to participate in your study. Participants may refuse because of fear of invasive procedures required, disillusionment with research, or poor health status. Some may have been discouraged by staff who have criticised the project.

As a part of the recruitment process, you need to have procedures in place to ensure that you avoid generating a biased sample. It is necessary to approach all of the selected potential participants at a suitable time, for example, when they are not heavily medicated. Explain the study in plain, simple language, avoiding the use of jargon. Most ethics committees require that you give the potential participant a statement to read that has already been approved. It is a good idea to give the potential participant time to consider participating in the study by leaving the information and coming back later for an answer. After the potential participant has consented to participate, you will need to get the consent form signed.

In making arrangements to collect your data in the clinical area it is wise to consider nursing care and other routines. With regard to individual clients you will need to consider their specific scheduled care and their conscious state. Be flexible in arranging times and rescheduling times for data collection if necessary.

Prior to collecting the data, it may be necessary to allocate participants randomly to treatment and control groups. For two groups, this can be done by a coin toss. Because you almost never end up with equal numbers of heads and tails, you will need to toss the coin about 20 per cent more times than the number of names you need to allocate. List the results of each throw. If you throw more heads than tails, say, you need to keep tossing and listing till you get enough tails. Between the first and last tail that you need, you may find too many heads, so you have to keep tossing and listing till you have equal numbers of heads and tails. You keep the part of the list that has the equal numbers and disregard the rest. You then match your list of heads and tails to your list of names to assign the participants to the two groups.

To cope with two or more groups, you can put all the names, or numbers representing participants, in a hat. The first name or number drawn out goes in the first group, the second into the second group and so forth. Another method is to write each name on a card, then shuffle the cards well and 'deal' them into as many groups as you need.

If you are using a list of random numbers or heads and tails, you allocate the participants according to your list. You can do this effectively by numbering envelopes and putting a slip in each envelope that tells participants which group they were assigned to. Each new recruit is given the next envelope in the sequence.

Researcher and data collectors

It is also necessary to prepare yourself and your data collectors for the data collection. You should ensure that anyone collecting data is sufficiently practised with the equipment and materials to ensure a smooth running process during the actual data collection. You can practise trial interviews or application of instruments on friends or colleagues. Multiple data collectors must practise until they achieve inter-rater reliability. Brief data collectors about procedures, but to prevent biased data do not tell them about an expected outcome.

In preparing yourself for data collection you should remind yourself to be cooperative at all times with the clinical area. Remember that you will be there as a guest and that you are a representative of your institution. Recognise that the client care takes priority over your research needs.

It is a good idea if you are a student or if you are acting as a clinical staff member to ensure that the research activity is covered by the professional indemnity insurance of your employer or university. This is particularly important if you are using any invasive equipment or if there is any potential for harm to the participants.

Make sure that any travel and accommodation arrangements are made well in advance.

EXERCISE

In your workplace you want to survey staff regarding aggression and violence towards them. List three ways you collect data:

1 _____
2 _____
3 _____

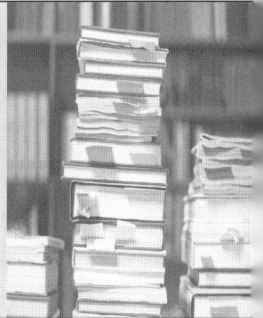

Preparation for data management

You will probably have to do some preparation for the management of your data once you get it; for example, learn how to operate any data analysis software, draw up coding sheets if you are using them, set up computer files for your data and allocate participant numbers to the data. Preparing for data entry also involves testing all of your procedures on the computer prior to entering real data.

The process of data collection

Data collection can take place using a variety of methods, which have been discussed in Chapter 8 and earlier in this chapter. Obviously, how you collect data will depend on which method you are using since different methods will require different techniques. You can safely anticipate that the data collection phase of the study will take longer than you expected and be more difficult than you anticipated, and will require adjustments during the process.

We will talk about some of the general principles of data collection and problems that may occur. We will then proceed to discuss some of the specific techniques of the more common quantitative methods, such as questionnaires, content analysis, structured observation, and using existing data sources. General observation and interviewing techniques will be discussed in Chapter 15 on qualitative data collection.

Managing equipment and materials

Various types of equipment can be used to collect quantitative data, depending on the design of the study, for example, biophysical instruments, audiotape recorders, videotape recorders and computers. Treatment and use of the equipment will vary, depending on what it is. Of course, all equipment should be treated with respect. Whatever hardware you are using, you must make sure that it is kept in top condition during the course of the data collection. It should be given whatever regular maintenance is suggested by the manufacturer. For example, recording heads on audiotape or videotape recorders should be cleaned regularly.

If you are using a computer in data collection, it is likely to be either a laptop into which you can type your data directly, or a computer that is an integral part of another instrument. A computer may also be interfaced with a bioinstrument so that the instrument inputs data directly into the computer. In a study by Berry et al. (2004) a computerised symptom and quality-of-life assessment tool for patients with cancer was used and found to be technically possible and to have a number of benefits over interview procedures.

Some of the advantages of computerised data collection are increased reliability and accuracy, ability to collect larger pools of data, and time and cost savings in recording and coding. The disadvantages are the need for increased space, a lengthy set-up time, focus on the machine rather than on the client and possible measurement error related to the computer.

If you are using computers during the process of data collection, you should ensure that the data are put in correctly and completely. You should also ensure that you have procedures in place to protect against loss at any time during the process. The computer must be protected against power surges if it is plugged into the mains; if necessary, use a surge protector in the line. If you are using batteries, make sure that the batteries give sufficient power for the period of data collection. Save the file at least every 10 minutes using an automatic save function if you have one. Make frequent backup copies of your files using whatever system you normally use, store them in safe places, and update them regularly.

Distribution of questionnaires

You can distribute questionnaires by several methods – the more personal the contact with the respondents, the higher rate of response you are likely to get, all else being equal.

You can deliver questionnaires personally to a nearby site. Then you can distribute them yourself to clients or nurses, or to a contact person to distribute for you. If you are using a self-selected convenience sample you can leave the questionnaires in a box with a flier asking people to take them. Personal delivery to the individual or the site may entail some travel costs to get to the group but this is balanced by a saving in postage.

Using a web-based or SMS-based survey design will deliver questionnaires in electronic format directly to either a participant's computer or mobile phone. This is obviously a very effective means of reaching people, and allows an easy means of responding to them.

If you are sending the questionnaires all over Australia or even overseas, postal delivery or email will be necessary. You can identify a contact person at the site to distribute them, and then send them to that person by post or email. Or you can send them individually by post or by email. You can even administer them by telephone or fax, which saves on the cost of postage but incurs the cost of a telephone call.

Whatever method you choose, you will need to be consistent in the distribution in order to even out external influences. That is, you should distribute them all using the same method and close together in time. You should send them all to the recipients' homes or all to their work, but not mix them.

If you are distributing your questionnaire by email to a list you will have no postage costs for either distribution or return but you may have sending and downloading costs if you are paying a commercial provider. You need to weigh the reduced cost against the quality of the sample. That is, the people on a list may not be representative of the characteristics of the population that you wish to sample. Instructions to people on email lists should include an instruction to return the reply to the individual researcher, not to the whole list. Your instructions should include in a prominent place the method of changing the address to the researcher rather than just hitting the reply button, which will send the reply back to the whole list. If the whole list can read the response, the confidentiality of the respondents is destroyed. If you send it out over the Listserver, everyone, including yourself, will get a copy but no-one will be aware of anyone but themselves receiving the information. Getting your own copy by email from a Listserver is a good way of checking that the message actually went out to the list.

If you are compiling your own list of email addresses to which you wish to send your questionnaire, it is a good idea to select the 'Blind CC' in the header of the email. This conceals the identity of other recipients of the questionnaire. In this case, of course, replies will come back directly to you as you have not sent them out over a Listserver.

Managing the site

If you are collecting data in the field, it is important to try to keep the site as conducive as possible to smooth data collection. Make sure there are no interruptions. Just before you commence an interview, take your telephone off the hook, turn off your mobile telephone and disconnect any beepers. Also ask your interviewee to turn off any mobile phone or beeper.

Collecting data on site can give rise to problems. The worst possible problem is a catastrophic change in the site during the time of data collection, for example a flood, fire, cyclone or earthquake destroying the site. Almost as bad are unforeseen institutional factors such as changes of policy that affect your study, industrial action, unplanned closure or re-organisation of a clinical area, transfer of cooperative staff out of the unit and transfer of uncooperative staff into the unit. If you are using available data, there may be a loss of charts that you were going to audit or the charts may be incomplete. Current trends in 'downsizing' mean changes in institutional structures are not unusual. However, if you are lucky, they will be planned long enough in advance for you to adapt to them. If a disaster happens, you will have to decide whether you have enough data to make a worthwhile study. Alternatively, if you have partial data, you could cut your losses and use the collected data as a **pilot study**, finding another site for the main study.

Managing the participants

The way to manage the participants during the data collection phase is to keep them onside. Treat participants well – you are dependent on them for your data. Remember, they are not compelled to participate and they can withdraw at any time. It is important to put participants at ease as much as possible during the data collection by introducing yourself, reminding the participant of the purposes and procedures of the research, and chatting briefly about other things just to break the ice.

There may be problems with the sample that has been recruited – it may be subject to participant mortality or loss of participants from the study. Some people agree to participate and then fail to show up for the interview or do not do the questionnaire. Try phoning the day before to remind them of the interview. Sometimes clients in the clinical field are transferred to another ward or facility or discharged before your study is complete. It is a good idea to maintain regular contact with clients and keep note of their home address so that if this happens you can arrange perhaps to collect the data later.

Even if participants complete the study, some produce unusable data, such as obviously flippant or insincere responses to interview questions, leaving lots of blanks on questionnaires or failing to cooperate with clinical procedures integral to your study. Any of these can render those parts of the data useless.

If these things happen and your sample gets smaller, you can spend longer to achieve an adequate sample, you can live with the smaller sample or you can re-evaluate your criteria. If you need to live with a smaller sample you must take the sample size into consideration when analysing the results.

Managing colleagues

The people on the data collection site must be managed as well. It is important to treat them well, because you are dependent on their cooperation also. Several ways of facilitating the study by interacting with the staff have been mentioned already in this chapter. It is important to continue these overtures and keep the staff onside. Perhaps make a contribution to morning tea or make other small gestures that show your appreciation for the opportunity to collect data.

Despite your best efforts, however, sometimes the staff will make it difficult for you to collect data. They can unwittingly do things that interfere with your data collection.

Even worse, they can sabotage your project. They can unintentionally or intentionally 'forget' to notify you of suitable prospective participants, they can schedule other activities that interfere with data collection or they can fail to carry out properly the procedures that are crucial to your research.

Sometimes staff factors outside their control interfere, such as horrendously busy spells, roster changes and so forth. If an increased workload occurs, naturally the staff will give a higher priority to the nursing care than to your research. Keep an eye out for these kinds of problems and deal with them by strategies such as educating the staff, inducting new people into the project, securing the support of local managers, taking over more of the data collection activity or modifying your protocols. It is important to give regular feedback to the staff concerning your project but do not give so much feedback that it influences your data in some way.

Managing the process

It is important to manage the process so that you get accurate, complete data. The importance of accuracy applies both to the measurement and to the recording of data. You or your colleagues as data collectors must be very well versed in the procedures to achieve this goal. Even then, unplanned errors can occur. You might forget to turn on the microphone of the tape recorder or you might overwrite an interview tape, thinking it is blank. Have procedures in place to prevent this sort of thing, such as routine checking and labelling of tapes before using them. In some methods, such as questionnaires, the accuracy will depend on the participant carrying out the procedure correctly, or giving the correct answers.

Sometimes researchers come up against a conflict of interest or ethical problem during the course of data collection. You might be trying to collect data as a participant observer and find that you have to choose between two functions that are both equally important. It has also been known for a researcher to discover an abuse of clients during the course of data collection. This poses a dilemma, because if the researcher blows the whistle, the institution and/or staff will probably cease to cooperate with the study and the data collection at that facility will be ruined. On the other hand, not to report the abuse would be unethical because it would harm the clients. Client safety must take precedence over research outcomes, but if it is possible to negotiate with the staff that the behaviour stops, the research project may be saved. See Chapter 5 for more discussion on this issue.

Keep track of events that may affect your data. We mentioned in Chapter 8 the threat to validity of historical factors. Sometimes unforeseen events could affect the staff on whom you are collecting data, for example, the death of a colleague or a favourite client. If this happens, you may need to suspend data collection until things have settled down.

Monitoring the process

In every project, no matter how small, it is important to keep track of the process: that is, to keep records of what steps you have taken. It is important to keep a written record, a logbook, so that you are not dependent on your memory. Memory can be unreliable, especially over the longer periods of time involved in a large project such as a thesis. Record-keeping can be done in a simple fashion for a small project by writing in an exercise book, ideally one with divided sections to keep track of the different parts of your project. For larger projects, it may be worth keeping records on a spreadsheet, or even a computer program designed for project management. You should record a 'diary' of your visits – dates, length, impressions and problems that you encountered. Record what data you collected on each occasion. Record your expenses for future reference, and keep receipts. These records will assist you when it is time to write up the procedures for the study.

Check the entries in the logbook regularly to make sure that things are going to plan. It is crucial to ensure that the appropriate steps of the data collection process, such as collecting protocols and making telephone calls, are carried out. It is important to document the arrival of data. It is also important to identify any intervening variables that have not been accounted for, and to monitor their effect or revise your data collection plan.

Aftercare

Your data collection process is not complete until you have taken care of the cleaning-up process. It is necessary to clean and repair any equipment and return it to its owner if it is borrowed. Leave the laboratory or clinical site at least as good as you found it, if not better. Thank the staff of a clinical site in some creative way, and offer to send a summary report of your findings and any publications that ensue.

One of the most important things to do is to prevent loss of data from natural disasters, such as flood or fire, or human intervention, such as theft. The usual way is to make a set of backups and store them away from the place where your data are held.

EXERCISE

If you are using a questionnaire to gather data, list three ways that you could distribute and collect it:

1 _____

2 _____

3 _____

Management of data and products of analysis
Logging the data

It is extremely important to keep good records of your data. Each piece of data should be clearly labelled and recorded. Each piece of data, whether it is a questionnaire, audiotape, videotape or rhythm strip, should be assigned some sort of code number or name to be used in all data pertaining to that item. A separate list of the code numbers and participant names, if any, should be kept in the logbook.

It is also important to monitor the quality and completeness of the data. Each piece of data should be checked for accuracy and completeness so that you can collect more data at the time if necessary.

Consider making a copy of all data, regardless of their format, and storing them in another secure place at a distance from the primary copy. This is important, at least until you have completed the objectives of the study, for example getting your degree. Making copies may be expensive, but it is less costly than collecting all of the data again if the originals are lost or destroyed.

A code book should be kept, either in an exercise book or on a computer program. The code book should show a map of the variables, including in which column they are in the database, the name used for each variable and element and, in the case of a program such as SPSS, how many columns each variable occupies. For more detail on the construction of code books, see Burns and Grove (2005).

Your original data must be stored in a secure place in the institution for a set period of time. This requirement of the NHMRC is implemented by the institutional ethics committee of the university, hospital, or other institution under whose auspices you are doing the project. You should be aware of the regulations of your institution. (These restrictions would not apply to storage of data for short undergraduate research courses whose purpose is to teach about research rather than to conduct actual studies. They would apply, however, to data for honours and postgraduate theses.) The main purpose of storing the data is to allow for investigation of fraud, should it be necessary. In any case, it is worthwhile to store data to enable further analysis. The period of time for which the data must be stored may vary from institution to institution but is usually five years after publication. Consult your supervisor about data storage.

Processing data for analysis

Some data do not require any processing because they can be analysed directly from their original form. Some data require a small amount of processing, for example writing code numbers on questionnaires. Some data require a large amount of processing, for example converting text units to numbers. Most methods of data collection require the researcher to transform the raw data in some way so that they can be transferred easily from the data source into a computer data analysis program. The principle is to process the data sufficiently to facilitate data analysis. The method of analysis will determine the preparation that will need to be done.

Some data that have already been put into a computer may not require any further preparation. For example, if you are using a database that has been input into a computer already you will only have to transfer the data into your own program for analysis. Similarly, some researchers can enter their data straight into a portable computer in the field or laboratory either directly from an instrument that is hooked up to the computer, or by means of the data collector typing the data into the computer keyboard. Questionnaires that have been prepared and responded to in such a way that they can be directly scanned into a computer can be entered into the computer easily. Burns and Grove (2005) provide a useful discussion of the issues around electronic scanning.

If the data are on audiotape, most researchers prefer to have the audiotapes transcribed into word processor text before analysing the data, particularly if they are analysing the meaning of the text. Transcription of audiotapes can be done by the researcher, a research assistant or a typist who has the requisite skills. If you are planning to do much of it yourself, it is well worth acquiring a dictaphone-type audiocassette player with foot controls and automatic rewind. These features allow you to keep your hands on the keyboard and retain your place in the tape when you pause.

If you are using videotapes, they will need to be edited and the shots you are using identified using a coding system.

Most questionnaires will require some coding. Coding is the process that usually renders the data into numbers that can be entered into your database in a form in which they can be analysed easily. Data can be from open-ended questionnaires that require a lot of researcher coding, to pre-coded questionnaires that require minimal coding. For example, on a pre-coded questionnaire, the respondent must tick one of four boxes, numbered 1–4, to answer a question. The researcher enters the number into that person's data entry for that question. To illustrate, the answer 'never married' could be given a code of '1', married '2', de facto '3' and divorced '4'. Actual numbers, for example the person's age in years, temperature or oxygen saturation, do not need to be coded. Sometimes data will be from open-ended questions on questionnaires or from text that is for content analysis. If you wish to quantify these data, you will have to develop a coding schema to handle it.

The process of coding can be done in two ways. The first method is to code directly from the data source. With questionnaires, some people like to write the code on each questionnaire and some prefer to code straight into the computer. The amount of transformation of data required depends on how the questionnaire has been constructed in the first place. If it is pre-coded by putting the numbers on the questionnaire, then there is little coding to do at this stage. The second method is to code the data onto a coding sheet and then enter it into the database from the coding sheet. Both of these methods have advantages and disadvantages. Coding directly from the data source is faster and avoids transcription errors that arise from the double-handling of the data, but is more prone to errors of data entry. The coding sheet method speeds up the data entry process and increases its accuracy but is more prone to errors of transcription during the coding process.

Direct data entry

If you are coding straight into the computer file, you must set it up first so that it will accept the data. A database file is usually a matrix of rows and columns, which intersect to form cells. Each row of the matrix is one person's data, while each column is one variable or answer to one question of the questionnaire. Thus, reading across a row will give you a participant's data, while reading down a column will give you every person's data on that one variable. You should head each of the columns with the variable name or its abbreviation to make it easier for you to recognise the variable. In addition, always put at the beginning of the row a participant number that is also on the raw data. Do not use the database row numbers instead of participant numbers. If you sort the data, the database numbers will not change with the data.

All programs will need to be instructed what your variable names are and what the values of the elements that comprise the variables are: for example, '1' equals 'never married' and so forth. Some data analysis programs let you type in the actual element name or part of it, such as 'n' for 'never married', 'm' for 'married', 'di' for divorced, 'de' for de facto and so forth. However, even though you type them in as names and they appear as names on the monitor, the computer stores them as numbers. It is useful to have a logical structure for the element labels of the variables, for example yes = '1', no = '0'. This will help later in interpreting your data correctly. It is particularly important where the variable has an underlying numerical structure, for example the Likert Scale. It is vital to keep to the same code as a pre-coded questionnaire when you are entering data in order to avoid errors in data entry. If necessary, you can recode the data later. An example of a print-out from a database is shown in Table 9.1.

When you have set up your data file in the computer, you are ready to enter the data. This is part of the drudgery of research, but a necessary part. You will have to decide whether to go for speed or accuracy.

Using coding sheets

If you are using a separate coding sheet, it is very important to make it the same structure as the computer file into which the data will be put, for ease of transfer. A blank coding sheet would look much like the print-out shown in Table 9.1, only without data.

It is crucial to check the finished coding sheet against the raw data. If there is only a small amount, you should check it all. If there is a large amount, you can check 10 per cent

Table 9.1 Print-out of data in database

Participant	Gender	Age	Marital status	Religion	Education
1	M	30	Married	Prot	Yr 10
2	F	25	Nevmar	RC	Yr 12
3	F	43	Div	Prot	Yr 12
4	F	64	Nevmar	Buddhist	Uni deg
5	M	36	De facto	Prot	TAFE cert/dip
6	M	29	Div	Nil	Yr 10
7	F	21	Nevmar	Muslim	Yr 12
8	M	19	Married	Nil	Uni deg
9	M	53	De facto	RC	Yr 12

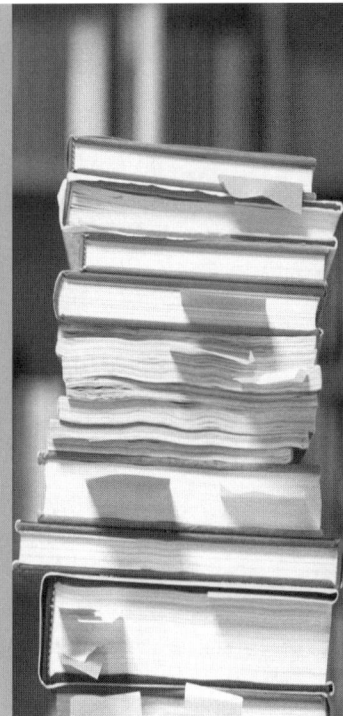

at random. If it is error-free, you could assume that the rest will probably be too, and decide to live with any errors.

During the processes of data coding and data entry, it is very important to ensure that they are done consistently. Changes can occur in the data because the data coder changed the code part way through coding or direct data entry. This should be resisted, but if it happens, the previous coding will have to be rectified so that it is consistent with the new code. Another source of disparity is the use of two or more different data coders. If this is the case, they should all be asked to code one section and the consistency of the coding should be checked. The accuracy rate should be one that you can live with, but it must be at least 90 per cent.

It is also extremely important to ensure accuracy during the process of data coding and data entry. If, for example, you have complicated procedures that require special care during coding and entry, you must check even more carefully. One example is that in a long questionnaire, the order of items may be reversed in half of the copies to control for respondent fatigue. Extreme caution must be exercised to make sure that all of the answers to each item are in the correct column.

Missing values are a problem that every researcher will have to deal with at some time. These occur where for some reason the data are missing: for example, a respondent has not given an answer for a question. If a whole section of data is consistently missing, you cannot enter any of it. For example, if you are collecting data on each of three days after childbirth, and most of the mothers have gone home on the second day, you can delete all data for the third day.

Some data analysis programs have a mechanism for handling missing values, giving them a code or not using that case in the data analysis. If your variable is numerical, it is important not to put zero for a missing value as this will lower the value of the mean. You can either leave it missing or put in the median value.

After the data have been entered into the computer, it is vital to proofread them. Your final results are only as good as your data. You can check them against the original source, or against the coding sheet if it has been proofread. There are various ways of doing this. One is to do it yourself; however, this does not eliminate potential for error. A better way is for two people to do it, one reading from the coding sheet and one reading from the computer print-out or monitor. Finally, some computer programs have a facility for double entry of data and checking both entries against each other and giving you a list of the mismatches. It is important to check the data for errors such as missing data, missing lines, or values that are higher or lower than those stipulated in the code.

Manipulating data

During the process of data analysis, it is almost always the case that you will want to change your data in some way. This can involve such operations as combining variables, recoding variables to change the values, applying a weighting to a variable and/or applying mathematical formulas. It is crucial to double-check that the conversion has been done correctly by checking the input with the output. If you have carried out these operations incorrectly, your data will be meaningless. Whenever you change your data, it is mandatory to note this in your logbook or record it in some way. Do not rely on your memory. When you have finished any changes and are satisfied with the result, it is imperative to make a fresh backup copy, renaming the file. Older versions of your data should be kept in an archive, either on a floppy disk or as hard copy. You should always keep backup copies of the original computer data as well as your working copy of the transformed data.

Managing the products of data analysis

When you begin to generate your data analysis, you will need to organise it in some way. A data analysis program will generate the analysis. Most programs generate output files that can be saved on your computer, or you can create a word processor file and copy the data analysis into it. These methods allow you to organise the data analysis and save it. You normally print the data analysis that you want to keep, either from an output or word processor file. The word processor file can also serve as a backup copy of the hard copy so that if you lose the hard copy you will not have to redo the analysis.

If you want to store hard copy of the data analysis, you will need to organise some sort of system. Normally, hard copy will be generated on ordinary A4 paper that can be put into an ordinary ring binder, possibly with plastic document protectors and section dividers if it becomes large enough to warrant separation into sections.

EXERCISE

Design a spreadsheet with columns and rows, where each column represents a variable and each row represents a participant. Think of four demographic variables (e.g. age, gender, residence, income) and four health variables (e.g. chronic illness, smoking, alcohol use, body mass index) that might be entered into this spreadsheet. What kinds of codes might be necessary to be able to enter these variables?

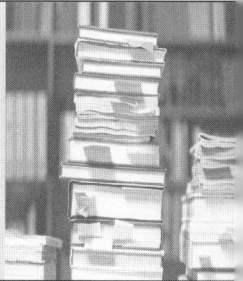

Pilot study

A pilot study is a mini-replica of a research project and is designed to test all aspects of it prior to commencement of the full study. It is a small-scale version of the study that goes in advance, incorporating all aspects of the procedures of the main study and providing guidance for the larger study. Thus, it is like a pilot ship, a small ship that navigates a difficult, dangerous or unknown route ahead of an ocean liner in order to lead the ship safely along its course. The pilot study can also be thought of as similar to the test piloting of a new aeroplane before production models are put into service. An example of a pilot study can be seen in Herrington, Olomu and Geller (2004), where salivary cortisol was collected from preterm infants in order to determine pain levels.

There is a difference in purpose, however, between a pilot study and a main study. The purpose of a pilot study is to identify strengths and weaknesses in the research plan in order to improve the main study, whereas the purpose of a main study is to develop knowledge. Also, the pilot study is carried out on a much smaller scale than the main study.

A pilot study should be carried out in such a way as to be as close as possible to the real thing. It should, if possible, be carried out in the actual setting in which the main study will be conducted. It should use the actual procedures proposed for the main study, including such things as obtaining informed consent. It should use the same type of participants.

As a researcher, you will need to consider whether or not a pilot study is necessary in your circumstances. Experienced researchers who are very familiar with techniques and have done previous similar research may be able to forego a pilot study. Most readers of this book, however, are unlikely to be in that category. The other exception is if you are a student doing a small undergraduate student project. The reasons for this are that the major purpose of such an exercise is to learn about research rather than to produce new knowledge, and that the time frame for this type of study is usually very short. However, in the real world of research, researchers do not do pilot studies frequently enough. This may be attributed to a small amount of perceived benefit for the amount of effort. As a researcher, you should incorporate at least one pilot study in the research plan of any substantial study. It may seem like a lot of fuss and bother to do a pilot study when one has designed the perfect research study with which nothing can possibly go wrong, but most researchers can tell you stories of studies – either where they did not do a pilot study and wished they had, or where they were glad that they did. It is a wise expenditure of time and money because it can save time and money later and prevent potentially devastating mistakes.

One major purpose of a pilot study is to assess the feasibility of the main study so that you can correct any problems. A pilot study will allow you to assess whether your study design is adequate. You can see whether the methodology is going to work. You can evaluate such things as the recruitment of participants, the sampling technique, the appropriateness and effectiveness of the procedures, the timeframe and the costs. You can also see whether the instruments are going to work, and if not, choose an alternative. You can see whether you need any extra equipment that you might not have anticipated. Testing the proposed study will help to identify any unanticipated variables and allow you to consider their impact on the study and ways of dealing with them. If the study design is not adequate you can repair it before you carry out the main study. It is not ethical to conduct studies that are badly flawed or to collect data that have no chance of being valid. The NHMRC requires that 'Every research proposal must demonstrate that the research is justifiable in terms of its potential contribution to knowledge and is based on a thorough study of current literature as well as prior observation, approved previous studies, and where relevant, laboratory and animal studies' (NHMRC 2001). A properly functioning ethics committee will not allow a research project to proceed where the design is obviously flawed.

Another major purpose of a pilot study is to allow the researcher or data collectors to practise with the equipment, techniques and procedures with actual participants, in the real setting. This will give confidence to the personnel conducting the research, allowing the main study to progress smoothly. It will also inspire confidence in the participants and allow multiple data collectors to achieve inter-rater reliability.

You can also assess the reaction of the people involved in the research project. You can see if your participants have understood the instructions and observe their reaction to the instruments. You can assess the efficacy of your recruitment procedures and you should find out how many participants you can expect to drop out. If it is a clinical project, you can also monitor the reaction of the staff in the setting and address any problems that arise, for example the impact of the project on any routines of nursing care. Finally, you can check the reaction of the researchers and data collectors to the project, addressing any problems that arise and incorporating any suggestions for improvement.

A pilot study will allow you to assess the adequacy of your data and adjust any instrumentation appropriately. You should enter your pilot data into your proposed data analysis program and assess the data entry procedures. You should analyse the pilot data, using the techniques that you propose to use in the main study, so that you can determine if you have collected the most appropriate form or level of data. You can save time and money if you revise or eliminate questionnaires that do not work.

After you have carried out the pilot study to the point of data analysis, you should evaluate your methodology. If you make major changes, you should do a second pilot study. Finally, you should write up the pilot study. The process of analysis involved will force you to evaluate the pilot study thoroughly.

The results of a pilot study are not normally included in the main results. The reason for this is that historical events and changes made between the pilot study and the main study may render the pilot data different from those of the main study and therefore unable to be incorporated into it. If there have been no changes and if you are short of participants, you may include the pilot data in your results.

It is also not customary to publish results of a pilot study; however, there have been some exceptions such as Brown (2003) and Thapar et al. (2004).

When you have carried out your pilot study and revised your research plan accordingly, you are ready to commence data collection for your main study.

Summary

In this chapter, we have covered the main points in the process of data collection and management. We have focused on strategies for managing equipment and materials, participants, staff and colleagues. We have looked at processing data, coding data, setting up computer files, data entry and managing the products of data analysis. We have explained the importance of running a pilot study as a 'dress rehearsal' for your main study. Having collected and processed your data, you can now take the next step of quantitative data analysis.

Main points

- Data are what the researcher collects in order to answer the research question. The data will be congruent with the design and there may be more than one form of data.
- In quantitative designs, data are almost always numbers or something that is converted to numbers.
- In preparing for data collection and management, the researcher sets up a data collection plan; selects and obtains the equipment and materials; prepares the participants, setting and self; and ensures arrangements for insurance, travel and accommodation are made.

- The researcher gains access to the site and the participants by securing written permission from gatekeepers where necessary.
- Immediately before collecting data, the researcher checks the equipment on site, and the site conditions. The gatekeepers and staff are also briefed.
- Data collectors are given the necessary training.
- Participants are recruited from relevant groups such as clients, the public and colleagues, with special care to cultural safety and language considerations. Plain language statements are given out and consent forms are signed before data are collected.
- In planning times of data collection, consider nursing care and other routines in the clinical area, be flexible in arranging times and reschedule if necessary.
- In preparation for data management, learn how to operate any data analysis software, draw up any coding sheets and set up computer files.
- Treat your equipment with respect, consider safety aspects and ensure regular maintenance.
- Questionnaires can be distributed by various methods, with personal contact offering the best response rates.
- When on site collecting data, ensure there are no interruptions; try to anticipate problems and forestall them.
- When dealing with participants, be polite, brief them, ensure good lines of communication and keep to your commitment of time.
- When dealing with your colleagues, be considerate, keep them informed and remember that client care takes precedence over research.
- Keep a logbook of visits and data collection procedures.
- After data collection, clean and repair any equipment, leave things as you found them and thank those who helped you.
- Implement sound procedures for handling, entering and analysing data and dealing with the products of data analysis. Ensure that you have backups.
- A pilot study is a small-scale, dress rehearsal for the main study, incorporating all aspects of the main study's procedures. It is done to find strengths and weaknesses of methods, to assess feasibility, to practise with equipment and procedures, to assess the reaction of researchers and data collectors, to assess the adequacy of data and to then adjust the methods appropriately.
- A pilot study should be done in an environment as close as possible to the real thing, in the actual setting for the main study, using the actual proposed procedures and the same type of participants.

CASE STUDY

You are interested in conducting a trial of an anger management program for young adolescent men.

Discussion questions:

1 Describe how you would obtain access to a data collection site for this study.
2 How could you allocate participants to groups randomly, so that they could be compared?
3 If you were using standardised questionnaires, how could you distribute and collect them?
4 What information should you enter into a logbook over the course of this study?
5 What would be the advantages of a pilot study prior to undertaking the main study? What might it tell you?

Multiple choice questions

1 Data are:
   a always numbers
   b numbers or words
   c the same as statistics
   d none of the above

2 In quantitative research, data are:
   a almost always numbers
   b often converted into numbers
   c collected to answer the research question
   d all of the above

3 The coding process includes:
   a creating categorical data from unstructured qualitative data
   b transcribing questionnaires into different languages
   c removing some data from a database for security reasons
   d all of the above

4 Code books are used:
   a instead of spreadsheets in some research
   b to keep a record of how data are transformed and handled
   c to present to ethics committees when the research is finished
   d so that participants can remain anonymous

5 Data collection cannot commence until:
   a ethics approval has been granted
   b consent by participants has been given
   c local gatekeepers have given permission
   d all of the above

6 Response rates to questionnaires are best when:
  a online surveys are used
  b reply-paid envelopes are provided
  c personal contact is made with participants
  d they are done via computers instead of paper
7 A logbook is used in research:
  a to keep names and contact details of all participants
  b to keep records of all expenses incurred in the research
  c to keep records of the research process and procedures
  d all of the above
8 Computerised data management allows:
  a data manipulation
  b quick data analysis and summary
  c easy presentation of findings
  d all of the above
9 Backing up a research database ensures:
  a data will not be lost
  b it can be accessed by others
  c no data are manipulated incorrectly
  d none of the above
10 Pilot studies may help to:
  a determine how difficult it is for participants to comply with protocols
  b determine the time needed for data collection with each participant
  c identify problems with the procedures
  d all of the above

Online reading

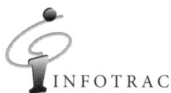

INFOTRAC

INFOTRAC® COLLEGE EDITION
Access information using the following keywords to retrieve information relating to quantitative methods:
➤ coding sheets
➤ data collection
➤ data entry
➤ logging data
➤ manipulating data
➤ participants
➤ pilot study
➤ processing data
➤ questionnaire
➤ site

References

Berry, D., Trigg, L., Lober, W., Karras, B., Galligan, M., Austin-Seymour, M. & Martin, S. 2004, 'Computerized symptom and quality-of-life assessment for patients with cancer part I: development and pilot testing', *Oncology Nursing Forum*, vol. 31, no. 5, 75–83.

Brown, D. 2003, 'Comparing different ulcer measurement techniques: a pilot study', *Primary Intention*, vol. 11, no. 3, 125–30.

Burns, N. & Grove, S. 2005, *The Practice of Nursing Research: Conduct, Critique and Utilisation*, Elsevier, St. Louis, Missouri.

Herrington C., Olomu I. & Geller S. 2004, 'Salivary cortisol as indicators of pain in preterm infants: a pilot study', *Clinical Nursing Research*, vol. 13, no. 1, 53–68.

NHMRC 2001, *Human Research Ethics Handbook: Commentary on the National Statement on Ethical Conduct in Research Involving Humans*, AGPS, Canberra.

SPSS 1999, *SPSS 10.0 Syntax Reference Guide*, SPSS Inc., Chicago.

Thapar, N., Warner, G., Drainoni, M., Williams, S., Ditchfield, H., Wierbicky, J. & Nesathurai, S. 2004, 'A pilot study of functional access to public buildings and facilities for persons with impairments', *Disability and Rehabilitation*, vol. 26, no. 5, 280–9.

CHAPTER 10

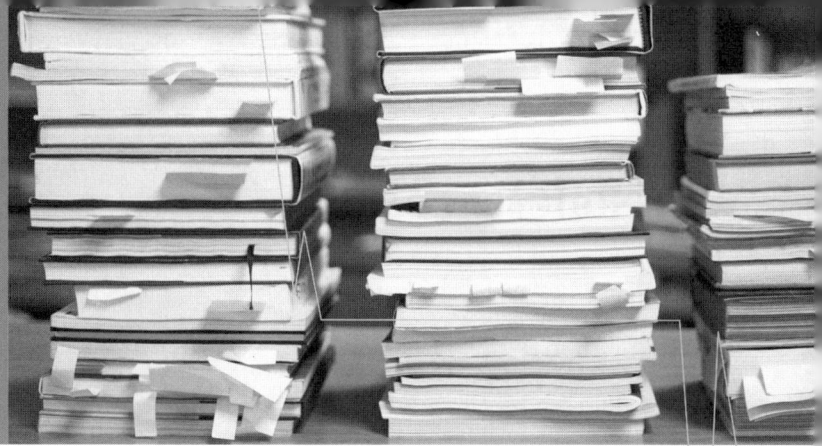

QUANTITATIVE DATA ANALYSIS

CHAPTER OBJECTIVES

The material presented in this chapter will assist you to:

- understand the difference between descriptive and inferential statistics
- describe the various types of data and scales of measurement
- interpret the meaning of common statistical tests
- choose an appropriate statistical test for an hypothesis
- describe patterns in your data.

Introduction to data

The purpose of this chapter is to introduce some beginning concepts of analysing quantitative data. Whether you actually carry out quantitative research or just read about it, you will need to know something about quantitative data analysis and how it is done. You will also need to understand something about statistics because researchers use them routinely to present information about quantitative data.

Data can come in many forms. They can be numbers, words or even objects. It is important to know what type of data you are dealing with as a researcher, because this will determine how you analyse them, and how you may or may not find answers to the research question you are asking.

Cases

In a research project, every participant is a 'case'. If you are studying cigarette smokers, every smoker in your research study is a case. Cases do not always consist of data about people. They might consist of data about hospitals, plots of land or streets. In international economic research, cases may be as large as whole nations. In molecular biology research, a case may be as small as a single gene.

Variables

The information we have in each case – the person's name and the number of cigarettes he/she smokes per day – are referred to as variables. They are called variables because their actual nature varies from case to case. One person might be 47 years old, for instance, while another is 28 – hence the variation. Because not all research is about people, some variables might relate to other types of cases, such as numbers of car accidents in the last year, crop yields, or numbers of dog attacks on postal deliverers.

Data

The value of a variable for a particular case is referred to as a datum (singular), and the values for all cases in a sample are referred to as data (plural). Data refer to the actual measurements taken, or information collected during the research. Data can have many different forms.

Types of data and scales of measurement

A scale is a 'measuring stick' or standard reference for comparison of measurements between cases. Measurement is the assignment of numbers or codes to observations of phenomena. Different types of data are measured on different scales. It is important to know exactly what type of data you are collecting and the scale on which you are measuring your variable because this will determine what type of data analysis you can carry out.

Data occur in two broad groups – qualitative and quantitative. Within these two groups there are a number of sub-groups of data types (Kermode 2004).

Before continuing with this chapter, you will need to reread the section in Chapter 8 on 'Scales of measurement' (see pp. 211–12).

Levels of measurement

As we move from purely qualitative and categorical 'measures' through interval to ratio scales there is an increasing amount of 'definiteness' about the relationship between any datum and another. This gives rise to the concept of 'levels of measurement', with categorical 'measures' as the lowest and ratio scales as the highest.

The mathematical basis of statistical procedures depends upon assumptions about the relationship between variable values. More precise or powerful statistical procedures are appropriate for data collected using higher levels of measurement.

The type of data analysis procedures you use depend on the type of measurement procedures you use. Data analysis procedures become more powerful as measurement procedures become more precise.

As data progresses along a continuum of precision, potential analyses progress along a continuum of power as follows:

Precision ranking	Level of measurement	Highest level of potential analysis
1	Ratio (continuous)	Parametric statistics
2	Interval (discrete)	Parametric statistics
3	Ordinal (ranked)	Non-parametric statistics
4	Nominal (categorical)	Descriptive statistics
5	Qualitative	Qualitative

Chapter 8 deals with the issue of data classification related to the use of parametric and non-parametric analysis. As measurement becomes more precise, analysis is able to become more sophisticated and more powerful.

An example of levels of measurement

Imagine you want to carry out research on cigarette-smoking behaviour. It may be possible to collect data across all five levels of measurement, as follows:

1   Qualitative level of measurement
         Why do you continue to smoke cigarettes?

2 Nominal level of measurement
   Please indicate which of the following symptoms you experience by ticking the
   appropriate boxes:
   ☐ Persistent cough
   ☐ Poor circulation to feet, legs and/or hands
   ☐ High blood pressure
   ☐ Sleep problems
3 Ordinal level of measurement
   Please rank in order (from 1 to 7) the importance of the following concerns you
   have for you own health:
   ☐ Diet
   ☐ Weight
   ☐ Cigarette smoking
   ☐ Alcohol
   ☐ Exercise and activity
   ☐ Sleep
   ☐ Stress
4 Discrete (interval) level of measurement
   Please indicate the number of days per week on average on which you
   smoke:_____
5 Continuous (ratio) level of measurement
   Please record your lung Vital Capacity (in litres) as measured by
   vitalograph:_____

EXERCISE

Write a question, which would require data to be provided about someone's weight, according to each of the following levels of measurement:

1 Qualitative:

2 Nominal:

3 Ordinal:

4 Interval:

5 Ratio:

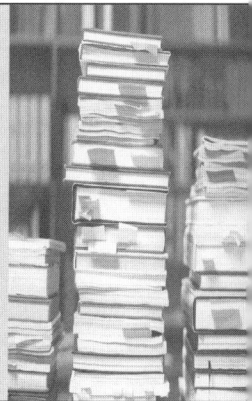

Quantitative data analysis

In quantitative data analysis, numbers are everything. Using numbers, you can describe amounts, proportions and patterns in the data. You can also test hypotheses by investigating the type and strength of relationships between variables. Quantitative data analysis can produce anything from simple sums to complex three-dimensional patterns.

Statistics

Quantitative analysis is done to generate statistics. A statistic is a summary description of information gathered through observation or measurement. It is a numerical summary of some phenomenon. Statistics can be found everywhere. Newspapers, for example, regularly report statistics, such as share indices, median house prices, average salaries, unemployment rates and cricket batting averages. Some statistics are simple, like counting the number of people in a population with measles. Others are quite intricate, like determining the statistical likelihood of high blood pressure causing a heart attack among all of the other factors known to be risk factors for heart attacks.

Most researchers now employ data analysis software to carry out statistical operations on their computer. These programs have enabled researchers to analyse data and generate statistics without the drudgery of knowing statistical formulae and how they work. But you must understand the language of statistics in order to be able to carry out the data analysis.

If you are developing a research project as a university student, it is wise to consult your lecturer or supervisor concerning statistical aspects of your project. You may be fortunate enough to go to a university or work for an institution that provides a statistical advice service. It is worth availing yourself of these services after you have done some preliminary reading on the subject.

Statistical inference

If a sample is representative of the total population (that is, it has similar overall characteristics to the total population of interest) we will be able to make inferences about the population from our sample data and the statistics we produce from it, such as the average number of cigarettes smoked per day. The process of statistical inference underpins the entire research process in most traditional approaches to health research. It depends on good sampling and good measurement.

Descriptive statistics

In writing up the results of a research project, you will probably want to describe the characteristics of the group or the sub-groups that comprise the group. For example, you may wish to give the total number in the group or the average score on a test. **Descriptive statistics** enable us to do that. We will now look at some statistics that describe and summarise data.

Sum

Frequently you want to know the total of something, for example, how many patients are in a hospital or come to a clinic. You do this by counting all of the elements to get their sum.

Suppose that you wanted to test an hypothesis that patients in the respiratory clinic where you work were more likely to be heavy smokers than light smokers or non-smokers. You could, through a chart audit, come up with the following list for one day's patients (Table 10.1).

By counting, you establish that there were 50 patients seen. This statistic is often given by the computer program in the course of other statistical analysis.

Table 10.1	Table showing clients who were heavy, light and non-smokers			
Heavy	Light	Non	Heavy	Heavy
Non	Non	Light	Heavy	Non
Light	Heavy	Heavy	Light	Light
Heavy	Non	Heavy	Light	Heavy
Heavy	Light	Heavy	Heavy	Light
Light	Heavy	Non	Light	Heavy
Heavy	Heavy	Light	Non	Light
Heavy	Light	Heavy	Light	Heavy
Light	Heavy	Non	Light	Non
Heavy	Non	Light	Light	Non

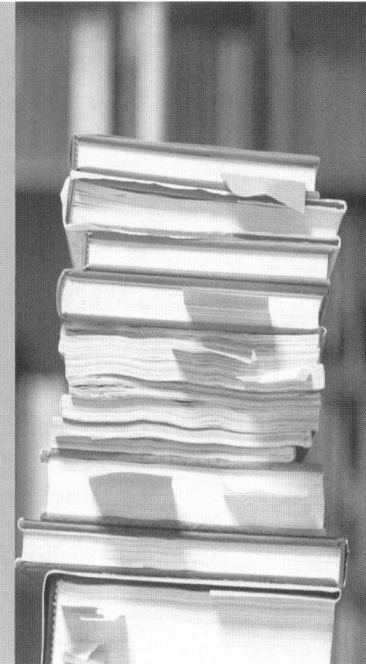

You may also wish to find out about the numbers in the different categories of smoking. To get this information, you must count the numbers of patients in the different categories to calculate the sum or total of heavy smokers to be 21, light smokers 18 and non-smokers 11. This tells you that on the day on which you collected your data more heavy smokers than light smokers or non-smokers were seen.

Percentage

A percentage is the proportion out of 100 that a group comprises. You obtain a percentage by taking the number, dividing it by the number of elements in the group and multiplying by 100. The beauty of a percentage is that it allows comparisons of groups. You cannot meaningfully compare a raw number of one group with a raw number in another group if the totals of the groups are different.

If you now want to establish what proportion of clients are in the three categories of smokers you would work out the percentage of the total clients in each category. By dividing each total by 50 and multiplying by 100, you find out that the proportion of heavy smokers is 42 per cent, the proportion of light smokers is 36 per cent and the proportion of non-smokers is 22 per cent. In the same way, you can also calculate that the proportion of smokers is 78 per cent. Again, a computer will give you this information.

Frequency distributions

If you have your data entered into a statistical computer program, you can get it to generate the number and percentage of each sub-group by generating a statistic called a frequency

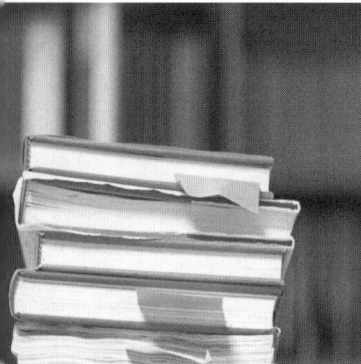

Table 10.2 Frequency table of categories of smokers and non-smokers

Bar	Element	Count	Percentage
1	Non	11	22
2	Light	18	36
2	Heavy	21	42

distribution table. This is a description of the components in a group. It tells you the number and percentage of elements in each sub-group of the main group. A frequency distribution statistic can also be used to generate both histograms and pie graphs by computer. The frequency distribution table for the client data will look something like Table 10.2.

This table tells you that there are 11 non-smokers comprising 22 per cent of the group, 18 light smokers comprising 36 per cent of the group and 21 heavy smokers comprising 42 per cent of the group.

Using graphics to show sums and percentages

In a research report, you can show categorical information more dramatically by means of a graphic illustration or figure called a histogram or bar graph. There is a trend towards using graphics to illustrate points in reporting information about data because graphics are easier to interpret than tables, thus illustrating the old saying that 'a picture is worth a thousand words'. Putting graphics into reports used to be constrained by the difficulty in generating them and the cost of printing them. However, computer programs can now generate graphics easily and the cost of reproducing them is decreasing because of modern printing processes.

Histogram and bar graphs

Histograms and bar graphs are figures that show the numbers in groups as vertical columns or horizontal rows, which allows for easy comparison of groups. The largest group will have the longest column or bar and the smallest group will have the shortest one. A bar graph shows discrete categories, such as types of injuries, while a histogram shows numbers in different categories of a range, such as income groups. In a bar graph there will be space between the bars, while in a histogram there is no space. Figure 10.1 (opposite) shows a bar graph of our group of clients broken down into its sub-groups of heavy, light and non-smokers.

Pie chart

A pie chart is another kind of figure that shows the proportions of sub-groups in a group. It divides the total 'pie' into its components, again allowing for ease of comparison. Figure 10.2 (opposite) shows a pie chart of the client data.

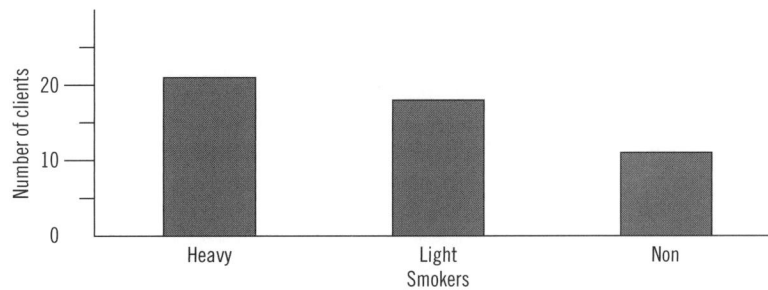

Figure 10.1   Bar graph of number of clients who are heavy, light and non-smokers

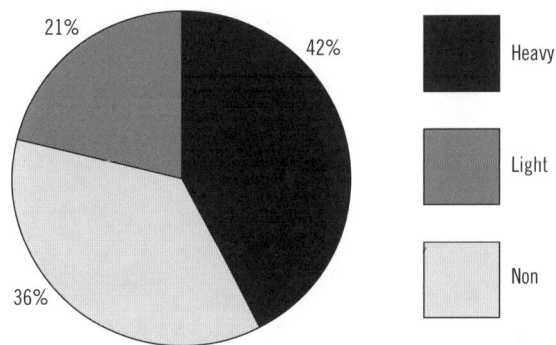

Figure 10.2   Pie chart showing types of smokers and non-smokers as percentages of the group

Table

Tables are one of the most common tools that a researcher uses when analysing data. A table is a meaningful presentation of numbers in rows and columns. Columns are the vertical arrangement of like numbers, and rows are the horizontal arrangement of like numbers. The intersection of a column and a row is called a cell. Each number will appear in both a column and a row, or a cell.

By analysing the clients in the clinic at the present time, you have taken a 'snapshot' of the data to see whether your hypothesis has any potential for a conclusion. However, you would not want to base your conclusion on data taken on only one day in case that day were atypical. You therefore decide to obtain data for a more extended period. You decide to take a random sample of one day per month and examine all of the clients on those specific days. Once again, you need to organise your data into some form that makes sense of it and allows you to see the patterns. You therefore decide to organise your data into a table showing the numbers of each group of smokers and non-smokers for each of the days that you have examined. You construct a table as follows, using the numbers that you have obtained (Table 10.3, overleaf).

Table 10.3   Table showing number of clients, by month, who were heavy, light and non-smokers

Month	Heavy	Light	Non	Total
January	21	18	11	50
February	18	9	8	35
March	14	10	6	30
April	19	14	10	43
May	20	9	15	44
June	7	6	3	16
July	9	6	7	22
August	10	6	9	25
September	11	9	9	9
October	15	9	6	30
November	16	16	12	44
December	15	7	10	32
Total	175	119	106	400
Total as %	44%	30%	26%	100%

Taking a look at your raw data, you see that there were 400 clients seen on the 12 selected days. Of these, 175 or 44 per cent were heavy smokers, 119 or 30 per cent were light smokers, and 106 or 26 per cent were non-smokers. This is the same pattern that you saw for the one day in January, so you can safely conclude that your January day was fairly typical. To see whether each day was typical, you would have to calculate the percentage for each group for each of the 12 days. You do this and construct Table 10.4. This allows you to compare the percentages of types of smokers and non-smokers for each month.

Notice that we didn't work out the percentages first and then calculate the 'average' from them. Try it: you will get 48 per cent for heavy smokers, for example, instead of the 44 per cent calculated from the totals. The reason for this apparent discrepancy is that averaging the percentages gives each month's result the same 'weight' or importance. In our example, the results for January are four times as important as those for June because we had four times as many observations. It is absolutely crucial to look at the raw data before transposing

Table 10.4 Table of percentages, by month, of smokers and non-smokers

Month	Heavy	Light	Non
January	42	36	22
February	50	27	23
March	48	33	19
April	42	30	24
May	45	20	35
June	48	30	22
July	41	29	30
August	38	25	37
September	40	30	30
October	50	30	20
November	36	36	28
December	48	22	30

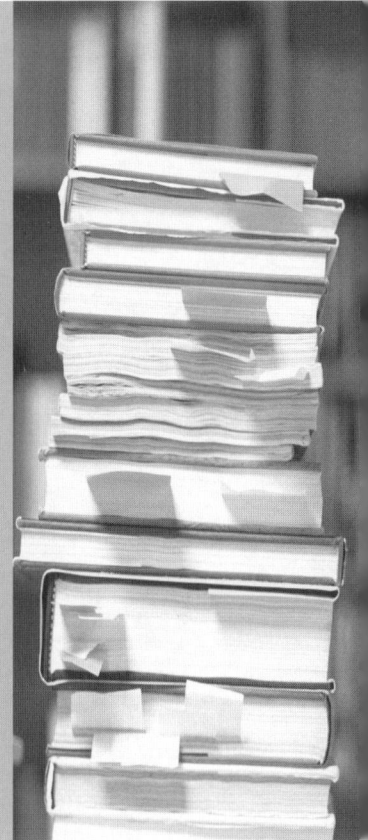

them to percentages. Otherwise you run the risk of drawing conclusions that misrepresent what happened. The information in the table of percentages can also be shown in graphic form (Figure 10.3, overleaf).

The graph shows that on every day examined, the percentage of clients who were heavy smokers was equal to or greater than each of the other groups. However, there is some fluctuation when different months are considered. The first day you measured in January may have had a fairly high proportion of heavy smokers compared to the other days. In order to find out how typical it was, you need to look at what the general picture is. This is explored in the next section.

Measures of central tendency

Measures of central tendency are the mean, median and mode. These are statistics that let us see what the most common scores in a group are, and how the group did as a whole.

The mean

The mean score of a group is the average, a concept with which you will be familiar. The mean is obtained by taking the sum total of the elements and dividing it by the number of

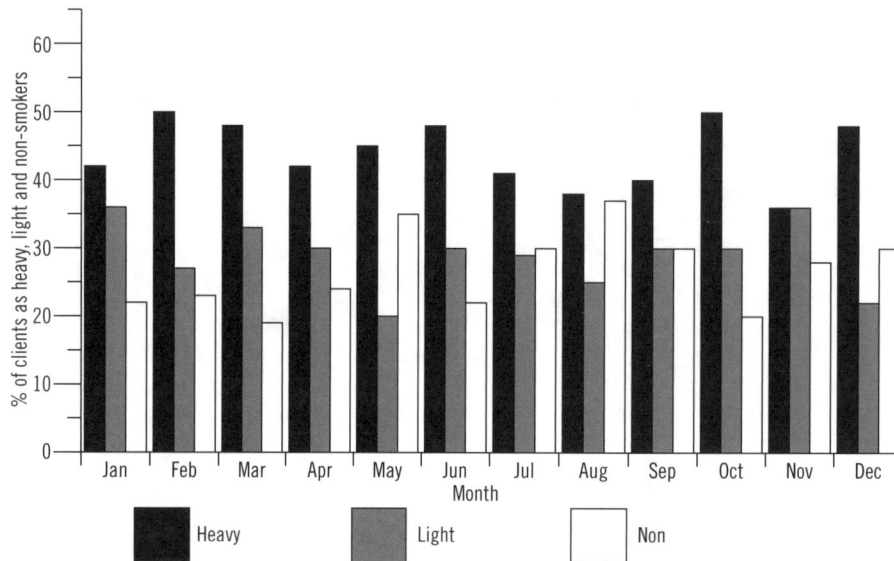

Figure 10.3   Bar graph showing the percentage of clients, by month, who were heavy, light and non-smokers

elements in the group. To continue our example, it would be helpful to compare the findings for January with the findings for the whole year. This would tell us whether January was a typical month for the percentages of sub-groups of clients. To do that, you calculate the average, or mean, percentage for the year for each sub-group. So, in this example, you divide the total number of clients seen by the number of days, or 400/12 = 33. The heavy smokers comprised (175/12 = 15)/33 = 44 per cent, light smokers comprised (118/12)/33 = 30 per cent, and non-smokers comprised (106/12)/33 = 26 per cent. You can now compare each month's percentage with the mean or average percentage and see how typical it was. January's figures were: heavy smokers 42 per cent, light smokers 36 per cent and non-smokers 22 per cent. Thus, you can conclude that January's figures were a bit over-average for heavy smokers, but under-average for light smokers and non-smokers.

The median

Another useful measure of central tendency is the median. This is the score in the middle. For an odd number of scores, the middle one is the median. For an even number of scores, the median is the average of the two middle ones. In the case of heavy smokers, if the data were rearranged from smallest to largest score, they would look like this:

36, 38, 40, 41, 42, 44, 45, 48, 48, 48, 50, 50.

Since this set of figures comprises an even number (there are 12 months in the year), the median would be the average of 44 and 45, the two middle scores, or 44.5. In this case, the mean and the median are very close.

You can calculate the median of the light smokers and non-smokers in a similar fashion.

The mode

The mode is the most frequently occurring score. In the case of heavy smokers, it can be seen easily that the mode is 48 since that score occurs three times in the data set. The mode is higher than the mean or the median for heavy smokers. You can calculate the mode for light smokers and non-smokers in the same way.

Measures of variability

Sometimes you want to see how the figures are distributed in a group of scores. Measures of variability help you to do this.

The range

The range is a number that reflects the spread of the scores. It is obtained by subtracting the lowest score from the highest score. To follow our example above, the highest number of heavy smokers is 50 and the lowest number is 36, so the range is $50 - 36 = 14$.

Standard deviation

The standard deviation is a number that is calculated from the data to show the amount of dispersion of the data. The standard deviation is the number that incorporates approximately one-third of the scores (34 per cent) above or below the mean. In the temperature data set, the mean is 37° and the standard deviation is 1. This means that one-third of the temperatures lie between 36° and 37°, and another third lie between 37° and 38°, or two-thirds are between 36° and 38°. If the data are normally distributed, then another 14 per cent are between two standard deviations above and below the mean, so that 96 per cent are between 35° and 39°.

If the temperatures were more tightly clustered about the mean, the standard deviation would be low. For example, in Figure 10.4 you can see that there are a lot of people

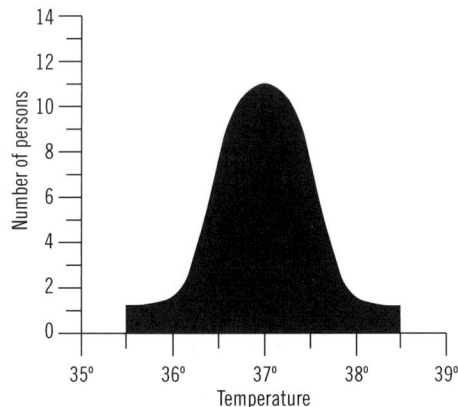

Figure 10.4   Graph showing temperature, low standard deviation

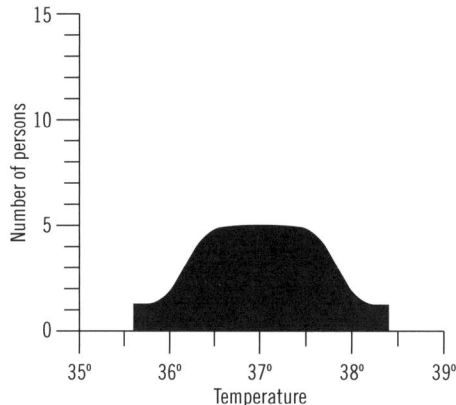

Figure 10.5 Graph showing temperature, high standard deviation

with a temperature on or around the mean temperature of 37°, whereas there are very few people at the extreme temperatures.

The standard deviation of these temperatures is 0.6 of a degree. This means that one-third of the observations fall between 36.4° and 37° and another third fall between 37° and 37.6°, and so forth.

On the other hand, if the temperatures were more spread out, the area graph would look like Figure 10.5.

You can see that there are fewer people with temperatures on or around the mean, and more at the extreme temperatures. The standard deviation for this set of data would be higher than the previous example because the temperatures are more dispersed.

Introduction to probability and hypothesis testing
Sampling distributions

The concept of sampling distributions refers to the characteristics of the curve which could be plotted from the means of sets of measurements taken from all possible samples of a population. It is the sampling distribution which underpins most of the techniques used in the statistical analysis of data. Sampling distributions tend to have certain key characteristics, and this chapter will deal with a number of these characteristics.

Central limit theorem

All inferential statistical procedures are based on the assumption that the data being used is based on a random sample taken from the population and therefore representative of the population data. To use **inferential statistics** with any validity, therefore, your data should be based on a random sample. Naturally, it is quite possible to draw a number of different random samples from a population and end up with data that is not identical from one sample to the next. In fact, if you drew an infinite number of random samples and took the mean of each random sample, the range of sample means would follow a 'normal' distribution. This phenomenon is known as the Central Limit Theorem.

The important thing about Central Limit Theorem is that it applies to the means of an infinite number of samples, not to the actual distribution of the parameter in the population. Very few things are normally distributed in nature, but the means of an infinite number of samples is normally distributed.

If, for example, you have 100 students in a class, and you took samples of 10 students and measured their average height, and you repeated this until you had exhausted the possible combinations of 10 students, you would have millions of average heights. If you plotted these on a curve it would represent a 'normal' or 'bell-shaped' curve. This distribution can be plotted graphically as a 'normal curve', and can be seen in Figure 10.6.

A 'normal' sampling distribution has the following characteristics:

- 68 per cent of scores will fall between one standard deviation either side of the mean.
- 95 per cent of scores will fall between 1.96 standard deviations either side of the mean.
- 99 per cent of scores will fall between three standard deviations either side of the mean.
- The total area under the curve represents the total population of possible values for the variable being examined.

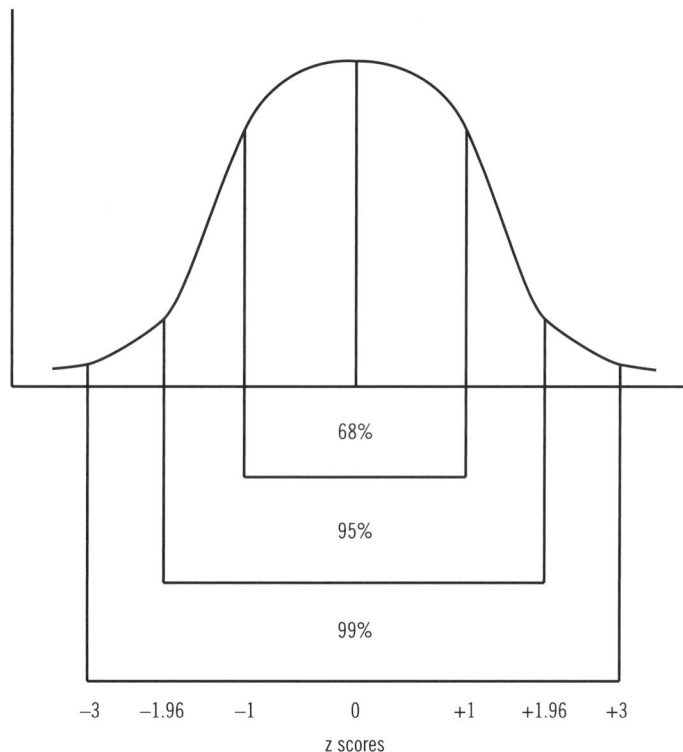

Figure 10.6   A normal curve

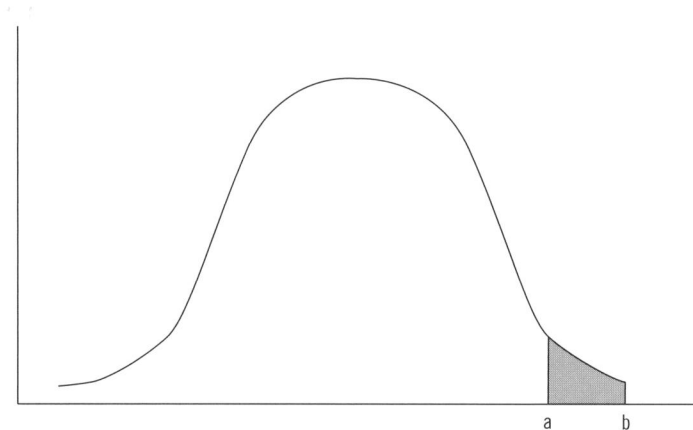

Figure 10.7 Probability and the sampling distribution

- It is possible to determine how many standard deviations from the mean a value is by calculating a *z score*. This tells you how many standard deviations above or below the mean the value is. The formula for calculating a *z* score is:

$$z = y - x \div s$$

where: y = the value under consideration
x = the mean of the distribution
s = the standard deviation of the distribution

- A *z* score of 1 means that a score is exactly one standard deviation above the mean.
- The probability of a sample mean having a particular value, or *z* score (*z*) which falls between two possible values (a & b), is equal to the area under the curve between the two values (where the total area under the curve is taken as 1.0). The value of this probability is calculated automatically by computerised statistics programs. The calculation of z scores is one of the techniques which is used when inferential statistics are applied to a set of data. Figure 10.7 represents how probability is derived from sampling distributions.

Checking the representativeness of a sample

It is possible to calculate the *Standard Error* of a sample mean to determine how representative a sample is, or to estimate the extent to which a sample might vary from the population. The Standard Error represents the size of a possible sampling error, based on the standard deviation and size of the sample. It gives the possible variation in the mean due to sampling error. The formula for calculating the Standard Error is:

$$Sx = sd \div \sqrt{n}$$

where Sx = Standard Error of the mean
sd = Standard Deviation of the sample
n = Size of the sample

It can be seen that the Standard Error is reduced by increasing the sample size. The larger n is, the smaller Sx is.

Hypothesis testing

When you use a set of data based on a sample of the population to make inferences about the characteristics of the population there is a certain amount of risk involved. For example, you might have accidentally obtained a biased sample, or tested the sample at a bad time. The data you get will therefore lead you to make incorrect decisions about your results. Inferential statistics uses the formal process of hypothesis testing to reduce this risk.

The errors you can make have to do with whether you wrongly accept or reject your hypothesis. Hypotheses are usually tested by stating them in reverse as null hypotheses and trying to prove them wrong. This is because it is not possible to actually prove anything using statistics, but you can statistically disprove it. For example, it is not possible to prove statistically the existence of two-headed wombats if none have ever been found. It is possible however, to disprove the existence of two-headed wombats by taking a set of observations of a sample of wombats and counting their heads. If 100 wombats are observed to all have only one head, we can reasonably assume that two-headed wombats do not exist. In the same way, research hypotheses are tested as null hypotheses because it is statistically easier to disprove something than to prove it.

If your research hypothesis was that 'there will be a significant difference in attitudes towards drug use between children in private schools and children in state schools', then your null hypothesis would be that 'there will be no significant difference in attitudes towards drug use between children in private schools and children in state schools'. If you measure these attitudes from two samples of children and then compare them, you can either accept or reject your null hypothesis. The key to hypothesis testing is the fact that your samples are truly representative of the population of interest from which they are drawn.

Type I and type II errors

There are two types of errors you might make when using inferential statistics:

- *Type I error* (alpha error) – this occurs when you mistakenly believe that you have found a significant result from a statistical test. In statistical procedures a null hypothesis is usually tested and wrongly rejected, leading to the acceptance of research hypothesis that is false. It usually occurs because of poor sampling. In other words, the sample is biased in some way, and the result was simply due to chance (Dawson-Saunders & Trapp 2001).

- *Type II error* (beta error) – this occurs when you mistakenly believe that you have not found anything significant, when it really does exist in the population of interest. In statistical procedures this is usually done by accepting a null hypothesis, which leads to rejecting a research hypothesis that is true. Once again, the result was due to chance, and probably based on a biased sample (Dawson-Saunders & Trapp 2001).

It is possible to quantify the likelihood that an error in judgement has been made using probability. Type I error is controlled by setting significance levels (p values). A p value of 0.05 means a 5 per cent probability of a type I error. Type II error is controlled by doing 'power' calculations, and setting a power level for the study. An 80 per cent power level means an 80 per cent probability that no error has been made. Both of these types of error are related to sample size.

Power is calculated to ensure that a sample size is large enough to find a significant difference between two or more groups, or association between two or more variables, if such a difference or association exists in the population. Power is expressed as $1 - \beta$. A 30 per cent probability of making a type II error (β) means a 70 per cent probability of not making the error. A power value of 0.70 or better is normally acceptable in most types of research.

Level of significance

The *level of significance* of the result is the term which describes the likelihood that an error in judgement has been made regarding the result. It is expressed as a probability, such as $p < .01$ or $p < .05$. This means that the probability of an error being made is less than 1 per cent (1 in 100) or less than 5 per cent (5 in 100). Whenever a statistical procedure is done a level of significance should be determined in order to qualify whether the result is statistically significant or not. The usual minimum accepted level of significance is $p < .05$ ($p < .01$ or $p < .001$ are much more significant). Such levels of significance are based on the size of the sample used, and computerised statistics packages will automatically determine them for you.

In a study of falls among the elderly it was found that males had greater deficits of ankle plantar-flexion strength and power, while females had greater deficits of knee extension strength and power and less walking speed (... $p < 0.05$ and $p < 0.01$)(Sieri & Beretta 2004). This meant that the researchers were confident that their results were statistically significant and that their findings could have occurred by chance less than 5 per cent or 1 per cent of the time in each respective type of deficit.

Degrees of freedom

An indication of sample size is obtained when calculating levels of significance and is referred to as *degrees of freedom* (usually $n - 1$, for the purpose of the calculations). It means the number of measurements which are free to vary and still give the sample the same mean score. Degrees of freedom is an important concept in the process of hypothesis testing because it affects the level of significance of a result, and hence the probability that an error in judgement has been made.

The term 'degrees of freedom' is closely related to the sample size. The size of the sample is closely tied to the level of significance of a result. You might, for example, correlate amount of cigarette smoking with stress and find a correlation of $r = .69$ (which is a moderately strong correlation). If your sample size was only 10 people, however, it would be unlikely to be statistically significant. You would have to say, therefore, that despite the moderate correlation, the result is not significant (because of the high probability of a type I error). If the sample size was 3000, however, the result would be most likely to be statistically significant.

One-tailed and two-tailed tests

If your research question requires you to compare for differences between two or more sets of data, you will use a procedure that determines whether there is any statistical difference between two sets of data. The level of significance you choose will allow you to determine the probability of your decision to accept or reject the hypothesis as being correct. For example, choosing a significance level of $p < .05$ means that there is a less than 5 per cent probability that the result was simply due to chance.

It is necessary, however, to identify whether your research hypothesis is directional or non-directional. This means whether you are interested in the direction of the difference, or simply whether a difference exists. For example, if your research hypothesis is that 'the mean blood sugar of diet-controlled diabetics will be no different to the mean blood sugar of insulin-controlled diabetics' then you are not interested in the direction of the difference – this is a non-directional hypothesis. If your research hypothesis was that 'the mean blood sugar of diet-controlled diabetics will be lower than the mean blood sugar of insulin-controlled diabetics', then you are stating a directional hypothesis.

You will recall that when the sampling distribution of the means of all the possible random samples drawn from a population is plotted it has the characteristics of a normal curve. It is then possible to determine what the probability of a value falling between two other values under the curve is by calculating the area under the curve between the two points as a percentage of the total area under the curve. When you use a non-directional hypothesis you want to find the probability of your result falling within the level of significance you have set for your test; in other words, whether your result falls in the area under the curve you designate as the 'rejection region', that is, the area in which a result forces you to reject your hypothesis.

The rejection region is defined by nominating a level of significance. The level of significance is expressed as a probability. The usual levels are $p < .05$ and $p < .01$. This means that the probability of the result falling in the rejection region is 5 per cent (5 in 100) or 1 per cent (1 in 100).

When your hypothesis is non-directional you will have a rejection region at either end of the sampling distribution. Each tail of the curve will have an area under it which is a rejection region. Testing a non-directional hypothesis is therefore called a two-tailed test. When your hypothesis is directional there will be a rejection region only under the end of the curve which relates to the direction of the hypothesis. Testing a directional hypothesis is therefore called a one-tailed test.

There are a range of statistical tables which automatically tabulate the probabilities of results falling in the rejection regions for a variety of inferential statistics and for both one-tailed and two-tailed tests. Computerised statistics programs will also automatically make these calculations.

It is important to nominate whether a one-tailed or two-tailed test of significance is being applied, as the result you get will depend on this decision.

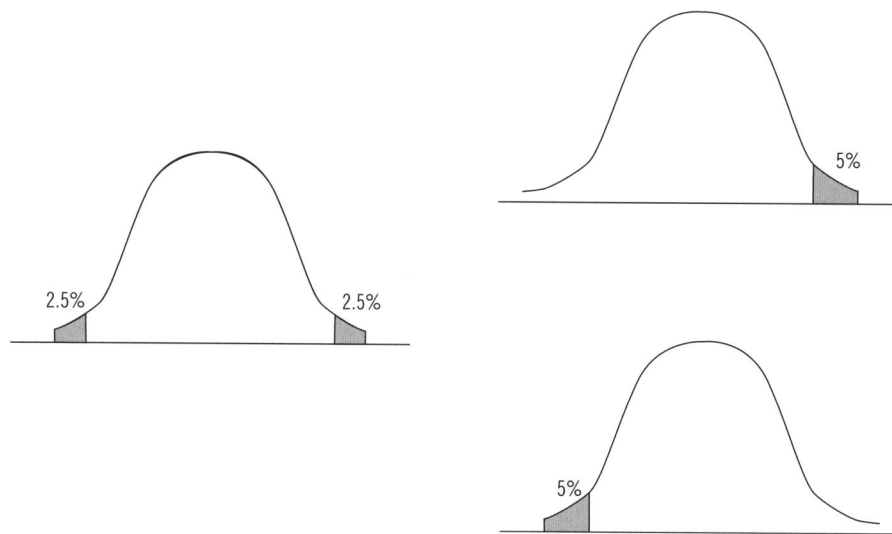

Figure 10.8 Rejection regions for one-tailed and two-tailed tests

There are three things you need to know to test an hypothesis:
- the size of the sample (degrees of freedom)
- the level of significance you have set (normally $p = .05$)
- whether the hypothesis is directional or non-directional (one-tailed or two-tailed test).

If you are doing your data analysis with a computerised statistics program, the computer will determine these things for you as part of its calculations.

Comparing for differences and associations

When using statistics to compare for differences (e.g. the difference in body fat between men and women) or to compare for associations (e.g. the association between dietary fat and total body fat), 'inferential' statistics are used to determine the differences. Inferential statistics have the following characteristics:
- They are used to make comparisons in order to find differences or associations between sets of data.
- They are used to make inferences about the population from which the sample data were extracted.
- They can be either parametric or non-parametric techniques.

Associations in one group
Correlation

Some research designs require the researcher to examine relationships between the characteristics of people in a group. For example, you might want to see if post-operative pain levels were higher for clients who had high levels of pre-operative anxiety than for those who had low levels. To do this, you would collect data on each person's anxiety and pain. If you had a numerical pain scale and an anxiety scale, you could investigate whether the amount of anxiety was related to, or correlated with, the amount of post-operative anxiety. You would perhaps expect that clients who scored high on the anxiety scale would also score high on the pain scale. However, it is possible that clients who scored low on the anxiety scale could score high on the pain scale. Finally, it is possible that there is no relationship between the two factors.

In order to test your hypothesis, you would need to look at the numerical relationship between the clients' scores on the two scales. To do this you would do a plot of each client's anxiety level along one axis of a graph (the X axis) and the pain score along the other axis (the Y axis)(see Figure 10.9). This concept can be shown pictorially by means of a scattergram, or a graph that shows each person's data as a point on the graph. Note that both variables must be numerical in order to use this test. Each client's datum for where the pain score intersects with the anxiety score will appear as one point on the graph. (You can find what each person's score was on both scales. Find a dot and draw a horizontal line from it to the Y or vertical axis and a vertical line to the X or horizontal axis.) The idea now is to 'fit' a straight line that best represents the data. You can do this 'by eye' or ask the computer program for the regression line, which is the fancy name for the best-fit straight line.

The graph in Figure 10.9 shows a positive relationship between anxiety and pain. Clients who had high anxiety levels also had high pain levels and clients who had low anxiety levels also had low pain levels. This means that anxiety is positively correlated with pain for this group of clients.

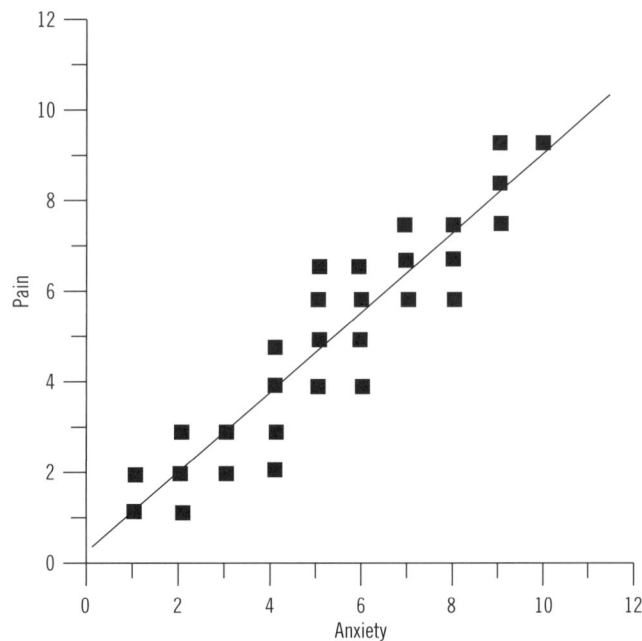

Figure 10.9 Scattergram showing positive correlation of pain and anxiety

The graph in Figure 10.9 also shows the regression line that has been fitted to the data by the computer program.

The extent to which the variables are related to each other is expressed as a correlation coefficient, the symbolic notation for which is an 'r' in italics. The 'r' value corresponds to the slope of the line. The most common correlation coefficient used in modern computer analysis is the Pearson Correlation Coefficient. The Pearson Correlation Coefficient has a range of scores from -1.0 to $+1.0$. The more strongly the two variables are correlated with each other, the farther the score will be from zero. A score of 0 in the middle represents no correlation at all.

$-1 \ -0.9 \ -0.8 \ -0.7 \ -0.6 \ -0.5 \ -0.4 \ -0.3 \ -0.2 \ -0.1 \ 0 \ 0.1 \ 0.2 \ 0.3 \ 0.4 \ 0.5 \ 0.6 \ 0.7 \ 0.8 \ 0.9 \ +1$

A helpful way to think of this is as similar to a pH scale. A pH reading at one end (14) is very basic, a reading at the other is very acidic (1) and in the middle it is neutral (7).

The Pearson Correlation Coefficient has the assumption that the data are normally distributed. If they are not, you would use a non-parametric test such as the Spearman Rank Order Correlation.

Figure 10.9 shows a strong positive relationship of pain and anxiety, with the participants' scores on one scale similar to their scores on the other scale. This result would give you a Pearson Correlation Coefficient of 0.92, which is a strong positive correlation.

If, on the other hand, you had a set of data in which the anxiety scores go up while the pain scores go down, you would see a different result, as Figure 10.10 shows.

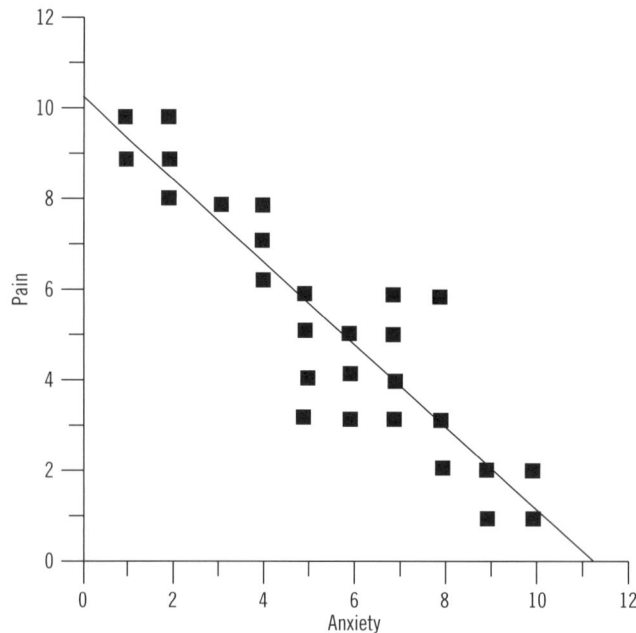

Figure 10.10 Scattergram showing negative correlation of pain and anxiety

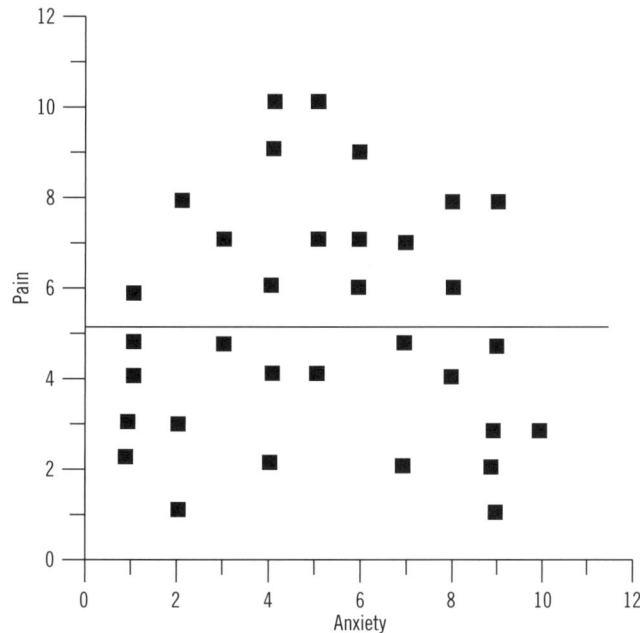

Figure 10.11   Scattergram showing no correlation of pain and anxiety

You can see in Figure 10.10 that the data points and the regression line run in the opposite direction to those in the previous graph. The high scores on the anxiety scale are matched to the low scores on the pain scale. Participants who were very anxious had a low level of pain after the operation. Conversely, participants who had high anxiety levels before the operation had low levels of post-operative pain. The Pearson Correlation Coefficient for these data is -0.9.

The third possibility is that there is no relationship between pain and anxiety. Figure 10.11 shows the lack of a relationship when anxiety is regressed upon pain.

Note that the scatter on this graph is random: there seems to be no relationship between anxiety and pain. The Pearson Correlation Coefficient on these data was near zero at 0.01.

Correlation and significance

At this point in discussing the statistical nitty gritty, things get a little sticky. In Figure 10.9 we saw a strong positive correlation spread over the whole range of possible responses. What if we had had only a few data and they were all grouped at one end, but showing the same 'best-fit line'? The 'r' value is the same (same slope) but our feeling about the reliability of the data is way down. Or what if the scatter is much wider? Again the slope of the best-fit line could be the same but we are not so sure of it.

At this point the statisticians give us an almost universally confusing table which relates the number of subjects in the study (the number of data points in this instance) to the value of 'r' that must be exceeded for it to pass a certain level of significance. The left-most column is usually headed 'degrees of freedom (df)' and for reasons we need not go into, is 2 less than the number of data points (so for our example 'F' or 'f' or 'df' is close enough to our number of data points, say 30). This determines which row of the table we use. It does not make sense to be too fussy here, provided you have more than a dozen points. We now compare our 'r' value (in this case 0.92) with the values in the 'F' or 'f' or 'df' = 30 row. If our value for 'r' is bigger (neglecting whether it is positive or negative) than the value in the column for our required level of significance, we have a winner! Fortunately, the computer program will work out the p value for us, taking the pain out of the process.

EXERCISE

List two sets of variables related to health where you think you could establish an association through use of a correlation coefficient. One set should demonstrate a positive association, while the other set should demonstrate a negative association:

1   Two variables that have a positive association with each other:

    i)   _____

    ii) _____

2   Two variables that have a negative association with each other:

    i)   _____

    ii) _____

Testing for differences in means of two groups of data

Independent groups t-test

Some research designs and hypotheses call for testing to see if there is a significant difference in two different groups' means on the same variable. For example, suppose that you were not satisfied to classify your mobile and immobile clients in a long-term care facility simply as constipated or not constipated. You want to compare the actual difference in numbers of bowel motions per week for the two groups. Again, you would collect your data on whether each client was mobile or immobile and also on the number of bowel motions for one week. You could then do an independent groups, or unpaired, t-test to see whether the mean number of bowel actions per week for the immobile clients was greater than that for the mobile clients. Your results might look like Table 10.5.

Table 10.5 Table showing unpaired *t*-test

Unpaired *t*-test: X: mobility and Y: bowel actions

Unpaired t-value			Probability
6.8			0.0001

Group	Count	Mean	Std. Dev.
Mobile	25	6.8	1.1
Bedrest	15	3.9	1.6

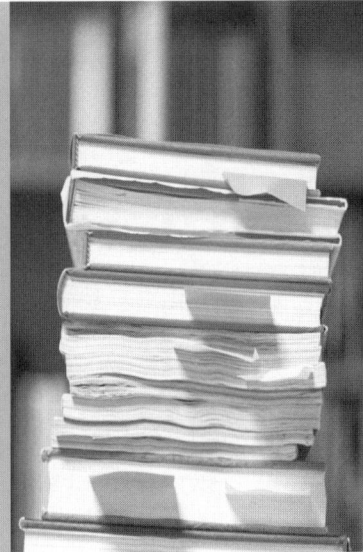

Table 10.5 tells you that you had 25 mobile patients, with 15 bedfast ones. The mean number of bowel actions per week for your mobile patients was 6.8, while for the bedfast ones it was 3.9. The results of the *t*-test tell you that this finding was statistically significant ($p = 0.0001$). This means that there was a probability of less than one in ten thousand that this result could have happened by chance alone.

The independent *t*-test rests on the assumption that your data for bowel motions are normally distributed; that is, they approximate the normal curve outlined earlier. If, however, your data were skewed, you would need to use a non-parametric test such as the Mann-Whitney U-test because it does not require a normal distribution. But how do you tell? The best way is to do a histogram to show the distribution of the data. If the data look skewed, it would be better to do the non-parametric test.

Paired *t*-test

Another test that can be done to find relationships in one group is the paired or one-group *t*-test. This test is done when you wish to compare two readings for each participant on the same variable. The paired *t*-test needs at least an ordinal level scale for this test; that is, it is done on data that are numerical. This test is useful where you have a pre-test/post-test design, or more than one post-test measurement. For example, suppose that you want to see whether pre-operative teaching results in less post-operative anxiety. You do a pre-operative pre-test of anxiety, an intervention of pre-operative teaching, and a post-operative post-test of anxiety. You then do a paired *t*-test to see if the post-operative anxiety scores are lower than the pre-operative scores. For example, suppose that your group of participants had a mean pre-operative anxiety level of 7 and the mean post-operative anxiety level was 4, i.e. a drop of 3. Table 10.6 shows the results for the paired *t*-test.

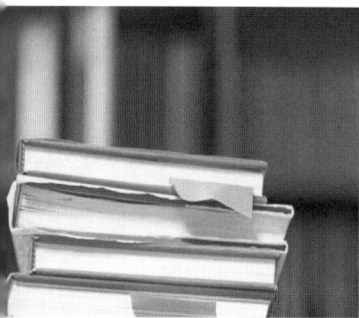

Table 10.6 Table showing results of paired *t*-test

Paired *t*-test	X: Pre-operation anxiety	Y: Post-Operation anxiety	
DF	Mean x–y	Paired t-value	Prob. (2 tail)
20	3	14	0.0001

The *p* value shows that these results were highly significant and that your hypothesis that the post-operative anxiety would be less after the intervention of pre-operative teaching is probably correct.

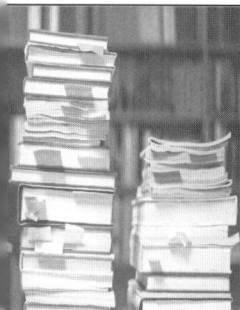

EXERCISE

Assume that you have two groups of people in a study. Describe one type of data you could collect for each group related to a single variable that would allow you to compare the two groups using a *t*-test:

variable:_____

type of data:_____

Chi square test and contingency tables

The chi-square test is a test for determining within-group relationships on nominal variables, that is, variables that are measured by categories rather than numbers. In a chi-square test, there are two variables, each of which is broken down into two levels.

Let us take a simple example. Suppose that you wish to look at the relationship between bedrest and constipation in long-stay clients. You hypothesise that those who are on bedrest are more likely to be constipated than those who are not. You collect data on 40 clients, classifying each one as either on bedrest or not, and constipated or not. Each person must be classified in both categories. Note that there are now four possible categories into which you can classify your clients. They can be constipated and on bedrest, constipated and not on bedrest, not constipated and on bedrest and not constipated and not on bedrest. You then do a chi-square test. If there were no relationship between bedrest and constipation, you might expect to have equal numbers of clients in each category, and your results might look something like Table 10.7.

However, if your hypothesis is correct and there is a relationship between mobility and bowel activity, your results might look like Table 10.8.

Table 10.7 Table showing chi-square: expected values

	Bedrest	Mobile	Totals
Constipated	10	10	20
Normal	10	10	20
Totals	20	20	40

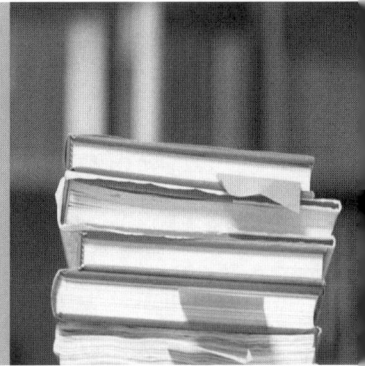

Table 10.8 Table showing chi-square: relationship between mobility and bowel activity

	Bedrest	Mobile	Totals
Constipated	14	6	20
Normal	5	15	20
Totals	19	21	40

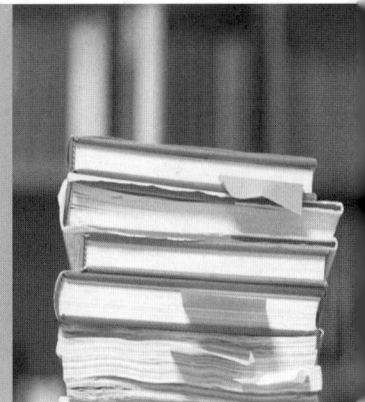

Just looking at Table 10.8, you can see that the clients who are on bedrest are constipated, and those who are mobile are not constipated.

The chi-square test will also give you information about percentages of clients in each category. By reading down the columns of the table in Table 10.9, you can see that three-quarters of the clients who are on bedrest are constipated and 71 per cent of those who are mobile are not constipated.

Another type of table looks at the percentages from the point of view of the other variable (see Table 10.10).

Table 10.10 tells you that 70 per cent of clients who are constipated are on bedrest and three-quarters of non-constipated clients are mobile.

A computer chi-square test will also give you a p value: in this case $p = 0.01$. This means that this result probably would have happened by chance alone only 1 per cent of the time and so the findings meet a 99 per cent level of confidence.

A contingency table is an expanded chi-square used where either variable has more than two categories. In the example above, you might want to break down the variables into finer categories. For example, mobility could be broken down to 'completely mobile', 'partially mobile' and 'bedrest'. Bowel activity could be broken down to 'badly constipated',

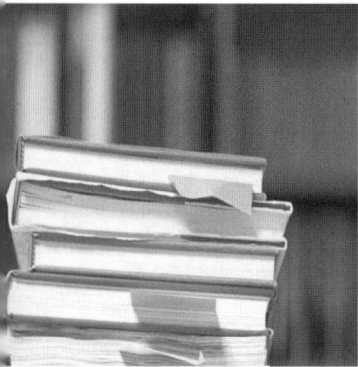

Table 10.9 Table showing chi-square column totals

	Bedrest	Mobile	Totals
Constipated	74%	29%	50%
Normal	26%	71%	50%
Totals	100%	100%	100%

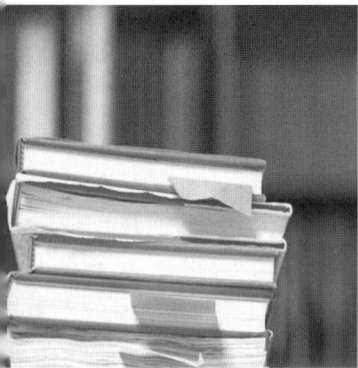

Table 10.10 Table showing chi-square row totals

	Bedrest	Mobile	Totals
Constipated	70	30	100%
Normal	25%	75%	100%
Totals	48%	52%	100%

'mildly constipated' and 'normal'. In this case you would have nine categories, with a 3×3 contingency table instead of the 2×2 table shown in Table 10.10. However, you would need many more participants to give enough data in each cell.

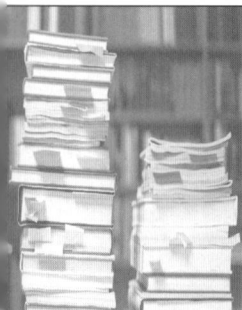

Testing for differences in means of more than two groups

Many research designs call for determining whether there is a difference in the mean score for more than two distinct groups. Suppose that you wanted to expand the earlier design,

Table 10.11 Table showing analysis of variance

One factor ANOVA: X: mobility and Y: bowel actions ($p = 0.0001$)

Group	Count	Mean	Std. Dev.
Bedrest	15	2.9	1.2
Partially mobile	22	5.3	0.8
Fully mobile	23	7.8	1.0

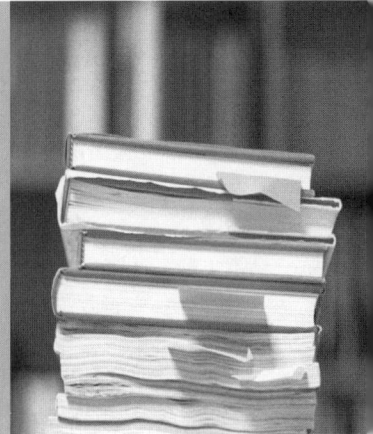

this time to look at the effect of three levels of mobility: bedfast, partly mobile and fully mobile upon the number of bowel actions. An analysis of variance (ANOVA) would allow you to determine whether the mean number of bowel motions per week was significantly different in the three groups. This test examines the mean scores and will detect whether there is a significant difference in them. The test actually detects whether there is more difference within each group than between the groups. Note that the independent variable, mobility, is nominal while the dependent variable, number of bowel actions, is numerical.

To do this test, you would need more participants since you are looking at three levels of mobility. Suppose you redid the study with more clients, classifying them as bedfast, partially mobile and fully mobile, again collecting data on the number of bowel motions for the week. Your results, using an analysis of variance, would look something like Table 10.11.

Table 10.11 tells you that you had 15 bedfast patients, 22 partially mobile patients and 23 fully mobile patients. It also tells you that there was a statistically significant difference in the mean number of bowel motions per week for the two groups. The bedfast patients had a mean of approximately three bowel motions per week, the partially mobile had a mean of 5 and the fully mobile had a mean of 8. This finding is statistically significant ($p = 0.0001$) with only one in ten thousand possibility that this finding would have occurred by chance. From these results, you would conclude that, all other things being equal, mobility makes a difference to the bowel activity of patients.

Again, if your data were skewed, you should use a non-parametric test. You could use the Kruskal-Wallis test for three groups. However, these data have a reasonably normal distribution, so a parametric test is indicated.

Methods involving more than one dependent or independent variable

It is not the intention of this chapter to teach you about complex statistical analysis. However, we want to introduce you to some advanced quantitative techniques so that you will recognise the terms if you see them in research reports. You can learn more about these techniques when the need arises by looking them up in books about statistics.

The advent of computers and statistical analysis programs has meant that ever-increasingly sophisticated techniques of data analysis have been demanded by researchers and devised by statisticians. The current complex techniques that we are about to introduce could not have been done by pen on paper or even by using hand calculators. This increased availability of sophisticated techniques has created a demand for research consumers to know something about them.

Creating complex statistics

Condensing data into scales: factor analysis

Some research projects use questionnaires that have a considerable number of items. Using the methods so far outlined, you would only be able to test your independent variables on each item individually. This would leave you with a large mass of data out of which it would be hard to make sense. One way of handling the data is to group the items into scales. In the context of a questionnaire, a scale is a group of items that are conceptually related. There are various ways of developing scales; one common way is factor analysis. All of the items can be entered into a factor analysis program. This program tests each item to determine with which group of items it belongs conceptually and clusters the related items into 'factors', or groups of items with a similar focus. The researcher can then treat each factor as one dependent variable.

Tests in which there is more than one independent variable

If a researcher wants to test the effects of two or more independent variables upon the dependent variable, more complex tests must be done. The researcher can test each independent variable individually using the techniques outlined earlier in this chapter; indeed this is one way to eliminate from the analysis variables that have little or no effect. However, individual analysis will not tell the researcher how the variables interact with one another and which has the most powerful effect. To do this, the researcher must use a test that will allow the entry of a group of independent variables into the analysis. Some of these statistical tests are described briefly below.

Multiple regression

If the independent variables are numerical and the dependent variable is also numerical, a more complex regression called a multiple regression can be used. For example, a researcher might want to analyse the relative effects of intelligence and socioeconomic status (SES) upon the ability of clients to learn information about diabetes mellitus. The researcher could administer an intelligence test (IQ) and a test of diabetes knowledge to the participants in the study and also determine their score on an index of socioeconomic status. The researcher could then use a multiple regression with the test of knowledge score as the outcome variable and the SES and IQ scores as the research variables. This would tell the researcher what effects SES and IQ have and whether they are linked.

Two-way and three-way ANOVAs

If there is more than one nominal-level independent variable and one interval-level dependent variable, the researcher would need to use a more sophisticated analysis of variance (ANOVA). A two-way ANOVA will handle two independent variables, a three-way ANOVA will handle three independent variables, and so forth. Continuing our earlier example, suppose that a researcher wanted to examine the effects of both mobility and gender on mean number of bowel motions per week in nursing home clients. The researcher would use a two-way ANOVA, with three levels of mobility and two levels of gender. If the researcher wanted to examine the effect of type of diet along with mobility and gender, a three-way ANOVA would be indicated.

Logistic regression

Log-linear analysis is a type of regression analysis in which all of the variables are measured on a nominal scale (Dawson-Saunders & Trapp 2001). Logistic regression examines the relative effect of more than one nominal-level independent variable upon a nominal-dependent variable. It is a kind of expanded chi-square. For example, a researcher might want to examine the effect of both gender and mobility upon whether or not clients are selected for placement in a particular nursing home. An example of this type of statistical analysis can be found in a study that examined the predictors of women's use of a breast cancer support service (Beckmann et al. 2003). The study found that women having mastectomies were much more likely to use the service, while older women and those with non-English speaking backgrounds were less likely to use it.

Discriminant analysis

Discriminant analysis is a technique that allows the researcher to use numerical independent variables to predict whether participants will belong to different groups. The independent variables must be interval level and the dependent variable is nominal level. For example, if a researcher wanted to see whether SES and IQ would predict whether a person was a smoker or a non-smoker, a discriminant analysis could do so.

Tests involving more than one dependent variable

Some research designs have more than one dependent variable. If the dependent variables are unrelated, they can be examined using separate ANOVAs. You will remember that an ANOVA allows only one dependent variable to be analysed at one time. If, however, the dependent variables are related in some way, they can be examined together, using more advanced statistical techniques. One of these is the MANOVA, or multivariate analysis of variance.

Summary of tests for comparing for differences

In Table 10.12 is a summary of those statistical tests that can be used to compare groups of data to see if there is a statistically significant difference between the groups. These tests will

Table 10.12 Table of tests for comparing for differences

	Nominal data (non-parametric)	Ordinal data (non-parametric)	Interval or ratopm data (parametric)
Two independent groups of data	Chi-square test	Mann-Whitney U-test	t-test (independent groups)
Two dependent groups of data	McNemar test	Sign test	t-test (dependent groups)
Three or more groups of independent data	Chi-square test	Kruskal-Wallis test	ANOVA (independent groups)
Three or more groups of dependent data	Cochran's Q test	Friedman two-way analysis of variance	ANOVA (dependent groups)

tell you if the mean of one group is higher than the mean of one or more other groups of data, other than by chance alone.

Summary of tests for comparing for associations

In Table 10.13 is a summary of those statistical tests which can be used to compare groups of data to see if there is a statistically significant association between the groups. These tests will tell you if one variable is associated with one or more other variables, other than by chance alone.

Want to learn more about statistics?

For further knowledge you can do some reading in basic books on statistics that have been written for health science students such as *Basic Statistics for the Health Sciences* (Bohneneblust 2000) or *Basic and Clinical Biostatistics* (Dawson-Saunders & Trapp 2001). You could also take a course in statistics.

Summary

In this chapter, we have looked at the various levels of data, the use of computers and various methods of analysing data using statistical analysis. We have looked at different ways of describing our data and of testing hypotheses, leading to conclusions about the validity of our findings. We have introduced the concepts of probability and type I and II errors. Finally, we have briefly introduced more complex statistical tests.

Table 10.13 Table of tests for comparing for associations

	Nominal data (non-parametric)	Ordinal data (non-parametric)	Interval or ratio data (parametric)
Two groups of data	Logistic regression or loglinear analysis	Spearman's Rank Order Correlation	Pearson's Correlation
Three or more groups of data	Logistic regression or loglinear analysis	Logistic regression or loglinear analysis	Multiple regression or factor analysis

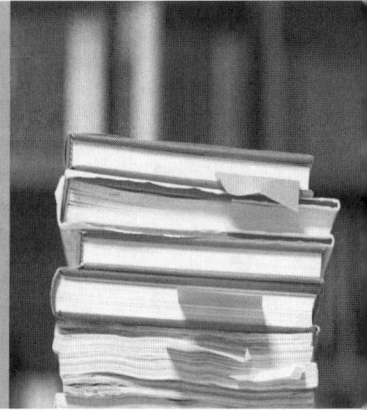

Main points

- Quantitative data analysis usually involves the use of statistics to describe the data, allow inferences about the relationships expressed in hypotheses and show the results of hypothesis testing.
- Nominal data are in the form of names or categories.
- Ordinal data are in the form of names or categories.
- Interval data can only be counted as whole numbers.
- Ratio data can be collected on a scale with infinitely small graduations of measurement, with an absolute zero.
- Descriptive statistics are those which describe a phenomenon.
- The main descriptive statistics are the sum, percentage and frequency count.
- Illustrations such as tables, bar graphs, histograms and pie graphs can be used to illustrate the composition of the data.
- Inferential statistics are those which allow us to make inferences about the population from which the data were collected, through a process of hypothesis testing.
- Parametric data are collected on at least an interval level scale, and are representative of the population from which they were collected.
- The statistics chosen will be appropriate to show the trend in the data and to test the hypothesis and will reflect whether the data are parametric or non-parametric, and the number and nature of the dependent and independent variables.
- It is important to avoid type I and type II errors when testing for significance by setting appropriate p values and determining appropriate sample size.

CASE STUDY

You are conducting a trial of an exercise program for residents in an aged-care facility in order to reduce injuries from falls. Your research is quasi-experimental, and you are comparing the incidence of falls in the treatment group to the incidence of falls in a control group. Listed below are the types of data you collect. For each one, indicate what scale of measurement it represents, and what test might be used to compare the two groups:

variable/data:	scale:	test:
Age in years		
Gender		
Weight in kg		
No. of falls		

Multiple choice questions

1   Descriptive statistics are used to:
   a   summarise data for variables
   b   provide an overview of the data
   c   give indications for further data analysis
   d   all of the above

2   Which of the following would be an example of an ordinal data?
   a   5.5 mmol/L blood cholesterol
   b   tallest person in the room
   c   annual income of $50,000
   d   blue eyes

3   Which of the following is a characteristic of ratio level data?
   a   it is always found as whole numbers
   b   it is a substitute for a word description of something
   c   it can be measured to any number of decimal points
   d   it is expressed as a rank

4   The middle score in a range of scores is called the:
   a   median
   b   percentage
   c   mode
   d   mean

5   The average of a set of scores is called the:
   a   median
   b   percentage
   c   mode
   d   mean

6   In which of the following cases would a *t*-test be appropriate?
   a   comparing blood sugar levels before and after exercise in a single group of athletes
   b   looking for an association between blood cholesterol and hours of exercise in a single group of office workers
   c   looking for a relationship between gender and use of sunscreen among school students
   d   none of the above

7   In which of the following cases would a chi-square test be appropriate?
   a   comparing blood sugar levels before and after exercise in a single group of athletes
   b   looking for an association between blood cholesterol and hours of exercise in a single group of office workers
   c   looking for a relationship between gender and use of sunscreen among school students
   d   none of the above

8   In which of the following cases would a Pearson's Correlation be appropriate?
   a   comparing blood sugar levels before and after exercise in a single group of athletes
   b   looking for an association between blood cholesterol and hours of exercise in a single group of office workers
   c   looking for a relationship between gender and use of sunscreen among school students
   d   none of the above

9   Which of the following tests could be used to compare the mean blood alcohol levels of four different groups of drinkers?
   a   chi-square
   b   ANOVA
   c   contingency table
   d   Spearman's Correlation

10   Which of the following is an example of a parametric test?
   a   *t*-test
   b   chi-square
   c   Mann-Whitney U-test
   d   Spearman's Correlation

Review topics

1   Describe the different scales and levels of measurement.
2   What are the commonly used descriptive statistics?
3   What is the purpose of hypothesis testing in statistical analysis?
4   What is meant by statistical significance?
5   What conditions are necessary to allow the use of parametric data analysis techniques?

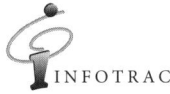

References

Beckmann, K., Abell, L., Ryan, M., Kirke, D. & Roder, D. 2003, 'Who uses the Breast Cancer Support Service (BCSS) in South Australia?', *Australian Journal of Cancer Nursing*, vol. 4, no. 1, 12–17.

Bohneneblust, S. 2000, *Basic Statistics for the Health Sciences*, Mayfield Publishing Co., Mountain View, California.

Dawson-Saunders, B. & Trapp, R. 2001, *Basic and Clinical Biostatistics*, 3rd edn, Lange Medical Books-McGraw-Hill, New York.

Kermode, S. 2004, *Getting Started in Health Research*, 2nd edn, Pearsons, Frenchs Forest.

Sieri, T. & Beretta, G. 2004, 'Fall risk assessment in very old males and females living in nursing homes', *Disability and Rehabilitation*, vol. 26, no. 12, 718–23.

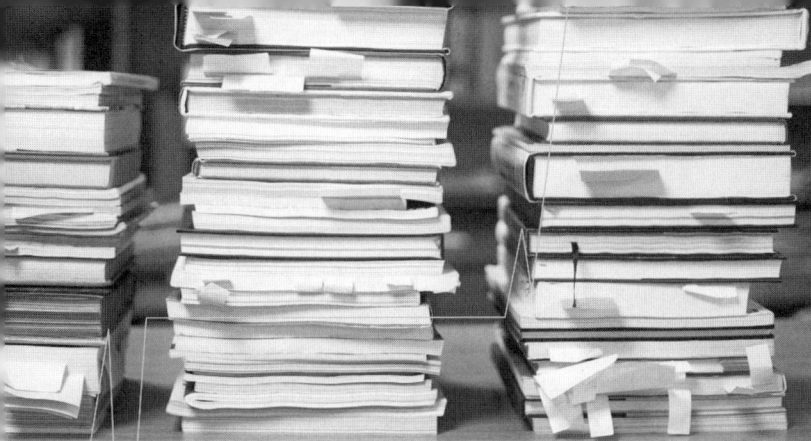

CHAPTER **11**

DETERMINING THE CLINICAL RELEVANCE OF QUANTITATIVE FINDINGS

CHAPTER OBJECTIVES

The material presented in this chapter will assist you to:

- keep track of your interpretations
- interpret relationship findings
- distinguish between causal and non-causal relationships
- distinguish between statistically significant and non-significant findings
- distinguish between statistically and clinically significant findings
- understand a selection of indicators of clinical significance
- search for the meaning in your findings
- relate the results of your study to theory, research and practice.

Introduction

You have collected and analysed your data. Now you are about to enter another phase of the research process: interpreting the results to make a coherent, meaningful interpretation of the findings. As a researcher, you are responsible for interpreting your findings. You will describe the findings, search for their meaning, draw conclusions from them, determine implications for practice and make recommendations for implementing any significant findings.

At some level, you may have started this process already if you have been doing some interpretation while you did the data analysis. Indeed, the processes of data analysis and interpretation are somewhat iterative. Some findings need immediate interpretation and some interpretations take you back to do more data analysis to answer questions that emerge from the data analysis.

Preparation

You are sitting at your desk with what will probably seem like an impossible amount of computer print-out to analyse. Where do you start? First of all, make sure that you are confident about the accuracy of the data analysis. In Chapters 9 and 10, we covered techniques to ensure accuracy. If you have followed the earlier suggestions, you will probably have accurate results. I re-emphasise this point because the value of your findings and the interpretation of the findings rests on the accuracy of your data analysis, which in turn rests upon the accuracy of the data and their input into the computer.

If you have not done so already, organise your material into logical groupings so that you can tackle one section at a time. Each project will suggest its own groupings to you. It is best to start with the purely descriptive data analysis output and then work up to the more complex analyses grouped according to your conceptual framework, hypotheses or questions. You may care to refer to Chapter 9 for suggestions on methods of organising your data analysis.

Some people like to keep track of their findings on a spreadsheet so that they can see the overall picture easily. Many people also find it useful to transform their findings into graphs to make it easier to interpret them. You can do this easily with a statistical analysis program.

As you interpret your data analysis and produce findings, it is best to start writing out your account of these, which will also serve as a preliminary draft of your research report. You can do this in a logbook, or type straight into the word processor.

Data reduction and summaries

One of the first things to do with a large pool of data is to reduce them into smaller and more useable summary statistics. The first thing usually done is to produce a set of simple descriptive statistics. These should usually include a frequency table for each variable, and a mean and standard deviation for each variable (where appropriate). It is sometimes also useful to generate cross-tabulation tables for any key variables you might want to compare.

Reducing your data into simple summaries allows you to 'eyeball' it and make decisions about more complex levels of data analysis which may follow.

Interpreting descriptive findings

In interpreting your data, it is also easier to start with the purely descriptive data analysis. In looking at the descriptive statistics, you should look first at the statistics for all of the sample before progressing to any sub-groups.

You can examine the results for your general descriptive variables such as age, sex and so forth. This will give you a profile of your sample. Then you can compare your sample with the known characteristics of the population to see how typical it was. This will reinforce the earlier point that it is important to plan your data analysis so that when you come to compare it with the population you actually have the correct data for the comparison. If your sample matches the population reasonably well on the major variables of interest in the study, you are probably fairly safe in generalising about the external validity of your results. Large samples tend to be less risky in terms of matching the population, but careful sampling and good participation rates can usually produce representative samples. For example, in the study by Johnson (2004), 1917 undergraduate students in three Chinese universities were surveyed, and the response rate was 89.7 per cent. There is not much risk of a biased sample in such a study.

If your sample is not similar to the population, or if it does not match on any one major variable of interest, you should not claim that your findings are valid for any group other than your sample. For example, if you collected data only on participants from urban areas, it would not be legitimate to claim that your results were typical of all clients in the country, or indeed the state. It is always better to err on the side of caution in generalising your findings.

Once you have looked at your descriptive data about the characteristics of the sample, you should also look at the descriptive data analysis about the variables you are investigating. For example, if you are relating the variable 'amount of tobacco smoking' to demographic data, you should also first look at the descriptive information about the smoking. This will give you a picture of the sample in relation to the major variables. Again, you can compare this picture with that of the population to look for its representativeness.

If you have created a questionnaire in which you have identified your first-round responders from your follow-ups it is useful to compare them on the various variables to see whether they are the same. If so, you can treat them as one group for the rest of the interpretation. If they are different, you will need to account for that in your interpretation of the findings.

If you are doing a clinical study or one that requires more than one data collection point, it is also useful to compare your drop-outs with your persisters on the demographic variables. This will tell you if your study has been affected by participant mortality.

Findings of association and difference

If your hypotheses have expressed associations between variables, or possible differences between groups, then these hypotheses will require testing for such associations and differences. Common differences that are examined are between males and females, control and experimental groups, and pre-test and post-test groups. You may or may not find differences in the dependent variable for the different groups. Sometimes you will want to compare the pre-test values for a control and experimental group to see if they were the same before the experiment. If not, the results of the experiment could be in doubt. Again, you need to look at the *p* **value** to decide whether to reject the null hypothesis or not (see Chapter 10 for details about the null hypothesis).

You also need to check that the results are not the result of some intervening variable. For example, suppose that you found that there was a higher rate of domestic violence in one racial group than another. The violence might not be related to the race as such, but an increased alcohol intake in that group.

A correlational study looks for an association between variables within one group. It can be positive; that is, when you have a high level of one variable, you have a high level of the other. Or it can be negative, in which a high level of one variable is accompanied by a low level of the other. Of course, you may find that there is no association. In Chapter 10, we looked at an example of these associations, so you may wish to refresh your memory by revisiting that section. To determine whether or not a relationship is statistically significant, it is necessary to determine whether the probability level is above or below the level of confidence that you set. Usually if the p value is below 0.05, we can say that the result is statistically significant at any rate.

In interpreting findings it is very important not to go beyond what the findings actually tell you. If you find a relationship between two variables, it means only that where you find one you find the other. It is very important not to assume that because one thing is related to another it is caused by the other. Both of the variables may be related to a third variable, for example, which may or may not cause the effect. For example, you may have found that there is an increase in body malfunction in people who live in a district that has a high-power transformer. It would be premature to conclude that high-power lines cause the malfunction. Perhaps the area that has a high-power transformer is a low socioeconomic area in which there is poor nutrition. It might therefore be the nutritional status of the people that underlies the malfunction, not the emissions of the transformer. Relationships such as these require further investigation before causality can be concluded.

Also, just because one thing is statistically related to another, there is not necessarily any meaningful relationship between the factors. For example, if you looked at the census data, you might find all sorts of correlations that were present but were not meaningful.

Causal relationships

In health research the two most important forms of evidence we are looking for are:

1   exposure/outcome relationships – this refers to how different types of exposures result in different types of health problems; for example, which risk factors are most important in the development of coronary heart disease

2   treatment/outcome relationships – this refers to how different types of treatment or intervention result in different types of health outcomes; for example, whether exercise

and diet are effective in reducing the risk of coronary heart disease, or improving the survival rates of people who already have coronary heart disease.

There are relatively few health problems where a direct cause and effect relationship can be seen. Microbial infections, poisoning and accidents are the best examples. Modern lifestyle diseases, however, have multiple risk factors which combine in different ways for different people. So it is not a simple 'cause-and-effect' relationship between one factor and one outcome. It is possible, however, to estimate the strength of the effect of each factor from well-designed research studies. In such cases it may be possible to estimate which factors have the strongest effect and which ones are not so strong.

You should be speaking about **causal relationships** only if you are sure that the one variable causes the other. In order for one thing to cause another, the causative factor must precede the effect. For example, a lightning flash always precedes electrocution from lightning. The two variables must also be specifically and strongly related to each other, for example, a micro-organism and a disease. When you have a patient with syphilis, you will always find the organism *Treponema pallidum* in the body. Finally, the relationship should be reasonable. For example, if you found that two things were related but it did not seem logical that one caused the other, you would probably conclude that the relationship was correlational rather than causal.

Usually causal relationships can be demonstrated only by an experiment in which a change in the independent variable can be shown to result in a corresponding change in the dependent variable. Even then, the experiment should be so highly controlled that the independent variable is the only factor that could have caused the result. A causal relationship will almost always require the examination of differences between a pre-test and a post-test on the same group to see if the manipulation of the independent variable resulted in a change in the dependent variable.

It is normally through experimentation (see Chapter 7) that scientists have built up knowledge about causes of diseases. However, sometimes if a statistical relationship is very strong and the other criteria are satisfied we can assume causality if it is not possible to experiment. Sometimes a disease in humans, for example, AIDS, is always linked to a specific micro-organism (HIV virus) that has been demonstrated to cause the disease in other primates. It would therefore be reasonable to assume that the micro-organism causes the disease despite the fact that you cannot do an experiment on people for ethical reasons. Tobacco smoking as a cause of cancer of the lung is another example of assumed causality from a naturalistic 'experiment' rather than from a controlled experiment. However, smoking tobacco always precedes the lung cancer, correlates strongly with the amount of tobacco smoked and the length of smoking, and produces cancer in animals. Furthermore, it is logical that inhaling an irritant into the lungs could disrupt cellular functioning. The case meets the criteria for causality so strongly that it is reasonable to assume that smoking causes lung cancer.

If your results suggest a causal relationship, you need to be suspicious of a placebo effect and be very cautious in your interpretation of them. It pays to use a placebo-controlled design to allow for the placebo effect. For example, Jorge et al. (2003) studied post-stroke patients to determine if the use of antidepressants improved survival. In order to be sure that the drug was producing an effect, they used a placebo with half of the participants.

They found that treatment with antidepressants for 12 weeks during the first six months post-stroke significantly increased the survival of both depressed and non-depressed patients.

Significance of findings – statistical versus clinical significance

The findings from any research study can be presented and interpreted in more than one way. Your study might have profound health care implications, for instance, but not have achieved **statistical significance** simply because of a small sample size. Likewise, you may have had a huge sample size and achieved a slight level of statistical significance. How should you make sense of these findings?

Interpreting or making sense of findings is perhaps the most important phase of the research process. It is at this stage of the process that you make an attempt to apply your findings to clinical practice, or to the theory out of which your study emerged. Research is the link between theory and practice, and it is at the point of interpretation that these links have to be demonstrated.

Non-significant findings

You first need to examine the findings to see whether they are significant. If they do not meet the criterion set previously for significance (usually $p < 0.05$) then the findings are not significant ($p < 0.05$) and the null hypothesis is not rejected. You are then faced with the task of explaining why they are not significant. Before reporting non-significant findings you should look for an alternative explanation for them. Perhaps they can be explained by an inadequate or biased sample, incorrect methodology, a design flaw, errors in measurement, data collection or analysis, or even some unforeseen event that affected participants. However, results that are statistically non-significant may still be important if they add to our knowledge, because the lack of difference is important.

Significant findings

If your findings are statistically significant, you get a rush of satisfaction. But wait! There are questions to be answered before you go and tell the world.

Are the findings pointing in the direction that you predicted? It is possible to have findings that are significant but that are the opposite of what you expected. Now you are left with the difficult task of explaining why, and you will have to critique your whole study to see if you can come up with an explanation. Before you do so, however, it is wise to check your data entry and analysis to see whether you carried it out correctly. For example, an incorrect step in recoding or omitting to recode a variable in the opposite direction could explain your results. If so, you are in the happy position of at least being able to fix your mistake and reinterpret the corrected data analysis. If not, you still have to explain why you got these results. If you are sure that your study was well designed and your methods were appropriate and carried out correctly, you might conclude that the theory is wrong.

Even if findings are statistically significant they may not be valid. It is therefore necessary to be cautious in the interpretation of statistically significant findings. You need to be sure that there is a continuity between your problem, theoretical framework, methodology, methods and findings. Remember, you also have to be certain that your findings have not been affected by any of the threats to validity that we discussed in Chapter 7. You must consider whether they could be accounted for by another explanation, such as a very large sample resulting in very small differences being statistically significant. Be careful not to mistake statistical significance for meaningful differences.

Indeed, you virtually need to do a critique of your own study, using the criteria in Chapter 3, so that you can evaluate the validity of your findings and be ready to defend your findings against criticism from colleagues. Of course, if your study problem, conceptual framework, design, data collection methods and data analysis were adequate, then your findings are likely to have internal validity. However, it is easier to see the flaws in the study in hindsight and some events cannot be predicted, so it is necessary to review the adequacy of every part of the study.

EXERCISE

You have completed a study of student health among Year 12 students at the local high school.

You measured the body mass index (BMI) of all students, and found the following results:

- *Female students*: mean BMI = 27.2; standard deviation = 4.2
- *Male students*: mean BMI = 25.1; standard deviation = 3.4
- *t*-test of mean BMI between males and females, $p = .02$

What do these findings mean?

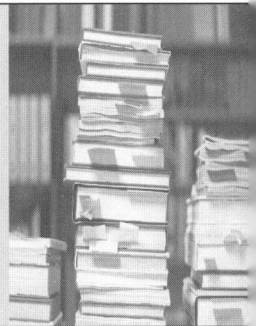

Difference between statistical and clinical significance

In interpreting research results, it is important to distinguish between statistical significance and **clinical significance**. Statistical significance is a difference in groups that is related to testing an hypothesis. It says only that the results probably could not have happened by chance alone. A small difference may turn out to be statistically significant, particularly if there are many participants. Clinical significance, on the other hand, is the strength of the 'effect' in your study. The 'effect' might be what happens when someone is exposed to a risk factor, or it might be the actual effect of a treatment on an existing condition.

There are a number of techniques used in epidemiology which help clinicians to determine the clinical significance of their findings. They include confidence intervals, odds ratios and risk calculations.

Confidence intervals

Confidence intervals are often used in health research to demonstrate the level of 'confidence' that a finding is true, and not the result of a sampling error. While *p* values tell us the probability that the result we have is a true estimate of the given statistic in the real population, they can vary according to the sample size and the actual effect size being measured (the size/strength of difference or association between two sets of measurements). In health research we are more concerned with the real strength of an effect, and not so much with the sample size needed to make it statistically significant. This refers to the 'clinical significance' of an effect.

Confidence intervals give us the range of likely estimates for an effect. p values are 'point estimates', that is, they tell us about the significance of a single point of measurement. The difficulty of relying on p values in clinical research is that they may obscure the clinical significance of a finding by relying totally on the statistical significance of a single point. A real health benefit or health problem may be ignored because the sample size was small, while a clinically insignificant result may be considered important simply because an extremely large sample produced a statistically significant result, based on a small effect level.

Confidence intervals are a way of discriminating between statistical significance based purely on p values and actual clinical significance of a result. A 95 per cent confidence interval will tell us where 95 per cent (19 out of 20) of the likely results would fall from all possible samples used. Confidence intervals are calculated as follows:

- Upper and lower limits are calculated to demonstrate 95 per cent confidence in the result, and these are then added and deducted from the mean to give the 95 per cent confidence interval.
- Formulae for confidence intervals:

$$\text{lower} = [\text{mean} + (1.96 \times \text{std. dev.})] \div \sqrt{n}$$

$$\text{upper} = [\text{mean} + (1.96 \times \text{std. dev.})] \div \sqrt{n}$$

(the number 1.96 in these formulae corresponds to a z score of 1.96 either side of the mean, which covers 95 per cent of the area under the normal curve; n is the size of the sample).

Odds ratios

An odds ratio refers to the ratio between the incidence of a health problem in a group of persons exposed to a risk factor, compared with the incidence of a health problem in a group of persons not exposed to a risk factor. An example is the rate of lung cancer in smokers compared to the rate of lung cancer in non-smokers. Imagine a hypothetical study of cigarette smoking and lung cancer produced the following data summary:

	Smoker	Non-smoker
Lung cancer	12	2
No lung cancer	88	98

Using the data in this contingency table you could make the following calculations:
- Odds of getting lung cancer if a smoker = (12/100) / (88/100) = 12/88
- Odds of getting lung cancer if a non-smoker = (2/100) / (98/100) = 2/98
- Odds ratio related to the risk of smoking and lung cancer = (12/88) / (2/98) = 6.68

Risk calculations

Risk and cause are not the same thing. Many modern lifestyle diseases, such as coronary heart disease, do not have a single cause. They are acquired by exposure to multiple risk factors including genetic predisposition, diet, exercise and cigarette smoking. No one risk factor 'causes' these types of disease, but some are more influential than others.

Understanding the importance of various risk factors in disease has become an important part of epidemiological research. Risk can be measured in two ways:

- Relative risk – the rate at which disease occurs in people who are exposed to a particular risk compared to the rate among those who are not so exposed; for example, the prevalence of lung cancer in smokers compared to the prevalence of lung cancer in non-smokers. From our previous table on cigarette smoking, this would be 12/2 = 6.0. This means that lung cancer would be six times more likely in smokers than non-smokers.

- Attributable risk – the difference between rates at which a disease occurs in exposed people and the rates at which it occurs in non-exposed people; for example, the degree of risk of acquiring lung cancer simply by smoking cigarettes. In other words, having subtracted the overall likelihood of getting lung cancer in the non-smoking population, how much risk can be attributed to cigarette smoking alone? From our previous table on cigarette smoking, this would be 12–2 = 10.0. This means that of all the deaths caused by lung cancer 10 out of 12 can be directly attributed to cigarette smoking.

EXERCISE

From your previous study of student health among Year 12 students at the local high school you produced the following results:

Female students:

- Mean Body Mass Index = 27 2
- Standard deviation = 4.2
- No. of females in the group = 37

What is the 95% confidence interval for these data?

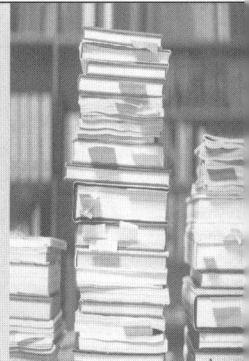

Mixed findings

Mixed findings occur when you have rejected some null hypotheses and not others, or some findings are in the direction of the hypotheses and some are not. It is important to consider each finding carefully in the light of the methodology and the theoretical framework. It may be that the different findings reflect different methods of measurement, or different data collectors, or a faulty theory.

Serendipitous findings

Serendipitous findings are findings that are unexpected. On most projects, most researchers cannot resist doing extra analyses if they have the data, just to find out what might be there.

Sometimes this will result in a finding that you were not expecting. Some of these findings may be useful and some may not. Serendipitous findings may go either in the direction of or against the hypotheses. Or they might be totally unrelated to the study but noticed by chance. A classic example is the story of the discovery of penicillin that resulted from Fleming's noticing that a culture plate contaminated with *Penicillium notatum* mould showed no growth around the bacteria. He concluded that the mould contained a bacteriostatic agent, and penicillin was born.

You need to consider very carefully how an unexpected finding could have happened – whether it is a spurious finding that occurred because of an error or whether it is genuine. If you think it is genuine, you need to arrive at an explanation for this finding. You should also consider the finding in the light of the theoretical framework. Serendipitous findings will usually need to be investigated further to determine whether or not they are valid, as another method may be more appropriate for a research project arising out of a serendipitous finding.

Searching for meaning within

In searching for meaning within the study findings, it is important to look at the patterns and connections in the total picture, as well as the individual parts of the findings. Often individual variables produce data, but when compared with one another, or clustered into groups for comparison, they can yield insights that were not evident when examining the individual variables.

In interpreting patterns in your findings, particularly if you have a complex set of findings, it can be useful to use a whiteboard or butcher's paper. By grouping the findings on the paper or board and looking at them and drawing links between them you can find the patterns in the findings. It is this conceptual mapping and synthesis that is the highest point of the interpretation of the results.

In searching for meaning, you need to go beyond a description of your findings and ask 'why did this occur?' or 'why did it not occur?' Any competent researcher can look at and describe findings. However, to make a meaningful commentary, you need to go beyond documentation or narration of the results and ask 'so what?' This involves interpreting for the research consumer the real difference that these findings make. This is a difficult step because it requires much thought and reasoning, and sometimes even intuitive leaps.

You need to relate your findings to the purpose of the study and the problem that you were investigating. Did they answer the study question? If so, how? If not, why not? If they answered some other question, then you have a serious threat to the validity of your findings.

It is important when interpreting findings to relate your findings to the conceptual framework you used to guide the study. This may be at the descriptive, correlational, comparative, explanatory or predictive level. Were your findings consistent with the theory? If not, why not?

You should also relate your findings to the results of previous research cited in your literature review. This is one of the areas that students find very difficult, because it requires a comparative evaluation and a synthesis. You need to have at least a simple concept map of previous research findings in order to see the relationships. What you need to ask yourself is how your results add to the total known picture about the findings on this topic. You need to decide whether they support previous findings or not. Again, it is also useful to group the previous findings according to an individual question or topic rather than on a study-by-study basis.

Searching for meaning beyond: implications, conclusions and recommendations

It is important to evaluate your study in terms of its implications for further theoretical development. Your findings may confirm the theory or part of it, may reject the theory or may make no difference one way or the other if they are not significant. Similarly, they may help to develop the theory further or they may help to critique the theory.

It is also important to evaluate your findings in terms of the implications for future research. It is rare for a study not to give rise to other questions that would need further research to answer them. In a study by Wright et al. (2000), for example, women's personal control in pain relief during labour was studied. In the study the rules the women believed applied to labour were found to change as a result of their labour. The authors were not sure, however, whether this was as a result of the labour itself or due to the influence of the midwives. Naturally, they recommended further study to be able to make this discrimination.

It is also important to evaluate your findings for the implications for practice, assuming they are clinically significant. If they are clinically significant, how can clinicians improve practice on the basis of your findings? What would the outcomes be for clients or their families if the practice were changed? What would the cost be in poorer client outcomes if the change were not made? A study by Eckert, Turnbull and MacLennan (2004) involved a randomised, controlled trial of immersion in water in the first stage of labour. They found that bathing in labour confers no clear benefits for the labouring woman but may contribute to adverse effects in the neonate. This has obvious implications for the advice given to women on methods of delivery during childbirth.

When you have addressed the implications, ask yourself what conclusions you can draw from your findings. Conclusions may be tentative or firm, depending on the certainty you have about the external and internal validity of your findings.

You should also consider what recommendations you would make, based on the findings, implications and conclusions from any significant and meaningful results. They can be recommendations for research, practice, theoretical development or testing, and education. These recommendations will follow naturally from the implications; indeed, they are an extension of the recommendations. Recommendations are very important because they are one of the major products of your research.

Summary

In this chapter, we have discussed how to go about discovering the meaning of your findings. This is the time when you examine your findings for validity and meaning both in terms of the question that you were trying to answer and the study's place in the bigger picture. Having done so, you are ready to move on to writing up the research report and disseminating it to the professional community.

Main points

- Researchers are responsible for interpreting their data accurately and objectively to convey to the audience a coherent, meaningful interpretation of the findings.
- Descriptive data are interpreted to give a picture of your sample and findings.
- Relationship findings and hypothesis testing are interpreted using p values.
- Causal relationships should only be inferred from an experiment.
- It is important to distinguish between findings that are statistically significant and those that are also clinically significant and can be used to influence practice.
- There are a range of indicators related to clinical significance which can be applied to your findings. They include confidence intervals, odds ratios and risk calculations.
- It is important to search for the meaning behind the findings and the relationships between the findings.
- Findings should be related to the theoretical framework and previous findings set out in the literature review.
- Findings should be considered for implications for further research, theory development and practice.
- Conclusions and recommendations should be formulated, based on the findings.

CASE STUDY

Examine the following table, taken from a study by Johnson (2004), in which Chinese undergraduate students were surveyed regarding their health behaviour practices:

Percentage of undergraduate university students aged ^{3} 18 years who reported having used tobacco, by gender, age, and hometown

Cigarette use

Category	Lifetime[†]	Lifetime daily[‡]	Current[§]	Current frequent[¥]	Cig. ever used
Gender	X2 – 172.8***	X2 –11.81**	X2 – 198.65***	ns	X2 – 57.48***
male	54.5	7.3	8.2	0.0	7.3
female	86.6	21.2	59.8	1.5	23.8
Age group	X2 – 9.43**	ns	X2 – 37.10***	ns	X2 – 23.53***
18–19 years	70.6	14.3	38.2	2.5	12.2
20–22 years	77.5	19.7	48.2	0.9	19.9
>22 years	79.2	26.3	60.1	1.2	26.8
Hometown	X2 – 34.32***	ns	X2 24.43***	X2 – 11.91***	ns
Urban/Suburban	69.7	20.2	40.6	2.8	18.4
Rural/Small town	83.7	18.0	54.2	0.0	17.6
Overall	75.2	19.8	44.7	1.5	18.1

(Continued)

s = non-significant, * p < .05
***p < .001
**p < .01
† Ever smoked at least one or two puffs of a cigarette.
‡ Ever smoked at least one cigarette every day for 30 days.
§ Smoked cigarettes on ≥1 of the 30 days proceeding the survey.
¥ Smoked cigarettes on >20 of the 30 days proceeding the survey.

Table source: Johnson 2004, pp.50–62

Questions related to the case study:

1 What do these findings say about the cigarette-smoking behaviour of males compared to females?
2 What do these findings say about the cigarette-smoking behaviour of students in various age groups?
3 What do these findings say about the cigarette-smoking behaviour of urban students compared to rural students?

Multiple choice questions

1 When interpreting statistical tests you should:
   a   only be concerned with p values
   b   not worry about the sample size
   c   ignore effect magnitude
   d   none of the above

2 Internal validity is dependent upon:
   a   whether the independent variable is really responsible for changes in the dependent variable
   b   whether your design accurately captured the effects of the independent variable
   c   the precision of the measurement taken in the research
   d   all of the above

3 Cause and effect relationships in health can be found as:
   a   exposures which lead to specific diseases
   b   treatments which lead to specific health improvements
   c   both of the above
   d   none of the above

4 External validity refers to:
   a   the extent to which the research is reproducible
   b   whether the participants were 'blinded' in the study
   c   whether the findings can be generalised to the population of interest
   d   all of the above

5   A *p* value of <0. 05 means:
     a   less than 5 per cent chance of an error in the outcome of the test
     b   more than 95 per cent chance of an error in the outcome of the test
     c   less than 5 per cent chance that the research is valid
     d   more than 95 per cent chance that the finding is wrong
6   Which of the following is a source of bias in health research?
     a   sloppy measurement
     b   confounding variables
     c   poor sampling
     d   all of the above
7   Which of the following are used to determine if a finding has clinical significance?
     a   the *p* value
     b   confidence intervals
     c   effect size
     d   all of the above
8   Odds ratios can be used to state:
     a   the likelihood of getting a health problem from undertaking a certain type of activity
     b   the likelihood of the findings in your research being wrong
     c   the chance that your sample was biased
     d   none of the above
9   Relative risk is calculated by:
     a   comparing the rate at which a disease occurs in exposed persons to the rate in non-exposed persons
     b   putting frequency data into a contingency table
     c   both of the above
     d   none of the above
10   The major difference between statistical significance and clinical significance is that:
     a   clinical significance cannot be measured
     b   clinical significance is more dependent on effect size
     c   clinical significance is only achieved with large sample sizes
     d   none of the above

Review topics

1   Distinguish between causal and non-causal relationships.
2   How do statistically significant and non-significant findings differ?
3   Describe two indicators of clinical significance.
4   What is meant by serendipitous findings?
5   Why is it is important to search for the meaning behind the findings and the relationships between the findings?

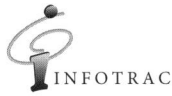

References

Eckert, K., Turnbull, D. & MacLennan A. 2001, 'Immersion in water in the first stage of labor: a randomized controlled trial', *Birth*, vol. 28, no. 2, 84–93.

Johnson, P.H. 2004, 'Priority health behavior practices among Chinese undergraduate students', *The International Electronic Journal of Health Education*, (www.iejhe.org), vol. 7, 50–62.

Jorge, R.E., Robinson, R.G., Arndt, S. & Starkstein, S. 2003, 'Mortality and poststroke depression: a placebo-controlled trial of antidepressants', *American Journal of Psychiatry*, vol. 160, no. 10, 1823–9.

Wright, M.E., McCrea, H., Stringer, M. & Murphy-Black, T. 2000, 'Personal control in pain relief during labour', *Journal of Advanced Nursing*, vol. 32, no. 5, 1168–77.

CHAPTER 12

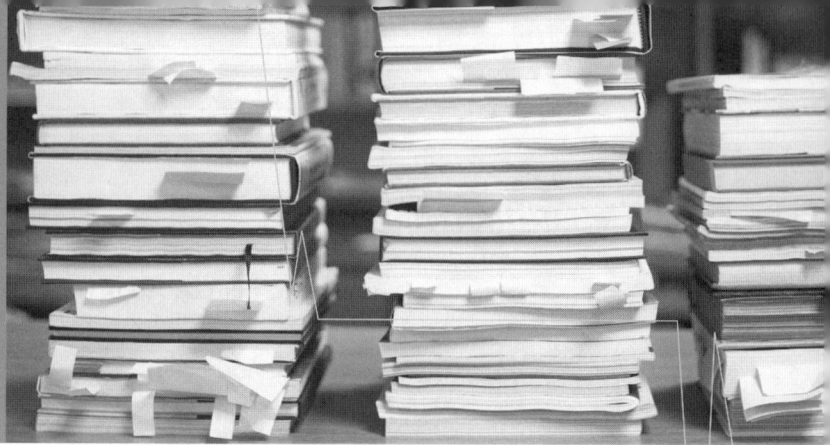

QUALITATIVE INTERPRETIVE METHODOLOGIES

CHAPTER OBJECTIVES

The material presented in this chapter will assist you to:

- describe research as a means of generating knowledge
- define epistemology and ontology
- clarify some common qualitative theoretical assumptions
- differentiate between quantitative and qualitative research
- describe postmodern influences on contemporary epistemology and ontology
- differentiate between interpretive and critical forms of qualitative methodologies
- describe postmodern alternatives for qualitative methodologies
- create flexible approaches to methodologies
- describe four qualitative interpretive methodologies in terms of their respective methodologies and methods
- recognise research examples of four qualitative interpretive methodologies
- generate potential research questions using these approaches.

Introduction

Research approaches provide the means of looking for answers to puzzles posed as research questions. The longest-standing questions that have perplexed humans are: 'What is true knowledge?' and 'What is the meaning of life?' These questions are epistemological and ontological respectively, and they are still being asked in modern-day research projects.

The history of the search for ideas through research approaches has been long and intensive. Therefore, this chapter builds the conceptual layers sequentially, by defining key terms, discussing research as a means of generating knowledge, clarifying some common qualitative theoretical assumptions, differentiating broadly between quantitative and qualitative research, describing postmodern influences, and showing you how qualitative research methodologies can be categorised into **interpretive** and **qualitative critical** forms.

Having clarified these foundational ideas, the chapter will show you how it is possible to create flexible approaches to methodologies because they can be used in various combinations. Exercises will help you to create your own flexible qualitative interpretive methodologies, to demonstrate the freedom you can enjoy in finding the best approaches to fulfil your research objectives. Examples of qualitative interpretive methodologies – **grounded theory, phenomenology, ethnography** and **historical research** – are described in terms of the key ideas contained within their respective methodologies and methods. Nursing and health research examples and potential research questions are presented so that you can consider the possibilities of using some of these approaches in research areas you might like to explore.

Research as a means of generating knowledge

The basic reason for doing research is to find new knowledge and adapt existing knowledge. The history of research is basically the history of ideas, or philosophy. It is not appropriate to go into a lengthy discussion here of the twists and turns in historical philosophical debate about finding knowledge. Suffice it to say that humans have adjusted their views over time to what constitutes research, and that it is, at this time, a relative matter, with no absolute answers.

From the time of Plato and Socrates and their contemporaries, through a time of dismal uninterest in philosophical thought in the Dark Ages, to the rebirth of knowledge in the Renaissance, humans have progressed through phases of observation and conjecture about people, the planet and the universe. Since the seventeenth century and Descartes, the scientific model has been the established approach, and there has been a reaction to that as the benchmark of all research in the last century or so, with the generation of multiple qualitative and postmodern research approaches. If you are interested in following these changes in depth, you would be advised to read an easily digestible form of philosophy in a book, such as Palmer (1988), before moving on to some of the heavier texts, such as Descartes (1970 trans.), Hume (1966, 1969, first published in 1739) and Barnes (1987). If these books excite you, you definitely need to consider studying philosophy!

The reason for raising these ideas about research as a means of generating knowledge is to have you consider from the start the possibility that there may be many approaches to finding knowledge through research that have merit, and that one kind should not necessarily be seen as being superior to another. Nurse-scholars such as Carper (1992) and Chinn and Kramer (1995) have expressed this idea succinctly in discussing the interrelatedness of four kinds of knowledge in contributing overall to nursing research.

Carper (1992) has described empirical, personal, aesthetic and ethical ways of knowing. Respectively, these basically have to do with science, personal insights, a sense of the beautiful, and moral judgements. Carper also made the point that these ways of knowing need to be integrated. This argument was taken up more strongly by Chinn and Kramer (1995), who contended that knowledge should not only be integrated, but that it should also be balanced. They posited that too much of one way of thinking and knowing about things can cause distortions, for example, too much empirical knowledge may result in control and manipulation; too much personal knowledge may result in isolation and self-distortion; too much aesthetics may result in prejudice and bigotry; and too much ethical knowledge may result in rigid doctrine and insensitivity to others. Using this reasoning, it seems fairly sensible to try to balance the kinds of knowledge generated and verified in research, to try to ensure that ideas, descriptions and explanations have the best chance of being well rounded and comprehensive.

Defining epistemology and ontology

Two words are inescapable in understanding how knowledge is generated: **epistemology** and **ontology**. Epistemology is the study of knowledge and how it is judged to be 'true'. Inverted commas have been used intentionally around the word 'true' to show that truth is, and has always been, an uncertain concept in philosophy. The search for what counts as truth has accounted for the various interpretations of new knowledge over time. It has always been important to argue the veracity of ideas before claiming their validity in counting towards the development of new or amended knowledge.

Ontology is the study of existence itself. Various authors have given their versions of 'the meaning of life' and their views have been debated thoroughly. For example, the philosopher Martin Heidegger (1962) considered that ontology and epistemology were one and the same thing. In other words, he argued that by understanding the nature of the existence of anything of interest, answers were supplied automatically to the very nature of knowledge itself. Whereas a diversion into ontological thought is not warranted now, you should be aware that it is a central focus of human thought and that it has relevance for nursing research.

Nurses and health care workers need to ask questions about knowing and existing, because the answers to such questions form the substance of their disciplines. Whenever researchers raise questions about what they know and how they know it is trustworthy knowledge, they are asking epistemological questions. Whenever researchers are asking about the nature of the existence of something or someone, they are asking ontological questions. Therefore, these words are relevant and integral to nursing and health research.

Some common qualitative theoretical assumptions

In this chapter, the word methodology is used to mean the theoretical assumptions underlying the choice of methods in generating a particular form of knowledge. Many philosophical traditions have contributed to research in that they have supplied theoretical assumptions about certain kinds of knowledge. For example, one of the bases of empirical/quantitative knowledge is that any knowledge that counts as truth should be free from the subjectivity of the researcher. In this section, we will examine some key theoretical assumptions that are common to various qualitative research approaches and that constitute some fundamental ideas about the nature of people as inquirers and research as a means of knowledge generation.

Qualitative research attempts to explore the changing (relative) nature of knowledge, which is seen to be special and centred in the people, place, time and conditions in which it finds itself (unique and context-dependent). Qualitative research uses thinking that starts from a specific instance and moves to the general pattern of combined instances (inductive), so that it grows from 'the ground up' to make larger statements about the nature of the thing being investigated.

The measures for ensuring validity in qualitative research involve asking the participants to confirm that the interpretations are correct, that they represent, faithfully and clearly, what the experience was/is like for the people acting as sources of information in the research. Reliability is often not an issue in qualitative research, as it is based on the idea that knowledge is relative and dependent on all of the features of the people, place, time and other circumstances (context) of the setting.

People are acknowledged as sources of information. Their expressions of their personal awareness (subjectivity) are valued as being integral to the meaning that comes out of the research. Qualitative research acknowledges that people and things may change according to their circumstances, so it is inappropriate to generalise research findings to the wider group of people or things being studied.

Differences between quantitative and qualitative research

It is a major oversimplification to say that the search for explaining human knowledge and existence has gone into two main streams, specifically quantitative and qualitative inquiry. However, this will be asserted here, for the sake of ease, and to prevent the need for following each and every detail and detour in past and present philosophical debate. Table 12.1 (overleaf) might be useful for you to consider some differences in quantitative and qualitative research.

The reason for caution in thinking of quantitative and qualitative research as being categorically different is that there may be some remnants of one in the other. For example, both approaches can use deductive and inductive thinking, and both require 'scientific' designs, in the sense that both must show they are systematic and rigorous. Caution is also necessary in trying to set both approaches up as irreconcilable alternatives.

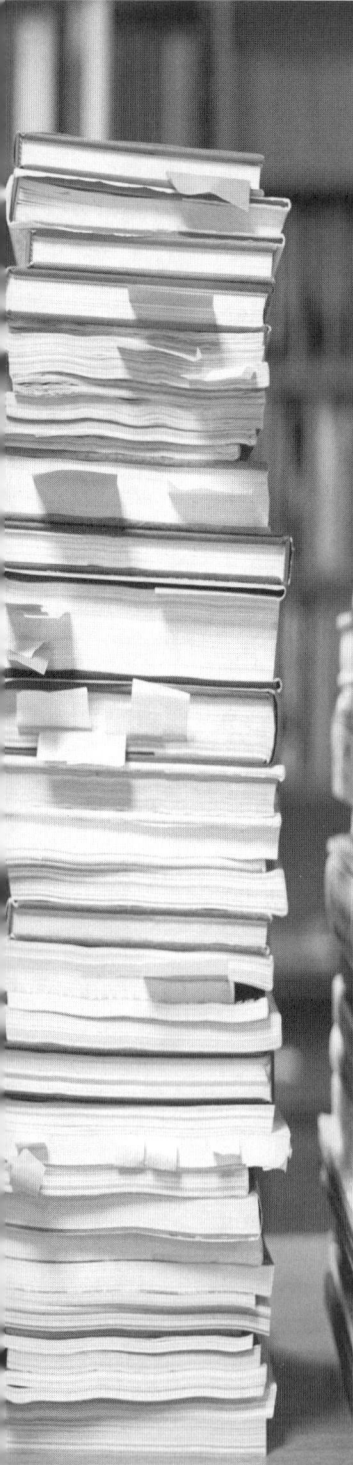

Table 12.1 Differences in quantitative and qualitative research (Taylor 1995)

Quantitative	Qualitative
Knowledge is	
absolute	relative
about finding cause-and-effect links	unique and context-dependent
deductive	inductive
Research questions are	
hypothesised	left open as tentative ideas
tested empirico-analytically	explored by a variety of means
analysed using numbers	analysed using language
interpreted as mathematical relations	interpreted as themes
Research conditions require	
validity through control of variables	participants' validation
reliability through test and retest	attention to context
objectivity without human distortion	valuing subjectivity
Problem areas for research	
are reduced to smallest parts	are part of the whole context
Findings	
are quantified in numbers	are qualified in words
need to be significant statistically	do not make absolute claims
can be predictive	provide insights to possibilities
claim to be generalisable	are specific to local phenomena
Outcomes include	
description, prediction and change	description, meaning and change

Some researchers (for example, Cox et al. 2003; Fitzgerald & Teale 2003–04; Gibson & Heartfield 2003; Ormsby & Harrington 2003; Wit, Chenoweth & Jeon 2004) have demonstrated that this is not the case, and that it is possible to combine qualitative and quantitative approaches and come up with richer research data and outcomes.

In summary, the features of empirico-analytical/quantitative research, also known as 'the scientific method', are to attain rigour in the reliability and validity of projects by using observational and analytic means to control and manipulate variables, and to produce objective data that can be quantified to demonstrate the degree of statistical significance in cause-and-effect relationships. This sounds like a good idea, and it is – for research in which the rules of the scientific method can be applied uniformly. Problems become apparent when researchers decide that they want to ask questions about human knowledge and existence that are outside the 'observe and analyse' domain, and when they want to value people's intentions, ideas and emotions as part of the research process.

EXERCISE

Write two research questions each for imaginary quantitative and qualitative projects. What are the main intentions of both sets of questions? Can any of these questions be approached by mixed methods? Why?

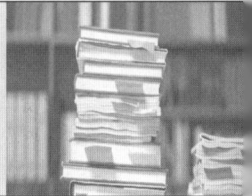

Postmodern influences on contemporary epistemology and ontology

Nursing and health research has had to take into account a radical critique of modernist (positivistic and post-positivistic) notions of epistemology and ontology. In other words, professions have been alerted to postmodern ways of thinking about what knowledge and existence might mean in an era that questions taken-for-granted quantitative and qualitative assumptions about 'truth' and 'being'. Although postmodern literature is vast, a handy guide to setting a foundation has been written by Rosenau (1992), who differentiates between a range of overlapping extreme to moderate forms of **sceptical postmodernism** and **affirmative postmodernism**. Even though Rosenau's book is dated, it still remains the best explanation I have located of the various writings on postmodernism, up until the time of its publication. I use Rosenau's work throughout this book because of its importance as an explanatory text for those of us who are not scholars in postmodernism and need a relatively easy guide to making sense of it all.

Rosenau (1992, p. 15) explains that the sceptical postmodernists offer 'a pessimistic, negative, gloomy assessment (and) argue that the post-modern age is one of fragmentation, disintegration, malaise, meaninglessness, a vagueness or even absence of moral parameters and societal chaos'. Contrastingly, affirmative postmodernists, while agreeing with the critique of modernity, nevertheless have a 'more hopeful, optimistic view of the post-modern age' (p. 15).

Extreme forms of sceptical postmodernism lambaste modernity to the extent that they leave no reasons for, or ways of, doing research because they claim authors use their authority as writers to control and censure readers; thus the 'death of the author' halts academic inquiry. The human as subject is rejected because s/he is a humanist product of modernity representing a subject–object dichotomy, and s/he is criticised 'for seizing power, for attributing meaning, for dominating and oppressing' (Rosenau 1992, p. 42). Effectively, these criticisms remove humans from the objects of their attention, such as asking or pursuing research questions. History is viewed as 'logocentric, a source of myth, ideology, and prejudice, a method assuming closure' (p. 63). This means that nothing that has gone before can be taken as fact or truth because of its association with human interpretation, rendering research methods and processes impotent as records of events over time. Time itself is rejected as chronological and linear, the modernity understanding of which is 'oppressive, measuring and controlling one's activities' (p. 63). Truth 'claims are a form of terrorism', that threaten and provoke, silencing those who disagree (p. 78), thereby making research tantamount to a terrorist activity. Words, images, meanings and symbols constitute a 'fixed system of meaning', and, as representations, they are rejected by sceptical postmodernists because they do not allow for diversity (p. 96). The inability to place (even tentatively) some faith in language renders researchers incapable of transmitting ideas gleaned by any research means. In summary, sceptical postmodernism leaves no reasons for, or ways of, doing research, thus making research endeavours unnecessary and impossible.

'All is not lost', however, as affirmative postmodernists allow room for different, less pessimistic interpretations, while still holding onto some central ideas. Affirmative postmodernists do not abandon the author completely, but they reduce the author's authority, so that s/he 'makes no universal truth claims, has no prescriptions to offer' (p. 31), and offers only options for public debate. This position allows researchers, as the authors of projects, to offer tentative insights for readers' interpretations and discussion. The human as subject returns 'not as the same subject banished' by sceptical postmodernists, but as a 'post-modern subject with a new non-identity', who 'will reject total explanations and the logocentric view that implies a unified frame of reference' (p. 57). This allows researchers to focus on humans as subjects, but in ways that do not make bold, broad theory claims. History is a source of criticism, but it is radically revised 'to focus on the daily life experience of ordinary people', akin to storytelling of small events on the margins of human existence, left open to constant questioning as possibilities rather than statements of fact and truth. Time is not linear or bounded, and truth is rejected as universal in favour of 'specific, local, personal and community forms of truth' (p. 80). This allows researchers to work with people's narratives to emphasise the relative nature of their self-understandings. Representation is permissible, but in improved political forms that assist oppressed minorities and women to find voice. This leaves room for participatory and emancipatory research that focuses on the specific circumstances of participants and finds multiple and contradictory personal and local solutions. In summary, affirmative postmodernism does not sever ties with organised research. Rather, it can influence projects by the application of redefined ideas about people and the sense they make out of their knowledge and existence.

Differences between interpretive and critical qualitative methodologies

There are many ways of categorising qualitative research; however, a useful and reasonable way is to think of them is as essentially interpretive or critical. Interpretive research is about making meaning and critical research is about causing change. Some examples of qualitative methodologies (used here as meaning 'the theoretical assumptions underlying the choice of methods') are presented in Table 12.2.

Table 12.2 Differences in interpretive and critical qualitative methodologies (Taylor 1995)

Qualitative interpretive	Qualitative critical
Grounded theory	Action research
Phenomenology	Feminist research
Historical research	Interpretive interactionism
Ethnography	Critical ethnography

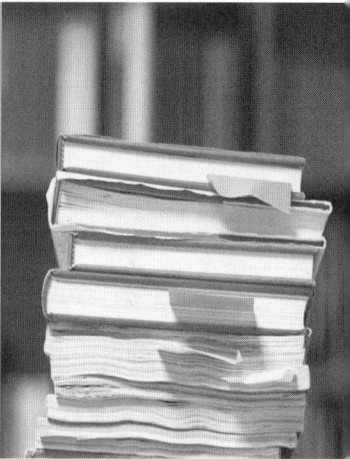

The major difference between interpretive and critical qualitative research is the main intention of what the researcher hopes to achieve through the research process. Interpretive research mainly aims to generate meaning, in other words, it tries to explain and describe, in order to make sense out of things of interest. Critical research aims to bring about change in the status quo, by working systematically through research problems to find answers and to cause change activity in light of those answers. In doing what they intend to do as their first priority, interpretive and critical researchers also manage to do other things; for example, they both generate meaning and they can bring about change, but they differ in the intensity of their intentions.

Postmodern alternatives for qualitative methodologies

Postmodernism does not fit into the categories of interpretive or critical qualitative research approaches, and by its own admission repudiates grand narratives and would not be seen as one itself. Yet it needs attention because it is related to interpretive or critical qualitative research by extending their ideas into greater realms of relativism, contradiction and **deconstruction**. Leaving aside sceptical postmodernism (which rejects the intentions, methods and processes of research), alternatives for qualitative methodologies exist, if one takes qualitative methodologies in this case to mean post-positivist (after quantitative) theoretical assumptions underlying the choice of research methods.

Grand theories (narratives) are rejected by postmodernists as statements that claim universal truth, and that can be applied in all like cases. As grand theories are indefensible; so are the research methods by which these theories can be developed and validated. The words 'strategies' or 'struggles' may be used in preference to the word 'method', which has typically taken on the meaning of the rules and procedures of modern science (the scientific method). By association, the whole idea of grand theories is suspect when the rules of rigour or trustworthiness are used to test the legitimacy or 'truthfulness' of knowledge.

The turn against absolute truth claims is pulled back from the brink of extreme relativism by affirmative postmodernists, who argue that some realities are brutal and some causes matter. Rape, poverty, violence, starvation and diseases are real, and the plights of women and other minorities matter. If it were otherwise, society would disappear into a moral morass and the vulnerable would be left to the wiles of more powerful groups, who would be left unchallenged to fulfil their own political intentions.

Extreme contradiction and deconstruction of texts negates and questions the thinking of all authors and leaves the way open for 'anything goes' to the point of creating multiple paradoxes, never-ending questions and a multiplicity of answers. The problem in this is best described by Rosenau (1992), who suggests that postmodern social science (by which nursing and health are influenced in their delivery of care):

> . . . rejects the Kuhnian model of science as a series of progressive paradigms and announces the end of all paradigms. Only an absence of knowledge claims, an affirmation of multiple realities, an acceptance of divergent interpretations remain. We can convince those who agree with us, but we have no basis for convincing those who dissent and no criteria to employ in arguing for the superiority of any particular view. Those who disagree with us can always argue that different interpretations must be accepted and that in a post-modern world one interpretation is as good as another. Post-modernists have little interest in convincing others that their view is best — the most just, appropriate or true. In the end the problem with post-modern science is that you can say anything you want, but so can everyone else. Some of what will be said will be interesting and fascinating, but some will also be ridiculous and absurd. Post-modernism provides no means to distinguish between the two (1992, p. 137).

EXERCISE

What does sceptical postmodernism mean for nursing and health research? Is research possible in this view of human knowledge and existence? Why?

Just as postmodernists reject paradigms as being legitimate solely on the basis of the claim that they are progressive in thought, researchers can choose to be influenced by postmodern ideas, but not constrained or directed by them. This leaves open the possibilities of multiple choices for researchers. They can choose to be influenced by postmodern variations of thought about human knowledge (epistemology) and existence (ontology) and adjust their projects to take account of the diversity, difference and contradiction of life on the margins as everyday ordinary history told in people's narratives and interpreted by them as their self-understandings. Researchers who do not choose postmodern influences can be guided by methodologies that tentatively claim the legitimacy of relative degrees of local theories that are trustworthy by virtue of their context-dependence and the ways in which they resonate with their readers. A detailed account of trustworthiness in qualitative research is given in Chapter 14.

Creating flexible approaches to methodologies

When you look at Table 12.2, you may be tempted to think that research approaches fit into neat categories that are either interpretive or critical, and that is simply that. However, I have represented the categories in Table 12.2 to give you a sense of stability, so that you can gain some awareness of where these approaches might reasonably be located. Having done that, I am now suggesting that, using postmodern thought, you can loosen up the methodologies, so that they move within and across categories, and you can group them into whatever combinations you choose that are helpful for your research purposes. Bear in mind, however, that even though you have 'postmodern licence' to mix and match methodologies, you need to have a sound rationale for doing this, especially for the benefit of selected audiences of your research, for example, thesis examiners or journal reviewers. In other words, it is simply not good enough to toss a number of methodologies together with no thought as to the fit of their philosophical assumptions, and then when the combination is judged to be tantamount to a 'dog's dinner', to claim that you have 'postmodern licence', without knowing how or why.

The flexibility in choosing **multiple methodologies** comes from an affirmative postmodern justification. This is the argument that researchers, as the authors of projects, offer tentative insights for readers' interpretations and discussion, and that multiple methodologies offer wider frames of reference with greater likelihood of generating many more options for public debate. Read the sections in this chapter for further justification for selecting mixed and **mobile methodologies**.

Previously, a purist approach dictated that certain methodologies fitted into particular paradigms, and that they could not be combined because they contain inherent theoretical contradictions that clash with one another. The rationale for a purist approach was, and still is, to some extent, that if you have carefully selected a single methodology, for example, grounded theory, it can adequately act as a vehicle to carry the data collection and analysis methods and will be sufficient to fulfil the research objectives. In today's research climate, it is possible to open up methodologies to creative combinations and move them along paradigmatic continuums, due to the extreme relative positions affirmative postmodernists take in relation to knowledge generation and verification.

Table 12.3 Mobilising qualitative methodologies

Examples	Potential mobility in 'paradigmatic' positions		
	interpretive	critical	postmodern
Action research	→→→→→→→→→→→→→→→→→→→→→→→→→→→→		
Ethnography	→→→→→→→→→→→→→→→→→→→→→→→→→→→→		
Feminist research	→→→→→→→→→→→→→→→→→→→→→→→→→→→→		
Grounded theory	→→→→→		
Historical research	→→→→→→→→→→→→→→		
Narrative	→→→→→→→→→→→→→→→→→→→→→→→→→→→		
Phenomenology	→→→→→→→→→→→→→→→→→→→→→→→→→→→→		

Table 12.3 shows how methodologies previously categorised into discrete paradigms in Table 12.2 can move across 'paradigmatic' positions. I have represented the word 'paradigmatic' in inverted commas to acknowledge that postmodernists would resist totalising words such as paradigm, which would represent composites as fixed and certain categories. You can see that most of the research methodologies in Table 12.3 extend across 'paradigmatic' positions, and this means that they can take on the theoretical assumptions of any of the positions. For example, action research may involve interpretive, critical and/or postmodern perspectives, depending on a specific project's intentions, methods and processes.

EXERCISE

In Table 12.3 you will notice that grounded theory does not extend into the critical and postmodern positions. Why is this the case? Look at the descriptions of this methodology and the explanation of the assumptions of the affirmative postmodern perception in this chapter, and reason grounded theory has not been extended beyond the interpretive position.

Combining qualitative methodologies

Just as it is possible to mobilise methodologies across 'paradigmatic' positions, it is also possible to imagine many combinations of methodologies, depending on the aims and objectives of your research. If you ascribe to a view that many methodologies offer more scope for multiple, broader, deeper and more relative interpretations, you can be creative in how you combine methodologies. For example, researchers have taken many combined methodological approaches including narrative and hermeneutics (Barton 2004), ethnography and phenomenology (Maggs-Rapport 2000), and critical, feminist and postmodern (Glass & Davis 1998).

Barton (2004, p. 519) used 'narrative analysis and the elicitation of life stories as understood through dimensions of interaction, continuity and situation'. The project was also informed by an understanding of the hermeneutic circle to create deeper layers of meaning for an Aboriginal epistemology. The mixed methodologies were useful in this project because Barton (p. 519) made 'a philosophical connection between two paradigms of thought – the hermeneutic circle and the Aboriginal sacred circle', which combined well with the oral tradition of storytelling used by Aboriginal people in British Columbia and the Yukon, Canada. By using narrative and the hermeneutic circle, Barton (p. 519) was able to 'coax open a window for co-constructing a narrative about diabetes as a chronic illness' and to 'adapt a methodology for use in a cultural context' that was totally inclusive of the participants' cultural perspectives.

Maggs-Rapport (2000, p. 219) acknowledged that although 'combining a number of methods of data collection and analysis within a single research study is common place, little has been written about the combination of two or more methodological approaches'. She suggested that 'methodological triangulation may be the key to telling a credible story whilst at the same time convincing the audience that data collection and analysis are carried out in a thorough and unprejudiced manner'. Maggs-Rapport (2000) used ethnography and phenomenology to achieve deeper levels of meaning of the work practices of district nurses in a large health authority in England. She argued that the mixed methodologies allowed her to fulfil the objectives of the project while demonstrating that attaining methodological rigour is possible when using a combined approach.

Although Glass and Davis (1998, p. 44) admit that 'the "merging" of feminism and postmodernism ... is contentious, offering a diversity of opinions that culminate for some scholars as binary opposing beliefs', they contend that both discourses are changing, making it 'timely to explore the contemporary debates by considering an integrated on-the-move feminist postmodern approach to nursing research'. While accepting as the main tenet of feminism that women are oppressed within patriarchal societies, Glass and Davis (p. 45) disrupt modernist feminism by presenting views in what they term 'the dissatisfaction debate' and 'the fragmentation debate' to arrive at the solution of 'an integrated turning point' in nursing research. The disruption refers to the questions they raise about feminism in light of postmodern thinking. This thinking is only possible within an affirmative postmodern approach, that, while dealing with relativities, difference and marginality, also acknowledges the important features of the grand narrative of feminisms that seek inclusiveness, social justice and action and to give voice to silenced women.

Although methodologies can be combined, this is not necessary if one methodology is sufficient to carry the needs of the project, in terms of the research methods and processes. The methodologies of grounded theory, phenomenology, ethnography and historical research will now be discussed as examples of qualitative interpretive research approaches. You may choose to use these methodologies alone or in combination. Each approach will be discussed in terms of methodology, methods, research examples and potential questions that you might ask, should you be considering such approaches for your nursing or health research interests.

Grounded theory

Grounded theory is named for its ability to start from the 'ground' of an area of interest and work up in an inductive fashion. It attempts to make sense of what people say about their experiences and to convert these statements into theoretical propositions that form a middle-range theory, midway between a grand (the sun is central in the solar system) and local ('I learn from reflective practice') theory. Middle-range theories are informative for specific contexts, offering possibilities for other people in similar circumstances. Grounded theory has differentiated through philosophical debate from its original form (Glaser & Strauss 1967) to later interpretations (Strauss & Corbin 1990, 1998). This section describes the methodology in terms of its two main forms: the methods of grounded theory, nursing and health research examples; and suggestions for research questions that may be raised using a grounded theory approach.

The methodology

Grounded theory is a qualitative interpretive approach that grew out of the symbolic inter-actionist tradition (Robrecht 1995). This, in turn, is a form of social psychology that is interested in how people interpret their roles and behaviours through words, symbols and language (Denzin 1989). Grounded theory is generated solely from the data and thus the participants' perspectives are reflected in the findings (Glaser & Strauss 1967). Existing theory is not imposed on the data, but it is utilised to support the emergent theory, creating possibilities for multiple theoretical frameworks to be applied to the research interest (Hutchinson 1986; Stern 1985).

Grounded theory is useful when little is known or experienced about the problem under scrutiny (Hutchinson 1986; Stern 1985). The approach identifies and relates factors that might be used to define and explain relatively unknown situations. Thus the methodology is based on the assumptions that problem identification and solution generation are within the realms of interpretive research. This means that practical solutions can be found to problems generated by nurses and health care workers.

The originators of grounded theory were Glaser and Strauss (1967), who later disagreed on certain theoretical areas of grounded theory, resulting in the publications of an adapted form of grounded theory by Strauss and Corbin (1990, 1998). McCallin (2003) suggests this sensible approach to choosing between the versions of grounded theory:

> In a small study, tight timeframes are common, hence extensive study of the theoretical issues . . . may not always be possible. While there are some differences methodologically on how the techniques and procedures are interpreted . . . the distinctions tend to be a matter of explication. For example, Strauss and Corbin (1998) provide a clear, explicit framework that is often reassuring for newer researchers. On the other hand, some researchers may be uneasy with such specificity, finding the clear-cut directions constraining, preferring to work with Glaser's more open version of the method (p. 205).

It is important to know the differences in the versions of grounded theory, especially if you are undertaking a large project or one that is being submitted for an academic degree. By reading about the differences in approaches, you can make a clear choice about whose version of grounded theory you will use to inform your project. This section will describe commonalities to give you an appreciation of how grounded theory is constructed as a research methodology and how you can apply it to projects that would be enhanced by a grounded theory approach.

The method

Glaser and Strauss (1967) used the term 'grounded theory' to refer to the generation of constructs (or theory) from the data, so that theory remains connected to or grounded in the data. As a research method, grounded theory involves searching out and relating factors to the research problem being studied.

The grounded theorist is involved in looking for processes, rather than being concerned with static conditions. Observational, interview and document-analysis methods generate data through a system of constant comparison until hypotheses are generated. Various modes of data collection may be used, for example, unstructured interviews, media items, personal observations and informal conversations. Of these methods, Swanson (1986) and Stern (1985) explain that an unstructured interview is considered the most fitting means to elicit the personal viewpoint of the participants, to preserve the flexibility required to find codes and categories and to clear up inconsistencies arising from the data. The interviews are transcribed by the researcher as soon as possible after the interview and data analysis commences within the first interview to facilitate the simultaneous collection, coding and analysis of the data, and to provide a focus for subsequent data collection (Glaser & Strauss 1967; Stern 1985; Swanson 1986).

For ease of learning about the fundamental ideas within grounded theory, the method will be described in terms of its common aspects. These include **theoretical sensitivity**, theoretical sampling, **constant comparative analysis**, coding and categorisation of data, theoretical memos and diagrams, literature as data sources and the development and integration of theory.

Theoretical sensitivity is a beginning point of seeking some clarity on the nature of the research area to sensitise the researcher and give insights into what might be possible (Glaser 1978), relevant or irrelevant (Strauss & Corbin 1990), while being careful to not impose meaning on what might emerge as the project continues. A literature review may be done as a preliminary look into the area being researched, but the insights complement, rather than direct, the grounded theory project. Grounded research requires researchers to eradicate or minimise their own preconceptions because personal biases can affect the data (Sandelowski 1986). Researchers' presuppositions about the area of interest are acknowledged at the outset and set aside to allow the data to speak for themselves. The word **bracketing** is used to describe this process; it comes from its use in mathematics, in which numbers are put to one side in brackets to be attended to separately. For example, people in the health field, such as registered nurses, physiotherapists, social workers and so on, need to acknowledge their previous knowledge and experience of any area so that they do not unwittingly impose their interpretations on participants' accounts of their experiences.

Theoretical sampling occurs as the project progresses. Initially, there will be purposive sampling, in which particular people fulfilling certain criteria, such as gender, age, professional experience, or experience of the phenomenon to be studied, will be recruited intentionally to the research. After the project is under way and the initial insights are forming, based on the emerging theory more participants may be recruited or questions may be become more focused in a process of theoretical sampling (Strauss 1987). As the codes and categories are starting to emerge, the researcher may need to return to the data, the participants and possibly to the literature, to extend categories and increase the depth of understanding of them (Strauss & Corbin 1990).

Constant comparative analysis is a flexible and open-ended feature of grounded theory (Charmaz 1990). The researcher works with the data from the beginning of the project in a process of analysis to constantly compare all new data that emerge from participants' accounts of their experiences, to identify similarities in codes and categories, and to facilitate conceptualisation of higher order categories by comparison of codes, categories and their properties. Interpretations and codes arising from the data analysis are clarified during the interview, or at a later time, and are substantiated during subsequent interviews. Indicators including causes, contexts, contingencies, consequences, co-variance and conditions are utilised to clarify the nature and validity of emergent categories and theoretical constructs (Corbin 1986; Stern 1985). Glaser and Strauss (1967) identified four stages in constant comparative analysis: comparing incidents applicable to each category, integrating categories and their properties, delimiting the theory and writing the theory.

Coding and categorisation of data occurs during constant comparative analysis to identify patterns and events in the data, akin to sub-themes in a qualitative analysis process. The codes create categories, akin to themes, when they are assembled into similar groupings. The coding occurs in three levels: open, axial and selective. Level I, open coding, occurs when the raw data are first given conceptual labels using words spoken by participants. This labelling occurs line by line to thoroughly reduce and analyse the data, and as the process becomes more familiar, open coding can occur in sentences and sometimes paragraphs (Strauss & Corbin 1990, 1998). Axial coding, also known as Level II or theoretical coding (Strauss & Corbin 1990), occurs when the data are put back together to form links to emerging categories. Selective coding at Level III identifies categories and attempts to make links with other categories through a cyclical process that moves between the levels of coding to sort the data into meaningful connections, from which a theory can be generated. Category saturation is reached when there are no new codes or categories identified during analysis of subsequent data. That is, no new ideas are raised in the data. This process results in the emergence of a core category, which appears frequently in the data, explains most of the variation in the data, links easily with all categories, and has implications for the theory, allowing it to become known and progress forward with maximum variation in the analysis (Strauss 1987).

Theoretical memos and diagrams are aids to the analysis process. Memos are notes and diagrams are drawings recorded by the researcher as memory aids and conceptual imagery tools that assist in generating categories at each stage of the analysis.

Literature as data sources are useful in grounded theory, but as with qualitative projects involving participants, they are not imposed on the data because the participants' accounts of their experiences are what the research reveals. Strauss and Corbin (1990) suggest the benefits of literature are to assist in theoretical sensitivity at the outset of the research, as a secondary source of data, to pose questions about the data, to be used in theoretical sampling, and as a means of validating the grounded theory.

The development and integration of theory occurs throughout the analysis with deep immersion in the data and through the processes of category reduction, selective sampling of the literature and of the data (Glaser 1978). Category reduction means clustering large amounts of categories and subsuming them until they are reduced down to their smallest number without losing their uniqueness. Selective sampling of the literature refers to integrating existing literature with the emerging codes and categories. Selective sampling of the data occurs when more data are collected form participants to test hypotheses and reveal the properties of the categories.

This section presented the common characteristics of grounded theory methods. If you are considering a grounded theory approach to your research, you would be well advised to return to some of the original writing to help you sort out the differences between the versions of grounded theory. You can then become conversant with the steps in the chosen method (see Glaser 1978; Glaser & Strauss 1967; Strauss 1987; Strauss & Corbin 1990, 1998).

Nursing and health research examples

Nurses and other health care workers in projects relating to their work and disciplinary concepts have used grounded theory. For example, research areas include working with homeless youth (Rew 2003), mental health practice and services (Gibb 2003; McCann & Clark 2003), and client control in health care (Fiveash & Nay 2004).

Rew (2003) was interested in studying the self-care behaviours and attitudes of homeless adolescents, because she recognised that homeless youth are vulnerable in terms of their health and the stressful lives they lead. She selected a grounded theory design suggested by Strauss and Corbin (1994), which she felt had the potential to reveal patterns of behaviour. Rew (2003, p. 235) wrote down initial preconceptions, values and beliefs about the population based on previous experience with them and from a review of the literature. After ethical clearance, she accessed participants through a street outreach program housed in a church basement, and then she audiotaped interviews with 15 homeless youth, asking two main questions: What helps you maintain healthy living as you do? and What would you like to tell me about how you take care of yourself? (p. 236). The constant comparative analysis method resulted in the emergence of the basic social process of:

> Taking Care of Oneself in a Risk Environment, (which) linked three categories together to form a descriptive theory of self-care for homeless youth. The three categories were: Becoming Aware of Oneself, Staying Alive with Limited Resources, and Handling One's Own Health ... Given that many adolescents who live on the streets have made a conscious decision to leave an abusive or dysfunctional family, this avenue may be perceived as freedom from the oppression they experienced at home (Rew 2003, p. 236).

Gibb (2003) used a grounded theory approach (Glaser & Strauss 1967) to elicit rural mental health nurses' accounts of their sole practitioner practice. The research interest was in how nurses accommodate their rural values and lifestyles with working alone in mental health settings. Participants were recruited from five rural health settings in New South Wales, and the data collection consisted of focus groups run with six nurses from each centre and interviews with three other senior community mental health nurses. A model of therapeutics was articulated based on 'a relationship of intense professional intimacy and trust against a context of geographical disadvantage and professional isolation'. The nurses in sole practice experienced 'unusually high levels of responsibility, professional ingenuity, powerlessness and the independent and risky character of bush life' (Gibb 2003, p. 243).

McCann and Clark (2004) used a Strauss and Corbin (1998) approach to study the role nurses play in increasing clients' willingness to access community health services. After ethical clearance, purposive sampling accessed three groups of participants, including nine young adult clients with schizophrenia, eight caregivers, and 24 community health nurses from three community mental health centres. Forty-four unstructured interviews were audiotaped in relaxed settings seeking information on what encouraged and deterred clients form seeking mental health services. Non-participant observations totalling 55 hours were also undertaken of nurses interacting with clients in the centre and private homes. The findings showed that:

> Several factors simultaneously encouraged and inhibited individuals initiating contact at mental health centres, and these had serious implications for care and treatment, and recovery. There were two client access pathways to care: a direct access pathway where individuals recognized signs of being unwell and sought help early, and an indirect access pathway where others, such as caregivers, general practitioners, police, and inpatient facilities initiated contact on the individual's behalf. Nurses used three strategies to enhance client and caregiver access to services: 'promoting favorable experiences to enhance approachability', 'using technology to promote access', and 'being available' (McCann & Clark 2003, p. 279).

Fiveash and Nay (2004, p. 192) wanted 'to identify how healthcare clients achieve and maintain a sense of control over their health'. They used a modified version of Strauss and Corbin's (1998) approach to grounded theory, after they reviewed literature relating to key definitions of control, locus of control, and control and wellbeing. Over a six-month period, 60 participants were interviewed. Other data sources included participant observation and document analysis of records, including nursing care plans, nursing notes, case histories, organisational charts, policies and procedures manuals, and annual reports. Health care clients 'moved from feeling vulnerable to having a sense of control through to being purposefully active' (Fiveash & Nay 2004, p. 192). The researchers proposed a model of purposefully activating, which 'involves the client in reflecting, being self-determiningly involved and finally normalizing' (p. 202).

Other grounded theory projects that you might like to locate and read are about challenging the handover (O'Connell & Penney 2001), the nurse's role in improving Indigenous health (Wilson 2003), surviving myocardial infarction (Webster, Thompson & Davidson 2003), role stressors and coping for perioperative managers (Schroeder & Worrall-Carter 2002), and hypertension control (Mohammadi et al. 2002).

Potential nursing and health research questions

There are many research questions you may pose that would be suited to a grounded theory approach. As grounded theory suits any area in which little is known, all you need to do is to scan your practice for puzzles and problems that need systematic research attention. The question(s) may be about anything at all, the knowledge of which can be communicated to you best by talking with people who know it well. To assist you in choosing some areas of possible exploration through grounded theory, begin with specific areas of nursing or health-related practice, and people/conditions/circumstances/events you would like to know about related to each of them.

For example, clinical settings may include an accident and emergency ward, a medical ward, a surgical ward, a paediatric ward, a community health clinic and so on. People of interest within these clinical areas may include patients, nurses and/or allied health staff. Conditions, circumstances and events may include a wide range of possibilities, such as specific interpersonal relationships and interactions, routines, procedures, rituals and policies. Any area of patient concern may be explored, such as reactions to illness and hospitalisation, the need for education, clients' perceptions of the efficacy of treatments and procedures, and so on. As you can see, the possibilities are many for interesting and practical research using a grounded theory approach, but remember that you are essentially interested in creating theoretical propositions about the area of interest, so that the results can be stated in a middle range theory to inform the specific research aims and objectives.

EXERCISE

Imagine an area that could be researched using a grounded theory approach. Write an aim, some objectives, and list some possible methods for data collection you could use. You may need to refer to other chapters in this book to help you with this exercise.

Phenomenology

A phenomenon is a thing, or entity. Defined simply, 'phenomenology' is the study of a thing. In the human sciences, phenomenology concerns itself with the study of things within human existence, because it acknowledges and values the meanings people ascribe to their own existence. Its prime intent is to discover, explore and describe 'uncensored phenomena' (Spiegelberg 1970, p. 21) of the things themselves, as they are immediately given. There are many kinds of phenomenology although they all propose to explore the nature of a thing directly, by going to its source (Spiegelberg 1976). Therefore, phenomenology will allow nurses and other health professionals to explore the **lived experience** of any person in their care and also the people with whom they work, in order to explain the nature of that existence (Being).

The methodology

Much has been written about the theoretical assumptions of phenomenology (Dreyfus 1991; Gadamer 1975 trans., 1976 trans.; Heidegger 1962; Hekman 1986; Husserl 1960 trans., 1964 trans., 1965 trans., 1970, 1980 trans.; Kockelmans 1967; Krell 1977). These references are fundamental reading when embarking on an in-depth study of phenomenology and the philosophy can be very dense and circular. However, if you are keen to get started, Spiegelberg (1976) is worth reading. He will give you a good introduction to the many kinds of phenomenology and point out some important differences between them.

There are so many approaches to phenomenology, it is difficult to know where to focus when considering theoretical perspectives. You might begin by looking at a few ideas of two well-known philosophers, Husserl and Heidegger, before reverting to some of the ideas of Max van Manen, who is a contemporary phenomenologist cited often in nursing circles. Be guided by the requirements of your project and by your research supervisor if you are undertaking an honours or postgraduate degree, because your project may be informed adequately by van Manen (1990), thus avoiding unnecessary detours into the complex philosophical positions of Husserl, Heidegger, Gadamer, Ricoeur and others (see, for example, Gadamer 1975 trans.; Giorgi 2000a&b; Heidegger 1962; Husserl 1960 trans.; Jones 2001; Kockelmans 1967; Langford 2002; Moran 2000; Ricoeur 1976).

Husserl (1970 trans.) suggested that it is necessary to suspend your ideas about what you know, when you try to see it as it really is. This phenomenological reduction, or 'bracketing', is supposed to be helpful in narrowing one's attention in such a way as to be able to discover rational principles underlying the phenomenon of concern. In contrast to this idea, Heidegger (1962) was concerned with 'Being-in-the-World'. Therefore, instead of trying to lay presuppositions to one side, Heidegger explored them as legitimate parts of finding out about the nature of a thing of interest. In other words, Heidegger suggested that humans live in a body and that the experiences of living in the world could give them clues to the nature of human existence.

Max van Manen (1990) applies a mixture of phenomenological concepts, for example, bracketing and the value of understanding lived experience. Derived from Husserl's work, bracketing means suspending one's own knowledge about a certain phenomenon. Lived experience refers to the knowledge people have of things of interest because they have experienced them through the daily activities of living their lives. Bracketing and lived experience are two of many key concepts that may underlie a phenomenological approach to research.

The theoretical assumptions presented in this section are simplistic explanations of relatively complex concepts. It should be remembered that if you want to undertake research informed by phenomenological thought, you will need to grapple at some time with these and other philosophical ideas. Even though the philosophy is challenging, the task is not overwhelming, as evidenced by the abundance of research claiming to be informed by phenomenological concepts (e.g. Austin, Bergum & Goldberg 2003; Beck 2004; Byrne 2001; Edwards & Titchen 2003; Hodges, Keeley & Grier 2001; Horberg, Brunt & Axelsson 2004; Langford 2002; Lauterbach 2003; Lindahl, Sandman & Rasmussen 2003; Maltby, Kristjanson & Coleman 2003; McCormack 2003; Milligan 2001; Nahalla & Fitzgerald 2003; Nasrabadi, Emami & Yekta 2003; Paech 2002; Peters 2003; Sadala 1999; Simons, Franck & Roberson 2001; Soderhamm & Idvall 2003; Sundelof, Hansebo & Ekman 2004).

The methods

Phenomenological methods differ according to the kinds of theoretical assumptions on which they are based. Some people advocate that there should be no structured steps in a method (Morris 1977; Psathas 1973; Schwartz & Jacobs 1979), while others, such as Patton (1980), feel that the inquiry must proceed as the experience unfolds, the only methodological consideration being that inquirers use some form of bracketing to minimise presuppositions.

Some authors claim that researchers need some framework to assist their inquiries and thus some adaptations of 'the phenomenological method' for analysing particular phenomena by intuiting, analysing and describing (Spiegelberg 1976) have been suggested. Some of these include the Van Kaam method (1959), the Giorgi method (Giorgi, Fischer &

Murray 1975) and the Colaizzi method (1978), and a method of transformation of interpretations (Langveld 1978). The methods range in specificity for guiding the researcher in a method which will uncover, supposedly, the nature of the phenomenon of interest.

Max van Manen (1990) developed a method that may be useful to you in understanding how to go about phenomenological research. It involves six steps:

1   Turning to the nature of the lived experience.
2   Investigating experience as we live it, rather than as we conceptualise it.
3   Reflecting on the essential themes which characterise the phenomenon.
4   Describing the phenomenon through the art of writing and rewriting.
5   Maintaining a strong and oriented relation to the phenomenon.
6   Balancing the research context by considering the parts and the whole.

Many of the so-called phenomenological methods leave prospective researchers wondering just what to do. Read as many examples of phenomenological research as you can, and access theses to see how research candidates have managed the methodological challenges and applied the methods and processes. For example, the six steps in van Manen's (1990) method still need to be interpreted by researchers and applied into a practical approach for collecting and analysing information. For example, a very simple reading of this method, in the order listed above, is:

1   Ask: What experience do I want to research? Access the people who can tell you about it from their experience, including yourself if it is also your experience.
2   The experience is told, as it is lived, straight from a spontaneous source of telling through thoughts on direct observations, stories and impressions, usually in creative writing, interviews, and any other ways of exposing fresh and immediate insights.
3   Ask: What is the nature of the phenomenon I am gaining from these accounts? Search the visual data sources such as transcripts, creative writing, photographs and so on for illumination on the essence of the directly expressed phenomenon (thing about which you wanted to know).
4   Describe the phenomenon through the art of writing and rewriting. This might mean working with participants' transcripts to create themes or exemplars, or it might mean working with your own writing to create clear, direct synopses if you are the person giving an account of your lived experience.
5   Keep your thoughts and attention on the phenomenon for richer and deeper insights, as they will come when the eloquent clarity of simplicity and directness illuminate the research interest.
6   All things (phenomena) exist in relationship with other phenomena, so keep this in mind when considering all of the features of the research setting, to which this phenomenon relates.

Researchers have selected various methods for collecting, analysing and verifying phenomenological-informed research. If you are thinking of using this approach, review the literature carefully, so you will be aware of the benefits and pitfalls. For example, Beech (1999, p. 35) wrote about the 'muddy waters of methodology as a novice researcher' when she shared her understanding and application of the concept of bracketing in her research. Other areas which have received attention in the literature are the authenticity and ethics of phenomenological research (Haggman-Laitila 1999), the development of a Gadamerian-based research method (Fleming, Gaidys & Robb 2003), methods using the phenomenology of Husserl and Merleau Ponty (Sadala & de Camargo 2002), data analysis methods (Byrne 2001; Priest 2002; Whiting 2001) and evaluating phenomenology in terms of its usefulness, quality and philosophical foundations (Annells 1999).

There are no absolutes when it comes to phenomenological methods; the very nature of phenomenology makes it a nebulous task that defies sure and certain methods for grasping and representing the phenomena. Heidegger focused on the meaning of Being (existence) and after writing dense and circular tomes (e.g. Heidegger 1962) he came to the conclusion that: 'Es ist es' – It is itself! So, if you are embarking on phenomenology, use the version you prefer, but be very careful about claiming that you have 'done phenomenology' – my position is that the best we can claim is to say that we have been 'informed by phenomenological thought'.

Nursing and health research examples

As there are many examples of published phenomenological research projects from which to choose, this section identifies international researchers' perspectives of using phenomenology in nursing and health research (Beck 2004; Maldonado, Efinger & Lacey 2003; Peters 2003; Sundelof, Hansebo & Ekman 2004).

Beck (2004) used the Internet and word of mouth to recruit a purposive sample of 40 mothers from New Zealand, the USA, Australia and the United Kingdom. Each mother 'was asked to describe the experience of her traumatic birth and send it over the Internet to the researcher' (Beck 2004, p. 28). The researcher was informed by the writing of Husserl (1960) in relation to bracketing, and she used Colaizzi's (1978) method of data analysis. Beck (2004, p. 30) described the ethical considerations, including negotiating access to mothers through 'Trauma and Birth Stress (TABS), a charitable trust located in New Zealand'. The criteria for inclusion in the research included mothers who had experienced birth trauma, and were willing to articulate their experiences, through writing and reading English. As postal mail was an option for returning their accounts, some mothers recruited through a seminar presentation did not have to be able to use the Internet to send their email responses.

Analysis of the mothers' stories brought forward four themes relating to birth trauma experiences: 'To care for me: was that too much to ask? To communicate with me: Why was this neglected? To provide safe care: You betrayed my trust and I felt powerless, and The end justifies the means: At whose expense? At what price?' (Beck 2004, p. 28). The discussion section of the research article aligned these mothers' experiences with others documented previously in literature, and from mothers' accounts of their birth trauma experiences, the researcher made these suggestions:

> During labour and delivery, clinicians should strive to enhance a woman's sense of control by offering her
> options when possible. Many events during the delivery process are, however, out of the control of both the
> obstetric care providers and the mothers. Obstetric care providers need to discuss with women the means

of their delivery, and not just the outcome. When the hopes for the best laid birth plans are dashed, women's unmet expectations regarding their anticipated birth process need to be addressed by clinicians. Mothers' perceptions of birth trauma can be based not only on the event, but also on their unmet expectations regarding the event (Beck 2004, p. 35).

Maldonado, Efinger and Lacey (2003) made a social research inquiry about shared perceptions of personal moral development, using a 'phenomenological approach' informed by a constructivist perspective (Denzin & Lincoln 1998; Schwandt 1998). Although the only phenomenological writing cited is Moustakas (1994) and the majority of the references are to an interpretive, constructivist position, the researchers appeal to constructivist intentions to reveal participants' perceptions of shared experiences. Thus they claim the methodology in the abstract as qualitative, and in the text as phenomenological. This research article is a good example of needing to be tentative about claiming a project as phenomenology, when in fact the most that researchers can claim is that it has been informed by phenomenological thought.

Methodological considerations aside, Maldonado, Efinger and Lacey (2003) used a survey of graduate students, open-ended interviews with selected leaders, and document analysis to investigate personal moral development. The methods section of the research article documents considerable detail in how the 14 selected 'moral leaders' were recruited to the study. While the details are too many to repeat here, the principle to note is in purposefully selecting those individuals who are thought to have lived the experience, and are therefore able to explicate the phenomenon. Using content analysis to identify issues and themes the researchers 'indicated that a number of important factors influenced the participants' moral development, including parents, spirituality, education/mentors/friends, and peak experiences' (Maldonado, Efinger & Lacey 2003, p. 8).

Peters (2003) used van Manen's (1990) approach to phenomenology to guide a project exploring women's experiences of *in vitro* fertilisation (IVF). The reasons for doing the research were based on the need for women seeking IVF to find voice and to feel empowered, and to 'add to existing knowledge of the phenomenon and generate understanding that may contribute to informing nursing practice' (Peters 2003, p. 258). After ethical approval, six women were recruited from infertility groups to the study who were 'without biological children, able to understand and speak English, willing to describe their experiences, and active participants on an IVF programme for approximately two to three years' (p. 259). The researcher collected data through audiotaping conversational one-hour interviews, using open-ended questions to promote free expression of experiences.

Five themes emerged from the transcripts, including Keeping Secrets, Why Me? Trying Different Avenues, Getting it Wrong and Being Let Down. Each theme was described using selected examples of the participants' accounts. Keeping Secrets refers to the need for secrecy relating to the cultural and religious implications of being infertile and seeking assistance, avoiding gossip and stigmatisation, and feeling that others would not understand. Why Me? relates to anxiety about not being a 'normal' woman capable of natural reproduction. Trying Different Avenues refers to 'women trying anything and everything to ensure a positive pregnancy result' (pp. 261–2). Getting it Wrong refers to how health professionals got it wrong during treatment, and Being Let Down 'encapsulates the disappointment felt by participants when IVF cycles proved fruitless' (p. 263). It is difficult to imagine the depths of these disclosures coming from 'objective' methods, such as structured questionnaires and/ or surveys, so phenomenological assumptions about human experience guiding the project's method were very relevant and informative in this research.

Swedish researchers (Sundelof, Hansebo & Ekman 2004, p. 13) used a 'phenomenological-hermeneutic method, inspired by the French philosophy of Paul Ricoeur' to 'illuminate the meaning of (the) caring relationship directed to the elderly' in district nursing. The 12 female district nurses recruited to the study were responsible for areas with populations of 1200 to 2000 people, and they worked in homes and outpatients clinics with people across the life span. The interviews invited narratives of situations in which nurses cared for an elderly patient. The audiotaped accounts were transcribed and were analysed according to a textual analysis method (Ricoeur 1976). This involved '(a) naïve reading, (b) structural analysis, and (c) comprehensive understanding' that required the researchers to interpret the text of the transcripts through a 'dialectical movement between the parts and the whole, and between understanding and explanation' (Sundelof, Hansebo & Ekman 2004, p. 14).

The researchers depict their naive understanding of the nurses' accounts as 'balancing between closeness and distance'. The structural analysis and explanation generated three main themes of 'balancing between being professional and being a private person', 'knowing the members of the local community' and 'togetherness'. The comprehensive understanding the researchers reached was that 'the meaning of (the) caring relationship in district nursing is friendship, which is presented in a caring communion and has its base in the local community' (Sundelof, Hansebo & Ekman 2004, p. 14).

Other examples of research using phenomenological approaches include those listed previously in this chapter in the last paragraph of the methodology section for phenomenology. Be careful to read the critiques of phenomenology also, as it has been argued that this methodology has been misapplied in nursing and health research (Crotty 1996, 1998). Responses have been made to the criticisms, and sound arguments have justified its use by researchers lacking formal philosophical education and qualifications (Barkway 2001; Corben 1999; Darbyshire, Diekelmann & Diekelmann 1999; Drauker 1999; Fleming, Gaidys & Robb 2003; Garrett 1998). As you can imagine, phenomenology is vast in its heritage, scope and applications, so ensure that you study it comprehensively if you are intending to understand it well enough to inform your project judiciously.

Potential nursing and health research questions

Any questions that ask: 'What is the nature of ...?' and 'What is it like to experience ...?' can be considered to be research interests that may be illuminated by a phenomenological approach. This means that researchers can raise questions about the nature and effects of their profession, in whatever practice and theory areas they choose. For example, research questions may be posed broadly or specifically, such as: 'What is a caring practice?' or 'What is the caring practice of X?' and 'How do clients perceive caring intentions?' or 'How do clients perceive the caring intentions of Y?'.

You might also want to know about what it is like for certain people to experience various phenomena, such as patients' experiences of particular illnesses, caring professionals' experiences of specific clinical practices, and/or relatives' perceptions of all phenomena related to being concerned about someone who is ill or hospitalised. For example, questions may be asked like: 'What is the nature of waiting for a diagnosis?' 'What is it like to experience chemotherapy?' The possibilities are many and varied for using phenomenological research in nursing and health, assuming you are aware of the various philosophical positions and you are convinced that phenomenology has the potential to inform your research aims and objectives by providing methods and processes for illuminating the phenomenon.

Exercise

Imagine an area that could be researched using a phenomenological approach. Write an aim, some objectives, and list some possible methods for data collection you could use. You may need to refer to other chapters in this book to help you with this exercise.

Ethnography

Much has been written about ethnography for application by health professionals (e.g. Allen 2004; Burns & Grove 1993; DePoy & Gitlin 1994; Germain 1979; Kanitsaki 1989; Leininger 1985; LoBiondo-Wood & Haber 1994; Rosenbaum 1989; Spradley 1980; Streubert & Carpenter 1995), but a comprehensive approach to ethnography in all of its forms and applications right up until its postmodern representations can be found in an edited text by Atkinson et al. (2001). This section draws on authors within this text, to apply ethnography to health care research. Atkinson et al. (2001, p. 1) acknowledge the 'commission to edit a Handbook of Ethnography is a well-nigh impossible task' because the field is broad and diffuse and defies exact and totally inclusive categorisation, and because of its associations with various anthropological and sociological perspectives. The admission of these difficulties means that a novice researcher needs to approach the terrain with caution. As with discovering the depth of meaning in phenomenological research, 'one size does not fit all' when trying on ethnographic perspectives to inform your research. Even so, the editors admit that ethnographic traditions share common features and they describe them as:

grounded in a commitment to the first-hand experience and exploration of a particular social or cultural setting on the basis of (though not exclusively by) participation observation. Observation and participation (according to circumstance and the analytic purpose at hand) remain the characteristic features of the ethnographic approach. In many cases, of course, fieldwork entails the use of other research methods too. Participant observation alone would normally result in strange and unnatural behaviour were the observer not to talk with her or his hosts, so turning them into informants or 'co-researchers'. Hence, conversations and interviews are often indistinguishable from other forms of interaction and dialogue in field research settings (Atkinson et al. 2001, pp. 4–5).

The methodology

This chapter has already pointed out that some methodologies traverse the entire span of the paradigmatic continuum between interpretive, critical and postmodern forms (Table 12.3). Ethnography is an example of this methodological versatility and mobility. For example, ethnography has been described in relation to health and medicine (Bloor 2001), education (Gordon, Holland & Lahelma 2001), science and technology (Hess 2001), children and childhood (James 2001), communication (Keating 2001), photography and film (Ball & Smith 2001), narrative analysis (Cortazzi 2001), feminism (Skeggs 2001), autobiography (Reed-Danahay 2001) and postmodernism (Spencer 2001).

Interestingly, although unsurprisingly, Bloor's 'ethnography of medicine and health' (2001, pp. 177–87) makes few references to ethnographic studies in nursing research. It chooses instead to interpret health through medical sociology within the social constructions of medical doctors (e.g. West 1993), institutions (e.g. Maines 1977) and organisations (e.g. Goffman 1961), and social phenomena pertaining to health, such as the lived experience of illness and the sociology of the body (e.g. Davis 1963) and dying (e.g. Sudnow 1967). In acknowledging Lawler's (1991) work as 'a very accessible ethnography of Australian nurses' body care work', Bloor (2001) writes that:

> Lawler deals with the intimate work which nurses undertake on a privatized body – not the least their responses to sexuality of male patients – and shows how body care is a practical accomplishment which is simultaneously invisible, neither a topic for social discourse nor nursing knowledge . . . (p. 182).

It is important to remember that ethnographic approaches are derived from anthropological and sociological sources. Even though medical versions may refer to sociological perspectives, renowned nurse ethnographers, such as Madeleine Leininger and Olga Kanitsaki, acknowledge the anthropological connections with ethnography. For example, Leininger, a noted American nurse anthropologist, defines ethnography as 'the systematic process of observing, detailing, describing, documenting, and analysing the lifeways or particular patterns of a culture (or subculture) in order to grasp the lifeways or patterns of the people in their familiar environment' (Leininger 1985, p. 35). Leininger (p. 238) coined the term ethnonursing, because it 'focuses mainly on observing and documenting interactions with people of how these daily life conditions and patterns are influencing human care, health, and nursing care practices'. Leininger defined **culture** as:

> a way of life belonging to a designated group of people, a blueprint for living, which guides a particular group's thoughts, actions and sentiments, all of the accumulated ways a group of people solve problems, which are reflected in the people's language, dress, food and a number of accumulated traditions and customs (pp. 48–9).

Similarly, Kanitsaki (1988, 1989, 1992, 1993), awarded the Order of Australia in 1995 for outstanding professional leadership in the field of nursing, especially in the area of multicultural care services, provides fresh and clear views of issues and challenges faced by nurses, who seek to consider transcultural aspects of their work. For example, in her research, Kanitsaki (1989, p. 102) described the importance of family to Greek people in Australia and how 'the rituals of eating, play, work, conversation, birth, baptism, marriage, health crisis, illness, death, and so on, are family rather than individual events'. These are important insights for nurses when Greek people are admitted to their nursing care, and within a wider perspective, research findings such as this are important to alert nurses generally to the need for culturally sensitive care of all people.

The method

Ethnography has adopted two basic research approaches from anthropology, emic and etic. Behaviours are studied from within the culture in an emic approach, and behaviours are studied from outside the culture and across cultures in a wider etic approach (Burns & Grove 1993, p. 72). For example, nurse-researchers interested in describing the culture of the people interacting in a particular clinical setting would take an emic approach, whereas a comparison of US and Australian nurse education institutions would take an etic approach.

Ethnographies can vary according to the scope and nature of the research. Leininger (1985) uses the practical distinction of 'maxi' and 'mini' ethnographies, so that large, comprehensive studies, and smaller-scale studies with a narrowed focus of inquiry, can be done.

In the matter of what to do (methods) and how to do it (processes), Bloor's specific chapter in Atkinson et al. (2001) relating to medicine and health is unhelpful, so I refer you again to a very dated, but exceedingly practical source (Burns & Grove 1993, p. 72), for the steps of ethnographic research:

1 Identify the culture to be studied.
2 Identify the significant variables within the culture.
3 Review the literature.
4 Gain entrance.
5 Immerse yourself in the culture.
6 Acquire informants.
7 Gather data.
8 Analyse data.
9 Describe the culture.
10 Develop theory.

The result of attention to these steps is a thick description of the culture of the group of people being studied, so that a deep understanding is gained of the activities and ideas that comprise the culture of that group. Of course, if you are taking a critical or postmodern approach to ethnography, you will need to read more widely to gain a sense of these methods and processes (e.g. Reed-Danahay 2001; Skeggs 2001; Spencer 2001). As always, it is a good idea if you are undertaking honours or postgraduate research to acquire copies of theses using the particular ethnographic approach you want to use. Copies of theses may be obtained through the various universities to which they were submitted for the award.

Nursing and health research examples

A review of literature shows that there are many published examples in peer-reviewed journals of ethnographic approaches to nursing and health-related research (Allen 2004; Cleary 2004; Juntunen, Nikkonen & Janhonen 2002; Kelly & Long 2001; Koskinen & Tossavainen 2004; Maggs-Rapport 2000; Lee 2001; Oliver & Butler 2004; Powers 2001; Savage 2004). Given the wide selection, this section features four examples by international health researchers from various professions (Draper 2003; Juntunen, Nikkonen & Janhonen 2002; Kenefick & Schulman-Green 2004; Marquis, Freegard & Hoogland 2004).

Draper (2003, p. 66) was 'guided by the principles of ethnography' and ritual transition theory to explore 'men's passage to fatherhood'. Draper (2003) explains that ethnography

> was chosen because of its ability to not only illuminate how the men made and marked their own individual transitions to fatherhood, but also to examine how this transition was influenced by the changing fathering practices in contemporary Western culture (p. 66).

Draper (2003) interviewed 18 first-time and experienced expectant men three times each over the course of their partner's pregnancy, twice during the antenatal period and once after the birth. She recruited the men through the National Childbirth Trust (NCT) in the United Kingdom, by a snowballing technique. The interviews were analysed for experiences of transition, within the main phases of pregnancy, labour and delivery and post delivery. The men all acknowledged a change of status, either from not being a father to becoming a father for the first time, or from being a father to becoming a father again. The feelings of changing status were accompanied by feelings of uncertainty of coping in changing circumstances during pregnancy and the projection to after delivery, of coping with the changed status of father.

Juntunen, Nikkonen and Janhonen (2002, p. 210) used an ethnographic approach informed by van Manen (1995) 'to explore the cultural care practised among the Bena in the Ilembula villages in Tanzania', in order to improve and maintain lay health care. The project is richly anthropological in nature, describing the setting's geographical location and the health system in the village of 5000 inhabitants as having 'its own government with health committees, primary health providers and traditional midwives' (p. 211). The data collection methods included interviews with 61 villagers, participant observation of village life, and personal working diaries. Detailed accounts are given by the researchers of the participants' demographics and the precise nature and duration of the participant observation and the use of working diaries. The researchers report that:

> respect has two main functions: it confirms unity and ensures wellbeing. Unity is important, and any violation against it is expected to be followed by a punishment, usually in the form of health deterioration.

The main respective activities ensuring unity are observed in communication patterns, obedience, sharing the hardships of life and innocence. Rituals focus on the living-dead ancestors and serve both to confirm unity and to ensure wellbeing (Juntunen, Nikkonen & Janhonen 2002, p. 210).

Kenefick and Schulman-Green (2004) used an ethnographic approach, informed by Fontana and Frey 1994, to describe the nurses' 'beliefs, values, and experiences related to assessing pain in nursing home residents', who were cognitively impaired (Kenefick & Schulman-Green 2004, p. 32). The data collection involved participant observation and semi-structured interviews with three key informants, who were in senior positions in a large nursing home in southern New England, USA. Unobtrusive participant observations were made of the setting, the nursing home residents and the nurses, and the researchers exemplified these aspects with selections of field notes, to paint a picture of nursing home culture:

Findings of this study demonstrated the centrality of comfort to caring practices. Nurses demonstrated elements of a standard of care ... (that) included (a) seeing the person as a unique individual, (b) picking up cues, (c) acting to decrease pain, (d) showing concern, (e) being involved, (f) comforting, (g) knowing the person, (h) keeping watch over, (i) monitoring, and (j) giving medications and treatments. The critical attributes of nurses' beliefs related to assessing pain in nursing home residents were (a) the importance of knowledge about both the individual resident and the field of nursing home nursing, (b) thoughtful analysis of resident problems, and (c) the difficulty of assessing the verbally impaired nursing home resident (Kenefick & Schulman-Green 2004, p. 36).

Marquis, Freegard and Hoogland (2004, p. 178) used an interpretive ethnographic approach to examine the 'experiences of family members who have previously been primary carers of residents of residential aged services to identify factors, which have encouraged them to remain involved in a caring role'. This project was a pilot study for a larger project, and it focused on identifying issues that foster family involvement in aged care. An aged care facility was selected with a positive reputation for family involvement in residents' care, and after the ethical approval process, five females and two males in caring roles were interviewed for their views on the influences on family involvement in the facility. The researchers chose a grounded theory analysis method, assisted by the QRS NUD*IST package to locate codes and categories (Qualitative Solutions and Research 1995). It is interesting that the researchers chose to name this methodology as ethnography, when they did not report on any field-note observations of the culture of the facility. The naming of the methodology seems to rest on the use of 'ethnographic interviews' (p. 179), although other data in the larger project may have been ethnographic in nature.

The researchers located seven common themes in the participants' accounts that described their satisfaction with family involvement in the facility, including:

communication styles, emotional support for families, staff compassion and special skills, recognition of staff as a care team member, provision of timely information, attention to resident autonomy and the availability of private family space (Marquis, Freegard & Hoogland 2004, p. 180).

For further examples, you can read an abundant and easily accessible source of ethnographic research by locating the *Journal of Transcultural Nursing*, or follow through in accessing some of the references cited in this section.

Potential nursing and health research questions

You could use an ethnographic approach in research for any instance in which you want to get to know what the culture is like within a particular group. This could be from a broad, comprehensive 'maxi' approach if you have time and resources to undertake such an initiative, or a smaller focus, to fit in with constraints of time, funding, length of research degree and so on. Broader questions for a 'maxi' ethnography may be posed about comparisons between disciplinary practices in different countries or clinical settings, or care of specific cultural groups. 'Mini' ethnographies might frame questions about the people and practices in the culture of a ward or unit, and how they relate to nursing and/or health.

Remember, you do not have to undertake a project with an ethnic flavour to undertake ethnographic research. You could use this approach to study the culture of any group of people in any place, so in nursing this might be aged people in a nursing home, children in a ward, or nurses in a specialist unit. In health-related projects, you could research your particular interests within any institution or organisation, wherever people relate to one another in social and cultural settings. If ethnography serves your research purposes, and you need close and systematic observation and description of people and their customs, symbols, rituals and habits of daily life, the choice is entirely up to you. Don't forget also that you are not tied to interpretive approaches to ethnography, as it is possible to combine methodologies and to give your ethnographic research critical and postmodern perspectives.

EXERCISE

Imagine an area that could be researched using an ethnographic approach. Write an aim, some objectives, and list some possible methods for data collection you could use. You may need to refer to other chapters in this book to help you with this exercise.

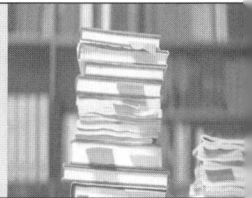

Historical research

History documents the events and trends of human activity as they have taken place over time. History is a form of research because its methods seek to discover new knowledge about what has happened in times past in relation to specific portions of time and foci of interest. Allemang (1987, p. 2) contends that history is 'all that has been thought and said and come to be since human beings inhabited the planet'. This being so, there is wide and deep potential for the generation of historical knowledge.

Yuginovich (2000, p. 70) suggests that history 'is probably a stronger force than language in the moulding of social consciousness' and that it is inextricably connected with power and political systems. Interestingly, this would not be denied by sceptical postmodernists, who would argue that the immersion of history in power is one of the reasons it should be discounted as it represents bias, domination and oppression (Rosenau 1992).

The methodology

Certain theoretical assumptions are forwarded as to the value of historical knowledge, including the need for the representation of historical accounts through interpretation. The retrospective nature of the documentation of history has been open to the interpretations of the historian, because 'facts, events, ideas, institutions and societal trends do not speak for themselves, but must be interpreted by a human mind hard at work trying to analyse the continuity, diversity and change involved in the complex interrelationships that characterise human history' (Ashley 1976, p. 30).

The issue of how to represent the past objectively has been a perplexing question for some historians, given that only remnants of the past exist (Dray 1978, 1980; Iggers 1971). Such clues to the past are through documents, art works and artefacts, memorabilia and the oral tradition.

Historical research and historiography are terms used interchangeably in nursing literature (Daisy 1991; Sarnecky 1990; Sorensen 1988). Sarnecky (1990, p. 2) claimed that 'most nurse historians define historical research from the standpoint of process', which are the ways in which the researcher 'subjectively synthesises and weaves together a diversity of facts'.

The compilation of a valid history relies on the legitimacy of its sources. The two kinds of historical sources are primary and secondary (Schafer 1980). Primary sources are provided by the original sources of the information, such as participants and observers. Secondary sources are all other accounts, once removed from participation.

According to Yuginovich (2000) history is of political significance, as she claims that:

> Against a background of an expanding and increasingly literate electorate, history has come to be seen as a unifying element in any country's political culture. To know about the past is to know that things have not always been as they are now and by implication that they need not always be as they are now. History has a social role in a society that requires an understandable past in order to learn and progress or to become whatever it is that is aimed for both on an individual as well as a national level ... does history have value as a body of independent knowledge? (p. 70)

In answering generally in the affirmative, she describes the form of historical research she uses as historical comparative research 'that reconstructs what occurred from available evidence but cannot have absolute confidence in the reconstruction because it depends on the survival of accurate data from the past and must take into account the bias or contextual meaning of the original recorder of the original data' (Yuginovich 2000, p. 72).

The methods

A systematic set of steps is advocated in doing traditional historical research, fashioned on the rules and procedures of empirical science (Schafer 1980) including: defining a topic by using an hypothesis or a set of questions, locating texts and compiling a bibliography, researching other sources, analysing and compiling information, and writing a research report. The researcher decides on the appropriate means of presenting the data. The completed historical research document may appear deceptively simple to the reader, who is unaware of the painstaking work needed to create the final product of historical research. The intention is to reconstruct from primary and secondary sources, with due attention to a rigorous research process, a faithful historical account of the area of interest that can be judged to be an accurate and 'truthful' record of events over time.

Historical comparative research is a form of historical research that compares social arrangements and policies in various societies, and explores the differences (Goldstone 1998). As such, the method is useful in studying commonalities, uniqueness and long-term changes in entire social systems. Researchers using this method employ an inductive process similar to grounded theory and akin to fieldwork in that they begin with the data and analyse information to build up to theories about relationships and silences (Neuman 1994). Silences are the significant historical events that have not occurred through a repression of possibilities and people's ability to speak out about injustices (Skopcol 1995). Historical comparative research method is guided by a set of specific characteristics (Goldstone 1998). It needs to be recorded with careful attention to sequence, comparison, contingency, origins and sequences, sensitivity to incompatible meanings, limited generalisation, association, part and whole, analogy, and synthesis (Neuman 1994).

Another form of historical research is oral history, which provides 'a picture of the past in people's own words' (Robertson 1990, p. 2). Oral evidence is gathered from a primary source whose accounts act as raw historical data, that can stand alone as their own account, or be synthesised with other sources for further analysis and interpretation. The benefits of oral history include the validity of the primary oral source as the person who has lived the experiences, and the potential for the historian to cross-check interpretations with the person providing the oral history. Plummer (1983), however, notes that oral history has been viewed by some historians as marginal, suspect and trivial because it deals with accessible people in recent times, it relies on people's accounts of the past that may be coloured by the present, and huge amounts of data may be gathered for no useful purpose. Even so, others (Candida Smith 2002; Crane 1997; Tonkin 1992) disagree and promote oral history as a means of 'writing the individual back into collective memory' (Crane 1997, p. 1372).

Reflective topical autobiography is an autobiographical method which can be used by nurses to retrace the events of their lives and the sense they have made of them through reflection. Johnstone (1999, p. 24) suggests that this form of historical research 'is an important research method in its own right, and one which promises to make a substantive contribution to the overall project of advancing nursing inquiry and knowledge'. She explains that '"re-visioning" of an original topical self-life story demonstrates the enormous creativity of the reflective topical autobiographical method' and 'leaves open to the self-researcher the opportunity to return at will to his or her life story again to re-read, re-vision and re-tell the story in the light of the new insights, understandings and interpretations of meaning acquired through ongoing lived experience' (p. 25). Such a suggestion situates reflective topical autobiography in the interpretive paradigm in a place that integrates story-telling with history. Johnstone (p. 25) cautions that when 'utilised as a research method, the aim is not to render a "true" account of the self (as some researchers subscribing to the tenets of positivistic research expect . . .) but to render an account of the lived experience of self that advances shareable understanding of common human experiences'. In this aim, reflective topical autobiography contributes postmodern influences to the traditional practice of historical research (see the discussion of postmodern influences on contemporary research earlier in this chapter).

Nursing and health research examples

Historical research approaches have been undertaken in a variety of nursing and health care areas (e.g. Brush & Capezuti 2001; Fairman & McMahon 2001; Madsen 2005).

Brush and Capezuti (2001) used a social historical research approach to undertake a historical analysis of siderail use in US hospitals. Their specific objectives were to 'explore the social, economic, and legal influences on siderail use in 20th century American hospitals and how use of siderails became embedded in nursing practice' (p. 381). They traced their search for primary and secondary sources back to 1893, when Isabel Adams Hampton made it clear that a nurse 'who works over (beds) daily ought to be a fair judge of what is required in the way of a bed for the sick' (Hampton 1893, p. 75, in Brush & Capezuti 2001, p. 381). Primary sources included:

> medical trade catalogs, hospital procedure manuals, newsletters, photographs, and other archival materials from the New York Academy of Medicine, the College of Physicians in Philadelphia, and the Center for Study of Nursing at the University of Pennsylvania. Journal articles, government documents, published histories of hospital bed design, and nursing and medical texts provided additional sources of data (Brush & Capezuti 2001, p. 381).

In describing the implications for current practice the researchers described the debates over the past decade about siderails related mainly to reports of patients becoming entrapped and of siderail-related deaths. They listed claims that have been brought successfully against hospitals for siderail misuse and the goal of discouraging health care providers from using siderails routinely. They concluded that the acceptance of alternatives to siderails would need consensus from the key 'health care providers, hospital administrators, bed manufacturers, insurers, attorneys, regulators, and patients and families' (p. 385) and that the issue is a rich area for nursing research.

Fairman and McMahon (2001, p. 322) used 15 hours of interviews with nurse Florence Downs to document an oral history. 'Florence Downs is a well-recognized nursing leader, educator, editor, and scholar who helped shape nursing as an intellectual discipline' and she also wrote extensively on the research-practice nexus. The article described the first part of Florence's career from when she first decided to become a nurse to the early 1970s when she studied towards her doctorate at New York University. From the interviews the researchers:

gained a sense of how Downs constructed her conceptual universe of nursing, as well as the language and political effectiveness to overcome barriers confronting the intellectual growth of nursing mounted by other nursing leaders as well as traditional academic disciplines (Fairman & McMahon 2001, p. 322).

Madsen (2005) reviewed the emergence of nursing within Western society by describing the work of Florence Nightingale, before documenting nineteenth-century nursing in Australia and the development of contemporary trends and issues. Although the author does not account for her data sources, the reference list at the end of each chapter reveals literature, so this project appears to be a literature review of articles, books and reports relating to Australian nursing history. Madsen's (2005) chapters focus on professional nursing associations, nurse training, nursing and public hospitals, theorising nursing, the movement from patriarchy to partnership, community perspectives, nursing unions, the debate whether nurses are trained or educated, and the transition from etiquette to professional conduct. The monograph is a useful compilation of relevant literature and, as such, it provides insights into Australian nursing history.

Other examples of literature and historical approaches to nursing and health research are Bassett (1992), Cushing (1995), Durdin (1991), Hemmings (1996), Pearson, Taylor and Coleburn (1997), Russell (1990) and Silins (1993).

Potential nursing and health research questions

Any questions relating to exploring the facts, events, ideas and people's lives in history can be answered by an historical approach. In nursing, this means that the entire history of nursing is accessible through this approach. This creates incredible potential for nursing research projects, which may choose to focus on certain times in history to document the events and trends in nursing, or on specific people who have been of particular influence.

EXERCISE

Imagine an area that could be researched using a historical approach. Write an aim, some objectives, and list some possible methods for data collection you could use. You may need to refer to other chapters in this book to help you with this exercise.

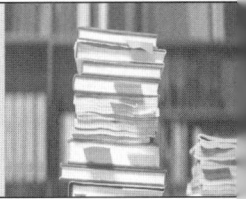

Summary

This chapter has described some qualitative interpretive research methodologies and some postmodern influences on them. It began by reminding you that research is a means of searching again for knowledge, as a basic premise on which all research is based. Generating knowledge is about using certain approaches to find information of a certain kind, which extends what is known, or says something new and different about what has been known previously. Some essential terms were defined, such as epistemology and ontology, in order to clarify some common qualitative theoretical assumptions about what constitutes useful and valid knowledge.

A broad differentiation between quantitative and qualitative research approaches assigned certain assumptions to either 'camp' and the caution was sounded that these artificial distinctions are not as clear-cut or poles apart from each other as they might at first appear. For ease of definition, qualitative research methodologies were categorised into interpretive and critical forms, the latter being the focus of the next chapter. In a postmodern world, distinctions such as paradigms and methodologies may have questionable use. However, they are presented here for you in your present role as a novice researcher, knowing that you have a vast body of research knowledge to work through that requires some categorisation into manageable parts for easier explanation and understanding. Even so, your attention was drawn to the possibility of mixing and mobilising methodologies, based on justification from affirmative postmodern ideas about knowledge and knowledge generation.

Four qualitative interpretive methodologies were described in this chapter, specifically: grounded theory, phenomenology, ethnography and historical research. They were described in terms of the key ideas contained within their respective methodologies and methods. Research examples and potential research questions were presented to allow you to consider the possibilities of using some of these approaches in research areas you might like to explore. You need to remember that the choice is yours. There are many approaches that you might take and the decision on a particular approach may be influenced by the research questions you are asking, and how you intend to answer them.

Main points

- Epistemology is the study of knowledge and how it is judged to be 'true'. Whenever nurses raise questions about what they know, and how they know it is trustworthy, they are asking epistemological questions.
- Ontology is the study of existence itself. Whenever nurses are asking about the nature of the existence of something or someone in nursing, they are asking ontological questions.
- Qualitative research attempts to explore the relative nature of knowledge, often by inductive processes and by valuing the subjectivity of people's experiences as being unique and context-dependent.
- Postmodern ways of thinking question what knowledge (epistemology) and existence (ontology) might mean by critiquing taken-for-granted quantitative and qualitative assumptions about 'truth' and 'being'.
- Interpretive research aims mainly to generate meaning by explaining and describing, thereby gaining insights into areas of interest.
- Critical research aims to bring about change in the status quo, by working systematically through locally generated research problems to find answers and create change in light of identified constraints.

- Postmodernism does not fit into the categories of interpretive or critical qualitative research approaches because it repudiates grand narratives and would not be seen as one itself. However, it is important for researchers as it encourages deconstruction that emphasises relativism, diversity, difference, contradiction and everyday ordinary history told in people's narratives and interpreted by them as their self-understandings.
- Grounded theory starts from the 'ground' of an area of human interest and works up in an inductive fashion to make sense of what people say about their experiences, and to convert these statements into theoretical propositions.
- Phenomenology ('phenomen - ology') is the 'study of things' within human existence, by discovering, exploring and describing the essence of phenomena through attending towards them directly.
- Ethnography provides a 'portrait of people' by describing and raising awareness of a group's cultural characteristics, such as their shared symbols, beliefs, values, rituals and patterns of behaviour.
- Historical research reconstructs from primary and secondary sources (with due attention to a rigorous research process) an accurate and 'truthful' record of events over time, thereby amending previous knowledge and discovering new knowledge in relation to specific portions of time and foci of interest.

CASE STUDY

Angela works as a physiotherapist in a multidisciplinary team in a large city hospital. For some time now she has been considering undertaking postgraduate research with local university staff, who oversee a teaching and research centre in her organisation. Angela checked out her assumptions about what postgraduate research entails, and an academic working in the centre told her that she would be eligible to enter into a Master by Research program, based on her qualifications, research experience and publication record. While the study itself was not a daunting prospect for Angela, deciding on how to research her chosen area gave her some concern. She noticed in her work that elderly women are often not listened to when they approach members of the health team and that they are seldom given adequate emotional support when they receive negative news about their health status. Therefore, in her research, Angela wants to 'give voice' to elderly women, and to sensitise staff to their unique needs. Angela is aware of her potential to mix and mobilise methodologies to explore the issue of the 'invisibility of elderly women to the multidisciplinary team'.

Generate some alternatives for a methodology, or a combination of methodologies, that could 'carry' Angela's project. What is the rationale for your choice? In other words, what can the methodologies offer Angela in terms of their theoretical assumptions about the kind(s) of knowledge she is seeking to generate?

Multiple choice questions

1 The study of the nature of human existence is:
   a   ontology
   b   epistemology
   c   philosophy
   d   scientology

2 Qualitative knowledge is:
   a   absolute
   b   relative
   c   deductive
   d   predictive

3 In qualitative research, subjectivity allows researchers to:
   a   maintain power and detachment
   b   control the subjects in the research
   c   generalise their research findings
   d   be immersed in the research

4 Qualitative interpretive methodologies:
   a   are fixed in categories
   b   show cause and effect
   c   can be combined
   d   permit generalisation

5 Qualitative interpretive methodologies can move across 'paradigmatic positions' because of the freeing potential of:
   a   affirmative postmodernism
   b   postmodern phenomenology
   c   sceptical postmodernism
   d   postmodern feminism

6 The research methods and processes of grounded theory are:
   a   deductive
   b   grounded
   c   cyclical
   d   inductive

7 In phenomenology, setting aside one's presuppositions is:
   a   bracketing
   b   'Being-in-the-World'
   c   understanding
   d   lived experience

8 Even though ethnographic approaches differ, they all are committed to the:

   a description of the essence of phenomena

   b creating historical accounts of events

   c developing middle range theories

   d exploration of social and cultural settings

9 Historical research:

   a creates fictional representations

   b favours indirect and ad hoc methods

   c documents events and trends over time

   d is always based on archival sources

10 A potential qualitative interpretive research question is:

   a How many Indigenous clients access health services?

   b What is the nature of experiencing recovery from illness?

   c How can marginalised people be given recognition?

   d What are the causes of confusion in the elderly?

Review topics

1 Why are epistemology and ontology relevant to researchers?

2 What research conditions are required in qualitative research approaches?

3 Discuss why the sceptical postmodern position disallows research.

4 Why is it possible to mix and mobilise qualitative methodologies?

5 Choose one qualitative interpretive methodology and write one question that would benefit from its use in a research project.

Online reading

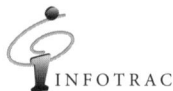

INFOTRAC® COLLEGE EDITION

When accessing information use the following keywords in any combinations you require to retrieve information relating to qualitative interpretive research:

➤ **Ethnographic**

➤ **Ethnography**

➤ **Grounded theory**

➤ **Health**

➤ **Historical research**

➤ **History**

➤ **Nursing**

➤ **Phenomenological**

➤ **Phenomenology**

➤ **Postmodernism**

References

Allemang, M.M. 1987, 'Oral historiography', *Recent Advances in Nursing*, vol. 17, 2–11.

Allen, D. 2004. 'Ethnomethodological insights into insider–outsider relationships in nursing ethnographies of healthcare settings', *Nursing Inquiry*, vol. 11, no. 1, 14–24.

Annells, M. 1999, 'Evaluating phenomenology: usefulness, quality and philosophical foundations', *Nurse Researcher*, vol. 6, no. 3, 5–19.

Ashley, J. 1976, *Hospital Paternalism and the Role of the Nurse*, Teachers College Press, New York.

Atkinson, P., Coffey, A., Delamont, S., Lofland, J. & Lofland, L. (eds) 2001, *Handbook of Ethnography*, Sage, London.

Austin, W., Bergum, V. & Goldberg, L. 2003, 'Unable to answer the call of our patients: mental health nurses' experience of moral distress', *Nursing Inquiry*, vol. 10, no. 3, 177–83.

Ball, M. & Smith, G. 2001, 'Technologies of realism? Ethnographic uses of photography and film', in P. Atkinson, A. Coffey, S. Delamont, J. Lofland & L. Lofland (eds), *Handbook of Ethnography*, Sage, London, 302–19.

Barkway, P. 2001, 'Michael Crotty and nursing phenomenology: Criticism or critique?', *Nursing Inquiry*, vol. 8, no. 3, 191–5.

Barnes, J. 1987, *Early Greek Philosophers*, Penguin Books, London.

Barton, S. 2004, 'Narrative inquiry: locating Aboriginal epistemology in a relational methodology', *Journal of Advanced Nursing*, vol. 45, no. 5, 519–26.

Bassett, J. 1992, *Guns and Broaches: Australian Army Nursing from the Boer War to the Gulf War*, Oxford University Press, Oxford.

Beck, C.T. 2004, 'Birth trauma: in the eye of the beholder', *Nursing research*, vol. 53, no. 1, 28–35.

Beech, I. 1999, 'Bracketing in phenomenological research', *Nurse Researcher*, vol. 6, no. 3, 35–51.

Bloor, M, 2001, 'The ethnography of health and medicine', in P. Atkinson, A. Coffey, S. Delamont, J. Lofland & L. Lofland (eds) 2001, *Handbook of Ethnography*, Sage, London, 177–87.

Brush, B.L. & Capezuti, E. 2001, 'Historical analysis of siderail use in American hospitals', *Journal of Nursing Scholarship*, vol. 33, no. 4, 381–5.

Burns, S. & Grove, N. 1993, *The Practice of Nursing Research: Conduct, Critique and Utilisation*, W.B. Saunders Company, Philadelphia.

Byrne, M. 2001, 'Understanding life experiences through a phenomenological approach to research', *AORN Journal*, vol. 73, no. 4, 830–2.

Candida Smith, R. 2002, 'Analytic strategies for oral history interviews', in J.F. Gubrium & J.A. Holstein (eds) 2002, *Handbook of Interview Research: Context and Method*, Sage, Thousand Oaks, 711–31.

Carper, B. 1992, 'Fundamental patterns of knowing in nursing', in L. Nicholl (ed.), *Perspectives on Nursing Theory*, 2nd edn, vol. 1, Lippincott Co., Philadelphia.

Charmaz, K. 1990, 'Discovering chronic illness: using grounded theory', *Social Science and Medicine*, vol. 30, 1161–72.

Chinn, P. & Kramer, M. 1995, *Theory and Nursing: A Systematic Approach*, 4th edn, Mosby Year Book, St Louis.

Cleary, M. 2004, 'The realities of mental health nursing in acute impatient environments', *International Journal of Mental Health Nursing*, vol. 13, no. 1, 53–60.

Colaizzi, P. 1978, 'Psychological research as the phenomenologist views it', in R.S. Valle & M. King (eds), *Existential Phenomenological Alternatives for Psychology*, Oxford University Press, New York.

Corben, V. 1999, 'Misusing phenomenology in nursing research: identifying the issues', *Nurse Researcher*, vol. 6, no. 3, 52–66.

Corbin, J. 1986, 'Qualitative data analysis for grounded theory', in W.C. Chenitz & J.M. Swanson (eds), *From Practice to Grounded Theory*, Addison Wesley, Menlo Park, California.

Cortazzi, M. 2001, 'Narrative analysis in ethnography', in P. Atkinson, A. Coffey, S. Delamont, J. Lofland & L. Lofland (eds), *Handbook of Ethnography*, Sage, London, 384–94.

Cox, H., Henderson, L., Andersen, N., Cagliarini, G. & Ski, C. 2003, 'Focus group study of endometriosis: struggle, loss and the medical merry-go-round', *International Journal of Nursing Practice*, vol. 9, no. 1, 2–9.

Crane, S. 1997, 'Writing the individual back into collective memory', *American Historical Review*, vol. 110, 1372–85.

Crotty, M. 1996, *Phenomenology and Nursing Research*, Churchill Livingstone, Melbourne.

Crotty, M. 1998, *Foundations of Social Research: Meaning and Perspective in the Research Process*, Allen and Unwin, Sydney.

Cushing, A. 1995, 'An historical note on the relationship between nursing and nursing history', *International Journal of Nursing History*, vol. 1, no. 1, 57–60.

Daisy, C. 1991, 'Searching for Annie Goodrich', *Western Journal of Nursing Research*, vol. 13, no. 3, 408–13.

Darbyshire, P., Diekelmann, P. & Diekelmann, N. 1999, 'Reading Heidegger and interpretive phenomenology: A response to the work of Michael Crotty', *Nursing Inquiry*, vol. 6, no. 1, 17–25.

Davis, F. 1963, *Passage Through Crisis: Polio Victims and Their Families*, Bobbs-Merrill, Indianapolis.

Denzin, N.K. 1989, *The Research Act*, McGraw Hill, New York.

Denzin, N. & Lincoln, Y. 1998, *The Landscape of Qualitative Research: Theories and Issues*, Sage, Thousand Oaks.

DePoy, E. & Gitlin, L. 1994, *Introduction to Research: Multiple Strategies for Health and Human Services*, Mosby, St Louis.

Descartes, R. 1970, *The Philosophical Works of Descartes*, E.S. Haldane & G.R.T. Ross (trans. ed.), The Cambridge University Press, Cambridge, UK.

Draper, J. 2003, 'Men's passage to fatherhood: an analysis of the contemporary relevance of transition theory', *Nursing Inquiry*, vol. 10, no. 1, 66–78.

Drauker, C. 1999, 'The critique of Heideggerian hermeneutical nursing research', *Journal of Advanced Nursing*, vol. 30, no. 2, 360–73.

Dray, W. 1978, 'Point of view in history', *Clio*, vol. 7, 265–83.

Dray, W. 1980, *Perspectives on History*, Routledge & Kegan Paul, London.

Dreyfus, H.L. 1991, *Being-in-the-world: A Commentary on Heidegger's Being and Time*, Division 1, The MIT Press, Cambridge, Massachusetts.

Durdin, J. 1991, *They Became Nurses: A History of Nursing in South Australia 1863-1980*, Allen and Unwin, Sydney.

Edwards, C. & Titchen, A. 2003, 'Research into patients' perspectives: Relevance and usefulness of phenomenological sociology', *Journal of Advanced Nursing*, vol. 44, no. 5, 450–60.

Fairman, J. & McMahon, M.M. 2001, 'Oral history of Florence Downs: the early years', *Nursing Research*, vol. 50, no. 5, 322–8.

Fitzgerald, A. & Teale, G. 2003–04, 'Health reform, professional identity and occupational sub-cultures: the changing interprofessional relations between doctors and nurses', *Contemporary Nurse*, vol. 16, no. 1–2, 9–19.

Fiveash, B. & Nay, R. 2004, 'Being active supports client control over care', *Contemporary Nurse*, vol. 17, no. 3, 192–203.

Fleming, V., Gaidys, U. & Robb, Y. 2003, 'Hermeneutic research in nursing: Developing a Gadamerian-based research method', *Nursing Inquiry*, vol. 10, no. 2, 113–20.

Fontana, A. & Frey, J. 1994, 'Interviewing: The art of the science', in N. Denzin & Y. Lincoln (eds), *Handbook of Qualitative Research*, Sage, Thousand Oaks, 361–76.

Gadamer, H.-G. 1975 trans., *Truth and Method*, G. Barden & J. Cumming (eds), Seabury, New York.

Gadamer, H.-G. 1976, 'The universality of the hermeneutical problem', in *Philosophical Hermeneutics*, D.E. Linge (trans. ed.), University of California Press, Berkeley, California.

Garrett, C. 1998, 'Michael Crotty's phenomenology and nursing research', *Annual Review of Health Sciences*, vol. 8, 36–40.

Germain, C.P. 1979, *The Cancer Unit: an Ethnography*, Nursing Resources, Wakefield.

Gibb, H. 2003, 'Rural community mental health nursing: A grounded theory account of sole practice', *International Journal of Mental Health Nursing*, vol. 12, no. 4, 243–50.

Gibson, T. & Heartfield, M. 2003, 'Contemporary enrolled nursing practice: opportunities and issues', *Collegian*, vol. 10, no. 1, 22–6.

Giorgi, A. 2000a, 'Concerning the application of phenomenology to caring research', *Scandinavian Journal of Caring Science*, vol. 11, 11–15.

Giorgi, A. 2000b, 'The status of Husserlian phenomenology in caring research', *Scandinavian Journal of Caring Science*, vol. 14, 3–10.

Giorgi, A., Fischer, C.L. & Murray, E.L. 1975, *Duquesne Studies in Phenomenological Psychology*, Duquesne University Press, Pittsburgh.

Glaser, B. 1978, *Theoretical Sensitivity: Advances in the Methodology of Grounded Theory*, Sociology Press, Mill Valley.

Glaser, B. & Strauss, A. 1967, *The Discovery of Grounded Theory: Strategies for Qualitative Research*, Aldine, Chicago.

Glass, N. & Davis, K. 1998, 'An emancipatory impulse: a feminist postmodern integrated turning point in nursing research', *Advances in Nursing Science*, vol. 21, no. 1, 43–52.

Goffman, E. 1961, *Asylums: Essays on the Social Situation of Mental Patients and Other Inmates*, Doubleday, New York.

Goldstone, J. 1998, *Sociology and History: Producing Comparative History*, Working Papers in Economic History No. 108, Australian National University, Canberra.

Gordon, T., Holland, J. & Lahelma, E. 2001, 'Ethnographic research in educational settings', in P. Atkinson, A. Coffey, S. Delamont, J. Lofland & L. Lofland (eds), *Handbook of Ethnography*, Sage, London, 188–203.

Haggman-Laitila, A. 1999, 'The authenticity and ethics of phenomenological research: how to overcome the researcher's own views', *Nursing Ethics*, vol. 6, no. 1, 12–23.

Hampton, I. 1893, 'Nursing: its principles and practice', W.B. Saunders, Philadelphia, in B.L. Brush & E. Capezuti, 2001, 'Historical analysis of siderail use in American hospitals', *Journal of Nursing Scholarship*, vol. 33, no. 4, 381–5.

Heidegger, M. 1962, *Being and Time*, Harper & Row, New York.

Hekman, S.J. 1986, *Hermeneutics and the Sociology of Knowledge*, Polity Press, Cambridge, Massachusetts.

Hemmings, L. 1996, 'Vietnam memories: Australian army nurses, the Vietnam War, and oral history', *Nursing Inquiry*, vol. 3, no. 3, 138–45.

Hess, D. 2001, 'Ethnography and the development of science and technology studies', in P. Atkinson, A. Coffey, S. Delamont, J. Lofland & L. Lofland (eds), *Handbook of Ethnography*, Sage, London, 234–45.

Hodges, H., Keeley, A. & Grier, E. 2001, 'Masterworks of art and chronic illness experiences in the elderly', *Journal of Advanced Nursing*, vol. 36, no. 3, 389–98.

Horberg, U., Brunt, D. & Axelsson, A. 2004, 'Clients' perceptions of client-nurse relationships in local authority psychiatric services: A qualitative study', *International Journal of Mental Health Nursing*, vol. 13, no. 1, 9–17.

Hume, D. 1966, *An Enquiry Concerning the Principles of Morals*, reprinted from the edition of 1777, Open Court Publishing Company, La Salle, Illinois.

Hume, D. 1969 (first published 1739), *A Treatise of Human Nature*, Penguin Books, London.

Husserl, E. 1960 trans., *Cartesian Meditations: An Introduction to Phenomenology*, Martinus Nijhoff, The Hague.

Husserl, E. 1964 trans., *The Idea of Phenomenology*, Martinus Nijhoff, The Hague.

Husserl, E. 1965 trans., *Phenomenology and the Crisis of Philosophy*, Harper & Row, New York.

Husserl, E. 1970, *The Crisis of the European Sciences and Transcendental Phenomenology*, Northwestern University Press, Evanston, Illinois.

Husserl, E. 1980 trans., *Phenomenology and the Foundations of the Sciences*, Martinus Nijhoff, The Hague.

Hutchinson, S.A. 1986, 'Chemically dependent nurses, the trajectory towards self annihilation', *Nursing Research*, vol. 35, no. 4, 196–201.

Iggers, F. 1971, 'The new historiography in historical perspective', *Australian Journal of Politics and History*, vol. 17, 44–55.

James, A. 2001, 'Ethnography in the study of children and childhood', in P. Atkinson, A. Coffey, S. Delamont, J. Lofland & L. Lofland (eds), *Handbook of Ethnography*, Sage, London, 246–57.

Johnstone, M.-J. 1999, 'Reflective topical autobiography: an underutilised interpretive research method in nursing', *Collegian*, vol. 6, no. 1, 24–9.

Jones, A. 2001, 'A condensed history of the phenomenology: The first and second phases from Franz Brentano to Hans-Georg Gadamer', *Nurse Researcher*, vol. 8, no. 4, 65–75.

Juntunen, A., Nikkonen, M. & Janhonen, S. 2002, 'Respect as the main lay care activity among the Bena in Ilembula village in Tanzania', *International Journal of Nursing Practice*, vol. 8, no. 4, 210–20.

Kanitsaki, O. 1988, 'Transcultural nursing: challenge to change', *Australian Journal of Advanced Nursing*, vol. 5, no. 3, 4–11.

Kanitsaki, O. 1989, 'Cross cultural sensitivity in palliative care', in P. Hodder & A. Turley (eds), *The Creative Option of Palliative Care*, Melbourne City Mission, Melbourne.

Kanitsaki, O. 1992, *Transcultural Nursing: a Teaching Package for Lecturers*, La Trobe University, School of Health Sciences, Department of Nursing, Melbourne.

Kanitsaki, O. 1993, 'Transcultural human care: its challenge to and critique of professional nursing care', in Gaut, D.A. (ed.), *A Global Agenda for Caring*, National League for Nursing Press, New York.

Keating, E. 2001, 'The ethnography of communication', in P. Atkinson, A. Coffey, S. Delamont, J. Lofland & L. Lofland (eds), *Handbook of Ethnography*, Sage, London, 285–301.

Kelly, B. & Long, A. 2001, 'Ethnography: A suitable case for nursing?', *All Ireland Journal of Nursing and Midwifery*, vol. 4, 135–40.

Kenefick, A. & Schulman-Green, D. 2004, 'Caring for cognitively impaired nursing home residents with pain', *International Journal for Human Caring*, vol. 8, no. 2, 32–40.

Kockelmans, J.J. (ed.) 1967, *Phenomenology: the Philosophy of Edmund Husserl and its Interpretation*, Anchor Books, Doubleday & Co., Garden City, New York.

Koskinen, L. & Tossavainen, K. 2004, 'Study abroad as a process of learning intercultural competence in nursing', *International Journal of Nursing Practice*, vol. 10, no. 3, 111–20.

Krell, D.F. 1977, *Martin Heidegger: Basic Writings*, Harper & Row, New York.

Langford, I. 2002, 'An existential approach to risk perception', *Risk Analysis*, vol. 22, no. 1, 101–20.

Langveld, M.J. 1978, 'The stillness of the secret place', *Phenomenology and Pedagogy*, vol. 1, no. 1, 181–9.

Lauterbach, S.S. 2003, 'Phenomenological silence surrounding infant death', *International Journal for Human Caring*, vol. 7, no. 2, 38–43.

Lawler, J. 1991, *Behind the Screens: Nursing, Somology, and the Problem of the Body*, Churchill Livingstone, Edinburgh.

Lee, D. 2001, 'Accompany the sick (pei ban): A unique practice in Chinese hospitals by patients' relatives and friends', *Contemporary Nurse*, vol. 10, no. 3–4, 136–41.

Leininger, M. 1985, *Qualitative Research Methods in Nursing*, Grune and Stratton, New York.

Lindahl, B., Sandman, P. & Rasmussen, B.H. 2003, 'Meanings of living at home on a ventilator', *Nursing Inquiry*, vol. 10, no. 1, 19–27.

LoBiondo-Wood, G. & Haber, J. 1994, *Nursing Research: Methods, Critical Appraisal, and Utilisation*, Mosby, St Louis.

Madsen, W. 2005, *Nursing History: Foundations of a Profession*, Pearson SprintPrint, Australia.

Maggs-Rapport, F. 2000, 'Combining methodological approaches in research: Ethnography and interpretive phenomenology', *Journal of Advanced Nursing*, vol. 31, no. 1, 219–25.

Maines, D. 1977, 'Social organization and social structure in symbolic interactionist thought', *Annual Review of Sociology*, vol. 3, 235–59.

Maldonado, N., Efinger, J. & Lacey, C. 2003, 'Shared perceptions of personal moral development', *International Journal for Human Caring*, vol. 7, no. 1, 9–19.

Maltby, H., Kristjanson, L. & Coleman, M. 2003, 'The parenting competency framework: learning to be a parent of a child with asthma', *International Journal of Nursing Practice*, vol. 9, no. 6, 368–73.

Marquis, R., Freegard, H. & Hoogland, L. 2004, 'Influences on positive family involvement in aged care: an ethnographic view', *Contemporary Nurse*, vol. 16, no. 3, 178–86.

McCallin, A.M. 2003, 'Research: Designing a grounded theory study: Some practicalities', *Nursing in Critical Care*, vol. 8, no. 5, 203–10.

McCann, T.V. & Clark, E. 2003, 'A grounded theory study of the role that nurses play in increasing clients' willingness to access community mental health services', *International Journal of Mental Health Nursing*, vol. 12, no. 4, 279–87.

McCormack, B. 2003, 'A conceptual framework for person-centred practice with older people', *International Journal of Nursing Practice*, vol. 9, no. 3, 202–9.

Milligan, F. 2001, 'The concept of care in male nurse work: an ontological hermeneutic study in acute hospitals', *Journal of Advanced Nursing*, vol. 35, no. 1, 7–16.

Mohammadi, E., Abedi, H., Gofranipour, F. & Jalali, F. 2002, 'Partnership caring: a theory of high blood pressure control in Iranian hypertensives', *International Journal of Nursing Practice*, vol. 8, no. 6, 324–9.

Moran, D. 2000, 'Heidegger's critique of Husserl's and Bretano's accounts of intentionality', *Inquiry*, vol. 43, 39–66.

Morris, M. 1977, *An Excursion into Creative Sociology*, Columbia University Press, New York.

Moustakas, C. 1994, *Phenomenological Research Methods*, Sage, Thousand Oaks.

Nahalla, C. & Fitzgerald, M. 2003, 'The impact of regular hospitalization of children living with thalassaemia on their parents in Sri Lanka: A phenomenological study', *International Journal of Nursing Practice*, vol. 9, no. 3, 131–9.

Nasrabadi, A., Emami, A. & Yekta, Z. 2003, 'Nursing experience in Iran', *International Journal of Nursing Practice*, vol. 9, no. 2, 78–85.

Neuman, W. 1994, *Social Research Methods: Qualitative and Quantitative Approaches*, 2nd edn, Allyn and Bacon, Boston.

O'Connell, B. & Penney, W. 2001, 'Challenging the handover ritual', *Collegian*, vol. 8, no. 3, 14–18.

Oliver, M. & Butler, J. 2004, 'Contextualising the trajectory of experience of expert, competent, and novice nurses in making decisions and solving problems', *Collegian*, vol. 11, no. 1, 21–7.

Ormsby, A. & Harrington, A. 2003, 'The spiritual dimensions of care in military nursing practice', *International Journal of Nursing Practice*, vol. 9, no. 5, 321–7.

Paech, S.E. 2002, 'Making the transition from enrolled to registered nurse', *Collegian*, vol. 9, no. 3, 35–40.

Palmer, D. 1988, *Looking at Philosophy: the Unbearable Heaviness of Philosophy Made Lighter*, Mayfield Publishing Co., Mountain View, California.

Patton, M.G. 1980, *Qualitative Evaluation Methods*, Sage Publications, Beverly Hills, California.

Pearson, A., Taylor, B. & Coleburn, C. 1997, *The Nature of Nursing Work in Victoria, 1840–1870*, Deakin University Press, Geelong, Victoria.

Peters, K. 2003, 'In pursuit of motherhood: the IVF experience', *Contemporary Nurse*, vol. 14, no. 3, 258–70.

Plummer, K. 1983, *Documents of Life: An Introduction to the Problems and Literature of a Humanistic Method*, George Allen & Unwin, London.

Powers, B.A. 2001, 'Ethnographic analysis of everyday ethics in the care of nursing home residents with dementia: A taxonomy', *Nursing Research*, vol. 50, no. 6, 332–9.

Priest, H. 2002, 'An approach to the phenomenological analysis of data', *Nurse Researcher*, vol. 10, no. 2, 50–63.

Psathas, G. 1973, *Phenomenological Sociology: Issues and Applications*, John Wiley & Sons, New York.

Qualitative Solutions and Research 1995, NUD*IST (Non-Numerical Unstructured Data: Indexing Searching & Theorising), application software package, QSR, Melbourne.

Reed-Danahay, D. 2001, 'Autobiography, intimacy and ethnography', in P. Atkinson, A. Coffey, S. Delamont, J. Lofland & L. Lofland (eds), *Handbook of Ethnography*, Sage, London, 407–25.

Rew, L. 2003, 'A theory of taking care of oneself grounded in experiences of homeless youth', *Nursing Research*, vol. 52, no. 4, 234–41.

Ricoeur, P. 1976, *Interpretation Theory: Discourse and the Surplus of Meaning*, University Press, Fort Worth.

Robertson, B.M. 1990, *Guide to Oral History*, 2nd edn, Oral History Association of Australia (South Australian Branch), Adelaide.

Robrecht, L.C. 1995, 'Grounded theory: evolving methods', *Qualitative Health Research*, vol. 5, no. 2, 169–77.

Rosenau, P. 1992, *Post-Modernism and the Social Sciences: Insights, Inroads and Intrusions*, Princeton University Press, New Jersey.

Rosenbaum, J.N. 1989, 'Depression: viewed from a transcultural nursing theoretical perspective', *Journal of Advanced Nursing*, vol. 14, no. 1, 7–12.

Russell, R.L. 1990, *From Nightingale to Now: Nurse Education in Australia*, Harcourt Brace Jovanovich, Sydney.

Sadala, M. 1999, 'Taking care as a relationship: a phenomenological view', *Journal of Advanced Nursing*, vol. 30, no. 4, 808–17.

Sadala, M. & de Camargo, R. 2002, 'Phenomenology as a method to investigate the lived experience: a perspective from Husserl and Merleau Ponty's thought', *Journal of Advanced Nursing*, vol. 37, no. 3, 282–304.

Sandelowski, M. 1986, 'The problem of rigour in qualitative research', *Advances in Nursing Science*, vol. 8, no. 3, 27–37.

Sarnecky, M.T. 1990, 'Historiography: a legitimate research methodology for nursing', *Advances in Nursing Science*, vol. 12, no. 4, 1–10.

Savage, J. 2004, 'Researching emotion: The need for coherence between focus, theory and methodology', *Nursing Inquiry*, vol. 11, no. 1, 25–34.

Schafer, R.J. 1980, *A Guide to Historical Method*, The Dorsey Press, Homewood, Illinois.

Schroeder, M. & Worrall-Carter, L. 2002, 'Perioperative managers: role stressors and strategies for coping', *Contemporary Nurse*, vol. 13, no. 2–3, 229–38.

Schwandt, T. 1998, 'Constructivist, interpretivist approaches to human inquiry', in N. Denzin & Y. Lincoln (eds), *The Landscape of Qualitative Research: Theories and Issues*, Sage, Thousand Oaks.

Schwartz, H. & Jacobs, J. 1979, *Qualitative Sociology: A Method to the Madness*, The Free Press, New York.

Silins, E. 1993, 'Looking back by listening: reflections on an oral history', *Contemporary Nurse*, vol. 2, no. 2, 79–82.

Simons, J., Franck, L. & Roberson, E. 2001, 'Parent involvement in children's pain care: views of parents and nurses', *Journal of Advanced Nursing*, vol. 36, no. 4, 591–9.

Skeggs, B. 2001, 'Feminist ethnography', in P. Atkinson, A. Coffey, S. Delamont, J. Lofland & L. Lofland (eds), *Handbook of Ethnography*, Sage, London, 426–42.

Skopcol, T. 1995, *Social Revolutions in the Modern World*, Cambridge University Press, New York.

Soderhamm, O. & Idvall, E. 2003, 'Nurses' influence on quality of care on postoperative pain management: a phenomenological study', *International Journal of Nursing Practice*, vol. 9, no. 1, 26–32.

Sorensen, E.S. 1988, 'Archives as sources of treasure in historical research', *Western Journal of Nursing Research*, vol. 10, no. 5, 666–70.

Spencer, J. 2001, 'Ethnography after post-modernism', in P. Atkinson, A. Coffey, S. Delamont, J. Lofland & L. Lofland (eds), *Handbook of Ethnography*, Sage, London, 443–52.

Spiegelberg, H. 1970, 'On some human uses of phenomenology', in F.J. Smith (ed.), *Phenomenology in Perspective*, Martinus Nijhoff, The Hague.

Spiegelberg, H. 1976, *The Phenomenological Movement* (vols 1 & 2), Martinus Nijhoff, The Hague.

Spradley, J.P. 1980, *Participant Observation*, Holt, Rinehart & Winston, New York.

Stern, P.M. 1985, 'Using grounded theory method in nursing research', in M.M. Leininger (ed.), *Qualitative Research in Nursing*, Grune & Stratton, New York.

Strauss, A. 1987, *Qualitative Analysis for Social Scientists*, Cambridge University Press, New York.

Strauss, A. & Corbin, J. 1990, *Basics of Qualitative Research: Grounded Theory Procedures and Techniques*, Sage Publications, Newbury Park.

Strauss, A. & Corbin, J. 1994, 'Grounded theory methodology', in N. Denzin & Y. Lincoln (eds), *Handbook of Qualitative Research*, Sage, Thousand Oaks.

Strauss, A. & Corbin, J. 1998, *Basics of Qualitative Research: Techniques and Procedures for Developing Grounded Theory*, Sage, Thousand Oaks.

Streubert, H. & Carpenter, D.R. 1995, *Qualitative Nursing Research: Advancing the Humanistic Imperative*, JB Lippincott Co., Philadelphia.

Sudnow, D. 1967, *Passing On: The Social Organization of Dying*, Prentice Hall, Englewood Cliffs.

Sundelof, E.-M., Hansebo, G. & Ekman, S.-L. 2004, 'Friendship and caring communion: the meaning of caring relationship in district nursing', *International Journal for Human Caring*, vol. 8, no. 3, 13–20.

Swanson, J.M. 1986, 'The formal qualitative interview for grounded theory', in W.C. Chenitz & J.M. Swanson (eds), *From Practice to Grounded Theory*, Addison Wesley, Menlo Park, California.

Taylor, B. 1995, *Qualitative Research Data: What it can Offer Women's Health Centres*, Centre for Professional Development in Health Sciences, Southern Cross University, Lismore, NSW.

Tonkin, E. 1992, *Narrating Our Pasts: The Social Construction of Oral History*, Cambridge University Press, Cambridge.

Van Kaam, A.L. 1959, 'The nurse in the patient's world', *American Journal of Nursing*, vol. 59, no. 12, 1708–10.

van Manen, M. 1990, 'Beyond assumptions: shifting the limits of action research', *Theory into Practice*, vol. 29, no. 3, 152–7.

Webster, R., Thompson, D. & Davidson, P. 2003, 'The first 12 weeks following discharge from hospital: the experience of Gujarati South Asian survivors of acute myocardial infarction and their families', *Contemporary Nurse*, vol. 15, no. 3, 288–99.

West, C. 1993, 'Reconceptualizing gender in physician-patient relationships', *Social Science and Medicine*, vol. 36, 57–66.

Whiting, L. 2001, 'Analysis of phenomenological data: personal reflections on Giorgi's method', *Nurse Researcher*, vol. 9, no. 2, 60–74.

Wilson, D. 2003, 'The nurse's role in improving indigenous health', *Contemporary Nurse*, vol. 15, no. 3, 232–40.

Wit, E., Chenoweth, I. & Jeon, Y.-H. 2004, 'Respite services for older persons and their family carers in southern Sydney', *Collegian*, vol. 11, no. 4, 31–5.

Yuginovich, T. 2000, 'More than time and place: using historical comparative research as a tool for nursing', *International Journal of Nursing Practice*, vol. 6, 70–5.

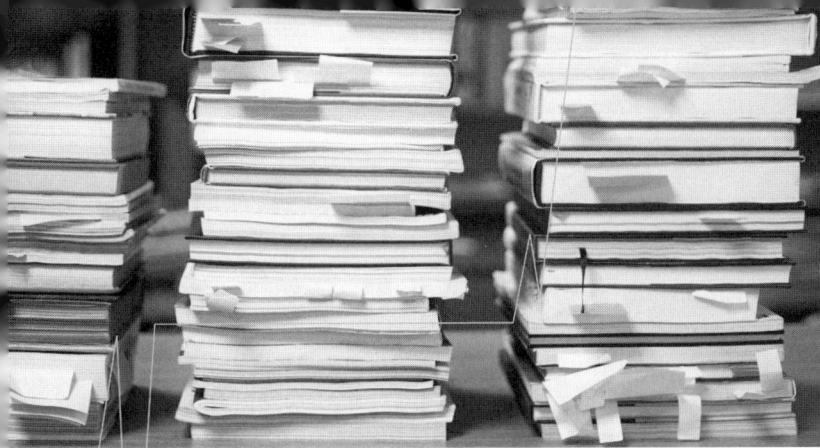

CHAPTER 13

QUALITATIVE CRITICAL METHODOLOGIES AND POSTMODERN INFLUENCES

CHAPTER OBJECTIVES

The material presented in this chapter will assist you to:

- clarify some common qualitative theoretical assumptions about the importance of critical research approaches

- differentiate between critical methodologies, poststructuralism and postmodernism

- define key terms associated with critical methodologies, such as empowerment, emancipation, hegemony and praxis

- describe through methodology, methods and research examples three forms of qualitative critical methodologies – action research, feminism and critical ethnography

- generate potential research questions using these approaches

- define key terms associated with postmodern thought

- describe research discourse reflecting postmodern influences.

Introduction

This chapter deals with qualitative research methodologies which have social change as their 'up-front agenda' and some postmodern thought which aligns with this aim. Whereas qualitative interpretive methodologies may bring about change as a consequence of raising awareness of social and political issues, critical methodologies begin with the stated objective of questioning the status quo in order to improve things. Therefore, critical research approaches have greater potential to address social and political issues in human life than interpretive approaches, which aim mainly to explore and describe.

In health care arenas, this means that critical approaches can address the power imbalances in disciplinary conditions, relationships and organisations, and turn upside down some taken-for-granted assumptions about the way things are, and the way they need to be. This is a crucial point to remember as you work your way through this chapter. Many of the circumstances in which health care workers find themselves can be attributed to events and influences over time. Due to the often subtle historical changes in the events inside and outside practice, clinicians may develop the impression that they cannot change their work conditions and relationships, and that little can be done about the social and political injustices they face as part of their chosen work.

Although not intended to be a precise placement, for the sake of seeing where it fits in the scheme of methodologies we can imagine that poststructuralism comes between critical social science and postmodernism. Following on from the work of Habermas (1972, 1973), other philosophers, especially Foucault (1990), reconceptualised key epistemological ideas such as power and knowledge, taking different viewpoints from critical social theorists. Some of these ideas are discussed later in this chapter and in Chapter 16.

Postmodernism reaches into all areas of life, and researchers can benefit from being aware of some postmodern ideas, even though sorting through and making sense of the masses of literature may be difficult. Rosenau (1992) is an author who has made the **reading** of postmodern thought easier for newcomers to the area, by her description of sceptical and affirmative forms. Sceptical postmodernism offers 'a pessimistic, gloomy assessment' and it argues that the postmodern 'age is one of fragmentation, disintegration, malaise, meaninglessness, a vagueness or even absence of moral parameters and societal chaos' (Rosenau 1992, p. 15). Such a position leaves little room for systematic inquiry through research. In contrast, affirmative postmodernists 'have a more hopeful, optimistic view' of the postmodern age (p. 15).

Researchers reflecting affirmative postmodern influences might agree in part with research approaches represented in this book as qualitative critical methodologies, inasmuch as they repudiate social constructions of power and domination. While espousing postmodern ideas, affirmative postmodernists may nevertheless be uncomfortable with extreme objectivity or relativism that requires an uninvolved and 'anything goes' attitude to questions of human knowledge and existence. For example, feminist postmodernists agree that men have had privileged status, but they are critical of not giving special authority to women's **voices** (Huntington & Gilmour 2001; Rogers-Clark 2002). Therefore, researchers reconciling their need to maintain a political consciousness for minority groups can choose a collection of methods influenced by affirmative postmodern thinking.

Common qualitative critical theoretical assumptions

In Chapter 12 you were introduced to the differences in interpretive and critical qualitative methodologies and some postmodern influences on them; the differences seem to be in knowledge-producing intentions. Whereas interpretive approaches mainly aim to generate descriptions and meaning, critical methodologies aim to address and change conscious and unconscious oppression and inequities in the status quo.

Critical methodologies are derived from some key ideas in critical social science, which emerged from the critical theory perspectives of the Frankfurt School of philosophers, who were intent on finding ways to improve social life after the defeat of left-wing working-class movements during the World War I (Stevens 1989). Early critical theorists of the 1920s, such as Horkheimer, Adorno and Marcuse, were also concerned with the dominance of positivistic science and the tendency to dismiss as unnecessary the questions of reason, which had long been the epistemological tradition of philosophers. The critical theorists reacted against the taken-for-grantedness of the supremacy of the empirical–analytical paradigm and its apparent inability to quell the rising unrest in world affairs.

The concern of the critical theorists was that science was being applied to human understanding with little appeal to social conscience. Objective facts, techniques and scientific rule-following had taken over subjective knowing, critical thinking and reason. The critical theorists considered that the ideology of science was tantamount to the ideology of the aggressors who were sweeping over Europe in the name of progress. Thus, critical social science was born out of reaction to social need as well as to epistemological dilemmas.

Some of the basic ideas of that time were that people need to feel, or be assisted to feel, the effects of oppression and to sincerely desire liberation. They must be able to see and understand their history and the effects of their false consciousness and realise that there are alternative ways of knowing and being. There must be a social crisis, which causes dissatisfaction and threatens the social cohesion of the group. The social crisis is illuminated through an historical account of the members of the group and the structural bases of the society. The accounts will bring enlightenment and the possibility of social transformation.

The criticism levelled against critical theory has been in relation to its idealism, in that the high aspirations of critical theorists have generally not been realised in relation to securing equity for oppressed groups. The powerful still tend to flourish, even in the centre of the most stringent reasoned reflection and critique. A postmodern criticism has been that politics intended to 'free the masses' is often reduced to superficiality by candidates in public office, rendering their representation unauthentic (Baudrillard 1983). However, it has been claimed that sociopolitical and cultural critiques, when effective, can have local effects and can bring changes over time (Culbertson 1981).

Essentially, the kind of knowledge that critical methodologies generate has the potential to be emancipatory; that is, it can free people from the conditions in which they are entrenched to something that can be better for them. The need for **emancipation** comes from the assumption that certain people may suffer oppression and constraints of some kind at the hands of other people and through the effects of the historical, social, political, cultural and economic circumstances in which they find themselves. Freedom from oppression comes from being aware that it is happening and in finding the motivation and means to do something about it.

Critical social science is of the view that collective social action can be successful in recognising and dealing with oppressive relationships, systems and conditions. Therefore, the critical research methodologies derived from critical social science apply to research that adopts this assumption about the nature and effects of power in human relationships. Critical research activity can be geared directly and strategically towards freeing people from forces and **agents** that cause human oppression and domination.

EXERCISE

Think about the work constraints that operate in your professional group. The constraints may be economic, cultural, historical, political and so on.

In what ways do you think that research based in critical social theory has a chance of changing your work conditions?

Invariably, critical methodologies involve research methods that encourage people to come together to share collaboratively, to bring forward their personal and collective concerns and to make group efforts for changes through their research. The intention is to decrease possible power differences between researcher and participants so that the people in the group take on co-researcher identities, thus attempting to own more equally their research problems, processes and outcomes.

Critical methodologies compared with poststructuralism

Following on from, and in response to, the limitations of the descriptive potential of interpretive qualitative methodologies, critical methodologies have taken on a change agenda through enlightenment, emancipation and **empowerment**. Beyond these still, lies poststructuralism, which focuses on **discourses** and discursive practices constituting power relations and knowledge. For example, critical social theorists analyse powerful cultural forces and the patterns of domination which maintain them, in order to free less powerful people from their false consciousness about the **hegemonic** nature of their oppression (Fay 1987; Giroux 1983). The implications in this noble intention to emancipate are that people *are* oppressed and, relatively equally, the emancipator is sufficiently informed of the levels of the false consciousness of the people to be able to free the oppressed. Also implied is that the emancipation will lead to more favourable conditions devoid of other more subtle forces of domination. With these and other critiques in mind, recent critical theorists have moderated their grand claims for enlightenment, empowerment and emancipation to 'redress injustices of race, class, ethnicity, gender, sexual preferences, age, and ability' (Best & Kellner 1991; Giroux 1992; Jordan & Weedon 1995; Mohanty 1994).

Poststructuralists reject the idea that power is possessed as a source of domination over other people; rather, authors such as Foucault (1990) contend that power is exercised and it operates in all directions, not just 'from the top down'. As power is not possessed, it cannot be given to someone else in an act of empowerment and emancipation; thus empowerment needs to be 'context-specific and based on the micropractices of a particular setting' (Gore 1992).

Poststructuralism compared with postmodern thought

Poststructuralism and postmodernism are in some ways similar, and authors have tended to use the terms synonymously, but this is not strictly correct. Rosenau (1992) explains that:

> Most of what is written . . . with reference to post-modernism also applies to post-structuralism. Although the two are not identical they overlap considerably and are sometimes considered synonymous. Few efforts have been made to distinguish between the two, probably because the differences appear to be of little consequence . . . As I see it the major difference is one of emphasis more than substance: Post-modernists are more oriented toward cultural critique while the post-structuralists emphasise method and epistemological matters. For example, post-structuralists concentrate on deconstruction, language, discourse, meaning, and symbols while post-modernists cast a wider net. There also seems to be an emerging difference in the status of subject and object . . . The post-structuralists remain uncompromisingly anti-empirical whereas the post-modernists focus on the concrete in the form of 'le quotidien', daily life, as an alternative to theory (p. 3).

Bearing in mind that postmodernism 'is stimulating and fascinating; and at the same time it is always on the brink of collapsing into confusion' (Rosenau 1992, p. 14), it is important to realise that postmodernism is derived from many '-isms' creating divergent and contradictory forms reflecting partially their theoretical roots. For example, using the qualitative methodologies in this book as a case in point, some versions of postmodernism have sprung from the work of Nietzsche and Heidegger, connected here to qualitative interpretive research; other forms of postmodernism can be traced to the critical theorists Horkheimer and Adorno, connected here to qualitative critical research. As a consequence, postmodernism adopts the views of critical theory to suspect the validity 'of instrumental reason, modern technology, and the role of the media in a modern consumer society' (Rosenau 1992, p. 13).

Even given the historical connections to forms of knowledge named in this book as being foundational to qualitative interpretive and critical research methodologies, you need to remember that for many postmodernists, methodologies constitute in *varying degrees* grand or meta (master) **narratives** 'that claim to be scientific and objective, that serve to legitimate modernity and assume justice, truth, theory, hegemony' (Rosenau 1992, p. 85). The qualification of *varying degrees* lies in the opposition of qualitative interpretive research to the absolute nature of the rules of the scientific method and objectivity, and in the claims critical research methodologies make in fostering processes that oppose hegemony. In so doing, however, both the qualitative interpretive and critical research methodologies assume some authority in addressing issues of justice, truth and theory, and thus run counter to some postmodern thinking.

What does this mean for researchers who choose to adopt postmodern thinking in their projects? Cheek (2000) argues that postmodern approaches can be used in research. She suggests that, in keeping with postmodern thought, Foucault's perspectives of discourse, gaze and governmentality in relation to power (Foucault 1990) can be particularly helpful in exploring and analysing health care practices. If you are interested in what this means for your project, read more about Foucault's perspectives and how Cheek (2000) has applied these ideas in her own research. It is important to remember, however, that there are no prescriptive approaches and that research influenced by postmodern thinking should not be a 'case of attempting to replace one grand narrative with another' (Cheek 2000, p. 124).

In the absence of standard 'strategies' or 'struggles' (methods), researchers can enlist ideas derived from various sources, such as the approaches taken by Anderson, McAllister and Moyle (2002) and Gilbert (2003). These authors combine concepts in critical theory, such as liberation and emancipation, with selected postmodern ideas of technology and power. Some work of researchers applying poststructural and postmodern thought to their projects is presented later in this chapter.

You may notice that the words to which you have been introduced convey fairly familiar concepts. You may also notice that many of the ideas merge, so that they relate closely to one another and combine to bring about a common message, which is that change allowing freedom from relatively enduring oppressive forces is possible through collective social action and research activities.

Even though there has been a progression of thought in research in response to philosophical debates, this does not mean that all of the methodologies that went before poststructuralism and postmodernism are eradicated, inappropriate or not useful. If that were so, there would be no use for this book, and you would be caught in a philosophical 'straitjacket' that would take away your choices. Whereas you need to remain aware of the recent epistemological critiques and trends, you can still exercise your rights as a researcher to choose any approach that may be useful for the kinds of questions you are asking and the aims and objectives you have set for your project. In other words, there is no escaping the 'fact' that if you are to do research you need to be proactive as the **author** of the project, even in thinking up the ideas and setting the project into train, regardless of any recent philosophical thinking by which you may be influenced. With this in mind, we explore examples of qualitative critical methodologies including action research, feminisms and critical ethnography. In the section that follows, each of these approaches will be described in terms of its specific methodological assumptions and methods. Research examples for each methodology will be given and you will be encouraged to generate your own potential research questions using respective approaches.

Action research

As with the history of critical theory, action research grew out of the effects of a war, in this case, World War II (Chein, Cook & Harding 1948), and it had a social change agenda. Kurt Lewin (1946) first used the term 'action research' and in the mid 1940s he used group research process for community projects in postwar USA. Lewin's work is the basis of contemporary versions of action research including those forwarded by Australian educationalists such as Carr and Kemmis (1986) and Kemmis and McTaggart (1988).

As you might expect, action research goes to the site of the concern or practice, and works with the people there as co-researchers to generate solutions to the problems with which they are keen to deal. This form of research involves action, which is directed to showing the problems in the present situation and then facilitating improvements and sustaining changes.

The methodology

Most of the theoretical assumptions underlying action research can be traced to critical theory. McTaggart (1991, p. 25) makes the point that 'many authors in both Europe and Australia have used the theory of knowledge-constitutive interests proposed by the German critical theorist Jurgen Habermas (1972, 1973) to describe three different forms of action research: technical, practical and emancipatory'.

Technical action research aims to improve techniques and procedures by having practitioners work collaboratively to test the applicability of results generated elsewhere. For example, in nursing this could mean that a group of nurses might work together to research the effects of a new aseptic dressing procedure to ascertain its benefits. In other health care practices, the multidisciplinary team might work together to assess the usefulness of amended treatment practices for caring for people with diabetes.

Practical action research aims to improve existing practices and develop new ones. The emphasis here is on reflecting and interpreting to take deliberate strategic action. A nursing example might be that nurses decide to work together to look at the patterns of communication and interpersonal relationships in their ward and how these patterns might be improved to facilitate more effective nursing care. A multidisciplinary example might be that various health professionals work together on improving team dynamics in a particular clinical area.

Emancipatory action research involves a group of practitioners taking responsibility for freeing themselves from the constraints of their practice through understanding and transforming the political, social and economic conditions that keep them from doing their work as they would ideally choose. In nursing, this might mean that nurses would meet to consider and work on all of the factors within their work settings that stop them from giving effective nursing care. They would then work towards changing the constraints by working within and through the influential sources in the system. Similarly, multidisciplinary researchers might examine the competing discourses intrinsic to providing care to specific groups of clients.

The method

The method of action research involves four stages of collectively planning, acting, observing and reflecting (Dick 1995; Stringer 1996). This phase leads to another cycle of action, in which the plan is revised, and further acting, observing and reflecting is undertaken systematically (Reason & Bradbury 2001) to work towards solutions to problems of a technical, practical or emancipatory nature (Kemmis & McTaggart 1988).

If you are thinking of undertaking action research, you would need to find other researchers who are willing to work together over time on collective problems. The group would need to understand some basic principles of action research in terms of its intention to change existing conditions to make them better. Members of the group would also need to be willing to share the workload and responsibilities of the research project and assist one another to create a co-researcher process.

Having established the working rules of the group, attention would need to be given to maintaining the group processes, so that they continued to be facilitative and focused on the problems at hand. Cycles of action research could lead to further foci and members could keep an action research approach to their work for as long as they chose, given that clinical nursing practice is typically fraught with many challenges on a daily basis. Even though there are some underlying principles based on researchers working together through action research cycles, there is not one way of doing action research. Researchers are free to interpret the methods of action research differently, according to the needs of the collaborating research group. For example, I worked with nurses in their clinical settings (Taylor 2001; Taylor et al. 2002) and we generated an approach, which you may find useful. You will find a full description of the approach elsewhere (see Taylor 2006), but there are 13 basic steps.

The steps are to: find enough clinicians to form a research group; ensure the clinicians are ready to make a commitment to the research group; decide on a venue and a regular meeting day and time; write a brief research proposal; check on ethics approval processes in your organisation; get the project under way and decide on who facilitates meetings; share the business of the first two meetings in deciding on group rules and clarifying the nature and potential of action research; share time in reflection on the childhood influences which have helped to form your work values; share everyday practice stories about what is good and not so good about your work; identify the thematic concern(s), which are issues common to everyone; generate an action plan and begin the action research cycles; write a research report; and disseminate the findings. We will explore how this approach was used, in one of the research examples in the following section.

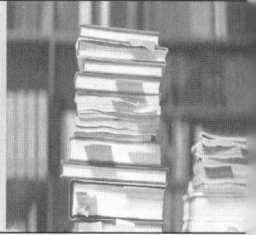

Research examples

Examples of action research approaches to clinical issues are Craig et al. (2004), Watson, Turnbull and Mills (2002) and Taylor et al. (2002).

Craig et al. (2004) improved the nursing management of patients with diabetes using an action research approach. Australian nurses working at a Sydney tertiary hospital recognised that a fixed regime for blood glucose levels (BGL) was unsuitable because of the need for flexibility in managing the types and frequencies of insulin in the acute care setting. Given this realisation, the aim of this 18-month project was 'to motivate nurses to upgrade their standard of care of dependent patients with diabetes mellitus (Type 1 or Type 2)' (Craig et al. 2004, p. 73).

The Clinical Nurse Consultant for Diabetes (CNC), the Diabetes Educator (DE), staff from the Acute Care Nursing Professorial Unit and staff from two specialty wards formed the research group. Two action research cycles were completed during the research meetings on 20-plus occasions at regular intervals. In relation to the research procedure, the

> CNC and DE undertook two observational audits on practice activities. The first audit was taken at the start of cycle one and the second sixteen months later towards the end of cycle two. Both audits recorded actual and documented times of BGL measurement, time of insulin administration, time from administration to meal and time of the documentation. The time meals arrived was charted. Data were recorded across three shifts, morning, afternoon and night, on five different days randomly selected within a fortnight on all patients with Type 2 diabetes mellitus (Craig et al. 2004, p. 74).

Cycle one began with the first practice audit. When the results were discussed in a group meeting, it was decided to develop collaboratively a new blood glucose chart designed to record in detail the actual times of BGL measurements in relation to patients' meals. During the cycle the CNC and DE provided education on the various types and actions of insulin and the importance of accurate documentation.

Cycle two began with the decision to continue using the new form while discussing practice issues. Feedback on the use of the form was gathered in a communication book. The two issues that emerged were that some nurses resisted altering the times of BGL measurements and others were reluctant to be involved in 'research'. During this cycle the patients' charts were reviewed frequently and the second audit was undertaken. The results were positive and can be read in detail in the research report. In summary, the researchers reported that:

> Eighty percent of the 42 ward nursing staff changed their practice in accordance with evidence used to guide the change, and endorsed the process as useful in helping develop practice. While all nurses used the new chart, some nurses did not consistently change in their practice behaviours with regard to BGL monitoring (Craig et al. 2004, pp. 74–5).

Watson, Turnbull and Mills (2002) evaluated the extended role of the midwife in the Northern Territory of Australia using participatory action research (PAR). The need for the research arose from a National Health and Medical Research Report (NHMRC) (1996), which highlighted service issues for midwives in Australia. Watson, Turnbull and Mills (2002) explain that some

> professional stakeholders may see the extended role of the midwife as threatening to their professional autonomy. What the extended role represents may also differ from hospital to hospital and country to country. Although the extended role of midwives within Australia may be formally acknowledged, recommendations are yet to be fully implemented for daily practice. Midwives from the United Kingdom, Europe and New Zealand already practice in an extended way on a day-to-day basis (p. 258).

The research aim was to 'evaluate the implementation of the NHMRC recommendations in two acute care hospitals in the NT: one a Central Australian hospital and one a Top End hospital' (Watson, Turnbull & Mills 2002, p. 258). For readers outside Australia, the authors clarify that the 'Top End' refers to 'the northern aspect' of the Northern Territory, and Central Australia refers to 'the desert region' of the Northern Territory (p. 258). This PAR evaluative research included the stakeholders, such as the mothers, midwives, Aboriginal health workers, medical officers and so on. This article focused on the first phase of the evaluation involving interviews with the midwives.

Five midwives from a Central Australian hospital and seven midwives from a Top End hospital agreed to participate. Interviews lasted 40 to 60 minutes and they were audiotaped for transcription and analysis. Four categories emerged from the data analysis: autonomy and responsibility; gaining in professionalism; it's better for the midwives; and it's better for the mothers. Essentially, the categories showed that midwives felt an increased sense of autonomy and responsibility in response to the extended role policy and standing orders; they linked the extended role to increased professionalism; and the extended role had benefits for midwives and mothers.

The researchers concluded that midwifery

> in Australia is an established profession. Yet when compared with their counterparts in the United Kingdom and New Zealand, midwives in Australia continue to practice with considerable limitations placed on their autonomy. This study has identified a need for further evaluation of this very important role within the context of midwifery and nursing practice, to ensure it is implemented and conducted in a way that

enhances the professional status and recognition of the role if the midwife in providing primary care of women during normal pregnancy and birth (Watson, Turnbull & Mills 2002, p. 263).

Taylor et al. (2002) explored idealism in palliative nursing care. The project used a combination of action research and reflective practice processes. Six experienced RNs identified their tendency towards idealism in their palliative nursing practice, which they defined as the tendency to expect to be 100 per cent effective all of the time in their work.

The nurses met weekly for one hour, for 21 weeks, to discuss clinical problems raised by them in their journal writing and discussion. Group processes were detailed by the researcher in minutes of meetings, and were confirmed weekly as faithful accounts by participants, thereby acting as participant checks for validation purposes. Four distinct research phases emerged: Phase 1, weeks 1–3, introductions; Phase 2, weeks 4–8, sharing practice stories; Phase 3, weeks 10–15, locating idealism and making an action plan; and Phase 4, weeks 16–21, putting the action plan into practice.

Participants collaborated in generating and evaluating an action plan to recognise and manage the negative effects of idealism in their work expectations and behaviours. The action plan included practical suggestions to apply to work situations before, during and after practice, a selection being:

Before practice

Realise that plans do not always work, so set realistic goals.

Recognise and label my own expectations and behaviour as idealistic.

During practice

Recognise and label my own expectations and behaviour as idealistic.

Own up to my idealism and tell the other person/people.

After practice

Review my practice by 'resetting my level of idealism, through feedback'.

Be satisfied with being the best I can be, which could be less than 100% on the day (Taylor et al. 2002, p. 329).

Participants expressed positive changes in their practice, based on adjusting their responses to their idealistic tendencies towards perfectionism. The project gave nurses a regular forum in which to discuss their reflections on practice and to generate an action pan to bring about change. The benefits of action research and reflection are that there are immediate, practical outcomes for participants because they can share their experiences with peers, work together on thematic concerns, and bring about local changes in their practice. Thus, the co-researchers experienced participatory research, while developing their reflective skills, and in this sense the research offered them personal and professional gains for their participation.

You may also like to locate other examples of action research (for example, Cheno-weth & Kilstoff 1998; de la Rue 2003; Keatinge et al. 2000; Koch et al. 2001; Koch, Kralik & Kelly 2000; Moody, Greenwood & Choong 2001).

Potential research questions

Research questions that may use action research are those concerns and issues raised by the research participants themselves, and/or someone else's questions, for example, those of a researcher or team of researchers that have been adopted by the research group for their collaborative research inquiry processes.

The potential is vast for raising research questions using action research, because any practice issue can be managed by this approach, especially if co-researchers are willing to take the time and effort to work together to find strategies and solutions. Action research projects explore practical problems, so they are totally useful by their nature.

If you want to consider possibilities for action research, begin by spending some time thinking about your work situation and the people and situations you face there.

EXERCISE

In what ways are the people and situations of your work setting problematic to you and your practice? Do other clinicians have similar concerns? Do you think others would be prepared to work with you to use an action research approach to working collaboratively through these problems? Ask them. You may find that you have made the first step towards setting up an action research project.

Feminisms

Feminism is a social movement concerned with women's issues and lives (Chinn & Wheeler 1985), and many kinds of feminisms reflect transitions over time in defining and addressing women's concerns, requiring multiple theories to explain the causes of women's oppression (Tong 1989). Examples of feminisms include liberal, Marxist/socialist, radical, poststructuralist and postmodern representations. Glass (2000, p. 357) states emphatically that 'there is no one feminism; feminism is feminisms' and describes three waves of feminisms.

First-wave feminism refers to events at the beginning of the twentieth century, which identified the lack of material benefits and production for women, the viewing of women as objects, the mistaken assumptions that women should not be thinking people with voices. The first wave also ushered in women's rights to vote and to be 'self-determining, enlightened and sexually liberated' (Glass 2000, p. 360).

The second wave includes liberal, Marxist, radical and lesbian feminists. Liberal feminism seeks equal rights within the existing social structures, through reasoning and equal educational opportunities for women. Liberal feminists seek to determine their social roles and 'compete with men on terms that . . . are as equal as possible' (Jagger 1983, p. 324). Critics of this approach argue that opportunities for education that privilege men negate women's attempts for equality and their ability to reason (Cheek et al. 1996), and that women's subjectivity is not addressed in gender differences in the development of reasoning (Bunting & Campbell 1990; Doering 1992).

Marxist/socialist feminism asserts that ownership of property and women is the basis of sexism and class division, and that women are oppressed within the family, motherhood, consumerism and class. This approach advocates the freedom to define one's own sexuality, equal sharing of child rearing and domestic roles, and the right to choose a family (Weedon 1991), thus addressing the relationships between the economy, family, class and gender (Seidman 1994). The ideas of Marxist/socialist feminism are influential in radical feminism.

Radical feminism withdraws from the dominant patriarchal system to replace it with 'woman defined systems, thought and culture' (Chinn & Wheeler 1985, p. 74). Critics who oppose radical feminism question a separatist stance, even though they may agree that women need to be free from the biological oppression of motherhood and sexual slavery, and the allocation of womanly work (Weedon 1991). Lesbian feminists 'espouse all of the values of radical feminists; however, they are concerned primarily with their sexual orientation in a feminist context' (Glass 2000, p. 362). Their issues involve 'not succumbing to male desire and rejecting heterosexuality per se' (Evans 1997, p. 362); therefore, they risk being doubly oppressed as women and lesbians.

The third wave of contemporary feminism, from the 1980s onwards, 'encompasses poststructural and postmodern feminisms' (Glass 2000, p. 363). Feminist poststructuralism responds to the idea that the division of feminisms into categories is problematic because the categories are arbitrary and socially produced (Delmar 1994; Gatens 1992) and the idea fails to address issues of power in language, subjectivity, social processes and institutions (Weedon 1991; Doering 1992). A feminist poststructuralist approach offers ways of identifying how language and discourse exercise power, showing how oppression operates by creating and affecting the possibilities for resistance (Weedon 1991), and of identifying women's participation in multiple discourses of everyday life (Davies 1994). Feminist poststructuralism allows women to recognise and change the cultural patterns of oppression inherent in dominant patriarchal society through constantly renewed ways of seeing and repositioning themselves.

Postmodern feminists espouse 'a philosophy that supports and values the social contextual experience and difference of unique individuals and rejects the generalisation of those experiences' (Glass & Davis 1998, p. 44). For example, third-wave feminists 'have become disgruntled with the generalising theories of women's oppression' (Glass 2000, p. 363) and question whether all women are oppressed equally, resulting in the same effects.

The methodology

Pervading much of feminist literature are the key ideas of embodiment, empowerment and emancipation. Embodiment refers to living in a particular body. In relation to feminism, it means living a life through adherence to, and activation of, certain feminist principles that value the individual and collective good of women. Empowerment and emancipation have been defined previously in this chapter, but in feminist research they are of particular relevance in using participatory research processes to work towards the attainment of women's power and freedom.

Living a feminist perspective is about understanding and applying certain principles of feminism to daily life, so that it shows in the way you live. Embodying feminism means that the person is open to others, and is prepared to listen and collaborate for the collective good of women. It also means being attentive to those conditions that dominate and oppress women through valuing women and their issues, concerns and experiences, and striving to create social change through critique and political action.

As can be seen from the three waves of feminism, different theoretical emphases have evolved over time, but they have not necessarily replaced each other sequentially. For example, some feminists may align with particular views preceding the third wave and see no reason for making postmodern adjustments in their thinking. However, feminist researchers agree that 'women are the major focus of feminist research from the beginning to the end of *whole* research projects' therefore feminist methodology 'concerns research *by* and *for* women … putting feminist theory into practice … by applying feminist principles directly from feminist premises' (Glass 2000, p. 368).

The methods

Feminist research uses methods that best reflect feminist principles and thereby ensure that all of the women involved are empowered by the research processes. In other words, feminist research not only emphasises *what* is done in terms of methods, but also *how* projects are done, in faithful reflection of feminist processes. Methods are not prescriptive, but they may include groupwork, storytelling, interviews, participant observation and so on, depending on the focus of the research interest. The main consideration is keeping to the important principles of feminist research, listed by Glass (2000, pp. 368–9), including the importance of a transforming and empowering focus, and research *with*, never *on* women, based on mutual respect and sharing: 'The researcher's values, beliefs and assumptions about who she is or her experiences are openly disclosed … as a means of equalising power relations' (Glass 2000, p. 369). Interpersonal interactions are 'based on equality, reciprocity, and promote mutuality amongst all women involved' (p. 369). Feminist research values women's unique experiences and stories and recognises and respects 'the inherent sensitivity in collecting data from women' (p. 369). Feminist research methods and design 'benefit the women involved either whilst actively participating in the research or in the longer term' (p. 369).

Research examples

Research projects using approaches informed by feminist principles are Hardin (2003), Meyer and de Oliveira (2003) and Armishaw and Davis (2002).

Hardin (2003, p. 209) was interested in the 'shape-shifting discourses of anorexia nervosa', particularly 'the circuitous relationship between individuals, the media, and discursive systems' that 'replicate and reinforce the act of self-starvation in young women'. A feminist poststructural methodology was used to expose how 'discourses and institutional practices operate to position young women who take up the subject position of wanting to be diagnosed as anorexic' (p. 209). Using the first person pronoun 'I', Hardin situates herself in the research by describing her research thus:

> Utilizing data from online accounts and individual interviews, I attend to the ways in which young women are institutionally positioned as 'anorexics' and the effects that those positions have on their behaviours, in addition to reinforcing institutional practices that construct anorexia nervosa. Questions addressed through this inquiry are: How do institutional practices create and continue to construct 'anorexia nervosa'? How do discourses operate to position young women such that they are either included and/or excluded into the category of 'anorexia nervosa'? What are the effects and consequences that emanate from these positionings? (Hardin 2003, p. 209)

Although Hardin's language may seem inaccessible at first, it has an inherent feminist poststructural/postmodern questioning process to it that seeks to go behind what first appears, to take a closer look. The research reported here was written as a Foucauldian discourse, meaning that anorexia nervosa was the focus not only as an object of interest, but also in the sense of how anorexia is 'constituted by the discourses' in which it emerges. This means that Hardin was interested in examining how anorexia nervosa is created and maintained by shaping agents, such as the media and organisations, so that women become 'types' or 'kinds' of people who starve themselves. After analysis of the messages women posted on online anorexia message boards, Hardin made the point that the media coverage has been so intense as to 'normalise' anorexia nervosa by 'glamourising' the subject, giving 'anorexics' ways of thinking and acting within the subject position of anorexia nervosa.

EXERCISE

Reread the above section on Hardin's research. Go to the relevant definitions in the Glossary and reread them also. Keep rereading until you feel that you are making sense of the way Hardin writes. You will start to notice how the postmodern language sounds and the patterns of thought it pursues.

Meyer and de Oliveira (2003) are Brazilian researchers who used a poststructural feminist historical-cultural approach to examine breastfeeding policies and the production of motherhood. They explain that in their research:

> Knowledges and practices that produce notions of maternity are problematized to argue that current political and economic arrangements have necessitated a redefinition of motherhood. This re-signification of motherhood has transferred to women the duty of solving an array of problems that were previously

considered the government's responsibility, in particular those related to the physical and emotional development of infants (Meyer & de Oliveira 2003, p. 11).

This research is interesting reading for mothers and midwives because it provides a strong argument that Brazilian women's bodies have become politicised by the government's insistence on promoting the positive aspects of breastfeeding on demand as a woman's responsibility to her child. The researchers were able to make this observation after a discourse analysis of a government document, a breastfeeding promotion guide, which was part of the National Program of Incentive to Breastfeeding (sic)(NPIB). The researchers also examined relevant newspaper articles published in Rio Grande do Sul, Brazil, in the year 2000.

Even though, on the face of it, many people would claim that breastfeeding is a good thing, the researchers argue that 'there are alternative ways of analyzing the issues and consequences of this contemporary emphasis on breastfeeding (Meyer & de Oliveira 2003, p. 11). From this statement the researchers move on to show how medicine and government have represented motherhood. Thus, the best or truest mothers have certain characteristics and functions against which all other mothers are judged. The researchers argue that the practices of signifying motherhood involve 'relations of power: the power to name, describe classify, identify and differentiate' ways of being a mother and a woman, thus including and excluding individuals and groups outside approved social practices (Meyer & de Oliveira 2003, p. 12). In other words, good mothers breastfeed on demand and not-so-good mothers do not.

Armishaw and Davis (2002) undertook a critical feminist exploration of women, hepatitis C (HCV) and sexuality. Their beginning assumptions were made explicit, that nurses may exhibit erotophobia and stigmatise patients with HCV. The researchers noted the silence in the literature of women's experiences of living with HCV, thus they decided to explore 'the question of whether living with HCV affected the sexuality of HCV women and if so, in what ways' (Armishaw & Davis 2002, p. 194).

The researchers chose a 'modernist feminist paradigm and used critical social theory as a tool that aimed for personal empowerment of the research participants' (Armishaw & Davis 2002, p. 196). In congruence with this aim, because 'the very act of speaking and being heard is, in itself, empowering' (p. 196), Judy Armishaw (the honours researcher) collected data via critical conversations and reflective journalling. After institutional ethical clearance, six women, all of whom 'turned out to be' lesbians, were selected using purposive convenience sampling. The women were over 18 years of age, had HCV, and had known of their HCV status for over two years.

The audiotaped conversations were listened to over and over again, and transcribed, and the researcher noted that during 'this period of intense familiarity common themes and an overarching analytical framework began to emerge from the data' (p. 197). The framework chosen was Gilligan's (1984) self-in-relations model of moral decision-making, because participants spoke of the risks within the dilemma of whether to disclose their HCV status to sexual partners. The themes were 'disclosure', 'the package' and 'transcending the package'. 'Disclosure' described the dilemma women experienced in not so much if, but when, to tell their sexual partner of their HCV status. 'The package' referred to the complexity of telling about HCV status in the sense of giving personal information to another and risking being 'boxed' into a stigmatised role, thus enduring being discredited by oneself and others. 'Transcending the package' included 'focusing in the positives of being positive, and having some positive experiences with disclosure' (p. 200).

The message to nurses was expressed thus:

> It is important that nurses be fully informed not only about HCV transmission, but also the moral complexity involved in decisions about to whom, why, and when to disclose a stigmatised health condition. Further to this, the research alerted nurses to be aware of how easy it is to see HCV positive people in a package and treat them in a discriminatory fashion based on personal prejudice, fear and ignorance (Armishaw & Davis 2002, p. 202).

Other research examples of projects influenced by feminist thought are Anderson and McCann (2002), Boughton (2002), Jackson and Raftos (1997), Jackson et al. (2005), Lumby (1997), Tuttle and Seibold (2002) and Walter, Davis and Glass (1999).

Potential research questions

If you are thinking of using a feminist approach to your research, you could begin by asking yourself some basic questions that relate to some underlying feminist assumptions. For example, you might ask yourself: 'What is it that I know that is of concern to women?' 'In what ways will this research attempt to value women's experiences?' 'How might this research increase the awareness of factors that oppress women?' 'How can this research assist women to create social change through critique and political action?' and 'How can postmodern thinking enhance my understanding of women's experiences and issues?' With these broad questions in mind, you need to consider specific areas of interest that may be best addressed by a feminist research perspective.

Questions may emphasise power relations between groups of clinicians and other members of the health care system. The focus might be on generating historical questions about the origins of healing that readmits women to its accounts. You might like to think of ways of working with women clinicians to address any issues of concern that they might have. You might prefer to start with a feminist process for research such as 'Peace and Power' described by Wheeler and Chinn (1989).

EXERCISE
What sort of work concerns could be managed best by a feminist research process in your health care setting?

Keep in mind the extent to which the possible research concerns reflect some fundamental principles of feminism such as those covered in this section (Glass 2000).

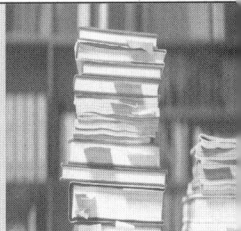

Critical ethnography

The meaning of critical ethnography connotes a hybrid of ethnography and critical social science. As you might imagine, critical ethnography not only has the exploratory and descriptive mission of an ethnography, but it also has the emancipatory aims of critical research approaches. This means that it can go further than descriptive or interpretive ethnography, which seeks only to describe the cultural features of a particular group of people in order to understand their symbols, rituals and practices.

The methodology

Critical ethnography began life as ethnography and added its critical component in response to a growing critique of the perceived inability of traditional ethnography to address political questions in research. With arguments similar to those raised against other interpretive research approaches such as grounded theory and phenomenology (Carr & Kemmis 1986; Fay 1975), ethnography has been criticised for failing to recognise that all human activity is political, that shared meanings are worked out through discourse, and that researchers are not exempt from subjectivity and bias (Angus 1986; Gitlin, Siegal & Boru 1989). For an ethnography to become critical it must be 'openly ideological, socially critical, overtly political, and emancipatory in intent' (Shannon 1994, p. 2).

The methods

Critical ethnography can create a dialogue with research participants so that they can examine the personal, political, social, cultural, historical and economic aspects of their contexts to develop local knowledge of use to their own situations. Therefore, critical ethnography is a reflexive research process that offers a means to reveal 'the complex micro politics of social relationships in the situation and the researcher's position within those politics' (Wellard & Street 1999, p. 133). In this way, critical ethnography goes beyond the surface features of social settings to uncover and examine the power relations and influences affecting and determining the nature and consequences of human behaviour. Even so, Smyth and Holmes (2005, p. 65) rightly point out that even though critical ethnography is being used increasingly, there is 'little advice as to what forms it may take, their applicability and their strengths and weaknesses'. Given this observation Smyth and Holmes (2005) recommend Carspecken's (1996) method of compiling the primary record, preliminary reconstructive analysis, dialogical data generation, describing systems relations, and systems relations as explanations of the findings.

EXERCISE

Locate a copy of Carspecken's method (1996; the reference is at the end of this chapter). After reading the resource, determine the extent to which it could help you set up a critical ethnographic approach to some of your work concerns.

Although there are no prescriptive rules to follow in planning and undertaking a critical ethnography, the methods used will be congruent with certain interests of critical inquiry, such as power and power relations. A critical ethnography will probably:

- focus on a setting in which specific day-to-day practices can be observed
- intend to bring about changes in the status quo by submitting the research area to constant and systematic political critique
- involve researcher–participant collaboration in open and honest communication and critical reflection
- attempt to acknowledge and deal with potential power differences and struggles between research participants
- generate a frank and critically aware discourse that allows participants to express their ideas, assumptions and concerns regarding the research process and the evolving aims of the research
- involve participants equally in actively engaging in problem-locating and strategy-solving within the agreed structures and processes of the research.

Given the nature of the principles of critical ethnographic research as listed previously, the methods to ensure that issues of power are addressed may include: group processes such as discussion and debate, participant observation, and reflective practice strategies such as keeping diaries, writing narratives and engaging in individual and group critiques.

Research examples

Although not described explicitly by the researchers as critical ethnographies, the following research examples show how critical social principles of power identification, examination and critique have been used to examine patient satisfaction (Rankin 2003) and the 'chain of command' in a nursing home (Jervis 2002).

Rankin (2003) conveys a critical ethnographic intention in researching patient satisfaction in Canadian health care by using an approach described by Smith (2001) as an institutional ethnography. Smith, a sociologist, 'is interested in how knowledge and power are related' (Rankin 2003, p. 57), so the research process is essentially a critique of institutional power and power relations within an ethnographic approach. Rankin critically analysed one instance of 'text-based management' in the form of a hospital patient survey that aimed to evaluate patient satisfaction. The researcher visiting a relative in a Canadian hospital and locating the instructional evaluation document established the ethnographic part of the project. The 'critical' part of the project was in the extensive analysis and critique to which the researcher subjected the patient satisfaction evaluation document.

The main argument in Rankin's critical ethnography is that much effort is put into creating and completing patient satisfaction forms, while the business of resourcing quality care is not managed well. After a thorough critique of the document and a study of the management environment, the researcher concluded:

> Official knowledge about the status of Canadian health-care is a product of health management constituted through particular textual practices... Faced with multiple demands, such as accreditation

standards, competitive funding cultures, and increased public/professional pressures for accountability, hospital administrators are socially organised to develop interests in 'quality assurance' programmes, such as patient satisfaction that track, measure and provide data to increasingly vigilant stakeholder groups . . . This approach to knowledge contains a fatal flaw — the experiencing subjects (the patient and her (sic) family) are dropped from the account, while organizational categories and relevancies get inserted (Rankin 2003, p. 65).

The second example of a critical ethnography is 'working in and around the "chain of command" in a nursing home' (Jervis 2002). Even though the researcher describes the project as ethnographic and it includes the application of some grounded theory ideas in the analysis, the focus on power and hegemonic practices places this project well within a critical ethnographic approach. The paradigmatic language of critical theory is shown clearly in the abstract of the article, where the researcher (Jervis 2002) explains:

Using ethnographic methods, this project explored power relations among nursing assistants and nurses in an urban nursing home in the United States. Factors contributing to tensions among nursing staff were stigma attached to nursing homes and those who work in them, as well as the long history of class conflict and power struggles within the discipline of nursing. The latter struggles, in turn, reflected nursing's quest for professional status in the face of medicine's hegemony over health-care. Ultimately, these factors coalesced to produce a local work environment characterized by conflict — and by aides' resistance to nurses' domination (p. 12).

The researcher undertook 21 months of participant observation in a 78-bed, for-profit nursing home, considered by many people to be a 'good' institution. The project also included audiotaped interviews with 14 residents and 16 staff members, and medical record reviews for the 14 participating residents. The researcher described a staff hierarchy and chain of command of 'royalty', nobility' and 'peasants', reflecting the trajectory of power within this hierarchy' (p. 14).

The top management staff enjoyed the perks of autonomy, job satisfaction and status, while workers such as nurse-supervisors described the challenges of excessive paperwork, supervision, and the stigma of working in aged care. The 'peasants' on the bottom of the hierarchy, the nurse assistants, described the effects of policies developed by the top staff that resulted in exploitation and racism. The nurse assistants also criticised the nurse-supervisors for their laziness, hypocrisy and domination, all of which the nurse assistants resisted through industrial sabotage and limiting work, questioning the chain of command, focusing on residents, avoiding enmeshment with higher level staff, and finally 'voting with one's feet' by resigning.

These examples demonstrate the powerful potential of critical ethnography to unmask organisational and personal agendas, and having exposed them, to raise the possibilities for awareness and change. Another example of a critical ethnography is Wellard and Street's (1999) research into home-based dialysis, that identified the issues of families involved in the home care of a person with end-stage renal disease.

Potential research questions

A critical ethnographic approach may be taken for any research interest that involves becoming familiar with rituals and practices with the intention of being politically provocative in order to challenge the accepted understandings and established power sources in the culture. Because it has emancipatory potential, critical ethnography can be used in any setting that will inform clinicians about the influences and constraints operating against nurses in their work. For example, co-researchers may work together to raise their awareness about work circumstances that may benefit from a critical appraisal in places such as wards, clinics, administrative offices, schools, universities and community settings.

If you want to consider possibilities for a critical ethnographic study, begin by thinking about your clinical setting and some of the rituals and practices that you may have noticed there.

> ### EXERCISE
> In what ways are work rituals and practices taken for granted? To what extent are clinicians aware of the taken-for-grantedness of aspects of their work? Are there political struggles in your workplace, either 'in the open' or on a hidden level? Is there any interest among colleagues in working together to set up systematic politically active research processes and methods to raise awareness, questions and critique about selected practices in the culture?

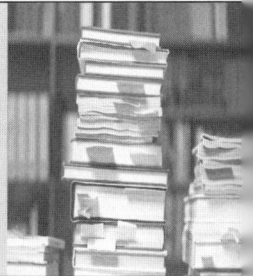

Research discourse reflecting postmodern influences

This section deals with research discourse reflecting postmodern influences, rather than 'postmodern research' per se, because my reading of various postmodern ideas leads me to suspect that to write and speak of the latter would constitute an oxymoron. It would be a contradiction in terms to claim that 'postmodern research' per se exists or could exist, because to construct a form called 'postmodern research' would be the same as constructing a grand narrative, which is antithetical to postmodernist claims for the plurality, diversity, relativity and multiplicity of truth.

All of the approaches described in this section, specifically action research, feminism and critical ethnography, constitute grand narratives, as they are based on certain assumptions about how knowledge is gained and verified through research methods and processes. The discourse arguing the legitimacy of grand narratives creates various positions. For example, some feminist scholars believe that the emancipatory impulse of feminism is silenced by postmodernism (Benhabib 1995; Farganis 1994); therefore postmodernism has no value in advancing the interests of women as members of oppressed groups. In nursing, Kermode and Brown (1995) have argued that failure to recognise the grand narratives of capitalism and patriarchy have left uncontested these issues as sources of power. However, there are researchers who have held onto important aspects of a 'grand narrative' while integrating what they see as compatible aspects of postmodernism (Fahy 1997; Glass & Davis 1998; Hall 1999).

There are examples in this chapter of research influenced by poststructural and postmodern thinking (Hardin 2003; Meyer & de Oliveira 2003). Another example is research undertaken by Langridge and Ahern (2003), which explored issues surrounding advanced nurse specialisation (ANS) and education. The researchers used a mixed methodology, because they claimed that:

> Intentional phenomenology and postmodern discourse analysis were necessary to our study because they each dealt with the perspective of a phenomenon characterised by contradictory and opposing realities. Husserlian phenomenology of the advancing nurse specialists was limited because it did not provide sufficient information about the social and political context in which nurses were experiencing the phenomenon. We therefore carried out an additional study using postmodern discourse analysis of ANS stakeholder interviews and triangulated the results (Langridge & Ahern 2003, p. 32).

In choosing to combine phenomenology with discourse analysis the researchers created a 'critical phenomenology', which had the potential to go beyond description of the phenomenon to a critique of all the determinants of the context. In a postmodern research era it is possible to combine methodologies, as long as you are clear about what each methodological addition offers to the project. We have moved beyond a 'purist' view of finding the best possible methodology for a project and staying with that, to making a selection of possible methodologies to create greater potential for wider readings of 'truth' from various **texts** and discourses.

EXERCISE

Create your own flexible qualitative critical methodologies with postmodern influences. Think of a research area or question that requires a broad view to explore it openly and comprehensively. It might help to imagine a complex situation that combines human communication, power and organisational expectations.

What methodologies are possible approaches for exploring your area/question? Why?

The co-author's postscript to postmodernism

It is important that you do not gain the impression that postmodernism is another methodology – because it is not. Researchers need to be careful to qualify postmodernism as *informing* research, rather than claiming that they are undertaking postmodern research per se. As a co-author of this book, I have put myself in a position of authority to present to you research processes you can use in your projects. In the various chapters of this book I have given you my own reading of scholars' writing and this may be in direct opposition to your or someone else's interpretation as a **reader** of the text. My dilemma resides in putting myself in a position of legitimate authority as a co-author of this book. Even so, as a teacher and researcher I put myself in a position of legitimate authority every day of my working life. The roles dictate that I take a position of authority as teacher and researcher so other people can learn from what I have to say and what I embody. My response to this dilemma of my modernist authority as co-author is moderated by postmodernist ideas of offering multiple ideas, and highlighting possible contradictions, while providing paradigmatic maps for you that make sense of the vast terrain of research. In this sense, I offer teaching as a form of guidance and hope that my explanations offer you choices for understanding complex and novel texts. You are the ultimate reader of your life and of this book, because in a postmodern sense, you interpret these texts for yourself.

Summary

This chapter dealt with qualitative research methodologies that have political awareness and social change as their 'up-front agenda'. Critical research methodologies have an active intention to question the taken-for-granted aspects of a culture in order to change it positively. Critical approaches can address the power imbalances in working conditions, relationships and organisations, and question assumptions about the way things are and the way they need to be.

The chapter also clarified some common qualitative theoretical assumptions about the importance of critical research approaches and defined key terms associated with critical methodologies, such as empowerment, emancipation, hegemony and **praxis**. Three forms of qualitative critical methodologies were described, specifically action research, feminisms and critical ethnography in terms of their methodologies, methods and potential for raising and dealing with nursing research questions of a political nature. Critical social theory, poststructuralism and postmodernism were compared briefly, and research and projects were presented that have used various postmodern ideas in their approaches.

Main points

- Critical research approaches address social and political issues in human life, and they can address the power imbalances in working conditions, relationships and organisations, and turn upside down some taken-for-granted assumptions about the way things are, and the way they need to be.
- Critical methodologies generate emancipatory knowledge that has the potential to free people from the oppressive conditions of their entrenched historical, social, political, cultural and economic circumstances, to something that can be better for them.
- Critical methodologies involve research methods that encourage people to come together to share collaboratively, to surface their personal and collective concerns and to attempt to own more equally their research problems, processes and outcomes as co-researchers.

- Even given the historical connections of qualitative interpretive and critical research methodologies to postmodernism, many postmodernists argue that these methodologies constitute in *varying degrees* grand or meta (master) narratives that assume some authority in addressing issues of justice, truth and theory, and thus run counter to some postmodern thinking.
- Action research goes to the site of a concern or practice, and works with the people there as co-researchers, to generate solutions to problems (thematic concerns) with which they have agreed to deal, through action cycles of systematically and collectively planning, acting, observing and reflecting.
- Feminism is a social movement concerned with women's issues and lives and many kinds of feminisms such as liberal, Marxist/socialist, radical, poststructuralist and postmodern representations, reflect transitions in defining and addressing women's concerns.
- Critical ethnography uses reflexive research processes that have exploratory, descriptive and emancipatory aims, to create a dialogue with research participants so they can go beyond the surface features of their social settings to uncover, examine and begin to deal with, the power relations and influences affecting them.
- 'Postmodern research' cannot exist per se, because to construct a representation called 'postmodern research' would be tantamount to constructing a grand narrative, which is antithetical to postmodernist deconstruction that supports the plurality, diversity, relativity and multiplicity of truth claims.
- As qualitative critical approaches constitute grand narratives, various responses to postmodernism from nursing researchers have been that the emancipatory impulse is silenced by postmodernism; grand narratives such as capitalism and patriarchy are left uncontested as sources of power; and that it is possible to retain important aspects of a 'grand narrative' while integrating compatible aspects of postmodernism.

CASE STUDY

We met Angela in Chapter 12. Angela works as a physiotherapist in a multidisciplinary team in a large city hospital. Angela has been accepted into a Master by Research program, and she has decided that she wants to 'give voice' to elderly women, and to sensitise staff to their unique needs. Angela's research area of interest is 'The invisibility of elderly women to the multidisciplinary team'. After reading about methodologies, Angela has decided to use a feminist approach, but she is noticing in her reading that there are many kinds of feminism. Angela is in a quandary and she asks you to help her understand what methodological combinations are open for her to use with feminism. To prepare yourself to talk with Angela, ensure you can answer these questions:

1   What kinds of feminism are there and why are there so many forms?
2   What basic principles underlie all feminist research processes?
3   Can poststructuralism be mixed with feminism in a research approach? If yes, why and how?
4   Can postmodernism inform a feminist project? If yes, why and how?
5   Are there any limitations on what can be mixed with feminism as research methodologies and influences? If yes, what are they and why?

Multiple choice questions

1   Complex and unending interwoven human interrelationships that do not arrive at an end point or consensus are referred to as:
   a   deconstruction
   b   hegemony
   c   praxis
   d   intertextuality
2   Qualitative critical methodologies all agree on their 'up-front' agenda for social:
   a   power
   b   change
   c   stability
   d   voice
3   In qualitative critical methodologies the process of giving and accepting power is:
   a   empowerment
   b   emancipation
   c   praxis
   d   discourse
4   In postmodernism, people assumed to have authority and power, by virtue of their knowledge and skills, are:
   a   authors
   b   readers
   c   oppressors
   d   agents
5   Collectively planning, acting, observing and reflecting are research phases characteristic of:
   a   critical ethnography
   b   action research
   c   discourse analysis
   d   feminism

6   The critique of events at the beginning of the twentieth century, which identified the lack of material benefits and production for women, and viewing of women as objects led to:
    a   first-wave feminism
    b   second-wave feminism
    c   third-wave feminism
    d   fourth-wave feminism

7   A wave of feminist philosophy that supports and values the social contextual experience and difference of unique individuals and rejects the generalisation of those experiences is:
    a   Marxist
    b   postmodern
    c   liberal
    d   socialist

8   An ethnography can only claim to be critical when it:
    a   involves women only
    b   creates rich descriptions
    c   intends to emancipate
    d   criticises cultures

9   Given the nature of critical ethnographic research, the data collection methods used will most probably include:
    a   discussion and debate
    b   participant observation
    c   reflective practice strategies
    d   all of the above

10   Which of the following research approaches/influences resists being labelled as a 'grand narrative'?
    a   feminism
    b   critical ethnography
    c   postmodernism
    d   action research

Review topics

1   What are the main philosophical features of critical methodologies?

2   In what ways has critical social theory been criticised, especially its weaknesses as applied to research approaches?

3   Why is postmodernism not another research methodology?

4   Describe the methodology and methods, and provide one research example, of critical ethnography.

5   What is the postmodern justification for combining multiple research methodologies?

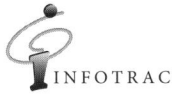

References

Anderson, C., McAllister, M. & Moyle, W. 2002, 'The postmodern heart: A discourse analysis of a booklet on pacemaker implantation', *Collegian*, vol. 9, no. 1, 19–23.

Anderson, J. & McCann, K. 2002, 'Toward a post-colonial feminist methodology in nursing research: exploring the convergence of post-colonial and black feminist scholarship', *Nurse Researcher*, vol. 9. no. 3. 7–27.

Angus, L. 1986, 'Research traditions, ideology and critical ethnography', *Discourse*, vol. 7, no. 1, 59–77.

Armishaw, J. & Davis, K. 2002, 'Women, hepatitis C, and sexuality: a critical feminist exploration', *Contemporary Nurse*, vol. 12, no. 2, 194–203.

Baudrillard, J. 1983, *In the Shadow of the Silent Majorities*, Semiotext(e), New York.

Benhabib, S. 1995, 'Feminism and postmodernism', in S. Benhabib, J. Butler, D. Cornell & N. Fraser (eds), *Feminist Contentions: A Philosophical Exchange*, Routledge, New York.

Best, S. & Kellner, D. 1991, *Postmodern Theory: Critical Interrogations*, Macmillan, London.

Boughton, M. 2002, 'Premature menopause: multiple disruptions between a woman's biological body experience and her lived body', *Journal of Advanced Nursing*, vol. 37, no. 5, 423–30.

Bunting, S. & Campbell, J.C. 1990, 'Feminism and nursing: historical perspectives', *Advances in Nursing Science*, vol. 12, no. 4, 11–24.

Carr, W. & Kemmis, S. 1986, *Becoming Critical: Education, Knowledge and Action Research*, Falmer Press, Lewes.

Carspecken, P. 1996, *Critical ethnography in educational research: a theoretical and practical guide*, Routledge, London.

Cheek, J. 2000, *Postmodern and Poststructural Approaches to Nursing Research*, Sage Publications, Thousand Oaks, California.

Cheek, J., Shoebridge, J., Willis, E. & Zadoroznyi, J. 1996, *Society and Health*, Longman Australia, Melbourne.

Chein, I., Cook, S. & Harding, J. 1948, 'The field of action research', *American Psychology*, vol. 3, 43–50.

Chenoweth, L. & Kilstoff, K. 1998, 'Facilitating positive changes in community dementia management through participatory action research', *International Journal of Nursing Practice*, vol. 4, 175–88.

Chinn, P.L. & Wheeler, C.E. 1985, 'Feminism and nursing', *Nursing Outlook*, vol. 33, no. 2, 74–7.

Craig, D., Donoghue, J., Seller, M. & Mitten-Lewis, S. 2004, 'Improving nursing management of patients with diabetes using an action research approach', *Contemporary Nurse*, vol. 17, no. 1–2, 71–9.

Culbertson, J.A. 1981, 'Three epistemologies and the study of educational administration', *Review, The University Council for Educational Administration*, vol. 22, no. 1, 1–6.

Davies, B. 1994, *Poststructural Theory and Classroom Practice*, Deakin University Press, Geelong.

de la Rue, M.-B. 2003, 'Preventing ageism in nursing students: an action theory approach', *Australian Journal of Advanced Nursing*, vol. 20, no. 4, 8–14.

Delmar, R. 1994, 'What is feminism?', in A. Herrmann & A. Stewart (eds), *Theorising Feminism: Parallel Trends in the Humanities and Social Sciences*, Westview Press, Boulder, Colorado.

Dick, R. 1995, 'A beginner's guide to action research', *ARCS Newsletter*, vol. 1, no. 1, 5–9.

Doering, L. 1992, 'Power and knowledge in nursing: a feminist poststructuralist view', *Advances in Nursing Science*, vol. 14, no. 4, 24–33.

Evans, M. 1997, 'Introducing contemporary thought', in N. Glass (ed.), *Speaking Feminisms and Nursing*, Polity Press, Cambridge, UK.

Fahy, K. 1997, 'Postmodern feminist emancipatory research: is it an oxymoron?', *Nursing Inquiry*, vol. 4, 27–33.

Farganis, S. 1994, 'Postmodernism and feminism', in D. Dickens & A. Fontana (eds), *Postmodernism and Social Inquiry*, University College Press, London.

Fay, B. 1975, *Social Theory and Political Practice*, Allen & Unwin, London.

Fay, B. 1987, *Critical Social Science: Liberation and Its Limits*, Polity Press, Cambridge, UK.

Foucault, M. 1990, *The History of Sexuality. Volume 1: An Introduction*, Penguin Books, London.

Gatens, M. 1992, 'Power, bodies and difference', in M. Barrett & A. Phillips (eds), *Destabilizing Theory: Contemporary Feminist Debates*, Polity Press, Cambridge, UK.

Gilbert, T. 2003, 'Exploring the dynamic of power: a Foucauldian analysis of care planning in learning disabilities services', *Nursing Inquiry*, vol. 10, no. 1, 37–46.

Gilligan, C. 1984, *In a different voice: psychological theory and women's development*, Harvard University Press, Cambridge.

Giroux, H.A. 1983, *Theory and Resistance in Education*, Heinemann Educational Books, London.

Giroux, H.A. 1992, *Border Crossings: Cultural Workers and the Politics of Education*, Routledge, New York.

Gitlin, A., Siegal, M. & Boru, K. 1989, 'The politics of method: from leftist ethnography to educative research', *Qualitative Studies in Education*, vol. 2, no. 3, 237–53.

Glass, N. 2000, 'Speaking feminisms and nursing', in J. Greenwood (ed.), *Nursing Theory in Australia: Development and Application*, Pearson Education Australia, Frenchs Forest, NSW.

Glass, N. & Davis, K. 1998, 'An emancipatory impulse: a feminist postmodern integrated turning point in nursing research', *Advances in Nursing Science*, vol. 21, no. 1, 43–52.

Gore, J. 1992, 'What we can do for you! What can "we" do for "you"?: Struggling over empowerment in critical and feminist pedagogy', in C. Luke & J. Gore (eds), *Feminisms and Critical Pedagogy*, Routledge, New York.

Habermas, J. 1972, *Knowledge and Human Interests*, Heinemann, London.

Habermas, J. 1973, *Theory and Practice*, Heinemann, London.

Hall, J. 1999, 'Marginalization revisited: critical, postmodern, and liberation perspectives', *Advances in Nursing Science*, vol. 22, no. 2, 88–102.

Hardin, P. 2003, 'Shape-shifting discourses of anorexia nervosa: reconstituting psychopathology', *Nursing Inquiry*, vol. 10, no. 4, 209–17.

Huntington, A. & Gilmour, J. 2001, 'Re-thinking representations, re-writing nursing texts: possibilities through feminist and Foucauldian thought', *Journal of Advanced Nursing*, vol. 35, no. 6, 902–8.

Jackson, D., Mannix, J., Faga, P. & Gillies, D. 2005, 'Raising families: urban women's experiences of requiring support', *Contemporary Nurse*, vol. 18, no. 1–2, 97–107.

Jackson, D. & Raftos, M. 1997, 'In uncharted waters: confronting the culture of silence in a residential care institution', *International Journal of Nursing Practice*, vol. 3, 34–9.

Jagger, A. 1983, 'Political philosophies of women's liberation', in L. Richardson & V. Taylor (eds), *Feminist Frontiers*, Random House, New York.

Jervis, L. 2002, 'Working in and around the "chain of command": power relations among nursing staff in an urban nursing home', *Nursing Inquiry*, vol. 9, no. 1, 12–23.

Jordan, G. & Weedon, C. 1995, *Cultural Politics: Class, Gender, Race and the Postmodern World*, Blackwell, Oxford.

Keatinge, D., Scarfe, C., Bellchambers, H., McGee, J., Oakham, R., Probert, C., Stewart, L. & Stokes, J. 2000, 'The manifestation and nursing management of agitation in institutionalised residents with dementia', *International Journal of Nursing Practice*, vol. 6, 16–25.

Kemmis, S. & McTaggart, R., (eds) 1988, *The Action Research Planner*, 3rd edn, Deakin University Press, Geelong, Australia.

Kermode, S. & Brown, C. 1995, 'Where have all the flowers gone? Nursing's escape from the radical critique', *Contemporary Nurse*, vol. 4, no. 1, 8–15.

Koch, T., Kralik, D., Eastwood, S. & Schofield, A. 2001, 'Breaking the silence: women living with multiple sclerosis and urinary incontinence', *International Journal of Nursing Practice*, vol. 7, no. 1, 16–23.

Koch, T., Kralik, D. & Kelly, S. 2000, 'We just don't talk about it: men living with urinary incontinence and multiple sclerosis', *International Journal of Nursing Practice*, vol. 6, 253–60.

Langridge, M. & Ahern, K. 2003, 'A case report on mixed methods in qualitative research', *Collegian*, vol. 10, no. 4, 32–6.

Lewin, K. 1946, 'Action research and minority issues', *Journal of Social Issues*, vol. 2, 34–46.

Lumby, J. 1997, 'Liver transplantation: the death/life paradox', *International Journal of Nursing Practice*, vol. 3, 231–8.

McTaggart, R. 1991, 'Principles for participatory action research', *Adult Education Quarterly*, vol. 41, no. 3, 168–87.

Meyer, D. & de Oliveira, D. 2003, 'Breastfeeding policies and the production of motherhood: a historical-cultural approach', *Nursing Inquiry*, vol. 10, no. 1, 11–18.

Mohanty, C.T. 1994, 'On race and voice: challenges for liberal education in the 1990s', in H.A. Giroux & P. McLaren (eds), *Between Borders: Pedagogy and the Politics of Cultural Studies*, Routledge, New York.

Moody, G., Greenwood, J. & Choong, Y. 2001, 'An action research approach to the development of a clinical pathway for women requiring Caesarean section', *Contemporary Nurse*, vol. 11, no. 2–3, 195–205.

Rankin, J. 2003, ' "Patient satisfaction": knowledge for ruling hospital reform – an institutional ethnography', *Nursing Inquiry*, vol. 10, no, 1, 57–65.

Reason, P. & Bradbury, H., (eds), 2001, *Handbook of action research: Participative inquiry and practice*, Sage, London.

Rogers-Clark, C. 2002, 'Living with breast cancer: the influence of rurality on women's suffering and resilience. A Postmodern feminist inquiry', *Australian Journal of Advanced Nursing*, vol. 20, no. 2, 34–9.

Rosenau, P. 1992, *Post-Modernism and the Social Sciences: Insights, Inroads and Intrusions*, Princeton University Press, New Jersey.

Seidman, S. 1994, *Contested Knowledge*, Blackwell Science, Oxford.

Shannon, S.J. 1994, 'Dilemmas of a feminist ethnography', Paper presented at the Discursive Construction of Knowledge Conference, Adelaide, South Australia.

Smith, D.E. 2001, 'Texts and the ontology of organizations and institutions', *Studies in Cultures, Organizations and Societies*, vol. 7, no. 2, 159–98.

Smyth, W. & Holmes, C. 2005, 'Using Carspecken's critical ethnography in nursing research', *Contemporary Nurse*, vol. 19, no. 1–2, 65–74.

Stevens, P.E. 1989, 'A critical social reconceptualization of environment in nursing: implications for methodology', *Advances in Nursing Science*, vol. 11, no. 4, 56–68.

Stringer, E. 1996, *Action Research: A Handbook for Practitioners*, Sage Publications, Thousand Oaks, California.

Taylor, B.J. 2001, 'Identifying and transforming dysfunctional nurse–nurse relationships through reflective practice and action research', *International Journal of Nursing Practice*, vol. 7, no. 6, 406–13.

Taylor, B.J. 2006, *Reflective Practice: A Guide for Nurses and Midwives*, 2nd edn, Open University Press, UK.

Taylor, B.J., Bulmer, B., Hill L., Luxford, C., McFarlane, J. & Stirling, K. 2002, 'Exploring idealism in palliative nursing care through reflective practice and action research', *International Journal of Palliative Nursing*, vol. 8, no. 7, 324–30.

Tong, R. 1989, *Feminist Thought: A Comprehensive Introduction*, Unwin Hyman, Sydney.

Tuttle, L. & Seibold, C. 2002, 'Ethical issues arising when planning and commencing a research study with chemically dependent pregnant women', *Australian Journal of Advanced Nursing*, vol. 20, no. 4, 30–6.

Walter, R., Davis, K. & Glass, N. 1999, 'Discovery of self: exploring, interconnecting and integrating self (concept) and nursing', *Collegian*, vol. 6, no. 2, 12–15.

Watson, J., Turnbull, B. & Mills, A. 2002, 'Evaluation of the extended role of the midwife: the voices of midwives', *International Journal of Nursing Practice*, vol. 8, no. 5, 257–64.

Weedon, C. 1991, *Feminist Practice and Poststructuralist Theory*, Basil Blackwell, London.

Wellard, S. & Street, A.F. 1999, 'Family issues in home-based care', *International Journal of Nursing Practice*, vol. 5, 132–6.

Wheeler, C.E. & Chinn, P.L. 1989, *Peace and Power: A Handbook of Feminist Process*, National League for Nursing, New York.

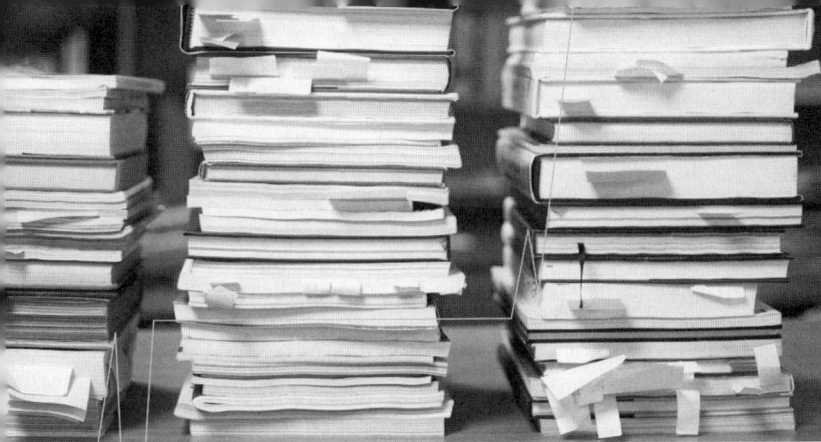

CHAPTER 14

QUALITATIVE METHODS

CHAPTER OBJECTIVES

The material presented in this chapter will assist you to:

- differentiate between methods, processes and methodology
- discuss the rationale for choosing congruent methods in qualitative research
- discuss the use of methods alone or in combination
- describe the central importance of contexts and participants in qualitative research
- determine 'rigour' in qualitative research
- discuss some data collection methods that may be used in qualitative research.

Introduction

There are many methodologies that underlie the generation of a variety of forms of knowledge, and there are many methods by which information can be collected. In qualitative research, usually there are attempts to ensure that the methods by which new information is collected are 'in tune' with the particular theoretical assumptions that underlie the kinds of knowledge that are being generated in the project. Being 'in tune' is another way of saying that methods and forms of knowledge need to be congruent, and for many qualitative researchers, **methodological congruency** is an issue they face as they plan research projects.

This chapter begins by differentiating between methods and methodologies, before exploring some of the issues around methodological congruency, the latter being an issue you may need to face if you think that the research questions you have might be answered well by a qualitative approach. You will then learn how to decide whether to select methods alone or in combination with other methods, and discover the importance of research contexts and people, because all the circumstances of the setting and the people within them have a great bearing on how interpretations are made in qualitative research.

Following this, a list of methods that may be used in qualitative research will be described alphabetically. You will see that the methods are many and varied, and in some cases they may seem quite creative and fun. Given that all the examples of methods are discussed briefly by way of introduction, you are directed to further reading, should you be thinking of using them in your research.

Differentiating between methods, processes and methodologies

When you read research texts and journal articles you will notice that authors use the words methods and methodologies differently and sometimes interchangeably. For example, methodology can mean the research design or plan for some researchers (Brockopp & Hastings-Tolsma 2003) or method can refer to the research approaches, such as phenomenology and grounded theory (LoBiondo-Wood & Haber 1994).

In this book, when referring to qualitative research, a distinction is made between methods and methodology. **Methods** are the means or strategies by which data are sought and analysed in a qualitative research project. For example, data collection methods may include interviews, participant observation, reflective journalling and so on. These methods include step-by-step guidance in what must be done to collect research information. Data analysis methods may include manual or computer program thematic analysis, which have a sequence of steps to ensure that the data are managed carefully to assist interpretation along the lines of the research approach.

Processes are *how* data collection and analysis methods are undertaken. Processes show the embodied values of researchers, such as respecting, being patient and thoughtful, honouring, acknowledging, and a host of other ways of being mindful of the human nature of the research. Qualitative projects are attentive to processes, because researchers are involved in projects, sometimes as co-researchers with participants, so attention is paid to how people relate to one another and to other ethical considerations to maintain the integrity of the research, researchers and participants. When thinking about research process the main questions are: 'How will I undertake these methods?' or 'How will I conduct myself as a researcher in this project?'

An excellent example of a research process is the 'Peace and Power' (Chinn & Wheeler 1995) group process. PEACE is an acronym for praxis, empowerment, awareness, consensus and evolvement, and the power is PEACE power through cooperation and valuing one another, not the dominant form of power as power-over. Therefore, the Peace and Power process fits well with methods that actively involve research participants, such as group work, and with methodologies that emphasise active collaboration with participants, such as feminism and action research. The particular features of the project will determine other research processes for data collection and analysis.

Methodologies are research approaches that may be chosen to act as overarching theoretical concepts for the selection of the methods. By this I mean that methodologies have within them certain theoretical assumptions about the nature of knowledge. As you may remember from Chapter 12, this is the same as saying that methodologies have certain epistemological assumptions.

EXERCISE

Refer to Chapter 12 and review the section that first introduced the word epistemology. What are the two main aims of epistemology? The following clue may help you to offer a correct answer to this question. Epistemology is the study of knowledge . . . and . . .

Examples of qualitative methodologies are listed in Chapters 12 and 13, and they include interpretive approaches, such as historical research and ethnography, and critical approaches, such as action research and critical ethnography. Refer to that section for further details on these and other examples that are described there in detail.

Therefore, the differentiation between methods and methodologies lies in their main functions. In other words, you choose methods for data collection and analysis based on the assumptions a particular methodology makes about the nature of knowledge generation and validation. For example, if you are interested in exploring the nature of patients' experiences of suffering by qualitative means, decisions are made about the project's aims and objectives, and from there the choices of methods and a methodology or methodologies become clearer.

Using the example of the nature of patients' experiences of suffering, many possibilities arise, depending on the specific nature of your research objectives. Methodologies that might suit the research area are narrative research, phenomenology and grounded theory, among others. All of these methodological examples describe theoretical assumptions about the nature of knowledge: narrative research values local knowledge within people's stories; phenomenology values knowledge that seeks to explicate human existence through the

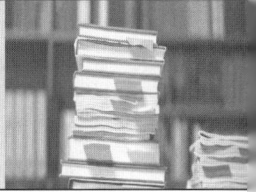

understanding of people's experiences; and grounded theory values the knowledge within middle range theories gleaned from people's accounts of their experiences.

Given a choice of methodology or combination of methodologies to suit the research aims and objectives, decisions need to made about the choice of methods. As you will see in this chapter, there are many possibilities for methods to fit with the theoretical assumptions of methodologies. In our example of exploring the nature of patients' experiences of suffering, methods that may be helpful are interviews, storytelling, reflective journalling and so on. Choosing congruent methods is a creative part of your research proposal process and it is the focus of the next section.

Choosing congruent methods

Methods are the ways or means by which new knowledge is collected and analysed, and they can include controlled trials, interviews, surveys, questionnaires, observation, field notes, historical documents and so on. For example, empirico-analytical methodologies include an assumption that knowledge is real and trustworthy if it is found through objective means, so the researcher will need to use methods that involve strict observation, manipulation and measurement of variables to produce new knowledge of that type. Therefore, for the quantitative researcher, a survey, questionnaire or controlled trial may be the most appropriate data collection method.

Conversely, qualitative methodologies are based on the assumption that knowledge that is real and trustworthy is found through paying attention to what people say and do in specific circumstances. Therefore, methods may be chosen that collect information that is language based and specific to people's particular experiences.

The word 'may' has been used to show that instances of matching methodologies to methods may not always be so straightforward and linear. Some researchers who have labelled their research 'qualitative' may use surveys and questionnaires, for example in an action research phase. Some 'quantitative' researchers may argue that they can 'qualify' quantitative data by using open-ended questions in surveys and converting the findings into numbers. This alerts you to the idea that matching methods and methodologies may not be as clear-cut as it seems at first, and there are instances when these arbitrary distinctions become blurred.

For many researchers who are using qualitative approaches to their work, issues of congruency are important. The attention to choosing congruent methods is based on the assumption that if a methodology is a set of theoretical assumptions, and a method is a means for generating a certain type of knowledge, then it seems reasonable to assume that there needs to be a degree of fit between the type of knowledge that is to be generated and the means that are available to achieve it.

If a qualitative research project is based on the assumptions that people are interpreters of their own experiences and that matters of their context and relationships are important components of how they can make sense of their experiences, the types of methods that are selected to reflect these assumptions need to be appropriate. For example, a research project that seeks to explore the lived experiences of nurses and patients would need to select some methods through which those people would have the best chance to express their experiences. In such a case, participant observation and participant interviews would be consistent with the epistemological (knowledge-producing and proving) assumptions.

The methods for the previous example could be argued as being appropriate because, through participant observation, the researcher has gone to the participants' own place of living and working to watch them on site and interact with them there. Through interviews, opportunities are given for people to express their experiences through language, experiences which may be different from those that could be represented in a prepared survey or questionnaire. In a forced-choice survey or questionnaire there may not be sufficient opportunity for a richer expression of variations in people's experiences. This is not to deny the likelihood that a very well-constructed, highly tested and amended questionnaire may not go some way in getting to the meaning of people's experiences, but most probably it would not allow for unique cases and unexpected responses that people may offer in a trusting conversation-like interview, that would give deeper insights into the area of interest.

EXERCISE

What is meant by congruent methods?

For each of the following methodologies, suggest congruent data collection methods and the reasons why these are most probably suitable:

Methodology	Possible methods	Reasons for suitability
Grounded theory		
Phenomenology		
Ethnography		
Historical research		
Action research		
Feminisms		
Critical ethnography		
Affirmative postmodernism		

Chapters 12 and 13 will help you to complete this exercise. Remember though that the methods are not strictly connected to any one methodology, so you may notice repetition in your choices.

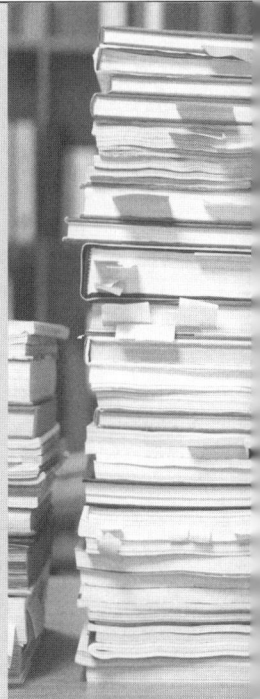

Using methods alone or in combination

You will soon realise that there are many research methods that can be used in qualitative research. You are encouraged to be as creative as you like in choosing them, as long as you can offer a rationale as to how they address the objectives of your project and fit with the theoretical assumptions of the methodology housing the project. You need to be able to give a reasonable explanation of your choice(s), because it is not a simple matter of haphazardly pulling a few methods 'out of a hat' and carelessly saying: 'These will do!'. You need to bear a few principles in mind when choosing methods that will best address all of the requirements of your project.

The first consideration lies in the nature of your project and what it intends to achieve. The objectives of a qualitative project, although sometimes stated broadly, need to be clear and to have some degree of containment, and when they are stated in this way, they give clues as to the choice of methods. For example, if you want to know about people's experiences of wellness, ask them to tell you, for example, through storytelling, interviews or focus groups. You could also encourage them to write a journal, or offer other creative means of describing their experiences, such as through art, poetry, metaphor and so on.

The second consideration lies in the choice of one or a combination of methods. It may be possible to use just one method of data collection, such as storytelling, or interviews, or focus groups. However, if you feel the data can be deepened and enriched further, you might make the decision to use a combination of methods. Remember that in agreeing to be involved in a project human participants are giving you their time and devoting energy to the research, so be thoughtful in what you choose as methods and the degree of participant involvement. It may help you to ask yourself whether a particular method or combination of methods justified in terms of a participant's age, gender, cultural and spiritual practices, health and wellness, availability, responsiveness to creativity, and so on.

The third consideration lies in mixing methods that may be seen by some researchers to not 'go well together'. It is important to remember that methods do not 'belong' exclusively to methodologies. For example, interviews do not 'belong' to qualitative research, as they can be used in quantitative research, especially if they are used in a 'structured' way. Surveys and observation methods can be used equally well in quantitative and qualitative research, depending on how they are designed and the extent to which they can provide description of human experiences and phenomena.

Decisions become less easy when certain methods are combined, such as open-ended interviews and randomised controlled trials. If the results and/or insights are contradictory, how will you reconcile them? Which method 'wins' the argument as to where the 'truth' resides? The inherent difficulty with combining open-ended interviews and randomised controlled trials is that they tend to represent different ends of the 'what counts as truth' continuum.

Open-ended interviews are like conversations, allowing participants to express themselves in a spontaneous 'flow of consciousness' and they fit with epistemological assumptions that 'truth' is relative and context-dependent. Conversely, randomised controlled trials are highly structured methods that minimise human bias and other confounding variables, and they are based on the epistemological assumption that objective and generalisable knowledge can be generated. This is not to prohibit the combination of any methods you might choose, but you should have a sound rationale ready for the consumers of the research, such as funding bodies and thesis examiners, if contradictions arise in your research findings with a mixed method approach.

Research contexts and participants

In its broadest sense, 'context' means the set of features specific to a particular setting, including the place, time and other specific circumstances. In relation to research, contexts are those features of the research setting that need to be taken into account when deciding to undertake and report on a research project. In qualitative research, it is important to acknowledge the features of the setting as having a bearing on how people might interact within them, so these contextual features are described clearly as part of the project report.

A general principle of qualitative research is that people are placed in time and space, and therefore they cannot help but be situated somewhere, and as such, they have some degree of involvement in their respective contexts. In other words, we have to be somewhere sometime and in relation to someone, even if it is ourself. Benner and Wrubel (1989, p. 82) claim that 'there can be no situationless involvement'. In other words, where people are placed has a bearing on how they will interpret their situations, and this is an important point to bear in mind when asking them to speak of their experiences. Applying this principle to nursing practice, nurses and patients will make sense of their experiences in relation to the situations they find themselves in, such as the ward or unit they are in, the time of day and their unique set of circumstances, including the social, political, economic, physical, emotional and spiritual aspects of their lives.

People are central in qualitative research, because as entities with language, they are the prime sources of information. People's experiences may seem insignificant to them because they may be regarded as simply part of living their lives, but qualitative research has an interest in commonplace experiences. It encourages people to delve into their experiences, and to realise that it is through their accounts that personal and practical knowledge may be generated for themselves and for others. For example, if we are to understand the meaning of illness and disease, it can be directly from the accounts of the experiencing people. If we are to understand and change the powerful constraints acting on nurses in health care organisations, we can work collaboratively with nurses in their practice settings. People are the key, because it is through the expression of their life stories that we come to understand their experiences.

Subjectivity refers to personal experiences and personal truths that may or may not have some resonance with other people's subjective experiences and truths. The 'subjective' knowledge that is generated through qualitative research methods does not make a universal claim to be true for everyone and for all things in all times and places, nor does it rely on proving things to be true through the objectivity of human senses. This means that my sense of 'truth' may not be your sense of 'truth', so I cannot make generalisations or absolute predictions based on my subjective stances. Subjectivity in qualitative research is linked inextricably with the relative nature of knowledge and the possibilities of understanding the complexities of human phenomena from the standpoints of the experiencing individuals. In other words, qualitative researchers value people and the accounts these people give of their experiences, because it fits with a relativistic view that knowledge changes and that understanding human existence resides in people's lives.

Qualitative research emphasises the central roles of the research context and people in generating knowledge that is personal and practical, and which comes from the perspective of people engaged actively in their lives. In contrast to research methods of an 'objective' nature, qualitative research values what people have to say about how they feel, what they believe and think, based on whatever information they have amassed as participants in experiencing life.

'Rigour' in qualitative research

In relation to research, '**rigour**' means the strictness in judgement and conduct that must be used to ensure that the successive steps in a project have been set out clearly and undertaken with scrupulous attention to detail, so that the results/findings/insights can be 'trusted'. This allows the project to be transparent in the sense that it can be scrutinised by others for evidence of methodological accuracy and worthiness. In other words, the interest is in whether the project's findings can be relied on as reflecting 'the truth' of the matter. 'Truth' appears here in inverted commas to denote its relative and uncertain status, in that the generation and verification of absolute truth is a debatable point in qualitative methodologies and in the postmodern era, in terms of whether it is actually possible.

In quantitative research, rather than referring to rigour in a general sense, the more specific words 'validity and reliability' would most probably be used. Validity refers to the extent to which the means used in the research to collect and analyse data do what they are supposed to do. Reliability refers to the extent to which consistent results can be achieved on repeated undertaking of the research project. These checking processes ensure that the strict rules and steps of the scientific method have been followed and reflected in the project. If the processes are judged to be accurate, the likelihood is greater that the research findings are 'true'. The criteria for rigour are related directly to the underlying assumptions of what constitutes knowledge and truth and how these are best generated and proven. Another way of stating this, is that criteria for rigour are related directly to the underlying epistemological assumptions.

EXERCISE

Refer to Chapter 12, so that you can review the differences between the assumptions underlying the use of quantitative and qualitative research approaches.

Why does it follow that the criteria for judging the rigour of quantitative and qualitative research projects must of necessity differ? Using that line of argument, why is reliability in the strictest quantitative sense not possible in qualitative projects?

Qualitative research is no less rigorous than quantitative research, but it uses different words to demonstrate the ways of making explicit the overall processes and worthiness of a project because it is based on different epistemological assumptions. As Emden and Sandelowski (1998) point out, issues of 'rigour' in qualitative research have gone through many 'translations', and this is especially so in nursing research. Please note that I use inverted commas around the word 'rigour' in relation to qualitative research, to denote the transition in meaning it has traversed from quantitative into qualitative methods, and the difficulties related to it in throwing off quantitative epistemological assumptions of measures for 'truth'.

Adjustments to imagining qualitative concerns about 'rigour' began with Guba and Lincoln (1981), who suggested the renaming of validity and reliability categories into trustworthiness to reflect the people-oriented nature of qualitative research. The reason for this is that the assumptions, methods and processes of qualitative research differ from quantitative research methods. Sandelowski (1986) took up this suggestion and applied it well to nursing. The criteria of credibility, fittingness, auditability and confirmability will be discussed later in this section.

Qualitative researchers (Beck 1993; Sandelowski 1986; Yonge & Stewin 1988) argued that it is unreasonable to judge a qualitative research project against the criteria designed for a quantitative investigation. For example, qualitative research works on the assumption that what is seen to be true may change, and it may reflect the features of the time, places and circumstances in which people find themselves. Also, quantitative research uses objectivity in searching for objective knowledge, whereas many qualitative research approaches acknowledge and intentionally use the subjectivity of research participants and value the subjective knowledge they offer.

Determining 'rigour' in qualitative research

Various means of determining 'rigour' in qualitative research have been suggested (Beck 1993; Denzin 1989; Hall & Stevens 1991; Meleis 1996; Sandelowski 1986). There is not one accepted test of 'rigour' in qualitative research, just as there is not one way of doing qualitative research, although the 'translation' of criteria now extends to postmodern thinking and the concept of goodness (Emden & Sandelowski 1998, 1999). This means that researchers must use the most appropriate means of assessing 'rigour' in qualitative projects, to reflect the methodological assumptions of the project.

For example, in some early feminist research 'rigour' was judged by the extent to which the project reflected 'dependability' and 'adequacy' (Hall & Stevens 1991). Stability and similarity across data collection methods and findings are the degree of dependability. Meaningful research outcomes reflect adequacy. Although dated by publication, these ideas can still act as a validating process for feminist research, given that they are situated in women's ways of knowing and research approaches.

According to Hall and Stevens (1991), areas contributing to 'rigour' are:
- reflexivity, by continually critiquing the research process
- credibility, by assessing the progress and outcomes through member checks
- rapport, experienced as open, trusting group dynamics
- coherence, by constantly confirming the research process
- acknowledging complexity in the research and its participants
- achieving consensus in decision-making
- addressing relevance to women's concerns

- attaining honesty and mutuality
- naming, using women's own terms and concepts, to denote the project's objectives, processes and outcomes
- achieving relationality, by forming collaborative interpersonal relationships to challenge ideas and respect differences.

It is important to select criteria for judging the 'rigour' of a project, based on the methodological assumptions of the approach you are taking. For example, even though Hall and Stevens (1991) attempt to ensure 'rigour' relevant for feminist research assumptions and processes, these criteria may have little or no relevance for qualitative researchers who do not place strong emphasis on collaborative relationships in research.

Burns and Grove (1997, p. 64) argued that 'rigour' in qualitative research is 'associated with openness, scrupulous adherence to a philosophical perspective, thoroughness in collecting data, and consideration of all the data in the subjective theory development phase'. They suggest that in order to be rigorous in qualitative research the researcher must be open to new ideas by being willing to let go of old ideas (deconstructing), and by examining many dimensions to form new ideas (reconstructing). Although deconstructing and reconstructing reflect the open, exploratory nature of qualitative research, these concepts do not provide potential qualitative researchers with actual steps in how to attain 'rigour'.

Sandelowski (1986) applied the ideas of Guba and Lincoln (1981) relating to 'rigour' in qualitative research in general to nursing research in particular. The categories for determining 'rigour' are credibility, fittingness, auditability and confirmability.

Credibility

Credibility means the extent to which participants and readers of the research recognise the lived experiences described in the research as similar to their own. If there is recognition of the phenomenon just from reading about it in the transcripts or research reports, credibility is achieved.

Fittingness

Fittingness refers to the extent to which a project's findings fit into other contexts outside the study setting. The term is also used to mean the extent to which the readers of the research find it has meaning and relevance for their own experiences.

Auditability

Auditability is the production of a decision trail, which can be scrutinised by other researchers to determine the extent to which consistency has been achieved in the project's methods and processes. A high degree of auditability would allow another researcher to use a similar approach and possibly arrive at similar or comparable conclusions.

Confirmability

Confirmability of a project is achieved when credibility, auditability and fittingness can be demonstrated. This relies on the confirmation of participants, whose subjectivity is valued as instructive in assessing the extent to which the project achieves neutrality from the researcher's stated biases.

These criteria for 'rigour' will appear quite different from those described in this book to ascertain reliability and validity in quantitative research. This is completely admissible, given that the two broad approaches have many differences in what constitutes truth and the best ways of finding it. Given the longer-standing positive reputation of quantitative research, and the tendency to judge qualitative research against quantitative criteria, Yonge and Stewin (1988, p. 65) present some challenges for qualitative researchers to:

- develop and use rules, terms and procedures to describe qualitative research processes accurately
- ensure that participants are actively involved in all phases of the research project, including being present at dissemination of the findings through presentations, and are informed of publication
- understand the purposes and implications of using terms such as validity and reliability
- tolerate uncertainty and confusion (particularly when pitted against an articulate positivist!) as a new language to describe the relevance of qualitative inquiry emerges
- recall that there is an essential difference between qualitative and quantitative methods of inquiry and that if both are to be mixed, the researcher must provide a sound rationale.

Denzin (1989) suggested using triangulation to create multiple references, which converge to draw conclusions that may be claimed as the 'truth'. He identified data, investigator, theory and methodological triangulation. Data triangulation uses multiple data sources, such as interviewing many participants about the same topic in a study. Investigator triangulation uses many individuals to collect and analyse a single set of data. Theory triangulation uses many theoretical perspectives to interpret data. Methodological triangulation uses multiple methods such as interviews, document analysis and observation. By using many triangulation sources as described, Denzin (1989) suggested that a data cross-checking system would ensure the 'rigour' of a project.

In keeping with the distinction drawn in this book between qualitative methodologies and methods, I suggest an amendment to Denzin's definitions of triangulation, and list them accordingly as data, investigator, theory, methods and methodological triangulation. The difference is in defining method triangulation as the use of multiple methods such as interviews, document analysis and observation, and of defining methodological triangulation as the use of multiple theoretical approaches, for example, feminism, ethnography and affirmative postmodernism.

Meleis (1996) designed process-oriented criteria for research or scholarship, with a cultural focus for marginalised or transitional groups. She described eight criteria for determining 'rigour', these being contextuality, relevance, communication styles, awareness of identity and power differentials, disclosure, reciprocation, empowerment, and time.

Contextuality demonstrates an awareness of the features of the research setting. Relevance refers to how well a project aligns to the research groups' interests. Communication styles judges the appropriateness of the researcher's communication with the participants. Awareness of identity and power differentials refers to the differences between power for researcher and participants and how these features have been acknowledged and redressed. Disclosure is the authentic representation of participants' experiences. Reciprocation is the identification and negotiation of mutual gaols for researcher and participants. Empowerment is the demonstration of power sharing, resulting in raised awareness and positive changes. Time refers to the establishment of flexible processes, especially in relation to trust. These criteria for judging 'rigour' could be used in any project in which there is a high degree of collaboration between researcher and co-researchers/participants (Meleis 1996).

Emden and Sandelowski (1998, 1999) have taken up Yonge and Stewin's (1988, p. 65) challenge to qualitative researchers, and have evolved their ideas for the 'conceptions of goodness in qualitative research'. In a thought-provoking two-part paper, they review the transformations of criteria in qualitative research, noting the renaming of various approaches as more distance from quantitative criteria for 'rigour' has been accomplished. In the first part the authors 'trace efforts to define "goodness" in qualitative research within various fields, including nursing' noting that they 'continue to reflect a search for order' (Emden & Sandelowski 1998, p. 206). In the second part of the paper, the authors describe the problematic shortfalls in 'rigour' and 'criteria' by applying postmodern thinking. They point out that criteria attempt to define and limit reality in the assumption that 'truth' is out there, waiting to be discovered, harnessed and applied to problems of explanation, prediction and control in the human world. Thus, 'criteria' *and* 'rigour' have an 'ancestry (that) can be similarly traced to positivism and its problems' (Emden & Sandelowski 1999, p. 3).

Emden and Sandelowski contemplate 'the demise of criteria' to show how authors have attempted to sever 'qualitative research from the tenets of positivism'. One approach has been of 'conceiving criteria not as definite rules but as ever evolving and open ended "lists" ' (Smith 1990, cited in Emden & Sandelowski 1999, p. 3). Another approach has been to use enabling conditions 'to do with dialogue, a community of interpreters, rhetoric, conversation, and imagination' (Schwandt 1996, cited in Emden & Sandelowski 1999, p. 3). Even so, Emden and Sandelowski (1999, p. 4) cite Lincoln (1995), who wrote: 'We are not ready to close down the conversation or to say farewell to criteria quite yet'. Emden and Sandelowski remind readers of the practical realities of keeping qualitative research 'alive as a coherent whole' and satisfying criteria of goodness for 'those required to make speedy judgements about the quality of qualitative work, such as members of human research ethics committees, funding bodies, and editorial review boards, as well as consumers and designers of the research in the first place' (p. 4).

In responding to the conundrum of goodness in qualitativeresearch in the postmodern era, Emden and Sandelowski (1999, p. 5) raise the possibility that 'uncertainty can be turned to advantage, and novel avenues of thought forged, whereby both the impracticability of the grand narrative is recognised, as well as the richness and value of local contexts and meanings appreciated'. This means that researchers can opt to integrate the best of the modern and postmodern worlds of research into ensuring goodness in their projects. Emden and Sandelowski also raise the courageous and baldly honest possibility of a 'criterion of uncertainty' not in terms of methodological weakness, but as an 'open acknowledgment that claims about our research outcomes are at best tentative and that there may indeed be no way of showing otherwise' (p. 5). However, they admit, that 'within all terms and usages, the criterion problem lurks' and that in a postmodern world that 'decries all such searches for order and meaning' it is 'never too late to ask . . . "Whose criteria?" "Criteria for what?" and "Why criteria at all?"' (Emden & Sandelowski 1999, p. 6).

Methods that may be used in qualitative research

In this section you are introduced to a variety of methods that may be used alone or in combination in qualitative research projects, according to the requirements of your research question or area. For ease of access, the methods are listed alphabetically. Bear in mind that methods are used to gather information considered most likely to be of assistance in fulfilling the aims and objectives of a research project. This means that they have been considered carefully and put into place and used with thoughtfulness in relation to what they may offer. Bear in mind also that if we are informed by postmodern thought, we might hold only as tentative any knowledge that comes about, no matter however carefully we undertake our methods. In other words, there are no perfect methods and methods may be useful now, but they do not guarantee 'truth' either for all time or even for a moment, as in human research of a qualitative nature, there are no 'foolproof' methods, nor is there a final absolute point in the search for undeniable 'truth'.

Archival searches

Archival information consists of original hard copies of aged documents such as logs, diaries, government agency agendas and minutes, reports, photographs, newspapers, books, private papers donated by families to the archives, and so on. Historians are well versed in archival searches with respect to what to seek and how to make the best of the information once it is gathered and copied.

This method involves going to archival repositories, such as purpose-built archival buildings and libraries, to seek specific research information of an historical nature. Archives are listed in telephone directories and/or contact details may be gained by phoning the information centres of country and city councils. There is usually a search fee to gain access to records, and photocopying charges apply. The cost of archival data collection should be itemised in project budgets, so that the cost does not become a problem for the overall management of the project. Remember also that once you are in among the archives your enthusiasm for finding treasures may get the better of you, so for the sake of time, effort and expense, keep your research focus in mind so that you do not become unduly sidetracked.

Categories of copied data can be sorted systematically into a favoured filing system, which can be accessed easily by yourself and other members of the research team. Boxes, hanging files, cupboards and shelves may store information in some practical order, such as by time, place or main content. Labelling items with full reference details, dates, times, sources and so on makes for easier management of the data when it is time for analysis.

For further information on how to do archival searches, refer to Streubert Speciale and Rinaldi Carpenter (2003). Examples of research projects using archival searches can be located in Chapter 12 in the section relating to historical research.

Artistic expression

Sometimes it might be appropriate in the research design to collect data in the form of a direct and creative demonstration of the participant's experiences through artistic expression, such as painting, drawing, montage, photography, poetry, dance, music, symbols, singing and so on. At times, the data may be accompanied by the creator's interpretations of the piece, or the data may stand as they are, to be interpreted by other means, such as through group discussion and/or the researcher's methods of interpretation.

Data collected through artistic expression may be particularly useful in research aimed at finding the experience of certain conditions/states/perspectives from the unique viewpoint of individuals. Participants may be invited to use a variety of artistic expressions to represent themselves and issues in their lives through creative images. Alternatively, as the researcher, you may decide to express some of your observations through an artistic medium, such as poetry, to add further richness to the other sources of data.

Careful storage and sorting of artistic data are important, because symbolic representations are best interpreted in relation to the person representing them. Therefore, items and their interpretive accounts must be stored together, labelled clearly and fully for later analysis if necessary. Details such as the artist's name or pseudonym, date, time, intention of the artwork, preliminary interpretational remarks and so on, may be useful in making sense of the contribution of any form of creative expression when applied as a research method.

Wikstrom (2002, p. 24) used visual art in relation to intuition in a project determining 'the degree to which student nurses in Sweden were able to predict responses of elderly women to 12 paintings'. She found the students used intuitive knowing to understand the situations and experiences of the elderly women and the researcher suggested that this method of data collection and interpretation may be a useful way for nurse teachers to develop student nurses' intuition skills.

In addition to using the artist's expression as a form of knowledge generation in itself, creative means may also be used when reflection is a part of a project. Taylor (2000) lists many ways in which artistic expression can aid reflection, and by association, assist research. These include writing, audiotaping, creating music, dancing, drawings, montage, painting, poetry, pottery, quilting, singing and videotaping. Any of these methods may be used alone or in combination. In the area of artistic expression, you are limited only by your own imagination, but remember the unlocking of creative potential needs to be related to the aims and objectives of your project, otherwise it may be fun but without practical application.

Case studies

A case study can be considered as a method or a design. In other words, some researchers focus on the discrete analytical means along the way (methods), while others look to the broader stream of events in the research project (design). On the whole, authors tend to agree that a case study is a research strategy that comprises an all-encompassing, comprehensive method and set of strategies (Burns & Grove 1997; Titscher et al. 2000; Woods 1997) that allow people, practices and phenomena to be described over time according to their contextual features (Fitzgerald 1999; Stake 1994; Yin 1994).

The case study method fully describes selected foci of research interest, such as individuals, in groups or institutions. The researcher uses a case study method to try to understand over time as much as possible about the area in focus, so the method is characterised by intensive analysis of all the determinants involved.

In planning a case study you need to consider your research questions and how you might best answer them. This may mean that you will need a variety of strategies in sequence that will ensure a comprehensive approach to the area of inquiry. As an illustrative case, consider a researcher (van Aken 2004) who wanted to explore the subjective experiences of people with moderate depression in relation to healing touch (Healing Touch International 2000). As she was not interested in proving that healing touch 'cures' depression, the researcher was not required to undertake an experimental design in which she could show statistically that healing touch alone was the healing factor.

After exploring the literature around case study and methodologies, the researcher realised that she could combine a case study approach with an overarching methodology of grounded theory, as the two are complementary in their intentions to explore an unknown area of inquiry inductively. Grounded theory also provides an analytical method and permits theory building, while a case study approach facilitates investigation and comparison over time of single (or collective) cases, using a variety of data collection methods. This being so, van Aken designed a project including five weekly healing touch treatments of one hour's duration. The first session involved assessment with the Beck Depression Inventory (Foreman 1997) to identify moderate depression, and the completion of the Healing Energy And Life Through Holism (HEALTH) tool (Healing Touch International 2000) for a holistic health assessment. The participants and researcher kept a reflective journal to record their experiences and the researcher also made case notes of participants' pre- and post-treatment responses. The final session included a further Beck assessment, an interview about each participant's subjective experience, and review of the data entries. The data were analysed by a constant comparative process with the aim of generating a theory (Strauss & Corbin 1990). From this case study, the researcher generated a middle range theory of emerging from depression and made recommendations as to the use of the theory in the provision of healing touch for people with moderate depression.

As there is no clear-cut way of doing a case study, it is really up to you as the researcher to set up a practical and systematic approach to gathering, recording, analysing and presenting information. For example, Solman, Conway and McMillan (2004, p. 159) used a case study design to explore nurses' experiences in a Cardiac Step Down Unit (CSDU). The researchers used 'focus groups, semi structured interviews, surveys, self-report, and observation' data collection methods and they found that 'the nursing care provided in the unit focussed on the provision of technology oriented rather than patient oriented care and that nurses experienced lack of role clarity about the care they provided' (Solman, Conway & McMillan 2004, p. 159).

De Wit and Davis (2004, p. 214) used 'an interpretive case study approach within a naturalistic paradigm' to explore nurses' 'understanding and experiences of learning about the effects of domestic abuse on the mental health of children and adolescents'.

Data for the case studies were collected using semi-structured in-depth interviews with four nurses working in one mental health unit. The analysis revealed three categories of education, resources and nurses' role and that 'nurses' knowledge and education about the effects of domestic abuse on the mental health of children and adolescents negatively impacted on nurses' ability to provide appropriate care' (De Wit & Davis 2004, p. 214).

Barnes et al. (2003, p. 14) used a case study design to evolve a 'picture of contemporary child health nursing services in Brisbane and surrounding areas'. The foci of their case studies were the child health centres in the metropolitan and suburban areas and the data for the case studies came from multiple sources, such as semi-structured interviews, observation, group discussion, focus groups and document analysis.

Given the examples above, you may be able to see that the case study approach you take will be entirely up to you, as long as you can show that the sequence of methods relate to exploring most directly and comprehensively the research questions and aims you have posed. You need also to consider issues of 'rigour' or trustworthiness (see this chapter), appropriate methods of data analysis (see Chapter 16) and interpretation (see Chapter 17). Read as widely as you can and see how other researchers have organised their case studies and be prepared to critique those methods and designs that could have been more creative and/or comprehensive in their approaches. Some examples to get you started are Wilkes (2003), Wellard and Rushton (2002) and Koch and Lyon (2001).

As with all research involving human participants, a case study requires ethical approval and the consent of all participants in each and every part of the case study in which they are involved. For example, if you are interested in undertaking a single case study about an exemplary woman who has survived cancer, you would need to think through all the usual steps of a research project. For example, what do you want to know, why, how, when, and for whose purposes? How will the case study be important to nursing and health? Having determined these ideas, you need to work with the person to set up a practical approach to recording her experiences. She might agree to having her stories audiotaped and transcribed. She might also agree to allowing you to spend some time with her in observation of her daily life, or she might have photographs and personal records that she will allow you to make public.

As you can see, the approach to a case study is open and creative, but this should not frustrate you if you have given the method sufficient thought and have planned it carefully with the people involved. The analysis and interpretation of the sections of the case study will depend on what is appropriate for the method used. For example, interviews and journal entries may require thematic analysis and the findings may be combined into a collective interpretation or retained as single case trajectories, depending on how the case study was set up. The people involved may want to offer their interpretations, some observational comment may be appropriate, and photographs and document analysis may add to the descriptive potential of the case study. The presentation of the case study may be as a journal article for publication, or it may be of sufficient depth and breadth to warrant publication in a book or monograph.

The last words on case studies are from Stake (2000), an expert in the method. He claims that:

> Case studies have become one of the most common ways to do qualitative inquiry, but they are neither new nor essentially qualitative. Case study is not a methodological choice but a choice of what is to be studied. By whatever methods, we choose to study the case. We could study it analytically or holistically, entirely by repeated measures or hermeneutically, organically or culturally, and by mixed methods – but we concentrate, at least for the time being, on the case (p. 435).

Fieldwork

Fieldwork occurs where the action is happening out in the 'field' of inquiry. Fieldwork methods may vary according to the intentions of the research, but they usually consist of combinations of observation, participation, documentation and analysis. A common form of data collection in fieldwork is the documentation of field notes. Field notes are selective notes made by the researchers to themselves that will form part of the data when the entire project is drawn together. They need to be made as soon as possible, so that the events are still fresh in the researcher's mind. Emerson, Fretz and Shaw (2001) describe field notes as 'a way of *representation* (author's emphasis) that is a way of reducing just-observed events, persons and places to written accounts'.

For example, if you want to do an ethnographic study of the inside culture and activities of a community health centre, part of the data would be notes that are written whenever it becomes necessary and/or advisable to capture the thickest possible description of what is happening, to whom, when, why, how and where. To save the effort of having to transfer the information later, a portable computer could be used to record the notes, making copies readily accessible.

If paper and pen are used for making notes, a system of careful storage is necessary to maintain the chronological and contextual order of the information. If computers assist the process, files should be identified easily and checked periodically to ensure that the disk is still operable. When the analysis phase begins, the records should be relatively complete and legible.

An alternative for researchers who prefer oral rather than written accounts is to use a portable audiotape system. In this way observations can be recorded rapidly and with the relative spontaneity of spoken words. All tapes should be identified with the date, time and general content of the recording, so that they can be organised easily for later analysis.

Fieldwork and observation/participation observation are related methods, in that fieldwork can be taken to mean broader activities such as those undertaken in ethnographic studies. Here, the emphasis is on the methods of observation researchers use when they are undertaking qualitative projects; for details see 'Observation/Participant observation' later in this chapter.

Research projects using field work are often classified according to a form of ethnography. For example, Koskinen and Tossavainen (2004, p. 111) used research diaries in which they documented field notes about their experiences of studying abroad 'as a process of learning intercultural competence in nursing'. They used a mixed method approach and combined the research diaries with group interviews, learning documents and background questionnaires. The researchers undertook an inductive content analysis to reveal that the exchange program as a context for learning intercultural competence 'was characterized by a problematic orientation phase, a study abroad phase that involved stressful but rewarding adjustments to intercultural differences and an inadequate re-entry debriefing phase' (p. 111).

Other projects requiring fieldwork include Oliver and Butler (2004), Kenefick and Schulman-Green (2004) and Johannessen (2004). Refer also to the section on field notes in Chapter 12 for descriptions of ethnographic research that require researchers to gather data in the 'field' of interest.

Focus groups

A focus group is a collection of people working together on a particular research issue. Just as research projects are directed at the fulfilment of tasks related to particular aims and objectives, so also focus groups have different foci. Fern (2001, p. 3) 'found it virtually impossible to derive a workable typology of focus groups' so he suggested theoretical and applied focus groups adapted to exploratory, experiential and clinical research tasks.

Exploratory tasks in applied research include 'creating new ideas; collecting unique thoughts; identifying needs, expectations and issues; discovering new uses for existing products or discovering new products; and explaining puzzles from … research' (Fern 2001, p. 6). Theoretical uses of exploratory tasks include 'generating theoretical constructs, causal relationships, models, hypotheses, and theories'. This means that a focus group may concentrate its collective intelligence on dealing purely with theoretical matters (p. 7). Experiential tasks for focus groups of an applied nature include people talking together to share 'life experiences, preferences, intentions, and behaviours', so that they can better understand 'individuals' language, knowledge and experience' in an intersubjective exchange (p. 7).

EXERCISE

The word 'intersubjectivity' has been used before in this book. Locate its meaning and write a sentence on how intersubjectivity relates to an applied experiential focus group.

In Fern's (2001, p. 8) categorisation of focus groups, an experiential focus group with a theoretical purpose can be used for triangulation and confirmation. Triangulation is used commonly to compare results across different methods. In this case, it is a form of theory confirmation, when individuals within focus groups can support or refute a theory or theories with reference to their own experiences.

Clinical focus groups are derived from marketing, and, in an applied form, this type of group meets to 'uncover individuals' motives, predispositions, biases, and prejudices'. For theory applications, clinical tasks of focus groups may be to uncover 'relationships between motives, beliefs, attitudes, and behaviours'. The difference between the two subsets of these focus group tasks are 'whether the focus group is to be used for planning strategies and programs, which are to effect applications, or to be used in theory development' (Fern 2001, pp. 9–10).

From all of the above, we can glean the basic ideas that focus groups differ according to their purposes, and that they have specific purposes and that is why they meet. The people who attend are research participants who have given their consent to be involved in the project, having been deliberately invited for their knowledge and/or skills in the area to which the research relates. The group is facilitated by the researcher or by a research assistant with the necessary skills to keep the group focused on its aims and objectives. In some cases, researchers may use their grant monies to pay an expert skilled in running focus groups to facilitate the meeting or series of meetings.

The process usually involves a brainstorming session, in which the focus group members respond to questions and comments made by the facilitator and/or in response to group discussion. Responses are recorded on an object visible to the group, such as a blackboard, whiteboard, overhead transparency or butcher's paper. The facilitator calls for all spontaneous responses with 'no holds barred', then the group works together to collate and prioritise ideas to remove duplications, 'off the wall' remarks, or responses that are judged by the group to be of minimal help or relevance to the research question/aim/context.

Focus groups help research by getting a number of people together to solicit their contributions. This means that many ideas are collated, it is less expensive than individual interviews and, in some cases, the group can collaborate on analysing and interpreting the data. The disadvantages of focus groups are that the less vocal members can be overlooked if they are not 'drawn out' carefully by the facilitator, the responses may not be as rich and full as they might be in the privacy of an interview, and it is difficult to track an individual's perceptions among the group's responses, leaving the interpretations broad and relevant only to the collective responses of the group.

Researchers can use focus groups as their sole method of data collection, or they can use focus groups in combination with other methods. For example, Fitzgerald and Teal (2003–04) used focus groups after observations and questionnaires. They asked doctors, nurses and general staff questions about professional group interactions and reactions to organisational change, thereby identifying issues that could be pursued in individual interviews.

Griffiths et al. (2003) explored the needs of nurses caring for refugees, by involving 13 nurses in two focus group interviews and then undertaking two in-depth interviews with nurse managers. They found that the nurses 'had the necessary clinical skills but needed specific refugee health profiles and training in culturally competent and trauma-sensitive care' (p. 183).

Locate and read the article: Cox, Henderson, Andersen, Cagliarini and Ski 2003, 'Focus group study of endometriosis: struggle, loss and the medical merry-go-round', *International Journal of Nursing Practice*, vol. 9, pp. 2–9.

Make notes on how the researchers used focus groups in their research. What other methods were used in this project? How were both methods integrated to generate the project results?

Another article that is helpful from the perspective of a beginning focus group facilitator is Jamieson and Williams (2003), because they provide 'explanatory notes for the novice researcher' (p. 271) in how to use focus group methods appropriately to generate quality data.

Group work

Some researchers use group interaction processes through which to collect, sort and sometimes analyse data. As we have seen, a focus group is a group with a specific purpose, and the following ideas about group processes apply to focus groups. However, there are more research group configurations to consider than those that are focus groups per se. Research groups can be set up in varying numbers for differing purposes and given their own identities as the group evolves. For example, group processes are particularly suitable for collaborative research such as action research, feminist research or research that is informed by poststructural and/or postmodern ideas, because they involve groups of people working together to create shared meaning. In all of these cases, the underlying assumptions of the research are that people need to be empowered to find and use voice, multiple perspectives are valued, group members have agreed on the research problems and those members are the best people to solve the problems through their own collective processes.

It is advisable to think ahead about how to collect and sort these kinds of data, to ensure that the group processes are of optimal value. In other words, you will invite a purposive sample of people to gather together because they have the experiences needed to offer insights into the research topic. Group members need to become quickly conversant with the aims and objectives of the research, how they contribute to the project, and what they can expect to receive from being involved in the process.

When people get together they need some direction, otherwise they may have a tendency to talk over the top of one another, to break into separate chatting sessions, and generally to become confused about their contribution to the research. Facilitation of the group conversations is needed, and it can be by the researcher as a facilitator, or all of the group members may take a turn in facilitating by a 'rotating chair' process. Shy or inexperienced members can be encouraged to apply the skills of group facilitation, learning at first by modelling their behaviours on those of an experienced group facilitator. Skills in group processes are many and varied and you are advised to read beyond this text for suggestions on how to do this effectively.

The success of group processes often relies on how the group members interact with one another in ongoing communication patterns. Therefore, at the outset of the project it is important for members to speak openly within the group to express their preferences for how the group members will work together. For example, members may state that they want to be able to speak honestly, to be heard without interruption, and to be able to trust other members to hold in confidence information they disclose. The group can agree on the communication processes they want for the duration of the research and they can agree to act as peer 'modifying' agents, to identify disruptive behaviours within the group and to respectfully request explanations from members acting outside the agreed group communication processes.

A research group meets for the primary aim of generating data. You need to give some thought to how you will collect information within the group, in order to capture faithfully how the members of the group interact and what has been discussed and decided upon collectively. Some methods for collecting information may include note-taking, audiotaping, videotaping, or by collective review processes at the end of the session. A good idea is to encourage the group to generate ideas and for these to be written clearly on a whiteboard or an overhead transparency sheet as the meeting progresses, so that members can decide collectively on the main ideas, areas to be prioritised and areas for further action. It may be useful to create smaller groups and present the main ideas to the whole group at the conclusion, or group members may take responsibility for contributing to a brainstorming or ideas-collating exercise at the end of the session. Whatever occurs, it is important to gather in the most important ideas, so that the perspectives of the group can be represented adequately. It is also important that the group members validate their ideas by confirming that the interpretations that have been made reflect faithfully the meaning that was intended.

If group processes are to be used sequentially, say, for one hour per week for six months, a great deal of data will be generated and many twists and turns in the life of the group will need to be documented to represent the processes and outcomes. This may be the case in an action research project in which members are committed to regular meetings to work through action cycles. When groups meet regularly, it is a good idea to create some documenting processes. An idea is to have all group members keep a journal of events and their responses to them, and/or to maintain meeting agendas and minutes. I found both these processes to be very helpful in action research and reflective practice projects (Taylor 2001; Taylor et al. 2002), because the group confirmed the minutes each week as a form of data validation, and the information was present in the minutes when I came to the point of writing the final report and preparing a journal article.

Other examples of research projects that used group processes are Wit, Chenoweth and Jeon (2004), Poole and Mott (2003) and Gaskill et al. (2003).

Interviews

Interviews as data collection methods are many and varied and they often differ according to whether they are being used in a qualitative or quantitative research design. For example, qualitative interviews tend to be more like conversations than interrogations. Unlike quantitative research, in which you might reasonably expect to find a structured interview format resembling an oral survey or questionnaire, the epistemological assumptions of qualitative research favour a less structured approach. The reasons for this are that a qualitative interview is designed to encourage participants to tell their stories and relate their experiences in the deepest and richest way possible, bearing in mind inevitable project constraints such as time, transcription costs, interviewee ability as conversationalist and storyteller, and so on.

Gubrium and Holstein (2002) edited a comprehensive text: *Handbook of Interview Research: Context and Method*. To give an appreciation of the wide-ranging details encompassed in interview methods, the editors canvassed invited articles from experts on forms of interviewing, distinctive respondents, auspices of interviewing, technical issues, analytic strategies, reflection and representation. Within each of these parts are many helpful and practical details on the 'how, why, when, where, and with whom' of interviewing. The forms of interviewing most useful for qualitative research are chapters on the qualitative interviewing, in-depth interviewing, the life story interview, focus group interviewing and postmodern trends in interviewing. Given that this book is expensive to buy and you may need borrow it from an academic library, some key points and quotes from each of these chapters are reiterated here.

Qualitative interviewing arises out of conversations and attempts to make meaning from people's accounts of their experiences. Warren (2002) steps the reader through essential considerations in qualitative interviewing, such as designing the research, finding respondents, informed consent and setting up the interview, to highlight the complexities and the often unacknowledged human aspects of the method. Her views on the intersubjectivity of qualitative interviewing are encapsulated well in her statements:

> In the social interaction of the qualitative interview, the perspectives of the interviewer and the respondent dance together for the moment but also extend outward in social space and backward and forward in time. Both are gendered, aged, and otherwise embodied, one person (perhaps) thinking about her (sic) topic, questions, rapport, consent forms, and the tape recorder, not to mention feeling nervous. The other is (perhaps) preoccupied with her (sic) relationships outside the interview, pressing tasks left undone, seeking information, getting help, or being loyal. These are the working selves and others at the center of qualitative interviewing. And that is just the beginning (Warren 2002, pp. 98–9).

In his chapter on in-depth interviewing, Johnson (2002) explains that in-depth interviewing is chosen when researchers want to go beyond the depth usually available from other methods, such as surveys or focus groups, to explore more intimate and personal aspects of people's experiences. The goal of the in-depth interview is to allow the participants to give rich accounts of their experiences that lead others into a deeper understanding of those experiences. He suggests that researchers remain open to digressions from the main topic as the participant speaks and that the free flow of conversation is recorded on audiotape. He cautions about the possibility of emotional catharsis and being mindful of how 'deep' to go 'in probing informants' answers' (Johnson 2002, p. 114). There are ethical considerations of protecting individuals and communities to take into account, especially if the interview goes into deep, relatively uncharted territory and the participant is vulnerable emotionally.

Atkinson (2002, p. 125) describes the life story interview as when 'a person chooses to tell about the life he or she has lived, told as completely and honestly as possible, what the person remembers of it and what he or she wants others to know of it, usually as a result of a guided interview by another'. The interview can scan a whole lifetime or selected segments and eras and in this way it closely resembles a life history or oral history. In order to gather comprehensive stories, Johnson (2002) suggests researchers think of life story as having three distinct phases: first, the planning pre-interview phase in which the objectives of the interview and process are decided; second, the phase of guiding the person through the interview, telling the story on audiotape; and last, the phase of transcribing and interpreting the interview material. On the matter of interpretation of life story, Johnson (2002, p. 135) makes it clear that there are two kinds: 'those that are founded on a theoretical basis and those that emerge from personal frame of reference', and that researchers and their informants negotiate the kind of interpretation together.

Morgan (2002) traces the transition of focus group interviews from marketing into the social sciences and compares the merits of individual and focus group interviews. He discusses the challenges in conducting group interviews and urges continued vigilance in developing better methods of group facilitation. For example, he discloses that 'in my own moderating, I have a series of things that I do to encourage the process of sharing and comparing, including the open instructions that I give, the kinds of questions I use and the way that I manage my own interaction with participants'. From this disclosure, it is possible to infer that there are no absolute prescriptions for success in focus group interviews, and that improvements in the process are through reading other people's experiences and being self-reflective and willing to change one's own practices.

Fontana (2002) offers a postmodern reading of postmodern trends in interviewing. She makes many salient points about the 'postmodern sensibilities and interviewing', including that:

> The boundaries between, and respective roles of interviewer and interviewee have become blurred as the traditional relationship between the two is no longer seen as natural.
>
> New forms of interviewing are being used as interviewer and respondent(s) collaborate together in constructing their narratives.
>
> Interviewers have become more concerned about issues of representation, seriously engaging questions, such as Whose story are we telling and for what purpose?
>
> ... Respondents are no longer seen as faceless numbers whose opinions we process completely on our own terms. Consequently, there is increasing concern with the respondent's own understanding as she or he frames and represents an 'opinion.'

Traditional patriarchal relations in interviewing are being criticized, and ways to make former unarticulated voices audible are now at center stage.

The forms used to report findings have been hugely expanded. As boundaries separating disciplines collapse, modes of expression from literature, poetry, and drama are being applied.

The topic of inquiry-interviewing has expanded to encompass the cinematic and televisual. Electronic media are increasingly accepted as a resource in interviews, with growing use of e-mail, Internet chat rooms, and other electronic forms of communication (Fontana 2002, pp. 162–3).

In summary, the *Handbook of Interview Research: Context and Method*, edited by Gubrium and Holstein (2002), is a comprehensive text, well worth your close attention, should you be thinking of using interviewing as a method in your research.

When you read books and articles about interviewing, you may notice many descriptors for qualitative interviews in the literature, such as in-depth (Beale, McMaster & Hillege 2004–05; Carolan 2004–05), semi-structured interviews (Downie, Clark & Clementson 2004–05; Ronaldson & Devery 2001) or conversational style (Jackson et al. 2004–05; Taylor et al. 2001). Some researchers may not specify a type of interview (Calabretto 2004–05). The type of interview specified gives you clues as to the way in which the questions were prepared and asked. For example, a semi-structured interview will have guiding questions asked of all participants, with room to move based on how the participant is responding, whereas an open-ended, conversational interview will pose an open-ended invitation to talk at the outset and leave it to the participant to weave a response, with the researcher coming back to prompting questions if the participant needs encouragement in continuing. We have already discussed in-depth interviews above.

When researchers 'label' a qualitative interview it is essential to indicate as clearly as possible the processes that were used, especially in the part of the project report that describes methods and processes. For example, interviews may be focused or non-directive, depending on how the participant is invited to respond. Some guiding questions may be necessary to keep a clear direction in a focused interview, but it is very important that the questioning does not extend to a long list, as depth of responses may be sacrificed for breadth of coverage. If you have many questions to ask in rapid-fire sequence, consider a survey, as this can cover a lot of material, with many people, in a relatively short time.

When a research participant is interviewed with an invitation to tell a story, the researcher's directive may be as simple as 'Tell me about your experience of . . . ' or 'I understand that you have experienced . . . . Can you tell me about that please?' Some lead-up conversation may be necessary to settle the storyteller emotionally, and to ascertain that s/he is clear about the focus of the research and how the story can contribute. The plain language statement and the consent form handed out prior to the beginning of the research can indicate all of the necessary information about the project and the participant's involvement. Participants may also be given a list of guiding questions that will be asked to engage the interviewee in a storytelling and/or conversational process. When an interviewee requires prompts, simple encouraging words may help, such as: 'What happened then?', 'Where/

when did that happen?', 'How were you involved?' or 'How did that make you feel?' As with all good communication, listening attentively and responding appropriately are important skills for unfolding effective conversations and stories. Don't underestimate the power of silence. If you remain silent it gives the participant a chance to think and to speak without haste and pressure.

In summary, qualitative interviews can be structured with a list of set questions to be asked, or they can be relatively unstructured with little more than an invitation being issued by the researcher for the participant to talk about an area of interest. In between both end points is a semi-structured interview, a conversation in which the researcher invites the participant to talk, encouraging a free flow of words and ideas but at the same time keeping the person relatively on track in the conversation if s/he has a tendency to wander off the point.

The best way to collect interview data is on audiotape, although video may be advisable in cases in which non-verbal cues are important. Buy reliable tapes to minimise the risk of data loss. To prevent loss of data you might also prefer to make backup copies of the tapes and store them in a different place from the originals. The audiotapes can be transcribed to form written text for analysis, or they may be replayed, to allow for the recognition of themes. If participants are shy of the audiotape machine, a time of general talking with the player on may be necessary in order for people to feel less conscious of it. If anxiety prevails about the use of the audiomachine, it may be necessary to take notes, although this method may take up your attention and energy, and you may miss important content details and voice inflections.

Interview transcripts generate lots and lots of data that must be managed systematically. If you are an organised sort of person, this will come easily to you. If you tend towards the haphazard end of the continuum, you might like to get the advice of a practical person who can set you straight on how to organise your sorting and filing system so that data are not misplaced or otherwise mistreated.

In the absence of an organised and practical person, here are some hints that might help you. The transcripts are most easily managed on computer disk. Make a copy of each transcript, transfer it to a separate well-functioning computer disk and store it in a different place to prevent loss. Keep a main copy of the transcript either on a floppy disk or the hard disk of the computer, and ensure that any alterations made to the main document are also made to the copies. This will help you to keep all of the work current, thereby preventing confusion as to which is the most recent working copy. It also means that if there is a computer glitch or the floppy you are using deteriorates, the information loss will only be as extensive as the last updated disk copy. Consider procuring a filing cabinet with hanging files for hard copies, foolscap folders, and a lockable computer disk container with plenty of disk labels. Some forethought in organising the storage of your data will prevent a lot of concern and chaos later.

If you do not have access to computer facilities, you may be using typed hard copies of transcripts. There is a similar need for caution in storing and filing these forms of data. Make multiple copies of the hard copies. Ensure they have all of the identifying details written on them. Keep a list of all the transcripts according to participants' actual names and pseudonyms and lock this away so that anonymity is maintained. Store the typed transcript copies in a paper filing system such as manila folders, and keep a copy in a different location to minimise the risk of loss.

Journal keeping

The journal form of data collection is useful for research in which researcher and participants are conversant with, and willing to indulge in, reflective writing for the purposes of the research. It may be just like keeping a diary that sets out the events of the day and reactions to them, such as in a journal you keep about being a research student. A journal of this nature might record your impressions of your meetings with your research supervisor, the joys and pains of being a researcher, and any thoughts, insights and inspirations you have along the way.

You might also find it useful to record information about your role in the research and how you manage being a nurse researching some aspect of nursing or health. Thus, a journal used in this more focused way may help you to reflect on your experiences of having multiple roles and responsibilities, while noticing the issues in everyday practice from the perspective of an interested participant observer divorced temporarily from the busyness of work.

Another way of using a journal is to enlist the cooperation of participants in keeping one for information gathering. You may also keep a reflective journal of your experiences as a co-researcher sharing equally in group processes. If you choose to use this method of data collection, you need to ensure that participants are willing, able and eager to write reflectively. The literature is clear that people benefit from coaching in order to reflect effectively (Conway 1994; Greenwood 1993). You may need to build some time into your project to coach participants in the methods and processes of reflection. These skills can be acquired, especially if you want them to go beyond descriptive accounts of their personal stories to making sense of their experiences. I suggest that you refer to my book on reflection for nurses and midwives if you are serious about making the best use of having participants and co-researchers keep journals (Taylor 2000).

In using a journal all participants need to be clear about the objectives of the activity, otherwise many words may be written that may have little hope of informing the research. So often, ideas can wander so far off the point of a project that the richness of the information is compromised. This does not mean that there is no room for discussion and journalling tangential to the project's main interests, but you should be careful to ensure that precious time given so generously by the participants is used to its best advantage, as a sign of respect for their contributions.

Journals may be private or semi-private, and therefore participants may decide on what they choose to divulge for the research data. Group processes or discussions with individuals can clarify expectations about the use of journal entries as data. Participants need to agree to disclosing material in the amount and level of privacy they choose. Indeed, there may be excerpts that are so deeply personal that they are known only to the writer, who may use them as aids for working through personal and professional issues. Areas that can be shared publicly can be spoken about in meetings and/or photocopied for incorporation into research reports and papers using pseudonyms.

The amount of material that can be generated will depend on the objectives of the exercise and the amount of disclosure that is required, but journal keeping is likely to amass a substantial amount of information that needs to be sorted in some way, in order for it be useful. Photocopies of the 'public domain' journal entries can be made, after words and phrases are adapted as ethical safeguards to reduce the risk of identifying people and places. Interpretations will be most useful if they are made by the person doing the writing, in collaboration with another person, possibly the researcher, who acts as a critical friend, asking constructive questions to bring out the richness of the content.

For further information on keeping a journal for the purposes of using critical reflection on practice for yourself or prospective research participants, you might like to read Street (1995, pp. 147–71). This is a comprehensive step-by-step account of how to set up and maintain a journal so that it is useful for more than personal reflection. The method and process Annette Street describes can help nurses to make sense of their practice and work in ways to change those parts of it that they would like to change. Alternatively, if you need a simple-to-follow 'recipe book' approach to when, why and how to keep a journal and do reflective practice, refer to my book, as mentioned previously (Taylor 2000, 2006).

Research projects that have used reflective journaling as a method of data collection include Tuckett and Stewart (2003) and Hewitt (2003).

EXERCISE

Locate and read one of the references cited above and notice what kind of reflective writing the researcher used and their impressions of the relative merits of journal keeping as a method of data collection.

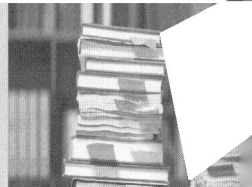

Literature searches and reviews

Part or all of a research project may involve searching for literature. Literature features in applied research as background data when it is used to show how the findings relate to published accounts of the same area of interest. In pure research, the project may consist of literature entirely, such as in the scholarly critiques expected in philosophical or evidence-based projects that critically appraise the extant literature. Literature in the form of books and refereed journal articles is collected from all the likely sources and repositories, such as electronic and library databases. A detailed account of literature search and review skills appears in Chapter 4.

The review process involves a succinct and focused analysis to show the strengths, weaknesses, connections and gaps in what is written and how each writer contrasts to and/or augments other writers in the area. Some helpful questions to keep in mind, to ensure a thorough literature review are:

- What is the purpose of the literature review? In other words, what is the relationship between the literature review and the research questions?
- Who has written in the area? What social/occupational roles do they occupy?
- What has been written in the area? What key propositions have been made and do they fall into key areas? What has been seen as problematic and what solutions/strategies/actions have been proposed and/or tested in relation to the area of concern?
- How have other scholars received this material? Has this material been subsumed into existing paradigms? Has it challenged existing theories or does it reinforce present ideas?
- What research projects have been carried out in this area? What methods have been employed and were they appropriate for the research questions investigated?
- What are the major findings of the research projects?
- Are research findings across various studies consistent, conflicting or both?
- What debates have there been about the content (substantive) and approach (methodological) components of these projects?
- What have been the main issues in the debates?
- What important issues appear to be overlooked, and constitute gaps, silences and omissions?
- What are the common threads in the research issues, debates, findings and themes?
- How can these common threads guide an evaluation of the knowledge that has been gathered to date, and how they can be informative for further inquiry?

If your literature review is under the special scrutiny of a discourse analysis, you need to use an even deeper level of examination, by asking questions as listed in Chapter 16 under 'Discourse analysis'.

Literature may be collected in piles and bundles, but it is of little use if it is not managed well. It is a good idea to create a running bibliography on computer disk, which keeps a record of the referencing details of the literature and the main ideas within it. If lists and descriptions are kept on computer disks, they can be cut and pasted readily into the research document. If computer technology is not available, coloured cardboard cards can be used to store information in secure filing boxes.

Some published reviews of literature include Brooks et al. (2004), Davidson (2003–04), Duke and Street (2003), Usher et al. (2003), Laws and Bradley (2003) and Lewis, Pearson and Ward (2003). These articles have been through a peer-review process and judged to be of a high quality according to their ability to fulfil criteria for writing a good literature review similar to those presented in this section. One of the best ways to hone your skills in writing a strong literature review is to read as many as you can of a high standard highlighted in refereed articles.

Often we can manage descriptive reviews of literature that inform readers of the main themes and findings of research. It is quite another skill to write a 'punchy' critical review that goes beyond description to other factors, such as to be effective in identifying gaps, silences, contradictions, and deficits in application of methodological, methods and processes aspects of the research.

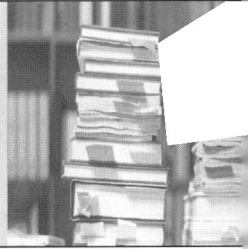

Member checks

A member check is a procedure used within qualitative research methods to ensure that participants validate their contributions to the overall project, as a source of determining the trustworthiness or validity of the project. This might mean that researchers invite participants to check various parts of the project to see whether the researcher is reflecting and interpreting their contributions in the way the participants intended. On a practical level, this means that participants might be given transcripts of their own interviews to ensure that the information is complete and accurate, or comment may be sought on the way in which the researcher has interpreted various themes in the data.

Even though it is good practice to use member checks in qualitative research, be aware of some of the likely scenarios that may arise. For example, people have a tendency to speak in broken sentences, adding redundancies, such as 'ums', 'ahs' and 'you knows'. When they receive a transcript full of these kinds of grammatical glitches, they may be embarrassed at best, and want to withdraw their contributions at worst. Be prepared for this eventuality, and if there are no methodological contradictions, tidy the transcript without changing the meaning of the words, or warn the reader to be forgiving of their use of spoken language, given that it is fairly typical of us all to speak in this way.

Also be clear about what the participant is checking. There are many reasons for giving a transcript back to participants, and some intentions may need to spelt out clearly. A transcript may be checked before or after analysis and the participant needs to be given directions in their part of the process. For example, you may ask them to check the content of the transcript to ensure that the conversation is as they remember. Alternatively, you may invite them to add or delete information they deem necessary, or to give their opinion on whether the interpretations and insights of the analysis are 'in tune' with their reading of the transcript. If there are certain functions you do not expect the participant to perform in relation to member checking, make this clear, and ensure that all provisos have been communicated previously in the plain language statement that accompanied the consent form they signed before they became involved in the project.

Mixed methods

A mixed method approach enlists whatever methods are considered useful for the attainment of the project's objectives. Usually, when researchers refer to 'mixed methods' they generally mean methods that would ordinarily be used in one paradigm, mixed with methods ordinarily associated with another paradigm, for example, mixing questionnaires (usually seen as being helpful for quantitative data generation) and semi-structured or in-depth interviews (usually seen as helpful in generating qualitative data).

The reasoning behind a decision to use a mixed method approach has already been covered in this chapter in the section relating to methodological congruency. It is important to bear in mind that a method is not uniquely connected to a methodology and that as long as you can justify your decision to the thesis examiners or research consumers, you are at liberty to choose whatever combinations of methods you prefer. Having made this point, the selection of a combination of methods needs to be carefully undertaken. It is not a matter of 'a dollar's worth of mixed lollies' approach, in which you select the attractive options, but rather it requires an approach that takes into account the various constraints of the project, such as participant cooperation and researcher skills, and mutual concerns, such as time, effort, enjoyment, applicability, ethical justification, and so on.

The decision to use mixed methods may also be taken on political grounds, in the sense that it may be wise to collect quantitative and qualitative data, based on the tendency of some funding bodies to award empirical designs, or to appease the expectations of health agency ethics committees, who use quantitative research as their yardstick for quality and evidence. Decisions for mixed methods may also be taken due to the breadth, depth and overall scope of a study, in order to include as many participants/subjects as possible and to represent their experiences as fully as possible through numerical and language-based means.

A cursory review of some Australian-based refereed journals (*Collegian, Contemporary Nurse* and the *International Journal of Nursing Practice*) shows that there has been an increasing tendency since 2001 to publish results of mixed method projects. Whether mixed methods projects are on the uprise due to funding opportunities, scope of projects, the need for evidence-based practice, the demands and expectations of organisations, or other factors not imagined here, is open to debate. For whatever reasons, nurses are using mixed method research more frequently, and combining methods to collect quantitative and qualitative data is becoming more prevalent.

Examples of research that used mixed methods are Cox, Henderson, Wood and Cagliarini (2003), Fitzgerald and Teale (2003–04), Gibson and Heartfield (2003), Ormsby and Harrington (2003), and Wit, Chenoweth and Jeon (2004).

Observation/Participant observation

Types of observation vary according to the research approach. They can be structured or relatively unstructured, and they can be solely by observation or by varying degrees of participant observation.

Structured observation, requiring strict attention to objectivity through checklists of events and behaviours, is most probably inappropriate in qualitative research generally, because there is no intention to standardise data collection conditions, as would be the case with empirico-analytical research. However, there may be some need for this type of observation as part of a larger issue-based participatory action research project, when the observation component of an action cycle has a particular intention to identify predetermined categories of events and behaviours (Keatinge et al. 2000). If you are interested in using structured observation refer to Chapter 8 in this book.

In unstructured observation, the researcher observes a context systematically and carefully, but with no predetermined categories in mind. The observation is done with open-mindedness as to what may occur, keeping in mind the central purposes for being there as stated in the research objectives. The researcher's attention is drawn to what is happening, where, when, how, why and with whom, without actual involvement in the setting as a participant. This means that the observation periods are flexible in relation to the place in which the observation of the people and events occurs, as well as the time of day, length of time, and expectations about the aspects to be observed. Observations are documented as field notes that describe the broad features of the setting. This kind of observation is useful for an ethnographic project, in which the researcher is present in the setting as an unobtrusive observer (Emerson, Fretz & Shaw 2001; Oliver & Butler 2004).

As it would suggest, participant observation is about getting involved in the action in a setting, while observing the details within it. Sometimes it is necessary to spend some time in a particular setting to see what happens there. There may be different reasons for observing the area, including getting to know who and what comes and goes, finding out about the routines, seeing how people interact with one another, and so on. For example, participant observer phases may be needed to gather data in ethnographic research, or observation may form part of the data collection phases of research that is not necessarily ethnographic, for instance in action research.

As nurses are working daily in health care settings, they have full access to the area as employees, and thus they are in a good position to become participant observers of their own work, such as when they become reflective in their practice and/or use reflective processes in their research projects. For example, in two different studies, nurses used participant observation to ascertain the effectiveness of an action plan they generated through an action research and reflection project. The first project relates to dysfunctional nurse–nurse relationships, in which nurses devised an action plan for identifying bullying behaviours improving nurse–nurse relationships (Taylor 2001), and the second project relates to palliative nurses exploring their tendencies towards idealism (Taylor et al. 2002). In both projects, nurses used participant observation in their working time to be actively engaged in reflective practice and the fulfilment of the research objectives.

Observation and participant observation usually involves watching and attending systematically to a setting, then retreating for some time to write up the impressions. If the data are written directly into a word-processing system it will save a lot of time in typing them up for later analysis. If there are no technological aids such as computers, impressions can be spoken into an audiotape or written into a logbook or some other permanent record system.

It is important to be fully aware of why you are acting in the role of a participant observer, so be familiar with the aims and objectives of the project in which the method is occurring. You need to be 'loitering with intent', so to speak, or actively engaged in work in some cases, so that you can 'tune in' intentionally to those areas of the context most directly related to your project. As with all human research, you need to be aware of ethical considerations.

You need to be aware of the people who have given their consent to be observed during interactions and to exclude anyone who has not consented. Attending to ethical issues means not only having informed consent to observe people, but also changing names and identities of people and places to pseudonyms to maintain privacy and anonymity.

Having gained consent it is important to 'blend in' as much as you can, so that people are unaware or become less aware of your presence, except in specific cases where you need to make your presence known for ethical or methodological reasons. Done well, participant observation is not conspicuous and therefore has less chance of disrupting the usual features of the setting. It may take a little time to settle into the situation before the actual work of observation begins. This allows people a chance to get used to having you around in a researcher capacity. Even if you are researching your own work area, people may feel self-conscious if they know you are doing research (which they will, because you are ethically bound to tell them and to gain their consent to observe them).

You may be involved in the interaction to varying degrees. For example, you may be assisting in making a bed or washing a patient, but as a researcher on a designated project, you will most probably not have responsibility for patient care. Exceptions to this will be when nurses decide to do action research projects and use their own practice as an area of inquiry and reflection.

You will need to develop a watchful approach to what is happening around you. Learn to 'tune in' and see as many details as possible in the situation. Use a systematic approach to watching and documenting what you see. For example, think carefully before you write field notes about:

- Who was involved?
- What was the nature of the interaction?
- What were the sights, sounds and smells?
- What happened?
- When did it happen?
- What were the outcomes (effects) of the interaction?

Write the field notes as soon as possible after the interaction. It is not advisable to write during the interaction as it important to be active, but not intrusive in the interaction. Also, it gives an unconcerned and thoughtless image if you stand there writing on a clipboard or in a book while busy nursing activities happen around you. It is quite cumbersome and artificial to collect data notes and descriptions in the course of participating in the setting, so a better alternative is to retreat periodically to write up impressions before rejoining the action for further phases of participant observation.

The data are best written in a richly descriptive form, and they read easier if they are written in the present continuous tense, for example, '*I take a wash bowl to the bed and the other nurse draws the curtains around the bed, as Mr Green suddenly holds his chest and winces with pain*'.

When you write notes, be as descriptive as you can. Don't worry about grammar or spelling, as these are minor glitches which can be fixed easily later. Concentrate on describing the situation as comprehensively as you can so you and others reading your account can understand what happened, why, when, to whom, and with what outcomes (effects).

Ensure that you have a selection of interactions occurring over time with the people involved; thus various people will be involved over many shifts or times of day. Participants need to be assured that you will not use their names on the accounts and that other identifiable information will be hidden. You can be careful in this respect as you write, by referring only to 'the nurse', 'the patient', 'the relative', the doctor', and so on.

In sorting the data it is important to gather the information in some kind of permanent storage system, such as a computer disk, and ensure that each description of the setting is labelled according to the date, time and other important details that may have some bearing in the later analysis. In qualitative research, field notes may count as data to be analysed or process notes to document the research progress, so it is feasible and advisable to use them in the text of research reports, journal articles and conference presentations when disseminating your results.

Photography

Harper (2000) described the use of visual methods in sociology, such as still photographs, film and video, arguing convincingly that they are empirical data. He cautions the reader, however, that he does 'not claim that these images represent "objective truth." The very act of observing is interpretive, for to observe is to choose a point of view' (p. 721). Harper's view reminds us that in qualitative research, photographs, or any other sources of data or methods of data collection, do not represent truth in themselves, but rather they give us the potential to amass enough information to make tentative and relative interpretations.

Photographs can be highly significant sources of data, assuming that you have permission to take and store them. In some health care settings, such as hospitals and private clinics, clients may want to have their identities hidden. Also, organisations may have strict rules about the use of cameras and videos, with respect to the anonymity of their clients and the workplace. Remember also that certain groups of people, such as Indigenous people, may have strong cultural taboos about having their images caught on camera. There may be potential for violating sacred beliefs by using photographs. Because of the risk of the researcher's unwitting insensitivity to certain people and/or institutions, always check thoroughly each and every time before you assume it is appropriate to use photography.

Photographs can be taken that represent the features of the research setting and/or participants. For example, if a project involved exploring the routines of a nursing home, other sources of data such as participant observation and interviews could be augmented well by selected pictorial images. Photographs could be sorted into categories and labelled accordingly, and the best images, in terms of the most descriptive photos, are chosen for inclusion in the research report. Details of the photographs could also be analysed to contribute to informing the research questions.

An example of using photographs in research is a project by Turner and Cox (2004), in which they used photography and in-depth interviews to describe the phenomenon of hope. Participants were supplied with a disposable colour film camera with a built-in flash and asked to 'imagine that they were being paid to mount a photographic exhibition of hope … to take pictures that in their view showed hope' (Turner & Cox 2004, p. 18). The photographs sparked conversations and stories embedded in metaphors that raised participants' awareness of the meaning of hope.

Moving pictures captured in video or DVD technologies can offer more scope and dimension than still photographs for data, so their value as sources of data is self-evident. The same precautions apply to videotaping and DVD as have been outlined for photography. It is imperative that ethical clearance is gained before videotaping and DVD begins, and that participants give consent for their involvement. Exceptions to this may be in the use of video or DVD as a compilation of personal data of an archival nature that may be used in an autobiography or oral history, when the researcher is the focus of the project.

Also, do not underestimate the amount of knowledge and practice that is needed to produce videos or DVDs which look professional and which record sound and movement well. Even with care in the recording phase, the video/DVD may need considerable editing to extract the extraneous details associated with the production glitches. If you are considering these media, check out some of the traps for beginners, by consulting someone conversant with videotaping or DVD, or by enrolling in a media unit through your local university or technical college.

The videos and DVDs need to be labelled clearly, or have specific identifying information recorded at the beginning of the taping, to ensure that the information is represented in its correct context. It may also be necessary to cross-reference information in the written report or thesis with particular sections in the video or DVD, so that viewers are made aware of the objectives for using the media and how they relate directly to your research intentions.

Storytelling

Researchers have tended to use the words 'story' and 'narrative' interchangeably. When Wiltshire (1995, p. 75) examined the use of the terms 'story', 'narrative' and 'voice' within health care, he pointed out that the words have been used synonymously in relation to telling stories and he claims that they all have therapeutic dimensions. Polkinghorne (1988) is more precise, differentiating a story as a single account reviewing life events in a true or imagined form, and a narrative as a scheme of multiple stories 'that organises events and human actions into a whole' (p. 18).

Whether as a single story or as in the organising scheme of a narrative, data for qualitative research can be gathered easily and effectively through having people relate accounts of their experiences relevant to the research. It is an effective way of involving people in research, because it is not unusual for people to think that they have little to offer research projects, and some people may feel intimidated by the thought of participating. However, people may respond to the invitation to tell a story.

For example, if you want to find out about how patients perceive care, they can be encouraged to tell a story about it. The lead-in to encourage the story could be as simple as: 'Please tell me about a time in which you were happy with the care you received here'. Alternatively, another story may be encouraged by the lead-in: 'Please tell me about a time in which you were not pleased with the care you received here'.

The story can be recorded on audiotape for later analysis, but some audiotape-shy participants may feel happier about writing their stories and adding illustrations. In some cases, stories may be enacted in traditional ways – dance, rituals – and other creative means, such as poetry, music, singing and film. If creative means are used, it is important that the artist is the interpreter of her/his own story, the accounts of which are stored by a recordable means to which the artist agrees.

As with all effective communication, if a storyteller has optimal conditions for speaking, the likelihood of a rich and deeply thoughtful story is enhanced through listener silence and attention. Once the storyteller has clear parameters for the story, resist the impulse to interject, unless the narrator is wandering right off the track and looks like being lost in irrelevancies. Look back in this chapter to 'Interviews' for further comments on how to encourage participants to tell their stories.

In storing and preparing data from transcribed stories, some considerations are noteworthy. It is important to label the tape containing the story according to the participant's pseudonym, and with the date, time and other contextual features of note. If many stories are stored on a single audiotape, use a numerical code on the label and keep and prepare a list of corresponding names and pseudonyms on computer disk or hard copy files. This prevents data confusion and ensures that each participant's story is attributed to the experience of that person, even though particular identities remain hidden. Set up a filing system and lock audiotapes, floppy disks and hard copies of stories away securely, as required by ethical procedures. You need to make a hard copy of each story to return to participants to validate their accounts.

For further reading on storytelling and narrative inquiry refer to Atkinson (2002), Graham (2002), Martin-McDonald (2003) and Walker (2002).

Summary

This chapter demonstrated the point that there are many methods by which information can be collected. In qualitative research, researchers usually ensure that the research methods and forms of knowledge are congruent, so for many qualitative researchers, methodological congruency is an important issue as they plan research projects. This chapter differentiated between methods and methodologies, and explored some issues around methodological congruency. It stressed the importance of carefully selecting methods alone or in combination with other methods, to suit the research contexts and participants, because they have a great bearing on how interpretations are made in qualitative research. Criteria for assessing trustworthiness and data collection methods for qualitative research were described.

Main points

- The attention to choosing congruent methods is based on the rationale that if a methodology is a set of theoretical assumptions, and a method is a means for generating a certain type of knowledge, then it seems reasonable to assume that there needs to be a degree of fit between the type of knowledge that is to be generated and the means that are available to achieve it.

- The objectives of a qualitative project, although sometimes stated broadly, need to be clear and to have some degree of containment, and when they are stated in this way, they give clues as to the choice of methods.
- It may be possible to use just one method of data collection, such as storytelling, or interviews, or focus groups; however, if the data can be deepened and enriched further, a combination of methods can be used.
- Although methods do not 'belong' exclusively to methodologies, a sound rationale is required for choosing them, especially if contradictions arise in research findings of a mixed method project.
- A general principle of qualitative research is that people are placed in time and space, and therefore that they cannot help but be situated somewhere, and as such, they have some degree of involvement in their respective contexts.
- Qualitative researchers value people and the accounts these people give of their experiences, because it fits with a relativistic view that knowledge changes and that understanding human existence resides in people's lives.
- Qualitative research is no less rigorous than quantitative research, but it uses different words to demonstrate the ways of making explicit the overall processes and worthiness of a project, because it is based on different epistemological assumptions.
- Qualitative researchers use the most appropriate means of assessing 'rigour' in qualitative projects, to reflect the methodological assumptions of the project.
- The categories for determining trustworthiness in qualitative research are credibility, fittingness, auditability, and confirmability.
- Credibility means the extent to which participants and readers of the research recognise the lived experiences described in the research as similar to their own.
- Fittingness refers to the extent to which a project's findings fit into other contexts outside the study setting and the extent to which the readers of the research find it has meaning and relevance for their own experiences.
- Auditability is the production of a decision trail, which can be scrutinised by other researchers to determine the extent to which the project has achieved consistency in its methods and processes.
- Confirmability of a project is achieved when credibility, auditability and fittingness can be demonstrated in a qualitative project.
- Investigator triangulation uses many researchers to collect and analyse a single set of data.
- Theory triangulation uses many theoretical perspectives to interpret data. Method triangulation uses multiple methods such as interviews, document analysis and observation.
- Methodological triangulation uses multiple theoretical approaches in one project, for example, feminism, ethnography and affirmative postmodernism.

- Archival searches are associated with historical research, because they involve the collection of data, such as original hard copies of aged documents.
- Data collected through artistic expression may be particularly useful in research aimed at describing the experience of certain conditions/states/perspectives from the individual's unique viewpoint.
- A case study is a research strategy that comprises an all-encompassing, comprehensive method and set of strategies that allow people, practices and phenomena to be described over time according to their contextual features.
- Fieldwork methods may vary according to the intentions of the research, but they usually consist of combinations of observation, participation, documentation and analysis.
- A focus group is a collection of people working together on a particular research issue.
- Group processes are particularly suitable for collaborative research such as action research, feminist research or research that is informed by poststructural and/or postmodern ideas, because they involve groups of people working together to create shared meaning.
- Qualitative research interviews encourage conversations, such as unstructured interviews, semi-structured interviews, in-depth interviewing, the life story interview, focus group interviewing and postmodern trends in interviewing.
- The journal form of data collection is useful for research in which researcher and participants are conversant with, and willing to indulge in, reflective writing for the purposes of the research.
- The literature review process involves a succinct and focused analysis, to show the strengths, weaknesses, connections and gaps in what is written and how each writer contrasts to and/or augments other writers in the area.
- A member check is a procedure used within qualitative research methods to ensure that participants validate their contributions to the overall project, as a source of determining the trustworthiness or validity of the project.
- Usually, when researchers refer to 'mixed methods' they mean methods that would ordinarily be used in one paradigm, that are mixed with methods ordinarily associated with another paradigm.
- Types of observation vary according to the research approach, and they can be structured or relatively unstructured, and range from observation solely to varying degrees of participant observation.
- Photographs, films and videotapes can be highly significant sources of data, but they do not represent truth in themselves. Rather, they give researchers the potential to amass enough information to make tentative and relative interpretations.
- Whether as a single story or as in the organising scheme of a narrative, data from stories for qualitative research can be gathered easily and effectively through encouraging people to relate accounts of their experiences relevant to the research.

Case study

Carmel, aged 35 years, is an experienced clinical nurse working in an acute care setting while undertaking a Master by Research program part-time with a local university. She is planning a practice-based, qualitative research project with the guidance of a university supervisor, who is an experienced nurse, teacher and researcher.

Carmel is in the preliminary stages of her postgraduate research, and her supervisor has asked her to write a brief research proposal, as a first draft discussion document. In other words, at her next meeting with her supervisor, Carmel needs to be able to discuss her beginning ideas for all of the essential aspects of the project, with particular reference to the selection of data collection methods. (Refer to Chapter 6 for the features of a research proposal.)

To date, Carmel knows that she wants to research collaboratively with 10 other experienced nurses working in acute care settings, about the facilitating and constraining factors they experience that influence their ability to give effective nursing care. Carmel's interest in this topic came about because she is noticing that many of her colleagues are leaving nursing and/or 'burning out' with the demands of the job. She also wants to give the nurses a chance to voice those aspects of their work they find rewarding, so that is why she is including both facilitating and constraining aspects of the nurses' experiences.

The research aim is to explore with experienced nurses working in acute care their accounts of factors that help and hinder the delivery of effective nursing care. The objectives for the project are to: give nurses a chance to voice their experiences; identify facilitating and constraining factors in nursing work in acute care settings; and to begin to accentuate facilitation and positively change the constraints, thereby improving nursing practice and patient outcomes.

What data collection methods and processes seem the best choices to fulfil Carmel's research aim and objectives? For each choice, give a sound rationale as to why it is suitable. Also, provide a clear rationale for the combination of the methods and processes, bearing in mind the contextual features of which you are now aware in this case study.

Multiple choice questions

1   In the qualitative sections of this book, methodology refers to:
    a   a combination of methods used for data collection
    b   theoretical assumptions underlying the choice of methods
    c   how researchers use methods within a project
    d   the means and strategies by which data are collected

2 Qualitative researchers value people and the accounts these people give of their experiences, because it fits with a view that knowledge is:

a certain

b absolute

c static

d relative

3 In terms of assessing 'rigour', qualitative researchers reflect the methodological assumptions of the project by the use of:

a reliability measures

b goodness and auditability

c the most appropriate means

d validity and credibility

4 Credibility is:

a the production of a decision trail, which can be scrutinised by other researchers to determine the extent to which the project has achieved consistency in its methods and processes

b the extent to which participants and readers of the research recognise the lived experiences described in the research as similar to their own

c the demonstration of successful measures for ensuring reliability, validity, auditability and fittingness within a qualitative project

d the extent to which a project's findings fit into other contexts outside the study setting and the readers of the research find meaning and relevance for their own experiences

5 The use of multiple references, such as data, investigators, theories, methods and methodologies, which converge in research projects to draw conclusions that may be more confidently claimed as being trustworthy, is:

a rigour

b triangulation

c trustworthiness

d congruence

6 All-encompassing, comprehensive methods and set of strategies that allow people, practices and phenomena to be described over time according to their contextual features are:

a artistic expression

b archival searches

c case studies

d focus groups

7 Qualitative interviews encourage:

a conversations and stories

b structure and sequence

c standardised responses

d measurable findings

8 Member checking:
  a ranges from observation to degrees of participant observation
  b provides certainty as to the absolute truth of the research findings
  c ensures that participants validate their contributions to the project
  d refers to group processes that ensure collaboration and credibility
9 Combining questionnaires, surveys, in-depth interviews and storytelling is an example of a:
  a quantitative research design
  b positivistic method integration
  c qualitative research project
  d mixed methods approach
10 Qualitative methods:
  a are matched exclusively to qualitative methodologies, such as ethnography and action research
  b give researchers the potential to amass enough information to make tentative and relative interpretations
  c collect data that are guaranteed to provide accurate and generalisable results that define human experiences
  d provide superior epistemological findings that can be relied on to give the best accounts of human experiences.

Review topics

1 Why is it considered important to choose congruent data collection methods in qualitative research?
2 Discuss the advantages and disadvantages of choosing a mixed methods approach for data collection.
3 Discuss the development of the debates relating to 'rigour' in qualitative research.
4 Describe the types of interviews most conducive to generating rich accounts of human experience.
5 List the main features of a well-written literature review.

Online reading

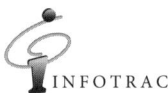

INFOTRAC® COLLEGE EDITION
To locate further literature relating to qualitative methods, use search words for your discipline, e.g. nursing, physiotherapy, occupational therapy etc, and combine them with:

➤ congruency
➤ contexts
➤ data collection
➤ methodology
➤ methods
➤ participants
➤ processes
➤ 'rigour'
➤ trustworthiness

References

Atkinson, P., Coffey, A., Delamont, S., Lofland, J. & Lofland, L. (eds) 2001, *Handbook of Ethnography*, Sage, London.

Atkinson, R. 2002, 'The life story interview', in J.F. Gubrium, & J.A. Holstein (eds), 2002, *Handbook of Interview Research: Context and Method*, Sage, Thousand Oaks, 121–40.

Barnes, M., Courtney, M., Pratt, J. & Walsh, A. 2003, 'Contemporary child health nursing practice: services provided and challenges faced in metropolitan and outer Brisbane areas', *Collegian*, vol. 10, no. 4, 14–19.

Beale, B., McMaster, R. & Hillege, S. 2004–05, 'Eating disorders: a qualitative analysis of the parents' journey', *Contemporary Nurse*, vol. 18, no. 1–2, 124–32.

Beck, C.T. 1993, 'Qualitative research: the evaluation of its credibility, fittingness, and auditability', *Western Journal of Nursing Research*, vol. 15, no. 2, 263–6.

Benner, P. & Wrubel, J. 1989, *The Primacy of Caring*, Addison-Wesley, Menlo Park, California.

Brockopp, D. & Hastings-Tolsma, M. 2003, *Fundamentals of Nursing Research*, 3rd edn, Jones and Bartlett, Boston.

Brooks, K., Davidson, P., Daly, J. & Hancock, K. 2004, 'Community health nursing in Australia: a critical literature review and implications for professional development', *Contemporary Nurse*, vol. 16, no. 3, 195–207.

Burns, N. & Grove, S.K. 1997, *The Practice of Nursing Research: Conduct, Critique and Utilization*, 3rd edn, W.B. Saunders, Philadelphia.

Calabretto, H. 2004–05, 'Emergency contraception: a qualitative study of young women's experiences', *Contemporary Nurse*, vol. 18, no. 1–2, 152–63.

Carolan, M. 2004–05, 'Maternal and child health nurses: a vital link to the community for primiparae over the age of 35', *Contemporary Nurse*, vol. 18, no. 1–2, 133–42.

Chinn, P.L. & Wheeler, S. 1995, *Peace and Power: Building Communities for the Future*, 4th edn, National League for Nursing, New York.

Conway, J. 1994, 'Reflection, the art and science of nursing and the theory and practice gap', *British Journal of Nursing*, vol. 393, 114–18.

Cox, H., Henderson, L., Andersen, N., Cagliarini, G. & Ski, C. 2003, 'Focus group study of endometriosis: struggle, loss and the medical merry-go-round', *International Journal of Nursing Practice*, vol. 9, no. 1, 2–9.

Cox, H., Henderson, L., Wood, R. & Cagliarini, G. 2003, 'Learning to take charge: women's experiences of living with endometriosis', *Complementary Therapies in Nursing and Midwifery*, vol. 9, no. 2, 62–8.

Davidson, P., Daly, J., Hancock, K. & Jackson, D. 2003–04, 'Australian women and heart disease: trends, epidemiological perspectives and the need for a culturally competent research agenda', *Contemporary Nurse*, vol. 16, no. 1–2, 62–73.

Denzin, N.K. 1989, *The Research Act*, McGraw Hill, New York.

Denzin, N.K. & Lincoln, Y.S. (eds) 2000, *Handbook of Qualitative Research*, 2nd edn, Sage, Thousand Oaks.

De Wit, K. & Davis, K. 2004, 'Nurses' knowledge and learning experiences in relation to the effects of domestic abuse on the mental health of children and adolescents', *Contemporary Nurse*, vol. 16, no. 3, 214–27.

Downie, J., Clark, K. & Clementson, K. 2004–05, 'Volunteerism: "community mothers" in action', *Contemporary Nurse*, vol. 18, no. 1–2, 188–98.

Duke, M. & Street, A. 2003, 'The impetus for the development of Hospital in the Home programs: a literature review', *Contemporary Nurse*, vol. 14, no. 3, 227–39.

Emden, C. & Sandelowski, M. 1998, 'The good, the bad and the relative: conceptions of goodness in qualitative research: part one', *International Journal of Nursing Practice*, vol. 4, no. 4, 206–12.

Emden, C. & Sandelowski, M. 1999, 'The good, the bad and the relative: conceptions of goodness in qualitative research: part two', *International Journal of Nursing Practice*, vol. 5, no. 1, 2–7.

Emerson, R.M., Fretz, R.I. & Shaw, L.L. 2001, 'Participant observation and fieldnotes', in P. Atkinson, A. Coffey, S. Delamont, J. Lofland & L. Lofland (eds), *Handbook of Ethnography*, Sage, London, pp. 352–68.

Fern, E.F. 2001, *Advanced Focus Group Research*, Sage, Thousand Oaks.

Fitzgerald, A. & Teale, G. 2003–04, 'Health reform, professional identity and occupational sub-cultures: the changing interprofessional relations between doctors and nurses', *Contemporary Nurse*, vol. 16, no. 1–2, 9–19.

Fitzgerald, L. 1999, 'Case studies as a research tool', *Quality in Health Care*, vol. 8, 75.

Fontana, A. 2002, 'Postmodern trends in interviewing', in J.F. Gubrium & J.A. Holstein (eds), *Handbook of Interview Research: Context and Method*, Sage, Thousand Oaks, 161–75.

Foreman, M. 1997, 'Measuring cognitive states', in M. Stromberg & S. Olsen (eds), *Instruments for Clinical Health Care Research*, 2nd edn, Jones and Bartlett Publishers, Boston.

Gaskill, D., Morrison, P., Sanders, F., Forster, E., Edwards, H., Fleming, R. & McClure, S. 2003, 'University and industry partnerships: lessons from collaborative research', *International Journal of Nursing Practice*, vol. 9, no. 6, 347–55.

Gibson, T. & Heartfield, M. 2003, 'Contemporary enrolled nursing practice: opportunities and issues', *Collegian*, vol. 10, no. 1, 22–6.

Graham, I. 2002, 'Leading the development of nursing within a Nursing Development Unit: the perspectives of leadership by the team leader and a professor of nursing', *International Journal of Nursing Practice*, vol. 9, no. 4, 213–22.

Greenwood, J. 1993, 'Reflective practice: a critique of the work of Argyris & Schön', *Journal of Advanced Nursing*, vol. 18, 1183–7.

Griffiths, R., Emrys, E., Finney Lamb, C., Eagar, S. & Smith, M. 2003–04, 'Operation safe haven: the needs of nurses caring for refugees', *International Journal of Nursing Practice*, vol. 9, no. 3, 183–90.

Guba, E. & Lincoln, Y. 1981, *Effective Evaluation*, Jossey-Bass, San Francisco.

Gubrium, J.F. & Holstein, J.A. (eds) 2002, *Handbook of Interview Research: Context and Method*, Sage, Thousand Oaks.

Hall, J.M. & Stevens, P.E. 1991, 'Rigor in feminist research', *Advances in Nursing Science*, vol. 13, no. 3, 16–29.

Harper, D. 2000, 'Reimaging visual methods: Galileo to Neuromancer', in N.K. Denzin & Y.S. Lincoln (eds), *Handbook of Qualitative Research*, Sage Publications, Thousand Oaks, California, 717–32.

Healing Touch International 2000, *Healing Touch Research Survey*, HTI, Denver.

Hewitt, B. 2003, 'The challenge of providing family-centred care during air transport: an example of reflection on action in nursing practice', *Contemporary Nurse*, vol. 15, no. 1–2, 118–24.

Jackson, D., Mannix, J., Faga, P. & Gillies, D. 2004, 'Raising families: urban women's experiences of requiring support', *Contemporary Nurse*, vol. 18, no. 1–2, 97–107.

Jamieson, L. & Williams, L. 2003, 'Focus group methodology: explanatory notes for the novice nurse researcher', *Contemporary Nurse*, vol. 14, no. 3, 271–80.

Johannessen, B. 2004, 'Norwegian nurses' choices to work with alternative/complementary therapy: how will this affect their professional identity?', *International Journal for Human Caring*, vol. 8, no. 2, 48–53.

Johnson, J.M. 2002, 'In-depth interviewing', in J.F. Gubrium & J.A. Holstein (eds), *Handbook of Interview Research: Context and Method*, Sage, Thousand Oaks, 103–19.

Keatinge, D., Scarfe, C., Bellchambers, H., McGee, J., Oakham, R., Probert, C., Stewart, L. & Stokes, J. 2000, 'The manifestation and nursing management of agitation in institutionalised residents with dementia', *International Journal of Nursing Practice*, vol. 6, 16–25.

Kenefick, A. & Schulman-Green, D. 2004 'Caring for cognitively impaired nursing home residents with pain', *International Journal for Human Caring*, vol. 8, no. 2, 32–40.

Koch, S. & Lyon, C. 2001, 'Case study approach to removing physical restraint', *International Journal of Nursing Practice*, vol. 7, no. 3, 156–61.

Koskinen, L. & Tossavainen, K. 2004, 'Study abroad as a process of learning intercultural competence in nursing', *International Journal of Nursing Practice*, vol. 10. no. 3, 111–20.

Laws, T. & Bradley, H. 2003, 'Transmission of health knowledge and health practices from men to boys among Aboriginal communities and non-Indigenous Australians: searching for evidence', *Contemporary Nurse*, vol. 15, no. 3, 249–61.

Lewis, M., Pearson, A. & Ward, C. 2003, 'Pressure ulcer prevention and treatment: transforming research findings into consensus based clinical guidelines', *International Journal of Nursing Practice*, vol. 9, no. 2, 92–102.

Lincoln, Y.S. 1995, 'The making of a constructivist – a remembrance of transformations past', in C. Emden & M. Sandelowski, 'The good, the bad and the relative, part two', *International Journal of Nursing Practice*, vol. 5, no. 1, 2–7.

LoBiondo-Wood, G. & Haber, J. 1994, *Nursing Research: Methods, Critical Appraisal, and Utilization*, 3rd edn, Mosby, St Louis.

Martin-McDonald, K. 2003, 'Being dialysis-dependent: a qualitative perspective', *Collegian*, vol. 10, no. 2, 29–33.

Meleis, A.I. 1996, 'Culturally competent scholarship: substance and rigor', *Advances in Nursing Science*, vol. 19, no. 2, 1–16.

Morgan, D.L. 2002, 'Focus group interviewing', in J.F. Gubrium & J.A. Holstein (eds), *Handbook of Interview Research: Context and Method*, Sage, Thousand Oaks, 141–59.

Oliver, M. & Butler, J. 2004, 'Contextualising the trajectory of experience of expert, competent and novice nurses in making decisions and solving problems', *Collegian*, vol. 11, no. 1, 21–7.

Ormsby, A. & Harrington, A. 2003, 'The spiritual dimensions of care in military nursing practice', *International Journal of Nursing Practice*, vol. 9, no. 5, 321–7.

Polkinghorne, D.E. 1988, *Narrative Knowing and the Human Sciences*, State University of New York, Albany.

Poole, J. & Mott, S. 2003, 'Agitated older persons: nurses' perceptions and reality', *International Journal of Nursing Practice*, vol. 9, no. 5, 306–12.

Ronaldson, S. & Devery, K. 2001, 'The experience of transition to palliative care services: perspectives of patients and nurses', *International Journal of Palliative Nursing*, vol. 7, no. 4, 171–7.

Sandelowski, M. 1986, 'The problem of rigour in qualitative research', *Advances in Nursing Science*, vol. 8, no. 3, 27–37.

Schwandt, T.A. 1996, 'Farewell to criteriology', in C. Emden & M. Sandelowski, 1999, 'The good, the bad and the relative, part two', *International Journal of Nursing Practice*, vol. 5, no. 1, 2–7.

Smith, J.K. 1990, 'Alternative research paradigms and the problem of criteria', in C. Emden & M. Sandelowski, 1999, 'The good, the bad and the relative, part two', *International Journal of Nursing Practice*, vol. 5, no. 1, 2–7.

Solman, A., Conway, J. & McMillan, M. 2004, 'Stepping out: education for cardiac recovery', *Contemporary Nurse*, vol. 17, no. 1–2, 159–66.

Stake, R.E. 1994, 'Case studies', in N.K. Denzin & Y.S. Lincoln (eds), *Handbook of Qualitative Research*, Sage Publications, Thousand Oaks, California, 435–54.

Stake, R.E. 2000, 'Case studies', in N.K. Denzin & Y.S. Lincoln (eds), 2000, *Handbook of Qualitative Research*, 2nd edn, Sage, Thousand Oaks.

Strauss, A. & Corbin, J. 1990, *Basics of Qualitative Research: Grounded Theory Procedures and Techniques*, Sage Publications, Newbury Park.

Street, A. 1995, *Nursing Replay: Researching Nursing Culture Together*, Churchill Livingstone, Melbourne.

Streubert Speciale, H.J. & Rinaldi Carpenter, D. 2003, *Qualitative Research in Nursing: Advancing the Humanistic Imperative*, 3rd edn, Lippincott, Philadelphia.

Taylor, B. 2000, *Reflective Practice: A Guide for Nurses and Midwives*, Allen & Unwin, Melbourne.

Taylor, B.J. 2001, 'Identifying and transforming dysfunctional nurse–nurse relationships through reflective practice and action research', *International Journal of Nursing Practice*, vol. 7, no. 6, 406–13.

Taylor, B.J. 2006, *Reflective Practice: A Guide for Nurses and Midwives*, 2nd edn, Open University Press, UK.

Taylor, B.J., Bulmer, B., Hill, L., Luxford, C., McFarlane, J. & Stirling, K. 2002, 'Exploring idealism in palliative nursing care through reflective practice and action research', *International Journal of Palliative Nursing*, vol. 8, no. 7, 324–30.

Taylor, B., Glass, N., McFarlane, J. & Stirling, K. 2001, 'Views of nurses, patients and patients' families regarding palliative nursing care', *International Journal of Palliative Nursing*, vol. 7, no. 4, 186–91.

Titscher, S., Meyer, M., Wodak, R. & Vetter, E. 2000, *Methods of Text and Discourse Analysis*, Sage Publications, London.

Tuckett, A. & Stewart, D. 2003, 'Collecting qualitative data: Part 11 Journal as method: experience, rationale and limitations', *Contemporary Nurse*, vol. 16, no. 3, 240–51.

Turner, D. & Cox, H. 2004, 'Hope: metaphorically speaking', *Australian Journal of Holistic Nursing*, vol. 11, no. 1, 16–24.

Usher, K., Holmes, C., Lindsay, D. & Luck, L. 2003, 'PRN psychotropic medications: the need for nursing research', *Contemporary Nurse*, vol. 14, no. 3, 248–57.

van Aken, R. 2004, Emerging from Depression: The Experiential Process of Healing Touch Explored Through Grounded Theory and Case Study, Unpublished PhD thesis, Southern Cross University, Lismore, New South Wales, Australia.

Walker, A. 2002, 'Safety and comfort work of nurses glimpsed through patient narratives', *International Journal of Nursing Practice*, vol. 8, no. 1, 42–8.

Warren, C. 2002, 'Qualitative interviewing', in J.F. Gubrium & J.A. Holstein (eds), *Handbook of Interview Research: Context and Method*, Sage, Thousand Oaks, 83–101.

Wellard, S. & Rushton, C. 2002, 'Influences of spatial practices on pressure ulcer management in the context of spinal cord injury', *International Journal of Nursing Practice*, vol. 8, no. 4, 221–7.

Wikstrom, B.-M. 2002, 'Intuition and visual art: student nurses' projection into experiences of elderly people', *Australian Journal of Holistic Nursing*, vol. 9, no. 2, 24–31.

Wilkes, L. 2003, 'Ethics on the floor', *Collegian*, vol. 10, no. 2, 34–9.

Wilkes, L. & Beale, B. 2001, 'Palliative care at home: stress for nurses in urban and rural New South Wales, Australia', *International Journal of Nursing Practice*, vol. 7, no. 5, 306–13.

Wiltshire, J. 1995, 'Telling a story, writing a narrative: terminology in health care', *Nursing Inquiry*, vol. 2, no. 2, 75–82.

Wit, E., Chenoweth, l & Jeon, Y.-H. 2004, 'Respite services for older persons and their family carers in southern Sydney', *Collegian*, vol. 11, no. 4, 31–5.

Woods, L.P. 1997, 'Designing and conducting case study research in nursing', *NT Research*, vol. 2, no. 1, 48–56.

Yin, R.K. 1994, *Case Study Research*, Sage Publications, New York.

Yonge, O. & Stewin, L. 1988, 'Reliability and validity: misnomers for qualitative research', *Canadian Journal of Nursing Research*, vol. 20, no. 2, 61–7.

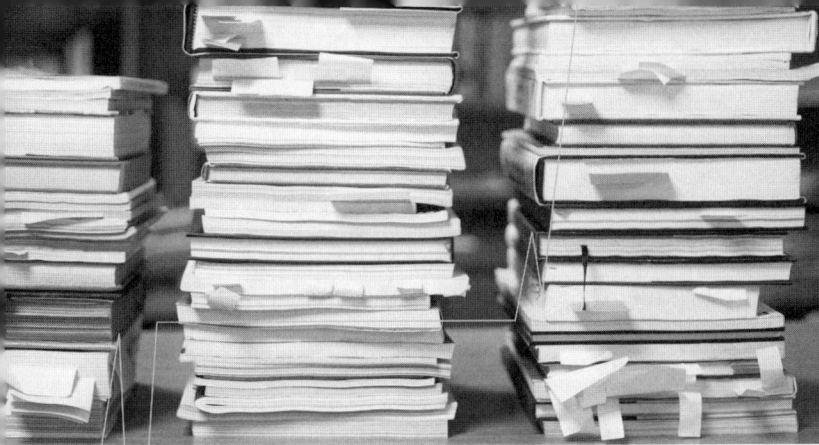

CHAPTER **15**

QUALITATIVE DATA COLLECTION AND MANAGEMENT

CHAPTER OBJECTIVES

The material presented in this chapter will assist you to:

- recognise forms of qualitative data, such as words, images and numbers
- discuss the usefulness of qualitative data in relation to context, lived experience, subjectivity and potential for change
- prepare for data collection by deciding on data forms and combinations
- use strategies for collecting the data
- recognise people, place and equipment pitfalls to avoid
- use collection hints for storing main copies and coding the data
- discuss the use of computers in collecting and storing qualitative research data.

Introduction

Research is about searching again; literally, *re-searching*, or looking again. This means that there has to be some agreed ways of going out and looking for, gathering in, and then storing the information until it is time to do something with it. You could, of course, just go out and look and make up your collection and sorting processes as you go along, but it is wise to have a plan and some well-tried strategies before you set out.

This chapter is about being practical and systematic in collecting and managing qualitative data. Some hints have been given to you already, in Chapters 12 and 13, about how to collect and manage data gathered using certain qualitative methods, so this chapter will continue the 'how to' theme of managing assorted practicalities in preparation for analysing the data.

We begin by discussing the forms of qualitative data, such as words, images and, to a lesser extent, numbers, and the usefulness of qualitative data in relation to context, lived experience, subjectivity and potential for change. This is followed by some strategies for preparing for data collection, and deciding on data forms and combinations. Then there are hints on pitfalls to avoid in the process and ideas for storing main copies and coding the data. Finally, there is some introductory discussion on the use of computers in collecting and managing qualitative data.

Forms of qualitative data

Qualitative research can offer many things to research inquiry in general, but probably the best features of its contributions lie in its stories and accounts of living, and the richness of meanings within its words. Qualitative research assists people to tell their stories about what it is like to be a certain person, living in a particular time, place and set of circumstances. This means that even the most ordinary people can do research, because if they can speak and tell stories about subjects they know best, such as their own life experiences, they can be part of qualitative research. The researcher invites them to share stories and from these stories, rich and useful data can be gleaned.

Words

The 'tools' or data for building new knowledge in qualitative research are mainly words, because they are the medium through which people express themselves and their relationships to other people and things, in and beyond their lives. As you discovered in Chapter 14, other data forms in qualitative research can include the demonstration and interpretation of artistic expression, such as painting, drawing, montage, poetry, dance, music, symbols and singing. Still photographs and videos may also be counted as data, but for the most part, qualitative research data are collected and stored in the form of words, whether they be from archival searches, case studies, field notes, group process outcomes, interview transcriptions, journal entries, literature searches, observation notes and/or written accounts of stories.

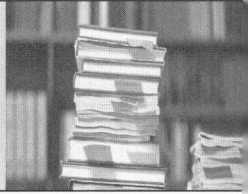

The usefulness of qualitative data

Qualitative data have a great deal to offer in the form of new and revised knowledge to researchers, through their deep and rich description of context, lived experience, subjectivity and potential for change.

Context

Qualitative data are bound to their particular context. As you may have read previously, 'context' means all of the features of the time and place in which people find themselves, and in which they locate their descriptions of things and people in their lives. People live their daily lives in the moment, yet they also remain connected to their past, and hopeful of their future. People cannot help but be placed in, and involved in, their particular time and place. In qualitative research, descriptions of contexts are useful in bringing forward new ideas about people's lives, their circumstances and the meaning they place on the events and phenomena around them. Qualitative data offer direct access to people's accounts of their experiences. Qualitative researchers consider participants' contextual appraisals as being worthy of inclusion as data in research projects.

Lived experience

Qualitative data can give researchers accounts of lived experience, which means how it is to live a life in regard to being someone or something unique. This implies that every human and every human situation is a lived experience. People live out their lives on a day-to-day basis in ways that are unique, and the level of conscious awareness of their existence may vary between people. Reflection is the key to making sense of human existence, because lived experiences accumulate and make sense as they are remembered. Thinking about what has happened and is happening to themselves and others, and of other phenomena of interest, gives people a sense of finding some meaning that is relevant to themselves and to others with whom it resonates. Therefore, qualitative data are gathered in word form to be available for analysis processes, which are congruent with the particular qualitative approach taken in the project.

Subjectivity

Qualitative data can take **subjectivity** into account. 'Subjectivity' means that which comes from the individual's sensing of inner and external things. Knowledge which comes from subjectivity does not make a universal claim to be true for everyone and for all things in all times and places; rather it refers to personal experiences and personal truths that may or may not be like other people's subjective experiences and truths. In the social world of daily life, humans take account of one another's sense of self and they share their experiences and personal truths through what is referred to as 'intersubjectivity'. When qualitative researchers are trying to understand the relationships between people, they take account of, and value, the intersubjectivity between people, as it is expressed to them in words as data.

EXERCISE

How does subjectivity fit with the postmodern idea of the importance of local narratives?

It might help to read other sections in this book on postmodernism, especially about how local, personal accounts of experience contribute to what can be considered 'truth'.

Potential for change

Gathering and analysing qualitative data has the potential for change in two main ways. In the qualitative interpretive research approaches, such as historical research and grounded theory, change can occur when people raise their awareness of something and make adaptations in their perceptions and/or actions to accommodate the new insights. In qualitative critical research approaches, such as action research and feminisms, the intention to bring about change is stated at the outset of the research, so that the methods used in the research ensure that there is a high degree of possibility for change to occur as a result of the projects.

Postmodern possibilities

While repudiating the grand narratives of qualitative interpretive and critical research approaches, postmodern thinking searches for meaning by questioning taken-for-granted assumptions about 'truth' and 'being'. Disciples of extreme forms of sceptical postmodernism would see no reasons for, or ways of, doing research, because they claim authors use their authority as writers to control and censure readers; thus the 'death of the author' halts academic inquiry. In effect, all data are as dead as the author, because words, images, meanings and symbols constitute a 'fixed system of meaning', and, as representations, they are rejected by sceptical postmodernists because they do not allow for diversity (Rosenau 1992, p. 96).

While affirmative postmodernists reduce the author's authority to offering options for public debate, they do not abandon the author completely. This position allows researchers as the authors of projects to collect data and offer tentative insights for readers' interpretations and discussion. In some readings of postmodernism, representation is permissible but in improved political forms that assist oppressed minorities and women to find voice (Armishaw & Davis 2002; Hardin 2003; Meyer & de Oliveira 2003), leaving room for participatory and emancipatory research data that focus on the specific circumstances of participants and find multiple and contradictory personal and local solutions.

Preparing for data collection

Given the rich variety of qualitative data, it may seem difficult at first to decide what to gather and store for analysis. You need to remember that the data you collect and use will be related directly to the methods you use. This means that certain methods may produce words as data, while other methods may produce photographic images or some numbers. These are the forms of qualitative data described in the section above.

Deciding on data forms and combinations

How will you decide on the forms of data you want? Believe it or not, this can be a fun part of a project, in which you get to make some decisions about the best ways of doing things. It all gets back to some very simple, yet fundamental questions: 'What do I want to know?' 'Why?' 'How will I find out the information?' The answers to these questions give you the basis for deciding on forms of data that would serve best the aims and objectives of your project. Some examples may help you to grasp the point being made here.

For the sake of continuity, the distinctions will be used that were made in previous chapters of this book between interpretive and critical forms of qualitative research. For each methodology, some methods and forms of data will be suggested (see Table 15.1, overleaf). This does not mean that these combinations are the best or only ways of looking at choosing forms of data; rather they are meant to be guidelines only, so that you can be as creative as you like when you are making decisions of this nature in your research.

> ### EXERCISE
> Imagine a clinical question you would like to explore using a qualitative research approach.
> What data forms and combinations would best serve this question?

From this exercise in setting out some of the possibilities for using qualitative data forms, you may see that data forms are basically combinations of words, images and numbers, which act as pieces of information that need to be analysed and interpreted, with the research questions, aims and objectives in mind. Therefore, your choice of data forms will depend on the nature and intentions of the research and your willingness to use combinations of methods, which will in turn produce certain combinations of data. You have to be very clear about what it is you want to explore and why, before you can be confident that the methods you choose will give you the data you need to find some insights and answers to your research questions.

Deciding on what data to collect will be determined by why you want it and how reasonable and sensible it is to access it. Therefore, it is important to think about what it is you want to know and why, before you decide on what data you will collect and how. For example, it would make a great deal of sense to arrange to talk with the actual people concerned if you want to know about their first-hand accounts of their experiences, rather than relying solely on secondary sources such as literature. Alternatively, if you are doing historical

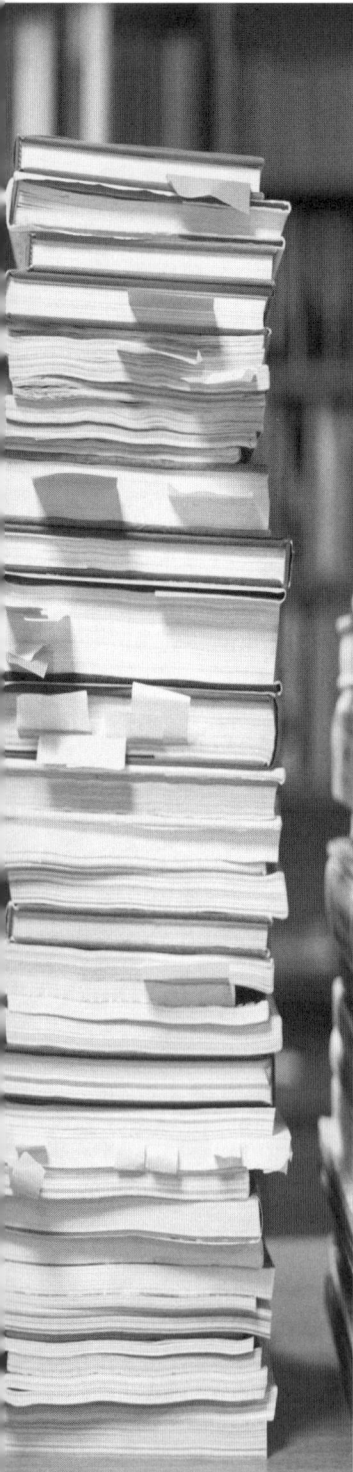

Table 15.1 Methodologies, methods and possible data forms

Methodology	Possible methods	Possible data forms
Interpretive research methodologies		
Grounded theory	Participant observation	Words, photographs
	Interviews	Words
Phenomenology	Participant observation	Words, photographs, video
	Interviews	Words
	Creative writing	Words
Historical research	Archival searches	Words, photographs
	Interviews	Words
	Document analysis	Words
Ethnography	Participant observation	Words, potographs, video
	Field notes	Words
Critical research methodologies		
Action research	Surveys	Words, numbers
	Questionnaires	Words, numbers
	Interviews	Words
	Participant observation	Words, photographs, video
	Group processes	Words
	Reflective journal	Words, drawings
Feminist research	Group processes	Words
	Interviews	Words
	Reflective journal	Words, drawings
	Surveys	Words, numbers
	Questionnaires	Words, numbers
	Creative expression	Words, painting, poetry, dance
Interpretive interactionism	Participant observation	Words, photographs, video
	Interviews	Words
	Group processes	Words
	Reflective journal	Words, drawings
Critical ethnography	Participant observation	Words, photographs, video
	Interviews	Words
	Group processes	Words
	Reflective journal	Words, drawings

research and all of the primary people sources have died, secondary sources such as relatives, friends and documents of various kinds may be your only data sources (unless you can convince the sceptics that you have communication with 'the other side').

Some qualitative approaches allow for a mixture of people and paper sources. In an oral history, for instance, you might like to augment the person's story of their life with some personal and public domain documents and photographs. These data not only add strength to the oral account, but may also give validation to what has been said, and add visual interest to the person's life story.

Having decided on the data forms that would best serve your research questions, aims and objectives, you need to spend some time thinking about how each of the data forms will be analysed and how the various forms of analysis will be integrated into producing interpretations that best express the findings of the research. Analysis will be dealt with in detail in Chapter 16. You need to realise at this point that thinking about possible ways of analysing data should begin around the same time that you are deciding on what forms of data to collect. The reason for this is that there is little point in collecting data that you do not know how to use, or which may have little or no relevance in fulfilling the aims and objectives of the research.

Strategies for collecting the data

Once you have decided on what kinds of data are needed, you then need to give consideration to how you will go about collecting them. The method of data collection may vary according to what you want to achieve in the research, and it can include single or multiple data collection methods. A selection of data collection methods was described in Chapter 14. You might like to refer to these before you continue.

Pitfalls to avoid

People problems

One of the greatest problems in any research is lack of communication. Essentially, qualitative research is people-oriented, so the best advice you can be given is that you have respect for, and be inclusive of, all the people involved. This means that before you step out to collect the data, you have observed certain basic steps, such as: you have full ethical clearance from the institutions involved; consent forms and plain language statements are prepared ready to read and sign; and people know you are coming and they know who you are, what you are doing, and what you expect from them in terms of their degree of involvement.

Sometimes you may find that you need to make several phone calls or write letters to confirm the details of the research and all of the arrangements. Even then, you may find that people do not show up, or you arrive and they have little or no idea of who you are and why you are there to talk with them. That is all right because contingency plans can be negotiated on the spot, and you can learn from those experiences to make your initial approach better the next time. As the researcher, you have the responsibility to be as clear and concise as you can be and to be prepared for any contingencies that may arise.

Place problems

Find a place to collect data that is conducive to the methods you are using. For example, if you are undertaking interviews, encourage participants to meet you in a quiet and private place so that they can speak freely and what they say can be heard clearly on the recording equipment. As a general rule, avoid busy places that have high traffic flows, banging doors and ringing phones, because they are not conducive to collecting data, unless, of course, it is the specific setting in which you intend to take field notes.

Make sure that the people in the setting who are not involved in the project know who you are and why you are there. It would be extremely unpleasant to be frogmarched out of a high security or 'closed to the public' area, which you had not gained permission to enter. If you cannot gain admission to restricted areas, negotiate another place in which to meet participants, or think of creative means by which data may be gathered. For example, once they understand what it is they are to do, and how and why, research participants may be willing to take active roles in collecting data. You may find they are willing to be involved in reflective practitioner methods, which allow them to develop critically aware means of assessing their workplaces and work practices. For example, they may be interested in keeping their own reflective journals and attending group meetings for regular discussion with you and the other participants.

EXERCISE

Think about an area in your workplace that might be considered 'off limits' to casual visits and to unannounced researchers. Plan an approach to this area, which could ensure entry and cooperation.

Equipment problems

If you are working with equipment such as audiotape recorders, tapes, videotape recorders and the like, make sure they work before you take them to your research setting. Many embarrassing and frustrating moments can be avoided by checking the energy levels of batteries, or having spares, or by buying good-quality recording tapes that do not get chewed up in the machine. When you arrive at your meeting place, set up the equipment and check that it works. If one power point does not work, try another. It is not always the case that the actual equipment is trying to sabotage your efforts. Other forces could be at work!

Collection hints

There is so much variety in qualitative data that it is difficult to speak in generalities about collecting it, but for the sake of avoiding undue repetition, we will try. One way to think of it is to remember that forms of qualitative data may be words mainly, images sometimes, and numbers occasionally or whenever mixed methods are used.

Have confidence in participants' contributions

Through experience, I have found that research participants in qualitative projects will do the best they can to give you their wholehearted accounts of their experiences, as long as they know what it is they have been asked to talk about and why. I have come to have confidence in participants' attention to the process, and I am astounded constantly by the generosity of their contributions. The researcher's part in this process is to be clear about the aims and objectives of the research (even if they are stated broadly). It is also important to be open to people, non-judgemental of their idiosyncrasies and life choices, and attentive to the basic rules and conventions of effective interpersonal communication.

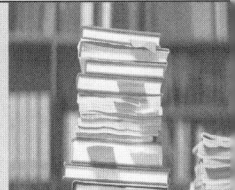

Know if you are collecting words, images and numbers, alone or in combinations

As noted previously, you are aiming to collect data in the forms of words, images and numbers, alone or in combinations. The kinds of methods that may produce words as data are participant observation, interviews, creative writing, archival searches, document analysis, open-ended responses in surveys and questionnaires, group processes and some forms of creative expression. Data as images may be produced through participant observation, archival searches and creative expression of artistic forms such as dance, painting and poetry. Qualitative research which uses mixed methods as part of the information-seeking processes may produce numbers as data through surveys and questionnaires. Ensure you know ahead of time the data forms you are collecting, so you can prepare appropriately for collecting them.

Choose the appropriate method

When using methods to collect words, images and numbers, you need to begin with some degree of confidence that the methods you are using will gather what it is you want. Going out with the inappropriate method is like going to fish for a shark with a tiddler line. It simply will not work, or if you do manage to 'land' something, it may be more trouble than it is worth. For example, if you are interviewing many participants for an hour, encourage them to agree to be audiotaped, because it will become an overwhelming process to try to capture their ideas by handwritten notes. Similarly, if non-verbal cues are important in understanding the participants' experiences, use video facilities that record all of the visual and auditory cues.

Check the usefulness of the method

All you need to do at this stage is to check, and possibly test, the validity of the method you are choosing. Ask a few friends to check over the way in which you intend to collect the data. For example, they may be willing to read through the questions you intend to ask or they may allow you to interview them. This trial run will not only allow you to see how you are coming across as a facilitator of the method, but it may also show you whether you are getting the information you want from the methods you are using. Use a checklist before collecting data.

You could also ask yourself some questions to check the ability of the method to gather the data you hope to gather. The reason you would be wise to ask yourself these questions is that they may help to ensure that the research will do what it intends to do, by means that are open and transparent to all of the people concerned. Questions may be:

- What am I exploring in this project? Why?
- What are my intentions for using this method?
- What kinds of data will it produce?
- Is the method likely to produce data that will contribute towards insights and answers to the research questions or general area of interest?
- Have I been as clear as I possibly can in telling the research participants who I am, why I'm requesting their involvement and how I would like them to contribute?
- Will I collect the information I actually want to collect; that is, will it be relevant to the project?
- What are my plans for analysis; that is, what do I intend to do to make sense of the data when I collect them?

Having decided that you are ready to go and collect the data, you need to be prepared on the day, being aware of possible people, place and equipment pitfalls to avoid.

EXERCISE

Apply the previous list of questions to the research question you imagined in the third exercise in this chapter.

Other practical hints

Some other practical hints to consider during the information-gathering sessions are to:

- introduce yourself and reiterate your gratitude for the participant's involvement
- spend some time in general talk, if necessary, to create a relaxed and open setting for the data collection
- label the data with the participant's name, time, date and setting for the collection
- keep to time – if you have told the participant that you will be taking a certain amount of time for the process, you must be aware of that, and negotiate with her/him if more time is needed
- maintain clear and open communication during the data collection

- check during the collection on the working order of any equipment you are using, to ensure that it is still doing what it is meant to do
- keep on track – this means that you need to keep focused on what it is you are doing, so the data you collect are what you want
- inform the participant when the end of the collection has come, and tell him/her what will happen next in the project, and how s/he is involved
- say 'Thank you!' and mean it, because participants' contributions to your research are an act of generosity on their part and you should acknowledge that sincerely.

Storing main copies: maintaining security and integrity

Data in the form of words, images and numbers may be stored as paper, computer disks or items of artistic expressions, such as paintings, poetry, and so on. It is no exaggeration to say that the data you collect are tantamount to a rich, raw resource; therefore, you need to treat them well to maintain their security and integrity. If you doubt this, ask some people with a PhD what they did in relation to the storage of their data. Some of the stories could be interpreted as the result of extreme anxiety related to the fear of loss of this precious information. Some researchers store paper and computer disks in the fridge, or the lining of curtains, or at a friend's house. These actions are rationalised in terms of the likelihood of theft, loss or destruction of data by fires, floods and all imaginable natural disasters. It is entirely up to you to decide what is appropriate for you in storing data.

Regardless of where you store data, they should be kept in locked storage. Security relates to ensuring that data are stored according to agreed guidelines. The NHMRC regulations for the storage of data dictate that they be stored in a locked area under the supervision of the researcher for five years after collection. Any copies of the data should be stored likewise.

Integrity refers to keeping data stored in such a way that they are maintained in their best state for use and possible review. Main copies are the 'heart' of the research; therefore, they need to be treated carefully. Transcripts, documents, photographs, computer disks, hard copies of items of artistic expression and other forms of data need to be stored in a safe place, away from potential threats such as dogs, cats, children, sun, rain, and so on. Treat the data as you would things of value to you, and their integrity should be assured. Check on their integrity from time to time and take steps to amend your storage plans if the data are not keeping as well as you intend.

Coding the data

Ethical requirements demand that data maintain the anonymity and privacy of the research participants and places. There are several ways you can do this.

Pseudonyms

You can ask the participants to suggest a pseudonym by which they would like to be known, and to select code names for organisations mentioned in the data. If they are hesitant to do this, you get the chance to make up names, and this can be fun, using the first names of friends and relatives. When the data are ready to be analysed, they can be organised according to the order in which they were collected, or according to the alphabetical ordering of the pseudonyms.

Numbering

A more impersonal way of coding the data for anonymity and privacy is to use a numbering system and to eradicate proper nouns, in relation to places. For example, the text could read: *'Participant 1 referred to her experience at the local hospital'*. Manual and computer codes may be used to hide the identities of participants and places. The researcher decides on the construction of the code, and then stores the main key to the code with the data in the locked area. Manual and computer codes can use letters, words or numbers, alone or in combination. It does not really matter what system is used, as long as it is logical and consistent throughout and has the potential to represent the data in their entirety.

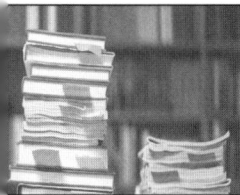

EXERCISE

Speak with qualitative researchers about the ways in which they code data to ensure participants' anonymity and privacy. Ask them why they have adopted these methods and what they do to ensure they store the main data copies safely.

Use of computers in qualitative data collection and management

Computers are incredibly useful in qualitative research because one of their main areas of expertise is in handling words through word-processing functions. Words can be written, amended, added and rearranged with ease by word processors in computers. Words are the most common data in qualitative research, and they need to be collected, stored, analysed and interpreted carefully. Computers can be useful in all of these activities.

Direct collection and storage system

Computers can be used as a direct collection and storage system, such as in field research for note-taking. It may be much simpler and more efficient to create field notes directly onto a disk than onto paper for later transfer to disk. Computer disks can be copied to ensure that there are backup versions of the data, and these can be accessed with relative ease at all stages in the research.

A means of smooth, creative thinking

Another interesting 'plus' about using computers in qualitative research is that they may soon allow researchers to take on smooth thinking processes while working with them.

That is, if you are a person who imagines that you think best by using paper and pencil, you might be surprised to find out how quickly you get over your first efforts at two-finger typing on the computer keyboard, to becoming 'at one' with the computer. I can attest to the usefulness of having research data on disk that can be arranged and rearranged and later 'cut and pasted' into a document. I was also impressed by the way I soon learned to think 'through' the computer as well, and even better than I had done before with my pencil in hand, poring over reams of paper. Try it. I hope you find it to be the case also.

Examples of computer systems

Any of the Apple and/or IBM-compatible computer word-processing systems are useful for qualitative research because of their ability to store and manage words. Some computers may also allow you to collect and store still or moving images, because they can be connected to audiovisual recording equipment and played through systems such as PowerPoint.

Disks

Computer floppy disks and CDs are sold by different companies for various prices. Be careful when buying them that they are of good quality and that they suit the computer you use. Check to see what symbol appears on the screen when you insert the disk because some may be formatted for one computer system only. For example, if you are a Macintosh user, some IBM-compatible disks may need to be formatted to Macintosh before you can store data on them without worries about opening the documents safely. Have a person who knows how, to 'step you through' converting the disk to a compatible form. Checking to ensure that the format is correct may prevent problems related to storing, reading and working with the material at a later date. Recently, floppy disk formatting has become less of an issue, because of the usefulness of CDs for data storage. Simply insert the CD and follow the instructions on your screen, or consult the guide that accompanies your computer.

Qualitative data analysis systems

Although there are many ways in which qualitative data can be analysed, there is a growing tendency to use computer systems solely, or as an adjunct to manual analysis techniques. Specific computer systems that have been used for analysis include the Macintosh word processing system Hypercard, Ethnograph (Siedel 1992) and NUD*IST (Qualitative Solutions and Research 1995). The strengths and weaknesses in using these systems will be discussed in detail in Chapter 16.

Data are usually entered into qualitative analysis systems in the form of transcripts containing sections of text prepared from the interviews, group discussions, researcher's notes and so on. The ways in which the various kinds of transcripts are prepared are specific to the requirements of the particular qualitative analysis system. Always check the instructions accompanying the system, or if that is not available, seek advice from a person who has used or created the system. You may prefer to attend a training course made available by the manufacturers/designers of the system, as this will give you a comprehensive overview of the operation of the complete package and provide you with a 'hotline' if problems arise.

Summary

This chapter intended to give you some practical and systematic strategies and hints for collecting and managing qualitative data. We discussed the forms of qualitative data, such as words mainly, some images, and the occasional use of numbers in mixed methods. Knowledge about human context, lived experience, subjectivity and potential for change were listed as the benefits in using qualitative data. These were followed by strategies for preparing for data collection, and deciding on data forms and combinations. Some hints were suggested on person, place and equipment pitfalls to avoid in collecting data and you were introduced to processes for storing main copies and coding data. Finally, there was some introductory discussion on the usefulness of computers in collecting and managing qualitative data. All of these areas may assist you in making the most sense out of the discussion on qualitative data analysis, which follows in Chapter 16.

Main points

- Research is about searching again, literally *re-searching*, or looking again, implying the need for some agreed ways of looking for, gathering in, and then storing the information until it is time to do something with it.
- Qualitative research can offer many things to research inquiry in general, but probably the best features of its contributions lie in its stories and accounts of living, and the richness of meanings within its words, which assist people to tell their stories about what it is like to be a certain person, living in a particular time, place and set of circumstances.
- The 'tools' or data for building new knowledge in qualitative research are mainly words, because they are the medium through which people express themselves and their relationships to other people and things, in and beyond their lives.
- Qualitative data can offer new and revised knowledge through their deep and rich description of context, lived experience, subjectivity and potential for change.
- Knowledge which comes from subjectivity does not make a universal claim to be true for everyone and for all things in all times and places; rather, it refers to personal experiences and personal truths, and the way humans take account of one another's sense of self and share experiences and truths through 'intersubjectivity'.
- Extreme forms of sceptical postmodernism would see no reasons for, or ways of, doing research, because they claim authors use their authority as writers to control and censure readers; thus the 'death of the author' halts academic inquiry.
- Affirmative postmodernists do not abandon the author completely, but they reduce the author's authority to offering options for public debate, thereby allowing researchers as the authors of projects to collect data and offer tentative insights for readers' interpretations and discussion.

- Qualitative data forms consist of combinations of words, images and sometimes numbers, which act as pieces of information that need to be analysed and interpreted with the research questions, aims and objectives in mind; therefore, be clear about what is to be explored and why, so the methods chosen will give relevant and appropriate data.
- Pitfalls to avoid in data collection include being aware of potential people, place and equipment problems that can be minimised by adequate foresight and planning.
- When collecting data have confidence in participants' contributions; know if you are collecting words, images and numbers, alone or in combinations; choose the appropriate method; check the usefulness of the method; and maintain effective and gracious communication throughout the interpersonal encounter.
- Data are rich, raw resources; therefore, treat them well to maintain their security and integrity.
- Code data with useful and uncomplicated pseudonyms and numbering systems.
- Computers can be used in qualitative data collection and management as direct collection and storage systems and to facilitate smooth, creative thinking.
- Specific computer systems for qualitative data analysis can manage large amounts of data tagged to participants' identities and dialogue, but they may not be able to find the finer nuances of meaning possible through manual methods.

CASE STUDY

You first met Carmel in Chapter 14. She is an experienced clinical nurse working in an acute care setting while undertaking a Master by Research program part-time with a local university. Carmel wants to research collaboratively with 10 other experienced nurses working in acute care settings about the facilitating and constraining factors they experience that influence their ability to give effective nursing care. The research aim is to explore with experienced nurses working in acute care their accounts of factors that help and hinder the delivery of effective nursing care. The objectives for the project are to: give nurses a chance to voice their experiences; identify facilitating and constraining factors in nursing work in acute care settings; and begin to accentuate facilitation and positively change the constraints, thereby improving nursing practice and patient outcomes.

In Chapter 14 you were asked to suggest data collection methods and processes to fulfil Carmel's research aim and objectives. You may have also provided a clear rationale for the combination of the methods and processes. It is now time to refine the project further and to plan for gathering data. Given that this is a clinical project with employees of the hospital, what aspects must Carmel consider carefully in gaining entry for clinical data collection? Also, given that the project relies on reflective processes, what kinds of data are the nurses likely to collect and how?

Multiple choice questions

1 The main 'tools' or data for building new knowledge in qualitative research are words because:
   a   qualitative researchers pride themselves on being good spellers
   b   words are better than numbers for demonstrating causal relationships
   c   human experience is described and defined through language
   d   qualitative researchers are not good at mathematics and statistics

2 In qualitative research, how it is to live a life in regard to being someone or something unique, is referred to as:
   a   context
   b   lived experience
   c   subjectivity
   d   postmodernism

3 Qualitative critical approaches have the potential for change because they:
   a   have a stated change agenda of mobilising direct political action
   b   demonstrate the relationship between cause and effect variables
   c   can allow change agents to predict and generalise future cases
   d   can raise people's awareness of areas that need to be different

4 Postmodern possibilities for research are present in an affirmative position, because:
   a   although the author's (researcher's) authority is reduced, the researcher is not abandoned completely
   b   they claim authors (researchers) use their authority to control and censure readers towards truth claims
   c   all data are as dead as the author (researcher), due to a 'fixed system of meaning' that inhibits human inquiry
   d   representations do not allow for diversity and thus halt academic inquiry and make all truth claims suspect

5 When conducting multiple interviews, the most effective method for collecting words is by:
   a   note-taking
   b   audiotaping
   c   photography
   d   videotaping

6 When you are collecting data from participants in qualitative research, a good practical hint is to:
   a   introduce yourself and reiterate your gratitude for the participant's involvement
   b   spend some time in general talk, to create a relaxed and open setting for data collection
   c   label the data with the participant's name, time, date and setting for the collection
   d   all of the above

7   In Australia, regulations for the storage time of human research data are set by the:
    a   REC
    b   HREC
    c   IRB
    d   NHMRC

8   In qualitative research, data are frequently coded by the use of:
    a   real surnames
    b   the participant's initials
    c   pseudonyms
    d   real middle names

9   If you have told the participant that you will be taking a certain amount of time for the data collection process:
    a   add one hour to allow for unforeseen circumstances
    b   change the time yourself within a reasonable range
    c   negotiate with her/him if more time is needed
    d   don't worry about it at all and just keep recording

10   NUD*IST is an example of a qualitative:
    a   researcher's summer retreat
    b   analysis computer system
    c   word-processing system
    d   reference storage system

Review topics

1   Given that words are the main forms of qualitative data, how are they best collected and stored?

2   Discuss how language conveys lived experience.

3   How can you ensure that your main data sources are stored safely?

4   Discuss how you will avoid the main people, place and equipment pitfalls when collecting qualitative data.

5   Discuss why effective communication is essential in collecting qualitative research data.

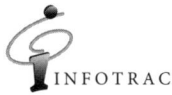

References

Armishaw, J. & Davis, K. 2002, 'Women, hepatitis C, and sexuality: a critical feminist exploration', *Contemporary Nurse*, vol. 12, no. 2, 194–203.

Hardin, P. 2003, 'Shape-shifting discourses of anorexia nervosa: reconstituting psychopathology', *Nursing Inquiry*, vol. 10, no. 4, 209–17.

Meyer, D. & de Oliveira, D. 2003, 'Breastfeeding policies and the production of motherhood: a historical-cultural approach', *Nursing Inquiry*, vol. 10, no. 1, 11–18.

Qualitative Solutions and Research 1995, NUD*IST (Non-Numerical Unstructured Data: Indexing Searching & Theorising), application software package, QSR, Melbourne.

Rosenau, P. 1992, *Post-Modernism and the Social Sciences: Insights, Inroads and Intrusions*, Princeton University Press, New Jersey.

Siedel, J.V. 1992, Ethnograph, Version 4.0, Qualis Research Associates, Corvallis, Oregon.

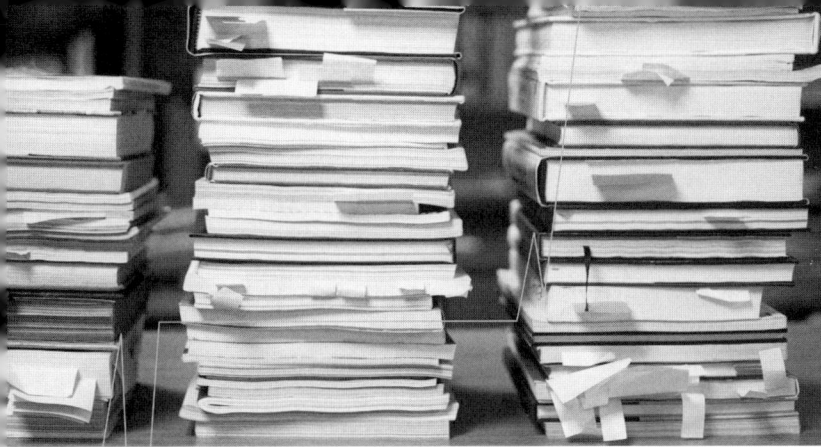

CHAPTER **16**

QUALITATIVE DATA ANALYSIS

CHAPTER OBJECTIVES

The material presented in this chapter will assist you to:

- consider some approaches for getting started in analysing qualitative data
- describe and use manual and computer-assisted methods of thematic analysis
- find explicit and implicit themes within the text
- describe narrative and discourse analysis
- be aware of benefits and constraints in using qualitative data computer analysis systems
- locate examples of completed qualitative analyses
- describe the analysis of images as qualitative data.

Introduction

The main data derived from qualitative research methods are words. In Chapter 14 you may have noticed that much reliance is placed on the trustworthiness of language. This is because language is the main way in which qualitative researchers make sense of the answers to the questions they pose in their projects about human phenomena. This reliance on language is in contrast to the main approach of quantitative research methods, which tend to trust the value of numbers as tools for analysis.

However, you may remember that things are not so 'black and white' as to assume that 'words equal qualitative' and 'numbers equal quantitative'. Be cautious about categorising research approaches too quickly into specific methods. Remember that qualitative researchers may also use a mixture of methods, and place their trust in words and numbers, to produce new or amended knowledge about a thing of interest to them.

In this chapter, we will deal with some practical hints for qualitative analysis. It will be assumed that words are the main data for analysis, and the chapter will deal most comprehensively with their analysis. A small part of the text will be devoted to the analysis of images as data. For help in how to analyse numbers as data, refer to Chapter 10, where it is dealt with most comprehensively.

You may find that research books and researchers are seldom useful in telling potential researchers how to undertake a method of qualitative analysis. I suspect that this is because it may all seem too simple if it is described step by step, or perhaps some researchers may prefer to hold onto the mystery and the power of creating complexities. So, for the most part, much of what follows is a compilation of hints and strategies that have worked for me over the years. I hope that you will find them helpful.

Approaches to analysing qualitative data

The good news is that qualitative research has 'come of age' in academia, and to a lesser extent in health care settings. For example, acceptance has come about in nursing because of debates of the 1960s and 1970s (Henderson 1964; Kratz 1978), the assertiveness about paradigmatic change in the 1980s and 1990s (Allen 1985; Chinn 1985; Goodwin & Goodwin 1984; Kermode & Brown 1995; Winstead-Fry 1980) and the postmodern age of valuing multiple discourses (Anderson, McAllister & Moyle 2002; Gilbert 2003; Glass & Davis 1998; Hardin 2003).

EXERCISE

Ask your colleagues about whether they think qualitative research is accepted as real research in your health care discipline. Ask them to explain their answer.

The coming of age of qualitative research

Be confident that qualitative research is *real* research. Qualitative research is judged by qualitative criteria and deemed to be of value by readers who understand and value the knowledge-producing and verifying assumptions of qualitative research.

EXERCISE

What are the knowledge-producing and verifying assumptions of qualitative research? It may help you to describe these criteria by reviewing the differences in quantitative and qualitative research in Table 12.1 in Chapter 12.

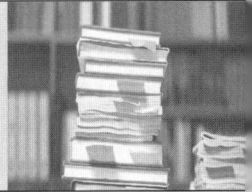

However, although qualitative research has come of age, that does not mean it is beyond critique. It is a positive measure of scholarship to welcome critique. Qualitative research continues to be criticised and even dismissed or invalidated by some researchers. Quantitative researchers may not know about the philosophical debates that questioned the use of the scientific method as the only way of generating knowledge in human inquiry. This means these researchers continue to use quantitative criteria for judging the worthiness of all research projects. For example, some human research ethics committees may be composed solely or mainly of members who are schooled only in quantitative research approaches. Understandably, these people question the worth of qualitative research on many lines, including its assumptions about knowledge, and sample size, subject selection, data collection and analysis methods.

Researchers who use qualitative approaches may also judge a project against the particular assumptions of their favoured theoretical orientation. For example, a researcher using a critical approach such as action research or critical ethnography may criticise an interpretive approach for failing to deal with issues of power and domination. In contrast, an interpretive approach may criticise critical qualitative research for being unduly dismal and sceptical and failing to fulfil its promises of emancipation.

Interestingly, even with the relative acceptance of qualitative research and the claim that it has 'come of age', another phenomenon has appeared in health care. Health care agencies in 'developed countries' around the world are embracing evidence-based practice (Courtney 2005; Dawes et al. 2005). As you may have discovered by reading Chapter 1 of this book, the data judged as the best evidence are quantitative in nature. This is related to the kinds of cause and effect research questions that are most urgent and thus important in health care, such as: What is the cause of this disease? What is the cure for this disease? So, even though the health care industry may be more open to qualitative research, it nevertheless continues to prefer quantitative research approaches that create data in numbers and mathematical relationships, that are deemed to be more objective and reliable than words and phrases.

The orientation of the qualitative researcher

It is suggested that you make a personal approach to qualitative research analysis with an attitude of respect for people, their experiences and words, and have confidence in finding meaning in them. Your attitude may not be this magnanimous at first, but with practice and experience, a respectful and confident attitude will develop over time. If you have chosen your methods wisely, and the research participants know what it is you want to know and why, the data you collect are likely to have some insights and answers to your questions.

Being ready physically and emotionally

Qualitative analysis requires that you read, look and listen to language with wakeful alertness. This means that you need to be feeling physically and emotionally fresh before you try to do the analysis, so choose a time of day when you know you are feeling the best. It might also help to use some sort of centring technique to get you into a mood that allows you to be fully present. For instance, if you meditate, spend some time relaxing with your particular technique.

If you are not conversant with meditation or other forms of relaxation, try this simple visualisation. Stand upright with your feet flat on the ground. Imagine that you are a tree. Feel your roots going deep into the ground. Feel the gentle wind in your branches. Allow yourself to experience this sense of stability for a few minutes of silence, and then, when you are ready, begin your work.

Getting started

The words you have collected may be stored in hard copies or on computer disks. How to take care of them has been discussed in Chapter 15. The time has now come to organise the data ready for analysis.

Make copies

Begin by making copies of all of the data, in whatever forms they are stored. Ensure that you keep the original copy to one side and stored carefully, with identifying details and the date written clearly on it. The duplicated copy can be labelled: 'Working Copy', to differentiate it as the copy on which the analysis will be done. Be sure to update and label copies as your work progresses, so that you do not become confused by differing versions of the same electronic document.

Decide on an organising system

Decide on a system for organising the paper or computer files. You may need to buy some manila folders or boxes to store paper files in their respective bundles, or you might need to code and name each computer file according to the content of data stored therein. The principle to keep in mind is the need to be practical and careful in getting the data ready for analysis. Choose an organising system that suits you best and be prepared to make adaptations to that system if it is not serving you well.

Have confidence in words as data

If you have been careful in the choice and implementation of the research methods, you can be fairly confident that within the words collected as data are the answers to the questions you have posed. If you have spoken with research participants who have responded well to the invitation to speak of their experiences and you have been careful to ask the sort of questions that will give them a chance to supply the answers you need to fulfil your research objectives, then you will probably be amazed and somewhat humbled at the magnitude and richness of the textual information which people will offer.

When you are collecting data, for example, by audiotaping interviews, you may not always be aware of the richness in the detail of what participants say. This might be because you are intent on listening to the account, or your mind is checking that the interview is progressing as intended. You might be pleasantly surprised to find that there is much more in the recorded words than you first thought.

EXERCISE

Using an audiotape, interview a friend for five to 10 minutes about a topic of your choice. Ensure the topic explores your friend's experience of something that can be analysed. For example, the topic may be: The experience of being healthy/unwell/fulfilled/hopeful/grieving/a research student/and so on.

The essential research question then becomes: What is the experience of . . . ? When you are both ready and the audiotape is recording, ask: 'Think of a time when you felt/were . . . Tell me about it please'. If your friend needs help to keep talking, give conversational prompts, such as: 'You were saying before that . . . Tell me more about that please'.

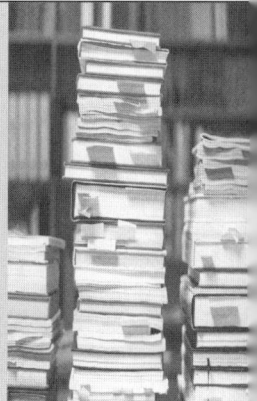

Methods of thematic analysis

One overarching approach to identifying the answers to research questions embedded in the data is a method called **thematic analysis**. As you might guess, thematic analysis simply means a method for identifying themes, essences or patterns within the text. In this case, text refers to the selection of words with which you are working. An interesting observation is that many researchers may talk about thematic analysis, but when it comes down to it, very few of them are able or willing to communicate to you just what it is they do to find the themes, essences or patterns within the text. Even when they tell you that they used a specific method (for example, Leininger 1985; Sarnecky 1990; Spradley 1979; Strauss 1987), and you go to the source and read about it, more often than not you may still be none the wiser as to how to actually go about doing the analysis. This chapter hopes to remedy that situation to some extent.

Methods appropriate to intentions

Qualitative analysis of words may be by either manual or computer-assisted means. The intentions of the analysis will determine what is done with the words. For example, researchers with exploratory and descriptive intentions may use analysis methods that produce groups of themes and sub-themes. Although there is no strict prescription, these methods are helpful because they allow a descriptive interpretation of human experiences. Practical guides for manual and computer-assisted methods of data analysis are described in this chapter.

Researchers with intentions to bring about changes may prefer critical analyses of discourses and the other economic, political, cultural, social and historical determinants. These analyses may involve thematic approaches, but with extra scrutiny to bring into awareness silences and gaps in the discourse, as well as issues of power and domination. Methods that provide analysis for qualitative critical research approaches based on critical social science, and for research influenced by poststructural and postmodern thinking, are described in this chapter.

EXERCISE

Transcribe the audiotape of the five- to 10-minute interview you undertook with your friend in the previous exercise. This process will work best if you use the pause button on the audiotape to play and type sections of text straight into a word-processing document in your computer. If you are not a speed typist, you will now see why the instruction was to keep the interview to five to 10 minutes, because transcribing takes time and effort.

Finding explicit and implicit themes within the text

It is one thing to tell you to find themes; it is yet another thing for you to feel confident that you can. Be aware also, that themes may be known by other names, but they are essentially the same thing. For example, in grounded theory, a sub-theme is similar to a code and a theme is similar to a category. Themes may also be called essences or aspects in approaches such as phenomenology. The following hints on how to find themes, however named, may help you, regardless of whether you use a manual or a computer-assisted method of thematic analysis.

Know what you are looking for

The first 'rule' when looking for themes is to know what you are looking for! It sounds so obvious, but it can be so difficult to remember. Before you start looking for themes, review your research proposal. What are the research project's aims and objectives? Keep those ideas firmly in your mind as you go about finding themes. Why? So that you will recognise a theme when you see one! It is easy to become sidetracked once you get in among the thick undergrowth of the data. Keep your aims and objectives in mind so you find what you set out to find.

Locate specific words for explicit themes

If you are searching for specific words or combinations of words, it is a relatively simple task to look for their appearance within sections of the text. The word 'health' for instance, will figure keenly in a discussion about health promotion. This is an **explicit theme**, in that it may float with relative ease to the top of a well of words when doing an analysis. Explicit themes are apparent because they provide direct answers to direct research questions, so they speak out loudly when you are reading, and unless you are becoming tired or otherwise uninterested, it is difficult to miss them.

Look closely for implicit themes

It is important to recognise that a theme will not always be stated as a direct word or words, or even as an easily recognisable concept. Take the example of health, for instance. People might talk about feeling 'good', 'well', 'happy', 'energised', 'bountiful', and so on. There may be no mention at all of health-like words, but rather a story, an innuendo, a hint, or a fine wisp of language that portrays a health-related situation.

So how will you recognise an **implicit theme**? You will recognise it because of the way it fits into the total context of what has been said. By now, you may be very familiar with the transcript, so you will be ever watchful for what it can tell you. An implicit theme may lie like a fine weave in the tapestry of the conversation. When you locate it you know that you have it, because its fine threads will be connected with other parts of the text and you will see where they began and where they finished. It will be a joyful discovery and it will fire you up to look for more.

Be sure it is a theme

How can you be absolutely sure that you have located an explicit and/or implicit theme? Well, how do you know it is a fish on the line when you go fishing? It is a similar problem. You will know you have located a theme because it bears resemblance to what you thought you might find; that is, it appears to have within it some features of the thing for which you are looking. It might not look exactly like the whole thing for which you are looking, but you will know that it is related because it comes up in front of your awareness in answer to the questions you have been posing as you analyse the text for signs of it. It is part of the pattern of answers you are intending to find within the text, and you know it is relevant because its identity is connected directly and sometimes indirectly to the stated research aims and objectives.

Now that you have some idea of how to recognise a theme when you see one, we will discuss two main ways of approaching thematic analysis; that is, through manual and computer-assisted methods.

EXERCISE

Review the previous section from the heading: Getting started. Prepare yourself and the transcribed document as suggested.

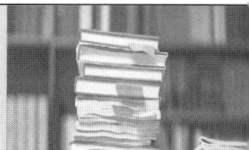

Manual approaches

Even in this age of technology, it is still reasonable to choose to analyse qualitative data by manual methods. It is entirely a matter of what you prefer and what is the best way for you to handle the data carefully and effectively. Qualitative research tends to produce a great many words stored on a lot of paper, so if you choose a manual method of analysis, you need to be sure that you are systematic about the way in which you handle the data. As mentioned previously, to chart a course through these data, you will need to document your analytical progress by a tagging system called thematic identification. It will show the pathway through which you made sense of the words and put them into some order for interpretation.

Review the research aims and objectives

The first thing is to remember why you have researched what you have researched. This is not only to give you a renewed sense of commitment to the project, but also to revive for you the main purposes of the research. What did you say you would do in the research? Why and how? Revisit the words you wrote in your proposal and centre on the key ideas to make sure you are clear about what it is that needs to emerge from the information you have amassed from the research participants. This means you will need to look again at the statements you made about the aims and objectives of the research, and keep these in mind while you are doing the analysis.

Read and reread

Having gained a refreshed and refocused view of the research objectives and strategies, begin by reading and rereading the text. As you may suspect, there is likely to be a lot of information in the transcripts, some of which is useful directly, and some of which may need to be stored away for another time. There are many ways to proceed at this point and these are some of them. Feel free to be creative in adjusting the following suggestions to suit yourself. Remember that there is no one way to do this, and that as long as you are clear about the research aims and objectives, you can adjust the analysis methods to fit the unique requirements of the project and its participants.

Make multiple copies

Number the pages of your transcript either sequentially from '1' onwards or using a number number (1-1, 1-2 etc.) or letter number (A-1, A-2 etc.) combination to number each transcript or each group of transcripts. Make multiple copies of the page-numbered transcripts. Ensure one copy is kept untouched as a guide. It is a good idea to put a large column on the left of the page in which to write notes about ideas that come to mind. You might like to have the audiotape of the interview playing as you read the transcripts, so that you can capture the intonations and emphases of the speakers' words.

Know the text thoroughly

Read the transcripts one by one. Be ready to pick up the nuances in the text. Endear yourself to the text so that you come to know it thoroughly. You may have to read it many times over to get to this stage of familiarity. As you attend to the text, remember the research question and/or objectives, so that your attention falls on the relevant words, phrases, sections of dialogue, and gross and fine connections between parts of the document.

Allow time for it to come together

Do not try to catch the whole of the meaning in an instant, or even in the first protracted sitting. Let the information percolate and incubate in your mind for a while. When you relax from reading, you may watch with interest as the connections start to pop into your mind, sometimes at the most inopportune moments – you may be at home involved in your family life and find your mind drifting to the research. Researchers sometimes speak of waking during the night and writing down an insight, or making a hurried note on a paper serviette in a restaurant.

The 'pile on the kitchen table' method

What you do next will depend on what you like to do when you 'play' with the intention of focusing your thinking. You can do the 'pile on the kitchen table' method, in which you cut out any sections of text that appear to be connected to a theme and arrange them in mounds. After you have amassed various groupings, try to reduce them into fewer groups, so that the essential themes that remain are those that cannot be subsumed into other categories without losing some of their meaning. Do not attempt this method near children, pets or open windows because accidents can happen at this point!

The 'colour coding' method

You might prefer the 'colour coding' method, in which you collect a wide range of coloured pens and go through the text marking in colour codes those words, ideas, sections and/or nuances that appear to be connected.

The 'changing font' method

You can work with a transcript to indicate relevant parts that seem to be parts of themes, by changing the font type and/or size. For example, all information relating to Objective 1 may be in Palatino 12 and all information for Objective 2 may be in Times 14. All you need to do is ensure you are aware of the font coding, so you can work effectively with the transcript later.

Finding the right word

When you have the kitchen table covered in piles, completed the colouring, and/or adjusted the fonts, go back to place a card containing a word or words on top of each pile or write a word or words in the column beside each colour or font to capture the main idea represented. List the words and review and then reduce the list so that similar ideas merge into groups. You have reached the limits of the reduction when you can no longer move ideas without losing some of their specialness in relation to the research. What remain (because they defy further movement into groupings) are the distinct themes.

The concise version of the manual thematic method

In point form, here is 'how to do' a manual thematic identification of research themes:
- Read and reread the text.
- Make multiple copies of the page-numbered transcripts.
- Ensure one copy is kept as a guide.
- Keep in mind the research question and/or objectives.
- *Either* cut out any sections of text that appear to be connected to a theme and arrange the cut-out bits in mounds, then try to reduce them into groupings that cannot be subsumed into other categories without losing some of their meaning; *or* use the 'colour coding' or 'changing font' method, marking in colour codes or fonts those words, ideas, sections and/or nuances that appear to be connected.
- Find a word or words to capture the ideas in each pile or to represent each colour or font.
- List all the words and review them.
- Reduce the list so that like ideas merge into respective groupings.
- You have reached the limits of the reduction when you can no longer move ideas without losing some of their specialness in relation to the research. These are your themes.

EXERCISE

Using the suggestions in the section above, and beginning with the heading: Manual approaches, undertake an analysis of your friend's experience. Try any or all of the methods suggested to analyse what the experience is like for your friend. When you have completed the manual analysis, show it to your friend to see if the themes resonate with her/him.

Computer-assisted approaches

If you are not into paper cut-outs, colouring in or changing fonts, you might like to try some computer-assisted and hard copy strategies for finding themes. Computers are helpful particularly to the qualitative researcher, because they have the ability to move mountains of words around documents with the greatest of ease.

Make a disk copy

Start by making a disk copy of the main text to be analysed. (If you have developed research neurosis, the chances are that you will have multiple disk copies stored all over your home or office!) Remember, if you have been clear with your participants about what you wanted to know from them, the chances are that they will have given you the information you need.

It will be all there in the transcripts. All you have to do is to locate these ideas in the participants' language.

Tidy the transcript

If you are working with a transcript of an interview, drop off any extraneous details from the copy, such as side conversations or comments not central to the research, and also 'ums', 'ahs' and 'ohs'. Some people are loath to drop these linguistic hesitations, but unless the research is looking at these things directly, say in a study of the lived experience of hesitation (this is a joke), they serve no purpose except to make the participant sound awkward, to impinge on the flow of language and to thicken the text with irrelevancies. If you feel nervous about dropping extraneous details, even on a copy, listen to your intuition, because it is probably trying to tell you that something lurks there that is far from extraneous. Remember though, that participants often read their own transcript for validation purposes. In my experience, many participants have remarked that they sounded awkward and unintelligent when every um and ah was left in their transcript for them to read.

Read and section

Start from the beginning of the sequence to be analysed and read through the text as it scrolls on the computer screen. You may have become very conversant with the information already through reading and rereading, so this is another chance for extra insight. As parts of the text relating to the research interests appear, section them off under a subheading that is relatively descriptive. As you progress through the document, you may find that 'sectioning' the document through the use of headings and subheadings can help you to organise the text and create connections between themes that are raised in one part of the text and reiterated in another part. In a practical sense, 'sectioning' is as simple as pressing the 'return' key several times to push a chunk of text several lines down to isolate it for separate consideration. This will provide some direction through the document and chart the course of ideas as they emerge from the information. Use your spontaneity to use creative subheadings, but keep the meaning as direct as possible to what appears underneath the subheading. The subheadings and general labels may contain some actual words that appear in the text or a short phrase that reflects most closely the explicit content and implicit meaning of the sectioned text.

Look for themes

As you work slowly and systematically through the scrolling document, look for explicit and implicit themes, as described previously. Explicit themes may pop up conspicuously, while implicit themes may hide away for a time. As you read sections of the text, ask yourself: 'What is this saying?' 'Is there anything here that relates to my research aims and objectives?' 'Is there anything here connected implicitly to what I have read before?'

It may be possible to locate themes straight away as you proceed through the analysis, or you may find sub-themes as you continue looking for explicit and implicit ideas. Sub-themes are related to main themes, and they are like subsections, or further elaborations on a theme. Do not become overly concerned at the first 'run through' about trying to find all there is to find, because some of the sub-themes and implicit themes may remain hidden until later. At this stage, do not even worry about whether they are themes or sub-themes, because you can sort that out later too.

Be aware of your feelings

As you go through the analysis, be aware of any emotions you may be feeling as the researcher. Analysis can be a fairly taxing and tiring experience, so be sensitive to how you are feeling, and why that might be. For example, do not become too disheartened if you think you are not finding enough. Sometimes one or two themes may be hidden in a mountain of data. Remember it is quality you are after, not quantity.

If the analysis process seems to be getting 'all too much' for you, it might be a good idea to take a rest from analysis for a while, and go outside for a walk, or create some space from the task until you feel fresh and ready again. Also, remember not to let 'your feelings get in the way'. This means that you must be diligent to ensure that the analysis is what the participants' accounts reflect, not what you are hoping to find. Another way of expressing this is: Don't impose your own biases upon the text.

Review after a break

When you return to the analysis, begin at the start of the document again, so that you can remind yourself of where you are and how you got there. It is a way of refreshing yourself about the context of the analysis before you go on to make further progress, or to finish a particular part of the analysis overall. Work through the document as described before, looking carefully for themes and 'sectioning' text into serviceable and practical chunks, until you come to the point where you consider you have analysed the document.

Be patient with the first run through

What you will have at this stage is a copy of the working document, which may have some headings, subheadings, themes and sub-themes, alone or in various combinations. In other words, it still looks a bit messy. Remember, it is the essence and basis of the final analysis. Now you need to tidy the working document and collate the actual themes.

Collate the themes

This is where a computer is useful, because you can copy all of the working document so easily, ready for its transformation. In order to collate the themes within the text you can copy the entire analysis of what you have just done (with its headings, subheadings, themes and sub-themes, alone or in various combinations). Paste that copy of the document into the end of the working document, so that you have the same document twice on one file. Alternatively, you might prefer to create a new file. This now means that you have the working document duplicated, so that you can make the next refinements.

Now, go through and drop off everything in the second, or duplicated copy of the analysis to date, except the subheadings, themes and sub-themes that you generated previously.

Review the list and concentrate on the research interest again by asking yourself: 'What does this say about the research interest?' The answers to this question, or others phrased in a similar vein, will give you the themes for the research. As you ask this question, look for connections between the words and phrases you see listed there. Do some of them look similar? Are they similar enough to be merged together without losing their essential identity? If yes, put them together. If no, leave them separate.

You keep going through this thinking, shifting and collating process until everything settles into the place it fits best, in relation to the original questions you posed in your project, and the aims and objectives you had in relation to them. When it has all come to its steady state, you have your thmes.

Name the themes

You can name the themes whatever you want. You have done the work, so this is your right and responsibility. Spare a thought, however, for the readers of your research by not making the theme names too obscure or exotic. Humour and/or simplicity are permissible in naming themes, so feel free to think creatively. Remember, though, to allow the name of the theme to reflect its nature, otherwise you could end up in the silly situation of naming the theme inappropriately, and this will be of little use to anyone trying to make sense of your project.

EXERCISE

Using the suggestions in the section above, and beginning with the heading: Computer-assisted approaches, undertake an analysis of your friend's experience. When you have completed the computer-assisted analysis, show it to your friend, to see if the themes resonate with her/him. Which analysis method do you prefer – the manual or the computer-assisted method? Why?

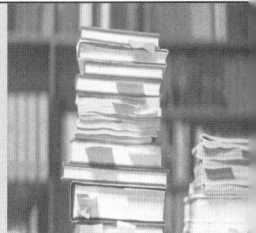

Combine to form common themes

The method of analysis thus far is useful for a single text analysis; however, if you have interviewed a number of people, you may want to analyse each transcript separately and then combine the group accounts to find common themes. This is just a simple matter of attending to each transcript as described above and making a document for each participant. Go through each document and attend to the analysis as described previously. When all of the documents have been analysed separately, if you want to combine them to find common themes, do this by duplicating the final versions of the separate analyses on a computer and putting them together in one file.

The aim of the collective analysis is to find the ideas that are different enough to remain in their own categories. If themes are similar, merge them. For example, if women say that they are happy, sad, confused and so on, these are all emotions. Incorporate these ideas under one heading of 'emotions' and be sure to include in your description of the theme, what the term means and what elements are included. In other words, you make your own definition of the theme based on what you have incorporated within it and what it has come to mean through the analysis process.

A good idea when naming common themes is to write a short phrase consisting of a verb and noun that reflects the participant's experience and is consistent with the project's focus. For example, when I asked people with arthritis how they managed their lives (Taylor 2001), they gave accounts that had within them themes that were indeed their daily strategies, such as managing mornings, ensuring personal comfort, keeping a positive attitude, doing housework, cooking meals, getting exercise, existing in day-to-day life, and so on.

The concise version of the computer-assisted method

The words taken to describe some ways of doing computer-assisted analyses are many, so to reiterate in point form:

- Make a disk copy of the main text to be analysed.
- Drop off any extraneous details from the copy, such as 'ums' and so on.
- Read through the text as it scrolls on the computer screen.
- Section the text off under subheadings that are relatively descriptive.
- As you progress through the document, make connections between themes that are raised in one part of the text and reiterated in another part.
- Collate the themes.
- Review the list while asking yourself: 'What does this say about my research interest?'
- Name the themes meaningfully.
- For multiple interviews analyse each transcript separately and then combine the accounts to find common themes.
- Define the themes and describe their components.

Other methods of text analysis

In qualitative research, words make up the texts, language and discourses that carry the meaning of human experience. Qualitative data analysis seeks to scrutinise and organise words in light of the research objectives and the particular methodological assumptions about the approach taken. Methods of data collection and analysis are not bound by methodologies; that is, a qualitative approach such as ethnography does not 'own' participant observation, and action research does not 'own' participatory group processes. Even though these two examples are known to use selected methods often, they do not always use them, nor do they exclude other possible methods. With this in mind, there are other analytic methods that can be used in a variety of approaches stretching across and beyond methodologies and research paradigms, such as **narrative analysis** and **discourse analysis**.

Narrative analysis

Storytelling is a popular method of qualitative data collection, for all of the reasons cited in Chapter 14. Making sense of the stories can be through a variety of methods (Labov 1972;

Linde 1993; Polanyi 1989), including thematic analysis as described in this chapter. If you are choosing a storytelling/narrative approach to your project, you are well advised to spend some time searching the literature for the particular approach you need to best suit your research questions, aims and objectives. For example, Cortazzi (2001, p. 385) suggests that narrative analysis in ethnography involves 'concern with the meaning of experience, voice, human qualities of personal or professional dimensions, and research as story'. Whereas, in analysing personal narratives, many approaches may be taken, for example, Riessman (2002) described analysing personal narratives as performance. She describes the analytic strategy thus:

> To make the process visible, we can analyse scenes in relation to one another, how narrators position characters and themselves, and we can 'unpack' the grammatical resources they select to make their moral points clear to the listener. Interpretation requires close analysis of how narrators position audiences, too, and, reciprocally, how the audience positions the narrator. Identities are constituted through such performative actions, within the context of the interview itself as a performance. Audiences, of course, may 'read' events differently than narrators do, resulting in contested meanings (Riessman 2002, p. 704).

Another way of looking at narrative analysis is to consider the ways in which stories told in interviews can be analysed. An interview can be converted to a story by amending the text to make the participant's words paramount. If you are considering creating stories from interview transcripts, a useful method of 'core story creation' is described by Emden (1998, p. 35), who suggests the following steps:

1   Read the full interview text several times within an extended timeframe (several weeks) to grasp its content.
2   Delete all interviewer questions and comments from the full interview text.
3   Delete all words that detract from the key idea of each sentence or group of sentences uttered by the respondent.
4   Read the remaining text for sense.
5   Repeat steps 3 and 4 several times until you are satisfied that all key areas are retained and all extraneous content is eliminated. Return to the full text as often as necessary to recheck.
6   Identify fragments of constituent themes (subplots) from the ideas within the text.
7   Move fragments of themes together to create one coherent core story, or series of core stories.
8   Return the core story to the respondent and ask: 'Does it ring true?' and 'Do you wish to correct/develop/delete any part?'
    Having created a core story, the next analysis task is emplotment, which is:

> a process of working with one or more plots of a story in such a way that the significance of the story is disclosed; that is, emplotment ascribes some sense to a story – at potentially different levels of complexity (Emden 1998, p. 36).

At the practical level of how to manage emplotment, Emden (1998) explains that she tracked the plots

aided by pencil and paper as I sought to keep track of the best fit possibilities between events as described by the participants and the emergent plot ... identified by me. This moving back and forth helped ensure that a preconceived plot structure was not imposed on events (p. 37).

In tracking plots, you could use pencil and paper, or you might prefer to mark the text with highlighter pens so that each story line through the transcript appears in a particular colour. Alternatively, if you are adept at reading from a computer screen, you may be able to convert sections of text in the same plot into a different font type and size, thereby indicating different tracks of various plots.

Searching carefully through text in this way will eventually locate sets of events that are common to all stories, that 'grasp together as one story' (Polkinghorne 1988, in Emden 1998, p. 37). Thus, the events as related by participants (storytellers) constitute the contexts of the stories, and the task of narrative researchers is to undertake an analysis that will 'make sense of all the events as one story' (Emden 1998, p. 37).

In summary, there are many ways of doing narrative analysis, just as there are many reasons and modes for telling stories. When you are intending to use a narrative approach in your research, explore the literature to locate descriptions of specific forms of narrative analysis. Then, you will be able to apply the most appropriate one to your research data.

EXERCISE

Audiotape yourself telling a story or a series of stories about an experience in your life which was of great significance to you. Remembering that interview transcription takes time and effort, decide on how long you will take to tell the story/stories and keep yourself to the allocated time.

Use the Riessman (2002) quote at the start of this section to inform your approach to analysing your personal narrative as performance. This means that you will analyse 'scenes' in relation to one another, how you position other characters and yourself in your story, the language you use to make your moral points clear, and the way you have written for whomever may read the story/stories.

Discourse analysis

Discourse and discourse analysis have different meanings according to the contexts in which they are applied. In a general sense, discourse means a series of written or spoken utterances with a formal and organised connotation, such as in a dissertation, lecture, sermon, conversation or text on a certain subject. In effect, discourses as systems of statements can be on any topic. In nursing and health care there are multiple discourses on the knowledge and skills clinicians need to practise effectively, such as evidence-based practice, practice guidelines, and various diagnostic approaches.

Also, the words discourse and discourse analysis are used in many ways in research reports. For example, in reporting their research about student nurses developing a professional identity in the workplace, Grealish and Trevitt (2005, p. 137) refer to 'academic and student discourse in the practicum'. By this reference they do not mean 'discourse analysis' in the Foucauldian sense used in this section. They are using discourse to mean what the participants said about their experiences. Their research used an interpretive methodology of constructivism to analyse focus group contributions. Therefore, even though discourse has become commonplace in recent research literature, be aware that the usage and meaning of the word can differ. You really will not know the specific meaning of the word until you look into how the researchers are using it in the context of their project.

Although opinions vary on the constitution of discourse analysis, a name appearing almost routinely in discourse analyses is that of Michel Foucault, a philosopher whose work has had a profound influence on researchers since the 1980s (see more about Foucault in Chapter 13). The method of discourse analysis used in this section is influenced by my 'reading' of the work of Foucault (1980).

Interpretations of some Foucauldian thought

The rules of discursive practices form and maintain discourses that in turn constitute power and knowledge relationships. For example, ethical requirements in research projects maintain the power bases of people on committees, who may favour particular design approaches and methodologies and thus obstruct the passage of those projects that do not fit the discourse judged by them to be important and appropriate.

Knowledge that counts as 'truth' is that which has won recognition in a culture as being successful and thus has gained and exercised power. For example, biomedical technology has been so highly successful in treating diseases that the powerful discourse of medicos has influenced other members of the health team to the extent that biomedical discourse is the benchmark by which effective patient management is judged. The power-knowledge of biomedical discourse is immersed in the culture of health care settings, especially those organised around hierarchies and bureaucracies that exercise the power of 'ownership' of human health care by experts.

Power can operate in many directions in micro-levels of a culture and people, through their knowledge, can change their subject positions to disrupt and challenge power relations. Therefore, power-knowledge not only maintains existing 'truth', but it can also shift, circulate, spread and change. For example, nurses and physiotherapists are not necessarily bound by biomedical discourses, as they too can exercise their power-knowledge by changing their subject positions in the health care team, as individuals capable of resistance against injustice.

EXERCISE

What are some of the rules of discursive practices (the way people talk and relate together) in your work setting? In what ways are these discursive practices maintained and how do they form and direct power and knowledge relationships?

A 'poststructural process'

A **Foucauldian-style discourse analysis** is a complex undertaking because it requires 'careful reading of entire bodies of text and other organising systems (such as taxonomies, commentaries and conference transcriptions) in relation to one another in order to interpret patterns, rules, assumptions, contradictions, silences, consequences, implications, and inconsistencies' (Powers 1996, p. 211).

If you are intending to use a Foucauldian-style discourse analysis you would be well advised to read widely in Foucault's writing (for example, Foucault 1972, 1975, 1978, 1979) and authors who have interpreted his writing (for example, de Lacey 2001; Giddings & Wood 2002; Holmes & Federman 2003; Morse 2001; Shakespeare 2003; Street & Kissane 2001). If you are considering a postgraduate research project at master's degree or PhD level, you need to immerse yourself in these and many other references, especially in relation to how Foucauldian thought has influenced your discipline's research. These suggestions are given in light of the idea that there is no particular way of doing a discourse analysis and if you are attempting to undertake a thorough process reflecting Foucauldian thought, you will need a comprehensive understanding of his discourse on knowledge and power.

Essentially, a discourse analysis asks questions about the knowledge and power inherent in all kinds of spoken and written life texts. Julianne Cheek (2000) offers a method of '*doing*' discourse analysis, so this will be used to highlight how you might go about doing something similar. She uses Parker's (2000) key features of research using discourse analysis, noting his contention that there is 'no set "recipe"' (Cheek 2000, p. 51) for analysing texts. Bear in mind that 'texts' may be interview transcripts, all kinds of academic and general publications, professional and public documents, and media sources such as films and videos.

According to Parker (2000), the first feature (phase, stage) of discourse analysis is the *introduction*, in which a literature review is done to position the project in relation to other research. Then, 'the types of questions/issues driving the research are discussed in order to contextualise the research' (Cheek 2000, p. 52). The second phase is *methodology*, describing the texts to be analysed, why these and not others were selected and how the selected texts will be obtained. For example, how will the interview be conducted and what type of articles will be collected? In the third phase, *analysis* occurs using 'a degree of intuition' and no set 'discursive frames' (p. 52); that is, using questions such as: 'What ways of speaking and thinking about the reality in question are not present and why might that be so?' (p. 52). In the last phase, *discussion*, 'analyses are linked to other material in the area in order to draw out points of discussion about the substantive area under scrutiny' (p. 52), and there is reflection by the researcher on her/his position on the issues raised.

You should note that in the third phase other questions could be raised to facilitate further discourse analysis of the textual comparisons, such as:

- What patterns and rules are present?
- How have the patterns and rules been constructed?
- What are the assumptions?
- What are the possible sources of these assumptions?
- What contradictions are apparent?
- What discourses are silent?
- What discourses are dominant?
- What are the consequences of the silenced discourses?
- What are the consequences of the dominant discourses?
- What are the implications of the discourse?
- What are the inconsistencies in the discourse?

In summary, research reports may use the words discourse and discourse analysis in many ways. One of the most accepted interpretations of discourse analysis, however, is to undertake a thorough analysis of texts using Foucault's ideas about knowledge and power. The main audience of this book is intended to be undergraduates in the health professions. If you are undertaking postgraduate research, you should pursue the whole area of discourse analysis very carefully, informed by wide reading in the philosophy of Foucault (1965, 1973, 1981, 1991) and other writers (for example, Fairclough 1992; Lupton 1992; McNay 1992; Powers 1996; Tamboukou 1999; Titscher et al. 2000), who suggest foci and strategies for intensive analysis.

Computer systems that manage qualitative data

Sometimes you may find that you can use manual methods of analysis in conjunction with a word search function on your computer. For Macintosh computers, Hypercard is a program that can be used to organise data in the analysis processes. There is no prescription as to what must be done, so feel free to do whatever you need to do to obtain the most comprehensive and thorough analysis that you can, so that the richest meanings can emerge.

Another avenue you might like to explore is the use of a computer almost exclusively to locate the themes for you through the use of qualitative data analysis systems. NUD*IST (Qualitative Solutions and Research 1995) and Ethnograph (Siedel 1992) are systems that can group and order the conceptual categories which have been decided progressively by the researcher. These are examples of computer systems that manage the qualitative data, with greater and lesser degrees of success depending on the aim of the researcher who is using them.

EXERCISE

Locate other examples of computer systems that manage qualitative data. It may help you to undertake a web search on Google, or to locate and read Weitzman's chapter on computers, in Denzin and Lincoln (2000).

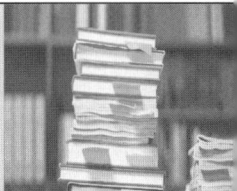

Benefits in qualitative data computer analysis systems

Computer software can help you analyse your qualitative data specifically by making notes, writing up, editing, coding, storing data, searching and retrieving, linking data, memoing, doing content analysis, making data displays, verifying conclusions, theory building, graphic mapping and report writing (Weitzman 2000). Generally, the main benefits of using qualitative data computer analysis systems are that they can manage large amounts of data and they are relatively easy to use.

Managing large amounts of data

Qualitative data computer analysis systems allow for whole transcripts and groups of transcripts to be merged and matched. This means that you have the potential to mix together all of the text and to do a collective analysis with ease. The added value of the systems is that they allow you to retrieve words and phrases from all of the combined transcripts that are connected to the context of the information. This means that sentences and phrases can be moved around the disk and located later, with their contextual features intact, which helps you to remember what words were said by whom, when and where. This is a very handy function for qualitative researchers who are making sense of large masses of words contained within the transcripts of high numbers of lengthy open-ended interviews.

Relatively easy to use

Systems are becoming easier to use as new versions appear on the market. They come complete with their own operating manuals for IBM-compatible or Macintosh computers. You may be able to access these systems through a site licence in an institution, or you can buy them directly from the manufacturers. Workshops run by the developers on how to use the systems are available, and it is advisable to avail yourself of them, and/or be assisted by someone who is proficient in using the particular system you have chosen.

Constraints in using qualitative data computer analysis systems

The main cautionary note in using qualitative data computer analysis systems is that the program will not do all the analytical work for you and the fullest interpretation may be missed because of the system's inability to locate implicit themes.

The system will not do all the work

Computer programs cannot do the analysis for you, as you might reasonably expect in quantitative statistical packages such as SPSS. A qualitative analysis system cannot read the data, do the analysis, and tell you what it means. This is because qualitative research data are words and the understanding of language relies on immersion by the researcher in the text. Even with computer assistance, the researcher is active in 'feeding in' the transcripts as text, locating the meaningful sections, naming and coding them according to their interpretive possibilities, and looking for finer nuances in meaning that a computer cannot detect.

Inability to locate finer nuances

When using any computer system for qualitative analysis, a cautionary note is that the resultant analysis and interpretation of the data are only as rich as the meaning that is tagged to the words, through a thorough analysis of the text. This means that the finer nuances of the text may be missed if the researcher relies entirely on the sophisticated word search ability of the system, and does not look between the words to find the implicit meanings within words, phrases and sections of text. In qualitative research, the richest and finest meanings may be hiding within the total context of the words, so that it is only through protracted and clear-minded attention to the text that these connections are made. It's a bit like relying on the spellchecker on your computer. It won't pick up words that are spelt correctly but used incorrectly. You (or some critical friend) must read all documents for errors that are beyond the 'ability' of the computer. In a similar fashion, you have to check the text to locate nuances the computer misses.

Examples of completed qualitative analyses

Before you embark on a qualitative analysis method, it may help you to look at completed forms that have been published. The main publication sources are books, journal articles, theses and published conference presentations.

Books about qualitative research

Books about qualitative research may be in the form of a teaching text, such as this book, they may be accounts of research that has been undertaken (Atkinson 2002; Benner 1984; Connor 2004; Lawler 1991; Taylor 2000; Tucakovic 2005), or they may be a combination of both (Atkinson et al. 2001; Denzin & Lincoln 2000; Gubrium & Holstein 2002; Reason & Bradbury 2001). Even though information in books dates quickly because of the time required for the publication process, books have the major advantage of generous word limits, thus making deep descriptions possible. Qualitative analysis processes are often non-linear, highly descriptive and dependent on readers understanding the context of people's experiences, so when you read qualitative books you have the best chance of 'getting inside' the researcher's analytical strategies.

For example, Judy Atkinson's (2002) book *Trauma Trails: Recreating Song Lines*, describes her research project that explored the transgenerational effects of trauma in Indigenous Australia. These stories in this topic and the sense Judy made of them could not be relayed adequately in a journal article constrained by a 5000-word limit. This is not only because of the risky nature of the stories, but also because of the research process of *dadirri*, which is a process of totally respectful and fully attentive listening to one another. When you read the book, there is no chapter that outlines the analysis per se, rather the analysis and interpretation are interwoven in the stories and in the sense the research participants made of them. Chapters 4 and 5 describe the trauma story and the healing story respectively, and the final chapter, Chapter 6, provides a model for community healing, to unite hearts and establish order. The totality of the research and its processes can only be fully appreciated by reading the book as a whole, because the stories of violence and healing cannot be reduced to brief outlines, or made into a convenience by being portrayed as concise themes.

Similarly, Marina Tucakovic's (2005) research book, *Nursing as an Aesthetic Praxis*, requires the luxury of a generous word limit to reflect the stories within her PhD project. Marina gives deep insights into her life and teaching experience, through the weave of stories, interpretations, extrapolations, and wisdom about the loving and healing essence of nursing and humanity. For example, stories, insights and literature provide a smooth transition from the 'paradigmatic position as process' to 'the void: the human being as an empty vessel' and 'aesthetics in nursing'.

The sequential flow of ideas moves on through careful writing about 'selfhood as energy', the 'ethics of health', 'the Human-being, creator energy', 'on thought and action in nursing', 'beauty and the body', 'the body as memory', 'the aesthetic in practice and curriculum', 'the body as temple', 'transformation through health care' and 'to love and to nurse'. As with Atkinson's book, there is no analysis chapter per se, rather the analysis and interpretations are interwoven in the participants' stories of learning and the researcher's experiences of teaching.

In summary, reading research books that describe projects in detail gives you the chance to see the finished project as literature, that is, as a literary work unlimited by the constraints of a reduced word count. The other advantage of reading research books of this nature is that they are not bound by the requirements of a research thesis or report, thus they are more likely to be reader-friendly and engaging reading.

EXERCISE

Locate and read a qualitative research book. How does the researcher/author present the analysis of the data?

Examples of research and thesis documents

You would be well advised to procure examples of research and thesis documents to give you a wide appreciation of the types of approaches that are possible. If you scan refereed journals that feature your discipline's research, you may find examples of qualitative research that clearly set out the methods of data collection and analysis. Some of the journal articles cited in the qualitative part of this book may give you some guidance as to how the researchers managed data analysis. However, journal articles are constrained by word limits, so you may need to contact the author(s) for deeper descriptions using the researchers' contact details supplied by the journal. You may have to access the original report or thesis document to glean practical assistance on how to go about the actual process of data analysis.

Often, libraries keep holdings of research theses for honours and master's degrees and PhD awards. Sometimes these theses have been copied onto microfiche or the full-text, hardbound copies are available for reading in the library. Some universities compile digital holdings of theses. Locate theses whose titles and abstracts suggest adherence to a particular approach, such as an interpretive or critical methodology, or suggest postmodern influences. The methods of analysis contained within these theses have been judged by examiners to be of a quality sufficient to warrant the academic award, so you can place a certain amount of trust in them as guiding documents. Realise, however, that there is no one best method of qualitative analysis and it is permissible to amend and re-create some methods, as long as you are consistent with the methodological assumptions of the research approach and describe your analysis method fully and clearly.

EXERCISE
In what ways are theses helpful to researchers, who must also produce a thesis document?

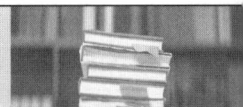

Research project presentations

Oral accounts of qualitative analyses may be given by researchers presenting their projects at professional conferences. In this case, you would be well advised to attend the presentation and seek the presenters out afterwards to request elaboration on how they managed the analysis component of their research design. Conference presentations may be published in a book of proceedings and these may be a good source of worked examples of research analysis. Even so, do not be afraid to use the contact details offered publicly to communicate with researchers who have worked through the vagaries of data analysis. Depending upon their interest and cooperation, you may learn a great deal from successful researchers willing to share their techniques and strategies for data analysis.

Adjust analytic methods with a rationale

Be energetic and thorough in seeking out examples of analytic methods, but remember that no one qualitative method is sacrosanct. Do not be afraid to adjust an analytic method. As a standard procedure for report writing, you need to explain what you did in the analytic stage as part of your rationale for the research methods. The main aim is to ensure that what you have done is defensible in respect of the methodological assumptions that you used to structure the research methods in the first place. For example, an approach influenced by affirmative postmodern thinking will be very open and exploratory in its analysis methods and tentative in reporting its insights. In contrast, a grounded theory approach may have set steps to follow, and you will need to provide a strong rationale for varying them in ways other than which the original authors intended.

The analysis of images as qualitative data

As words are the main tools of qualitative research, the analysis of them has taken up the largest part of this chapter. However, a discussion of qualitative analysis would not be complete without the acknowledgement of images as sources of qualitative data. You may remember that previously it was noted that some artistic expression, such as photographs, video and/or dance, may be admissible as data for qualitative analysis.

For the purposes of this chapter, the whole area of aesthetic judgement will be left to one side, as that is a highly specialised field in the arts which cannot be represented adequately here. Instead, the discussion will centre on the analysis of images that are generated by research participants as descriptive forms to augment or represent their personal expression of a phenomenon of research interest.

Analysis by the creator of the image

Images may be created by a researcher as photographs or videos, or they may be created by research participants as drawings, paintings and collages, as forms of expression to describe their experiences. This being so, it follows that the images would be analysed most accurately by the people who created them. This would mean that participants analyse and describe the images they created according to their intentions for creating them in relation to the research. Researchers would discuss with participants their analysis of the content of images and create a dialogue with them in making connections to the research aims and objectives. Therefore, the analyses of images as data are made in relation to the aims and objectives of the research and the intentions of the researcher and/or participant. The interpretations that result from the analysis of the images are what the person creating them says they are. These analyses and interpretations are admissible as they are relevant to the person involved; thus they add to the richness of the research findings. The research project report will need to show clearly that these analyses and interpretations are acknowledged as being those of the respective participants.

Summary

This chapter dealt with some practical hints for qualitative analysis. It was assumed that words are the main data for analysis, and the chapter dealt most comprehensively with their analysis. A small part of the text was devoted to the analysis of images as data. As I have found that most research books and researchers are seldom useful in telling potential researchers *how* to undertake a method of qualitative analysis, the chapter contained a compilation of hints and strategies that have worked from personal experience. I hope that you found them informative and that they continue to be helpful when you need to refresh your memory of them and put them into action in your own research.

Main points

- The orientation of a qualitative researcher undertaking the intellectual task of data analysis needs to include being ready physically and emotionally.

- Getting started in data analysis includes making copies, deciding on an organising system and having confidence in words as data.
- Qualitative analysis of words may be by either manual or computer-assisted means and the intentions of the analysis will determine what is done with the words.
- To find explicit and implicit themes within the text, know what you are looking for, locate specific words for explicit themes and look closely for the nuances of implicit themes.
- A theme bears resemblance to what you thought you might find, and it appears to have within it some features of the thing for which you are looking; that is, it is part of the pattern of answers you are intending to find within the text, and you know it is relevant because its identity is connected directly and sometimes indirectly to the stated research aims and objectives.
- A manual thematic analysis method is to read and reread the text; make multiple copies of the page-numbered transcripts (ensuring one copy is kept as a guide); keep in mind the research question and/or objectives; isolate (by cutting out or colour coding) any sections of text that appear to be connected to a theme; reduce the 'themes' to a word or two each and list them; and, finally, collect them into groupings until they cannot be subsumed into other categories/groupings without losing their specialness in relation to the research aims and objectives.
- A computer-assisted data analysis method is to make a disk copy of the main text to be analysed; drop off any extraneous details from the copy; read through the text as it scrolls on the computer screen; section the text off under a subheading that is relatively descriptive; make connections between themes that are raised in one part of the text and reiterated in another part; collate the themes; review the list while asking yourself: 'What does this say about the research interest?'; name and define the themes; and describe their components.
- Emplotment involves the researcher going carefully through text to track plots and locate sets of events that are common to all stories, then undertaking an analysis that will make sense of all the events as one story.
- Discourses are groups of ideas or patterned ways of thinking, writing and speaking immersed in social structures that constitute power and knowledge relationships.
- A discourse analysis asks questions systematically and thoroughly about the knowledge and power inherent in all kinds of spoken and written life texts, in relation to the nature and construction patterns and rules present, the kinds of assumptions and their possible sources, and the contradictions, silences, dominance and inconsistencies in the discourse.
- The main benefits of using qualitative data computer analysis systems are that they can manage large amounts of data and they are relatively easy to use. However, they will not do all the work for you, and the fullest interpretation may be missed because of the system's inability to locate implicit themes.
- Examples of completed qualitative analyses can be located in books, journal articles, theses and published conference presentations.

CASE STUDY

You first met Carmel in Chapter 14. If you have not been following Carmel's case study, go to the end of Chapters 14 and 15 and review her story so far. She is an experienced clinical nurse working in an acute care setting while undertaking a Master by Research program part-time with a local university. Carmel is using a collaborative approach with 10 other experienced nurses working in acute care settings, about the facilitating and constraining factors they experience that influence their ability to give effective nursing care.

After ethics clearance, Carmel set up a participatory action research (PAR) group which has been meeting for one hour per week for eight weeks. The PAR group has moved through processes to establish trust in the group, and at each meeting participants have been sharing journal entries in group discussions to locate a common issue in their work to research together.

After reflection and discussion, the group has identified a thematic concern of the use of power in the health care organisation. Many of their journal entries describe the downward push of power from management on their daily working lives. They decide to undertake a literature search to see what has been written about organisational power in hospitals. They also realise that power is exercised and maintained in their work settings within the culture of the organisation.

1   What key words should they use when seeking relevant literature?
2   What databases should they search?
3   What other organisational documents might be helpful?
4   If they decide to extend this part of the PAR into a discourse analysis, what approach/framework might they use to ensure the discourse analysis is thorough?

Multiple choice questions

1   Before undertaking qualitative research analysis, it is important to be ready physically and emotionally because:
   a   numbers and statistics are difficult to examine if you are tired and labile
   b   cause and effect relationships only become apparent with deep concentration
   c   you need to read, look and listen to language with wakeful alertness
   d   anything worth doing is worth doing well, especially when analysing data
2   The most useful organising system for your qualitative data is:
   a   the one that suits you best
   b   a set of manila folders

 c a bundle of paper files

 d a computer file

3 To find explicit themes within the text:

 a locate specific words

 b look closely for nuances

 c connect keywords

 d disregard irrelevancies

4 The first step in a thematic analysis is to:

 a read and reread the interview transcripts

 b make multiple copies of the data documents

 c allow time for the insights to come together

 d review the research aims and objectives

5 An example of a manual thematic analysis method is:

 a SPSS

 b NUD*IST

 c the 'colour coding' method

 d Ethnograph

6 Narrative analysis involves:

 a a variety of analytic approaches

 b one reliable analytic method

 c the interrogation of power

 d critique of literature and documents

7 According to Foucault, discursive practices:

 a are necessary and ideal in shaping people's compliance to power in organisations

 b form and maintain discourses that in turn constitute power and knowledge relationships

 c have no real effect on people or the way they choose to define and enact their daily lives

 d involve talking and acting in ways that create societies always mindful of people's needs

8 If a researcher needs to undertake a qualitative analysis on 200 interviews, s/he would be well advised to:

 a forget about it and change to a quantitative method

 b use the 'pile on the kitchen table' analysis method

 c look only for the explicit themes and disregard the rest

 d use a reputable qualitative data computer system

9 Research books are useful for describing qualitative analysis methods because:

 a they have generous word limits and less thesis format restrictions

 b they are durable, readily available and relatively inexpensive

 c they do not date as quickly as refereed articles and theses

 d researchers write them better to attract more book royalties

10 Images created by research participants such as drawings, paintings and collages, as forms of expression to describe their experiences, are best analysed by the:
a principal researcher
b thesis reviewer
c creator of the images
d report reader

Review topics

1 Discuss why qualitative research has generally 'come of age' in academia and in some clinical agencies.
2 Why is it advisable that your personal approach to qualitative research analysis is with an attitude of respect for people, and their experiences and words?
3 Describe the aspects of getting started when embarking on qualitative analysis.
4 Describe manual methods of thematic analysis.
5 Compare the benefits and limitations of using computer systems that manage qualitative data.

Online reading

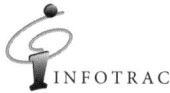

INFOTRAC® COLLEGE EDITION
When accessing information use the name of your health care discipline and the following keywords in any combinations you require to retrieve information relating to qualitative analysis:

➤ discourse analysis
➤ explicit themes
➤ Foucauldian discourse analysis
➤ Foucault
➤ images
➤ implicit themes
➤ interviews
➤ narrative analysis
➤ narratives
➤ storytelling
➤ text
➤ thematic analysis
➤ themes

References

Allen, D.G. 1985, 'Nursing research and social control: alternative models of science that emphasise understanding and emancipation', *Image: Journal of Nursing Scholarship*, vol. 17, no. 2, 58–64.

Anderson, C., McAllister, M. & Moyle, W. 2002, 'The postmodern heart: a discourse analysis of a booklet on pacemaker implantation', *Collegian*, vol. 9, no. 1, 19–23.

Atkinson, J. 2002, *Trauma Trails: Recreating Song Lines – The Transgenerational Effects of Trauma in Indigenous Australia*, Spinifex, North Melbourne, Australia.

Atkinson, P., Coffey, A., Delamont, S., Lofland, J. & Lofland, L. (eds) 2001, *Handbook of Ethnography*, Sage, London.

Benner, P. 1984, *From Novice to Expert : Uncovering the Knowledge Embedded in Clinical Practice*, Addison-Wesley, California.

Cheek, J. 2000, *Postmodern and Poststructural Approaches to Nursing Research*, Sage, Thousand Oaks, California.

Chinn, P.L. 1985, 'Debunking myths in nursing theory and research', *Image: Journal of Nursing Scholarship*, vol. 17, no. 2, 45–9.

Connor, M. 2004, *Courage and Complexity in Chronic Illness: Reflective Practice in Nursing*, Daphne Brasell Associate Press and Whitireia Publishing, Wellington, New Zealand.

Cortazzi, M. 2001, 'Narrative analysis in ethnography', in P. Atkinson, A. Coffey, S. Delamont, J. Lofland & L. Lofland (eds), *Handbook of Ethnography*, Sage, London.

Courtney, M. (ed.) 2005, *Evidence for Nursing Practice*, Elsevier Churchill Livingstone, Sydney.

Dawes, M., Davies, P., Gray A., Mant, J., Seers, K. & Snowball, R. 2005, *Evidence-Based Practice: A Primer for Health Care Professionals*, 2nd edn, Elsevier Churchill Livingstone, Edinburgh.

de Lacey, S. 2001, 'IVF as lottery or investment: contesting metaphors in discourses of infertility', *Nursing Inquiry*, vol. 9, no. 1, 43–51.

Denzin, N. & Lincoln, Y. (eds) 2000, *Handbook of Qualitative Research*, 2nd edn, Sage, Thousand Oaks, California.

Emden, C. 1998, 'Conducting a narrative analysis', *Collegian*, vol. 5, no. 3, 34–9.

Fairclough, N. 1992, *Discourse and Social Change*, Polity Press, Cambridge.

Foucault, M. 1965, *Madness and Civilization: A History of Insanity in the Age of Reason*, Pantheon, New York.

Foucault, M. 1972, *The Archaeology of Knowledge*, Tavistock, London.

Foucault, M. 1973, 'Spaces and classes', in *The Birth of the Clinic: An Archeology of Medical Perception*, Pantheon, New York.

Foucault, M. 1975, *The Birth of the Clinic*, trans. A.M. Sheridan-Smith, Vintage/Random House, New York (original work published 1973).

Foucault, M. 1978, *The History of Sexuality*, vol. 1: *An Introduction*, trans. R. Hurley, Vintage/Random House, New York (original work published 1976).

Foucault, M. 1979, *Discipline and Punish*, trans. A.M. Sheridan-Smith, Vintage/Random House, New York (original work published 1975).

Foucault, M. 1980, *Michel Foucault. Power/Knowledge: Selected Interviews and Other Writings*, Harvester Press, Brighton, England.

Foucault, M. 1981, 'The order of discourse', in R. Young (ed.), *Unlying the Text*, Routledge and Kegan Paul, Boston, 48–78.

Foucault, M. 1991, 'Orders of discourse', *Social Science Inform*, vol. 10, no. 2, 7–30.

Giddings, L. & Wood, P. 2002, 'Discourse analysis – making connections between knowledge and power: an interview with Debbie Payne', *Nursing Praxis in New Zealand*, vol. 18, no. 2, 4–13.

Gilbert, T. 2003, 'Exploring the dynamic of power: a Foucauldian analysis of care planning in learning disabilities services', *Nursing Inquiry*, vol. 10, no. 1, 37–46.

Glass, N. & Davis, K. 1998, 'An emancipatory impulse: a feminist postmodern integrated turning point in nursing research', *Advances in Nursing Science*, vol. 21, no. 1, 43–52.

Goodwin, L.D. & Goodwin, W.L. 1984, 'Qualitative vs quantitative research or qualitative and quantitative research?', *Nursing Research*, vol. 33, no. 6, 378–80.

Grealish, L. & Trevitt, C. 2005, 'Developing a professional identity: student nurses in the workplace', *Contemporary Nurse*, vol. 19, no. 1–2, 137–50.

Gubrium, J.F. & Holstein, J.A. (eds) 2002, *Handbook of Interview Research: Context and Method*, Sage, Thousand Oaks.

Hardin, P. 2003, 'Shape-shifting discourses of anorexia nervosa: reconstituting psychopathology', *Nursing Inquiry*, vol. 10, no. 4, 209–17.

Henderson, V. 1964, 'The nature of nursing', *American Journal of Nursing*, vol. 64, no. 8, 62–8.

Holmes, D. & Federman, C. 2003, 'Killing for the state: the darkest side of American nursing', *Nursing Inquiry*, vol. 10, no. 1, 2–10.

Kermode, S. & Brown, C. 1995, 'Where have all the flowers gone? Nursing's escape from the radical critique', *Contemporary Nurse*, vol. 4, no. 1, 8–15.

Kratz, C.R. 1978, *Care of the Long Term Sick in the Community*, Churchill-Livingstone, Edinburgh.

Labov, W. 1972, 'The transformation of experience in narrative syntax', in Labov, W., *Language in the Inner City*, University of Pennsylvania Press, Philadelphia PA, 352–96.

Lawler, J. 1991, *Behind the screens: nursing, somology and the problem of the body*, Churchill-Livingstone, Melbourne.

Leininger, M. 1985, *Qualitative Research Methods in Nursing*, Grune and Stratton, New York.

Linde, C. 1993, *Life Stories: The Creation of Coherence*, Oxford University Press, New York.

Lupton, D. 1992, 'Discourse analysis: a new methodology for understanding the ideologies of health and illness', *Australian Journal of Public Health*, vol. 16, 145–50.

McNay, L. 1992, *Foucault and Feminism*, Northeastern University Press, Boston.

Morse, K. 2001, 'Case in point? A parasuicide patient's recollections of being nursed: a discourse analysis', *Contemporary Nurse*, vol. 10, no. 3–4, 234–43.

Parker, I. 2000, 'Discourse dynamics: critical analysis for social and individual psychology', in J. Cheek (ed.), *Postmodern and Poststructural Approaches to Nursing Research*, Sage Publications, Thousand Oaks, California.

Polanyi, L. 1989, *Telling the American Story: A Structural and Cultural Analysis of Conversational Storytelling*, MIT Press, Cambridge, MA.

Polkinghorne, D.E. 1988, 'Narrative knowing and the human sciences', in C. Emden, 'A narrative analysis', *Collegian*, vol. 5, no. 3, 34–9.

Powers, P. 1996, 'Discourse analysis as a methodology for nursing inquiry', *Nursing Inquiry*, vol. 3, 207–17.

Qualitative Solutions and Research 1995, NUD*IST (Non-Numerical Unstructured Data: Indexing Searching & Theorising), application software package, QSR, Melbourne.

Reason, P. & Bradbury, H. (eds) 2001, *Handbook of Action Research: Participative Inquiry and Practice*, Sage, London.

Riessman, C.K. 2002, 'Analysis of personal narratives', in J.F. Gubrium & J.A. Holstein (eds), *Handbook of Interview Research: Context and Method*, Sage, Thousand Oaks.

Sarnecky, M.T. 1990, 'Historiography: a legitimate research methodology for nursing', *Advances in Nursing Science*, vol. 12, no. 4, 1–10.

Shakespeare, P. 2003, 'Nurses' bodywork: is there a body of work?', *Nursing Inquiry*, vol. 10, no. 1, 47–56.

Siedel, J.V. 1992, Ethnograph, version 4.0, Qualis Research Associates, Corvallis, Oregon.

Spradley, J.P. 1979, *The Ethnographic Interview*, Holt, Rinehart & Winston, New York.

Strauss, A.L. 1987, *Qualitative Analysis for Social Scientists*, Cambridge University Press, New York.

Street, A. & Kissane, D. 2001, 'Discourses of the body in euthanasia: symptomatic, dependent, shameful and temporal', *Nursing Inquiry*, vol. 8, no. 1, 162–72.

Tamboukou, M. 1999, 'Writing genealogies: an exploration of Foucault's strategies for doing research', *Discourse Studies in the Cultural Politics of Education*, vol. 20, no. 2, 201–17.

Taylor, B. 2000, *Being Human: Ordinariness in Nursing (adapted)*, Southern Cross University Press, Lismore, NSW.

Taylor, B. 2001, 'Promoting self-help strategies by sharing the lived experience of arthritis', *Contemporary Nurse*, vol. 10, no. 1–2, 117–25.

Titscher, S., Meyer, M., Wodak, R. & Vetter, E. 2000, *Methods of Text and Discourse Analysis*, Sage, London.

Tucakovic, M. 2005, *Nursing as an Aesthetic Praxis*, AuthorHouse, Bloomington, Indiana.

Weitzman, E. 2000, 'Software and qualitative research', in N. Denzin & Y. Lincoln (eds), *Handbook of Qualitative Research*, 2nd edn, Sage, Thousand Oaks.

Winstead-Fry, P. 1980, 'The scientific method and its impact on holistic health', *Advances in Nursing Science* (Jan.), 1–7.

CHAPTER 17

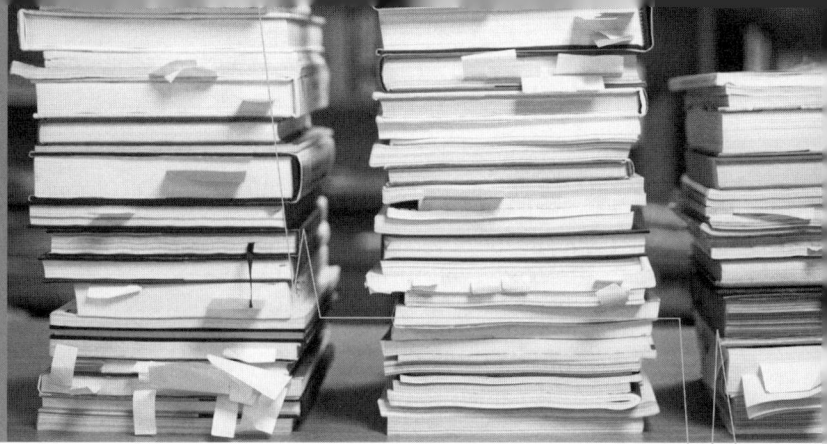

INTERPRETING QUALITATIVE FINDINGS

CHAPTER OBJECTIVES

The material presented in this chapter will assist you to:

- differentiate between analysis and interpretation
- acknowledge the relative nature of qualitative research interpretations
- relate varieties of findings to specific methodological approaches
- use qualitative interpretive and critical categories to make general statements about interpretive processes
- describe processes for synthesising qualitative interpretive and critical results
- identify postmodern influences on interpretation as another perspective for research.

Introduction

To some extent in qualitative research, **analysis** and **interpretation** appear to overlap, but they are not the same. There is a transition from a systematic review and analysis of the words and images (alone or in combination) to interpretive statements that can be made, revealing insights and relative answers to the areas being researched. In some cases, the transition is marked by step-by-step development of theory, for example, the structured approach of grounded theory (Strauss 1975). In other cases, such as phenomenological research, the transition from analysis to interpretation is not as structured, yet readers can locate analytic steps in the research process (Colaizzi 1978). Towards the postmodern end of the continuum, transitions may be relatively imperceptible, as analysis and interpretation blend and as relative and partial explanations are located, based on the multifaceted nature of human discourse and the tentativeness of the research questions.

There are many kinds of qualitative research; therefore, there are many means of analysing and interpreting the meaning emerging from them. This chapter introduces you to some of the ways in which the analysis phase of qualitative research leads to interpretation and theories/results/findings/insights/recommendations/implications. The reason for presenting all these words in this way is that language is important. In this part of a qualitative research project, language indicates the differences in various kinds of qualitative research and the assumptions that underlie them. As has been shown in other chapters of this book, it is very difficult to represent qualitative research approaches as a general group. Differentiation is required between different methods and processes of interpretation that are used, with basic assumptions about the nature of human knowledge in mind.

Although processes for interpreting analysed information vary according to research methodologies, for ease of reference and the sake of continuity this chapter will distinguish between them under the categories of interpretive qualitative research and critical qualitative research. This approach for categorising qualitative research was introduced in Chapter 12. The explanation was given then that even though the categories of qualitative interpretive and qualitative critical research are very broad, they nonetheless simplify what could be a very complex issue for new researchers. It is hoped that the qualitative interpretive and qualitative critical categories will allow you to make general statements about the various processes of interpretation that you may read about, or choose to use in your own projects. In addition, some discussion on postmodern influences on interpretation is offered, as another perspective for research.

Differentiation between analysis and interpretation

It is important to draw a distinction between analysis and interpretation, as they are separate yet related processes. In order to be able to make **interpretations**, data must be analysed thoroughly. However, just as there is often minimal practical help from literature in what to do to analyse, books and journals are also relatively silent on how to interpret the products of research analyses.

Qualitative researchers may find it difficult to explicate the actual methods and processes they use when they analyse and interpret research data. It is difficult to say why this happens – maybe the conceptual tasks are so simple that they seem self-evident, or maybe they are so complex as to be beyond comprehensive explanation. The conundrum of qualitative analysis interpretation is in contrast to quantitative approaches, in which confidence is placed in valid and reliable instruments that produce objective results as mathematical relationships. Even given the difficulty in working with words and language, qualitative researchers must attempt to set out the analytic and interpretive phases of the project for readers of the research.

EXERCISE

Locate two qualitative research reports published in peer-reviewed journals. There are many research examples in this chapter. Read the articles and examine the extent to which the researchers have described what they actually did in their respective projects to analyse and interpret the data.

Defining analysis and interpretation

Qualitative analysis and interpretation are related, yet they are different.

Analysis

Analysis involves reviewing research data systematically with the intention of sorting and classifying them into representational groups and patterns. After analysis, the data are organised from their raw state as words and images (alone or in combination) into groupings and symbolic forms that require explanation to ensure that the meaning is as clear as it can be.

Interpretation

Interpretation involves taking the forms of analysed information to another level or levels of abstraction, so that statements can be made about what they mean in light of the intentions, methods and processes of the research. This basically means that the analysed words and/or images are refined into more words and/or images that make the research outcomes more meaningful. In qualitative research, if the interpretations and explanations of the analysed data are not given, readers are left to infer their own conclusions. Sometimes, for example, in research influenced by postmodern thought, local stories may 'stand' as they are, with no attempt by the researcher to interpret them. This raises issues around interpretations from various perspectives.

Just as a work of art can be left open to multiple interpretations, so also can qualitative research findings. This is in line with the context-dependent and relative features of qualitative research approaches. For example, qualitative researchers and participants may place their unique interpretations on the data, having been actively involved in the project. Readers of the research may not necessarily agree with the researchers' and participants' interpretations, or they may posit other possible conclusions about the findings. This freedom to interpret or to leave interpretations open does not relieve qualitative researchers of their fundamental responsibility to be open and transparent in their methods and processes. Readers of the research need to be able to trace the methods and processes that were used in a project, so that they can audit the researcher's activities and/or have a sound rationale for their differing interpretations.

Analysis generally precedes interpretation

Generally speaking, analysis precedes interpretation, although some qualitative researchers, such as those using phenomenological writing, describe an intuitive grasp of the data, having focused on it so closely and thoroughly. Also, some qualitative researchers who use participatory research methods and processes with participants as co-researchers may experience spiralling and integrative processes in which analysis and interpretation blend and seem to become indivisible. Bearing in mind these and other possible exceptions to the rule, the approach taken here will to be to assume that interpretation occurs after a period of analysis, however protracted and by whatever means.

Interpretation requires immersion in the text

Language is the basis of qualitative research. Although images and numbers can also be part of qualitative analysis and interpretation, words are the main symbols from which meaning is derived. Because words are the main source of interpretation, many approaches require a high degree of familiarity with the text. Text was defined previously as the transcript and/or record of words. Text may be interview transcripts, field notes, historical documents, journal entries, summaries, audio recordings of group discussions, and so on. Essentially, in the sense in which it is used here, text can mean any sources of words that contribute to finding meaning in the research interest.

Invariably, qualitative interpretations of words and language require protracted time with the text to ensure that meaning is located and that it is as clear as possible to convey to other people. Therefore, qualitative interpretation is generally not a matter of putting data through a computer system to come up with statistical relationships for interpretation. Rather, analysis is usually through reading and rereading text, with manual or computer-assisted means. Interpretation follows after further reflection and validation by people such as other researchers, co-researchers, participants and peers.

EXERCISE

In Chapter 16, one of the exercises suggested that you audiotape yourself telling a story or a series of stories about an experience in your life which was of great significance to you. If you did not undertake the audiotaping then, do it now and transcribe the audiotapes(s). These 'raw data' are text, on which you can now work throughout this chapter in order to understand the difference between analysis and interpretation.

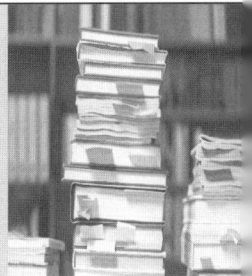

Qualitative research findings as relative interpretations

The findings of research projects will be disseminated to readers as trustworthy information. This is another way of saying that, to the best of their abilities, the researchers claim to share truthful findings. In Chapter 12 there is a discussion on what constitutes truth according to the major distinctions of quantitative (empirico-analytical) and qualitative (interpretive and critical) research traditions. The methods for knowledge generation, analysis, interpretation and validation differ according to assumptions about what constitutes new and/or amended truth and worthwhile knowledge. If you are unclear about these distinctions you may like to refer to this section in the early part of Chapter 12.

Interpretations as relative truth

Qualitative researchers agree that there is no way of guaranteeing absolute truth, because truth is relative, subjective, context-dependent and elusive. The idea that truth is relative may appear to leave open the whole issue of whether qualitative interpretations can be relied on as having some foundation for adding to knowledge. Even though truth is regarded as being relative, it is considered important to reveal it in its various forms. The main difference between qualitative and quantitative assumptions about knowledge in this regard is that the former do not seek to generate absolute, indisputable truths and facts. This is because they agree that the changing and complex nature of human existence does not permit research approaches to guarantee this kind of knowledge. Even so, qualitative researchers use various means of demonstrating the worthiness of their projects. For example, measures for ensuring validity may involve asking the participants to confirm that the interpretations are truthful for them. These issues are discussed in the section dealing with 'rigour' in Chapter 14.

EXERCISE

In Chapter 16, it was suggested that you analyse transcribed audiotapes of yourself telling a story or a series of stories about an experience in your life which was of great significance to you. If you did not undertake the analysis then, do it now according to the steps provided in Chapter 16. You can now work on this analysis to understand interpretation.

Interpretations by other names

Various words are used synonymously to mean interpretations. Qualitative research reports may use words such as theories, findings, results, insights, strategies, implications, examples of reflective awareness and changed practice, and so on. The words used may have been selected specifically to reflect the assumptions and intentions of the research methodology. That is because qualitative research is set up in different ways to fulfil different purposes. For example:

- a grounded theory approach may put forward interpretations as middle range theories (e.g. Fiveash & Nay 2004; Gibb 2003; McCann & Clark 2003; Rew 2003)
- a phenomenological approach may document insights or essences (e.g. Beck 2004; Maldonado, Efinger & Lacey 2003; Peters 2003; Sundelof, Hansebo & Ekman 2004)
- a feminist approach may describe competing discourses (e.g. Armishaw & Davis 2002; Hardin 2003; Meyer & de Oliveira 2003)
- an action research approach or a critical ethnography may report examples of reflective awareness and changed practice (e.g. Craig et al. 2004; Rankin 2003; Taylor et al. 2002; Watson, Turnbull & Mills 2002)
- a project influenced by postmodern ideas may document the presence of multiple and contradictory voices (e.g. Cheek 2000; Langridge & Ahern 2002).

The scope of interpretation

Most qualitative research approaches do not claim to generate interpretations that can be considered to be generalisable to the wider population. An exception to this is grounded theory, which sets out to make general statements in the form of middle range theories about what might be expected in similar circumstances.

Phenomenological approaches that provide insights might typically expect that interpretations will be useful for those people with whom they resonate. In other words, if readers of the research find it is relevant for them, then it has scope in being informative to them.

Action research approaches reporting examples of reflective awareness and changed practice have scope for local theories of practice. This means that the people who have participated in the project have realised local, personal truths that are relevant for them. The scope of the interpretations is broader when the people involved in the research influence other people, policies and practices in the wider setting.

Research using postmodern thought may not deem to offer anything concrete but to leave instead all ideas open as tentative, or make multiple interpretations and give authority to readers to make their own interpretations (Cheek 2000; Langridge & Ahern 2002). In some cases, key postmodern ideas, such as difference and voice, may be retained as the central core and integrity of a grand narrative (Glass & Davis 1998).

Qualitative findings in relation to methodological approaches

Qualitative findings will differ according to the underlying theoretical assumptions of the approach and the intentions of the research. There are many ways of categorising methodological approaches in qualitative research; however, they invariably lead to a great deal of detail and confusion. For this reason, the approach taken here will be to use the categories explained previously in Chapter 12 and 13.

A very simple and comprehensive way of thinking about kinds of qualitative research is to categorise them according to interpretive and critical forms and differences. Although categorisations of this kind have their shortcomings, they are useful for students who are trying to plot their way through a wide and deep range of ideas about research. As an important postscript, some possibilities will be considered of the diverse thought that postmodernisms offer.

Qualitative interpretive methodologies

Qualitative interpretive research methodologies intend mainly to generate meaning by exploring, explaining and describing things of interest in order to make sense out of them. Examples of these methodologies are historical research, grounded theory, ethnography and phenomenology. These methodologies are described in Chapter 12.

Qualitative critical methodologies

Qualitative critical methodologies aim to bring about change in the status quo by questioning aspects that are taken for granted. Through systematic political critique, these methodologies attempt to expose factors of control, oppression, power and domination and cause raised awareness and change activities. Examples of these methodologies are critical ethnography, feminisms, interpretive interactionism and action research. These methodologies are described in Chapter 13.

Similarities and differences

In doing what they intend to do as their first priority, qualitative interpretive and critical research methodologies also manage to do other things. For example, they generate meaning by looking closely at a phenomenon of interest. Also, they can bring about change.

The major difference between interpretive and critical qualitative research is in the main intention of what they hope to achieve through the research process. Interpretive forms are involved mainly with generating meaning. Critical forms concern themselves with change. Even though they both can bring about change, they differ in the intensity of their intentions and their choice of methods to do this. Critical methodologies are most intense in bringing about change. This is because they have an 'up-front' change agenda and they tend to use participatory research processes to realise their change intentions.

Qualitative interpretive and critical categories of interpretive processes

Processes for interpretation may differ according to what kind of qualitative research it can be considered to be; that is, whether it is essentially an interpretive (concerned mainly with meaning) or critical (concerned mainly with change) project. Some researchers may argue that they have combined methodologies across the interpretive and critical categories. In this case, they may need to use a combination of interpretive processes, appropriate to the assumptions, aims, objectives, methods and processes of the project.

Clarifying some preconditions for qualitative interpretation

A researcher may have made a clear decision as to the placement of a project in either the interpretive or critical methodology categories. Alternatively, the project may be placed in a combination of methodologies. In some cases a project may defy categorisation altogether into methodological groupings, for example, postmodern research. Regardless of the nature of the project, there are some general necessary preconditions for interpretation of which qualitative researchers are advised to be aware.

The need for congruency

Congruency is correspondence or agreement. In qualitative research, it means the fit or correspondence between foundational ideas and the activity phases of the research. Even though the phases of a project may be planned carefully at the outset, parts of the overall project may change over the course of the research. Therefore, before embarking on making sense of the analysed data it may be useful to take some time to reorient to the overall project. This will involve you asking yourself some questions to check on the congruency of the project's assumptions, aims, objectives, methods and processes.

Some questions which may be posed are:

Assumptions
- What ideas underlie this project about the nature of knowledge and how it is verified?
- What choices were made about selecting a paradigm in which the project would fit most appropriately?
- If no paradigm category was chosen then, does it matter now?

Aims and objectives
- What did I intend to research?
- Why did I want to research these things?
- At this stage, to what extent has the project fulfilled its stated purposes?

Methods
- What methods were chosen to gather the information?
- To what extent do the methods appear to be a good fit with the assumptions, aims and objectives of the research?
- To what extent did the methods gather the information required?

Processes
- How was the research undertaken in terms of the researcher-participant relationships?
- How was the research undertaken in terms of the overall management of the project?
- To what extent did the processes appear to be a good fit with the assumptions, aims, objectives and methods of the research?

Reasons for asking questions between analysis and interpretation

The reasons for asking certain questions at the transition from analysis to interpretation are to reorient to the overall project; to check on the degree of congruency between the assumptions, aims, objectives, methods and processes; and to prepare for the process of interpretation.

Reorienting to the overall project

In reorienting to the overall project, the researcher's memory is refreshed and an assessment can be made as to whether the project has progressed generally as anticipated to this point. If it has not gone as expected, it might be helpful to look at ways in which it has differed and locate the reasons why. It may be necessary to have this in mind when beginning the interpretation as this will help to sort out twists and turns in the data that otherwise may be confusing.

Checking on the degree of congruency

Congruency may not be an issue for some qualitative researchers, but it is worth bearing in mind that most qualitative research provides a theoretical basis for its choice of methodological approach, methods and processes (Atkinson et al. 2001; Denzin & Lincoln 2000; Gubrium & Holstein 2002; Reason & Bradbury 2001). However, because there are many qualitative approaches from which to choose, they do not all have the same assumptions about what constitutes knowledge and how to go about finding and verifying it. Supporters of having a theoretical basis might argue that researchers need to be clear about the degree of congruency within and between all the research phases, because it helps them prepare for interpretation and will provide a strong rationale for readers of the research as to what has been done, and why and how it has been done.

Preparing for the process of interpretation

When it comes time to move from analysis to interpretation, using the questioning exercise listed in this chapter may help you to determine the degree of congruency in the research to date. It will help you to focus thoroughly on the data. This intense focusing may help you to extract meaning that is congruent with the assumptions, aims, objectives, methods and processes of the research. It will also mean that some time will elapse between the analysis and interpretation phases of the research. This will not only give you time for thinking, but it will also permit time for reading and rereading so that there is deeper and deeper immersion in the data, in preparation for making sense out of it.

Processes for synthesising qualitative interpretive and critical results

In the strictest dictionary sense, processes are series of actions that produce changes or developments (as defined in *Collins English Dictionary* 1998). In qualitative research involving humans, however, the interest is not so much in the actions themselves but in how the actions are done through interpersonal processes. The processes for synthesising qualitative interpretive and critical interpretations happen as cognitive activities within the researcher. This interpretation process must happen for the researcher to make sense of the analysed data.

From analysis to interpretation

Being able to describe interpretation is tantamount to being able to describe cognitive processes, such as making intellectual leaps, connections, intuitive grasps, and so on. This makes interpretation a very difficult thing to describe on a biochemical and psychological level. Philosophers have taken different approaches to tackling the vexed problem of what it is inquirers do when they interpret, by addressing various forms of hermeneutics (Gadamer 1975 trans.; Habermas 1981). (Hermeneutics is taken here broadly to mean processes of interpretation.)

Hans-Georg Gadamer is one philosopher in the phenomenological tradition. Gadamer (1975 trans.) decided that all understanding is hermeneutical, because hermeneutics is the 'basic being-in-motion of There-being, which constitutes its finiteness and historicity and hence includes the whole experience of the world' (Gadamer 1975 trans., p. 323). This means that Gadamer reasoned interpretations were available to humans as beings in the world. He argued that things can be made apparent through understanding the nature of human existence. For him, the key to understanding existence is through language.

Gadamer contended that it is the task of hermeneutics to make distinctions between true and false prejudices by a process of effective historical consciousness. Gadamer suggested that effective historical consciousness was analogous to the I-Thou relationship in which openness to the other and willingness to be modified creates a dialogical relationship (Gadamer 1975 trans., p. 323). By this, he was advocating the need to be open to and surprised by what may emerge through interpretation.

For Jürgen Habermas, interpretation is more a matter of realising that knowledge is socially constructed through human interaction and that interpretation involves social, cultural, economic and political and personal dimensions. He proposed a kind of critical hermeneutics that:

> focuses on the communicative conditions under which meaning is produced and on power/justice dimensions of intended and unintended social consequences of interpretations. Critical hermeneutics has a commitment to both understanding and exposing how power imbalances and misunderstandings constrain and distort interpretations (Allen 1995, p. 180).

Habermas linked truthful interpretation to the idea of rational consensus gained through discourse. This means that people have the potential to create their own interpretations through non-coercive and non-manipulative rationality. He considered that people orient towards finding truth through daily communicative acts or speaking, and that ideal speech situations involve comprehensibility of the utterance, truth of the content, rightness of the performative content, and veracity of the speaker. This kind of rationality has been criticised by Bernstein (1978), who says that Habermas's idea of ideal speech is not real because it has not paid attention to people's choice and will, cultural diversity and language differences.

For the postmodernists, the whole idea of interpretation is open for debate. As Rosenau (1992) explains:

> Post-modernists recognise an infinite number of interpretations (meanings) of any text are possible because, for the skeptical post-modernists, one can never say what one intends with language, ultimately all textual meaning, all interpretation, is undecidable. Because there is no final meaning for any particular sign, no notion of a unitary sense of text, these post-modernists argue that no interpretation can be regarded as superior to any other. In its world of plural constructions, diverse realities, an absence of certainty, and a multiplicity of readings, post-modernism refuses to privilege one statement over another; all interpretations are of equal interest (p. 120).

Postmodern definitions of interpretation are influenced by deconstruction, which 'involves demystifying a text, tearing it apart to reveal its internal, arbitrary hierarchies and its presuppositions' (Rosenau 1992, p. 120). Deconstruction involves looking at the 'margins' of a text, to its contradictions, inconsistencies, and what is excluded, unnamed and concealed, not to unmask errors (as this would imply a search for truth) but to transform and redefine it. In this way, postmodernist deconstruction discloses tensions, but does not seek to resolve them, as this would give authority to the most correct interpretation. The consequence of postmodern deconstruction, therefore, is a never-ending critique of text to reveal its contradictions and to question the authority of the author.

Where does postmodern deconstruction leave researchers? If we are to take a sceptical view of postmodernism, we would be caught up 'in an infinite regress of deconstruction, where nothing is better than anything else' (Richardson 1992, p. 122). On a practical level, no research meanings would be viewed as defensible interpretations, providing no definite answers or even tentative guidance, reasonable for the moment. However, health care needs guidance in practice, education and management. In this postmodern world, trends towards evidence-based practice are paramount, and these favour quantitative measures and prioritise qualitative measures last as indicators of useful, 'truthful' interpretations.

So, is postmodernism interesting, but of no practical use for researchers? Debates have argued both cases. Kermode and Brown (1995) argue that postmodernism is not only of no practical use for nursing, but also that it can deaden our sensitivities towards capitalism and patriarchy, which may be left uncontested as sources of power and domination in postmodern times because of an 'anything goes' relativism inherent in postmodernism. In response, nurse-scholars and researchers argue that a narrow view of postmodernism takes account only of the sceptical literature and does not allow postmodernism to create wider and deeper possibilities for conceptualising and practising nursing (Cheek 2000; Glass & Davis 1998). On an optimistic note, a postmodern 'interpretation' leaves the reader in authority as the interpreter of any life text. In health care, that means making choices about what constitutes a particular discipline, while heeding caution about accepting unquestioningly all kinds of dominant discourses in grand narratives.

All in all, what is written about interpretation may provide cold comfort to a researcher who knows very little about philosophy and who simply wants to know how to go about interpreting qualitative data. The next section will attempt to break through the lack of direction to give clues to ways in which interpretation might be done. It will be done by raising some questions and suggesting some tentative answers. Examples of research will be given to demonstrate differences that will be noted in qualitative interpretive and critical research interpretations.

The assumptions underlying the listing of these suggested processes relate to differences in research relationships between researchers and participants. Qualitative interpretive methodologies involve participants by working with them in research processes, rather than doing research 'to' subjects. However, qualitative interpretive methodologies are not as mindful of participatory group processes and co-researcher status for participants as qualitative critical methodologies.

How do I go about the process of interpretation when I have used a qualitative interpretive methodology?

- Go through the exercise of asking yourself the questions listed in this chapter as preconditions for qualitative interpretation.
- Take some time away from the project. Take a walk, go on a holiday – in whatever way you prefer, give yourself some space. (This will depend on the time you have available to complete the project, of course!) 'Time out' will let the analysed data percolate through your mind.
- Although you are taking a rest from the project, notice any ideas that come up in your mind. Write them down, even if they seem insignificant.
- Remember that interpretation subsumes all the phases in the research that have gone before.
- Remember that the products of the analysis are incomplete in themselves. They only have fullest meaning when they have been described and explained through interpretation.
- Resume your work and reread the analysed data. Review how you came to make the themes/essences/categories.
- If you have already named any of the themes/essences/categories in the analysis phase, why did you choose those words? Are they still relevant? Would other words represent them more effectively?
- Clarify in your mind what the themes/essences/categories mean. Try writing down words and sentences that explain them to other people.

- If you are not a rapid writer and your thoughts are moving too fast, speak into an audiotape recorder and rephrase your thoughts over and over until you are sure you are saying what you mean to be saying. Commit the final version to writing.
- If you prefer vocalising your interpretations as they happen, ask a valued friend or colleague who is aware of the intentions of the research, to listen to you as you speak spontaneously about what you think the analysed data mean in light of the overall project. After you have finished the clearest possible explication of what you want to say, invite the person to ask questions and to be frank about any parts of your interpretations that did not seem to ring true to the overall intentions and phases of the project.
- Create definitions and explanations that represent most faithfully the clearest and truest meaning that you can extract from the analysed data.
- Ensure that you have created and explained links between definitions and explanations, that are congruent with the assumptions, aims, objectives, methods and processes of the research.
- Links between definitions and explanations need to be clear and your reasons for making them should be able to be traced by readers.

EXERCISE

Use the steps in interpretation described above to move from analysis to interpretation in your story or a series of stories about an experience in your life which was of great significance to you. How does your analysis differ from your interpretation of your story/stories?

For excellent examples of interpretation of research using interpretive methodologies, refer to the following projects:

Beck, C.T. 2004, 'Birth trauma: in the eye of the beholder', *Nursing Research*, vol. 53, no. 1, 28–35.
Fiveash, B. & Nay, R. 2004, 'Being active supports client control over care', *Contemporary Nurse*, vol. 17, no. 3, 192–203.
Gibb, H. 2003, 'Rural community mental health nursing: a grounded theory account of sole practice', *International Journal of Mental Health Nursing*, vol. 12, no. 4, 243–50.
Maldonado, N., Efinger, J. & Lacey, C. 2003, 'Shared perceptions of personal moral development', *International Journal for Human Caring*, vol. 7, no. 1, 9–19.
McCann, T.V. & Clark, E. 2003, 'A grounded theory study of the role that nurses play in increasing clients' willingness to access community mental health services', *International Journal of Mental Health Nursing*, vol. 12, no. 4, 279–87.
Peters, K. 2003, 'In pursuit of motherhood: the IVF experience', *Contemporary Nurse*, vol. 14, no. 3, 258–70.
Rew, L. 2003, 'A theory of taking care of oneself grounded in experiences of homeless youth', *Nursing Research*, vol. 52, no. 4, 234–41.
Sundelof, E.-M., Hansebo, G. & Ekman, S.-L. 2004, 'Friendship and caring communion: the meaning of caring relationship in district nursing', *International Journal for Human Caring*, vol. 8, no. 3, 13–20.

How do I go about the process of interpretation when I have used a qualitative critical methodology?

Given that critical methodologies have an emancipatory intent for groups of oppressed or otherwise disenfranchised people, the interpretive processes may often be shared by the people involved.

- Go through the exercise as a group, asking each other the questions listed in this chapter as preconditions for qualitative interpretation.
- Acknowledge the potential of group members to make a collective interpretation of the information, based on their active involvement in the collaborative project.
- Give the group the option of taking some time away from the intensity of the project. The time can be negotiated. This will depend on the time you have available to complete the project and on other factors the members may raise as being important.
- If the members decide to take time away from the project, suggest that during the time away they notice any ideas that come to mind. Ask them to write these down, even if they seem insignificant, so that they can be shared with others in the whole group.
- Resume or continue group meetings and decide on a way of reviewing the analysed data. Review how you came to make the decisions you made at the time of analysis.
- Remember that multiple interpretations of competing discourses are possible. There may be no easy answers to complex socio-political questions that have been raised by the research; rather, the group may be able to identify some tentative connections and interpretations related to interpersonal and institutional power relationships.
- Remember that the interpretations subsume all the phases in the research that have gone before.
- Remember that the products of the analysis are incomplete in themselves. They only have fullest meaning when they have been described and explained through critical appraisal and interpretation.
- If the group has already named any of the issues/themes/ideas/action cycles that were generated in the analysis phase, why did they choose them? Are they still relevant? Would other issues/themes/ideas/action cycles represent them more effectively now, in the light of further critique and new information?
- In an open group discussion clarify what the issues/themes/ideas/action cycles mean. Ask group members to write down words and sentences and explain them to other people. Invite them to share them with the other group members.
- It may be useful to have an audiotape recorder during the sharing of interpretations. Expose the interpretations to critique. Try to reach consensus on a shared and agreed set of statements about the interpretations. Note any possible alternative interpretations in light of the unique social, historical, economic, political, cultural and personal determinants of the research setting, intentions, processes and methods. Commit the final version to writing.
- You could also suggest that group members work in pairs to discuss individual interpretations. Suggest that they speak spontaneously about what the analysed data might

mean in light of the overall project. Encourage members to make the clearest possible explication of what they want to say. Suggest that they raise questions about interpretations and seek other possible explanations and conclusions. These are then shared with the whole group.

- As a group, create statements and explanations that represent most faithfully the multiple discourses that can be extracted from the analysed data.
- Ensure that you have created and explained links between the multiple discourses that are congruent with the assumptions, aims, objectives, methods and processes of the research.
- Links between the multiple discourses need to be as clear as possible and the linking should be argued carefully for the benefit of the participants and the readers of the research.
- Ensure that the final version of the overall interpretations represents all the group intend them to mean after full discussion and critical appraisal of the social, historical, economic, political, cultural and personal determinants operating in the research.

For excellent examples of interpretation of research using critical methodologies, refer to the following projects:

Armishaw, J. & Davis, K. 2002, 'Women, hepatitis C, and sexuality: a critical feminist exploration', *Contemporary Nurse*, vol. 12, no. 2, 194–203.
Craig, D., Donoghue, J., Seller, M. & Mitten-Lewis, S. 2004, 'Improving nursing management of patients with diabetes using an action research approach', *Contemporary Nurse*, vol. 17, no. 1-2, 71–9.
Hardin, P. 2003, 'Shape-shifting discourses of anorexia nervosa: reconstituting psychopathology', *Nursing Inquiry*, vol. 10, no. 4, 209–17.
Meyer, D. & de Oliveira, D. 2003, 'Breastfeeding policies and the production of motherhood: a historical-cultural approach', *Nursing Inquiry*, vol. 10, no. 1, 11–18.
Rankin, J. 2003, '"Patient satisfaction": knowledge for ruling hospital reform – an institutional ethnography', *Nursing Inquiry*, vol. 10, no. 1, 57–65.
Taylor, B.J., Bulmer, B., Hill, L., Luxford, C., McFarlane, J. & Stirling, K. 2002, 'Exploring idealism in palliative nursing care through reflective practice and action research', *International Journal of Palliative Nursing*, vol. 8, no. 7, 324–30.
Watson, J., Turnbull, B. & Mills, A. 2002, 'Evaluation of the extended role of the midwife: the voices of midwives', *International Journal of Nursing Practice*, vol. 8, no. 5, 257–64.

What will the interpretations look like?

- Interpretations will not look alike. They will differ according to the ways in which they were extracted from the data.
- Interpretations will bear a resemblance to the language of the methodologies that guided them.
- Interpretations may be represented as diversely as words, phrases, sentences, models, theories, action strategies, group summaries, and so on.
- Interpretations may be put forward to readers of the research as theoretical propositions, findings, results, insights, strategies, implications, and examples of reflective awareness, changed practice, multiple discourses, and so on.

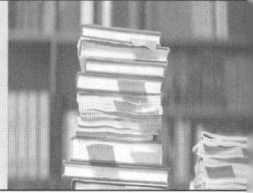

How will I know that the interpretations are relevant?

- Interpretations will have a high chance of being relevant if they can demonstrate methodological congruency. This means that they show that they are related directly to the analysed data, which in turn is related to the assumptions, methods and processes of the research.
- Interpretations have meaning only in terms of the research because they are specific to the research. Interpretations are context-dependent; that is, they are relative to the total set of circumstances that make up the research.
- Ways of checking relevance differ according to the methodological approach.
- The tests of relevance that are applied are particular to the approach taken.
- For further information on relevance refer to the section on 'rigour' in Chapter 14.

Interpreting the text in light of the literature

The need to do a research project may be based on a review of the literature review that confirms knowledge gaps or conflicting results. In contrast, if a researcher is interested in taking an inductive approach, such as that taken in grounded theory, the literature review may be delayed until during or after the data collection. Even so, at some point, qualitative researchers will go to the literature to see what it contains on an area of interest.

Interpretations may compare to or contrast with the results of other studies. Research reports may include a section in which the connections are spelt out clearly. If connections are found between the newly interpreted data and those already in the literature, qualitative researchers would not necessarily use this discovery to make a claim for the truthfulness of the interpretations. Rather, the similarities would be documented in the research report as a point of interest.

The other reason for consulting the literature is to provide a firm grounding for the interpretations in the methodological tradition of choice. For example, a phenomenological project may use certain concepts to show readers that the assumptions underlying the choice of methods and processes relate to the project; a feminist project will be guided by the literature relating to feminisms and feminist research processes, and a critical ethnography may cite references derived from critical social science to augment its questioning approach to the research interest. In each of these cases, the aim is to present the key ideas of the methodology to show the kind of knowledge it is capable of generating in research projects. Research reflecting postmodern influences may stand outside methodological categorisation on the basis that they represent grand narratives. Even so, researchers who are reflecting postmodern influences may appeal to literature that affirms key ideas, such as multiple voices, difference, fragmentation and deconstruction. For methods of narrative and discourse analyses, see the relevant sections in Chapter 16.

Summary

This chapter alerted you to the need to differentiate between analysis and interpretation in qualitative research. The relative nature of qualitative research interpretations was acknowledged, given that there is agreement in the methodologies that due to the complex nature of human relationships, there is no absolute and unchanging truth.

Interpretations differ according to specific methodological approaches. For example, qualitative interpretive methodologies tend to highlight context-dependent meanings and qualitative critical methodologies will tend to expose multiple interpretations associated with power relationships in socio-political settings. Postmodernism questions the whole idea of interpretation and definitions of interpretation are influenced by deconstruction, which involves looking at contradictions and inconsistencies at the 'margins' of a text.

As a practical guide for new researchers, processes were outlined for making qualitative interpretive and critical interpretations and some postmodern influences on interpretation were identified.

Main points

- Interpretation involves working with the forms of analysed information so that statements can be made about what they mean in light of the intentions, methods and processes of the research.
- Generally speaking, analysis precedes interpretation, although some qualitative researchers describe an intuitive grasp of the data, while others may experience spiralling and integrative processes in which analysis and interpretation blend and seem to become indivisible.
- Invariably, qualitative interpretations of words and language require protracted time with the text to ensure that meaning is located, that it is as clear as possible to convey to other people, and that it may also be validated by other researchers, co-researchers, participants and peers.
- Qualitative researchers agree that there is no way of guaranteeing absolute truth, because truth is relative and elusive; therefore, truth can change according to all kinds of context-dependent determinants associated with people, places, times and conditions in which it resides and from which it emerges.
- Various words are used synonymously to mean interpretations, such as theories, findings, results, insights, strategies, implications, examples of reflective awareness and changed practice, and so on, according to the assumptions and intentions of the research methodology.

- Most qualitative research approaches do not claim to generate interpretations that can be considered to be generalisable to the wider population, with the exception of grounded theory, which sets out to make general statements in the form of theories about what might be expected in similar circumstances.
- Research using postmodern thought may not deem to offer anything concrete, but to leave all ideas open as tentative, or make multiple interpretations and give authority to readers to make their own interpretations.
- Processes for interpretation may differ according to what kind of qualitative research it can be considered to be, that is, whether it is essentially an interpretive (concerned mainly with meaning) or critical (concerned mainly with change) project. Some researchers use a combination of interpretive and critical processes, appropriate to the assumptions, aims, objectives, methods and processes of the project.
- In qualitative research, congruency means the fit, or correspondence, between foundational ideas and the activity phases of the research.
- The reasons for asking certain questions at the transition from analysis to interpretation are to reorient to the overall project, to check on the degree of congruency between the assumptions, aims, objectives, methods and processes, and to prepare for the process of interpretation.
- For the postmodernists the whole idea of interpretation is open for debate, because postmodern definitions of interpretation are influenced by deconstruction. This in turn involves looking at the 'margins' of a text, to its contradictions, inconsistencies, and what is excluded, unnamed and concealed, not to unmask errors (as this would imply a search for truth), but to transform and redefine it.
- An affirmative postmodern 'interpretation' leaves the reader in authority as the interpreter of any life text. In nursing and health care, that means making choices about what constitutes the discipline, while heeding caution about accepting unquestioningly all kinds of dominant discourses in grand narratives.
- The process of interpretation in qualitative interpretive methodologies involves protracted reading and reflecting on the data to create definitions and explanations that represent most faithfully the clearest meaning that can be extracted from the analysed data in light of the descriptive intentions of the project.
- The process of interpretation in qualitative critical methodologies often includes collaborative group processes to sift through multiple interpretations of competing discourses to find tentative answers to complex socio-political questions involving social, historical, economic, political, cultural and personal determinants, in light of the descriptive intentions of the project.
- Interpretations will not look alike, as they will bear a resemblance to the language of the methodologies that guided them. They may be represented as diversely as words, phrases, sentences, models, theories, action strategies, group summaries, theoretical propositions, findings, results, insights, strategies, implications, and examples of reflective awareness, changed practice, multiple discourses and so on.
- Interpretations have a high chance of being relevant if they can demonstrate methodological congruency; that is, they show that they are related directly to the analysed

data, which are in turn related to the methodological assumptions, methods and processes of the research.

- Research projects reflecting postmodern influences may stand outside methodological categorisation on the basis that they represent grand narratives; however, researchers reflecting postmodern influences may appeal to literature that affirms key ideas, such as multiple voices, difference, fragmentation and deconstruction.

CASE STUDY

Carmel was introduced in Chapter 14. If you have not been following Carmel's case study, go to the end of Chapters 14, 15 and 16 and review her story so far. Carmel is using a collaborative approach with 10 other experienced nurses working in acute care settings. She set up a participatory action research (PAR) group and they have been meeting for one hour per week for eight weeks. After reflection and discussion the group has identified a thematic concern of the use of power in the health care organisation. The PAR group has undertaken a literature search to see what has been written about organisational power in hospitals. Members also have been reflecting on their own practice and sharing their stories in PAR group meetings.

1   In what ways might the PAR group analyse its practice stories?
2   Who could possibly make the interpretations of the practice stories, when, how, why, and with whom?
3   In what forms would these PAR interpretations most likely be represented?

Multiple choice questions

1   Interpretation involves:
   a   reading research data to create codes and categories from participants' accounts of their experiences
   b   working with the forms of analysed information so that statements can be made about what they mean
   c   thematic analysis approaches that systematically identify and name themes and sub-themes
   d   collecting and collating research data for systematic sorting, coding, categorising and analysis
2   Interpretation requires immersion in the text because:
   a   words and language are the bases of qualitative research
   b   numbers and statistics are the bases of qualitative research
   c   cause and effect relationships are the bases of qualitative research
   d   thinking and reading are the bases of qualitative research

3 When qualitative researchers say that truth is relative, they mean that truth:

    a can be fabricated by some creative researchers

    b is certain and can be found after test and retest

    c is fixed, absolute and measurable by scientific means

    d can change according to context-dependent determinants

4 Although most qualitative research approaches do not claim to generate interpretations that can be considered to be generalisable to the wider population, an exception is:

    a phenomenology

    b postmodernism

    c critical ethnography

    d grounded theory

5 Thinking influencing qualitative research that all ideas are open as tentative, that multiple interpretations are possible and that readers have authority to make their own interpretations is:

    a phenomenological

    b historical

    c postmodernist

    d ethnographical

6 In qualitative research, processes for interpretation:

    a are always predictable according to the assumption that truth is fixed and certain

    b may differ according to what kind of qualitative research it can be considered to be

    c always claim to be considered to be generalisable to the wider population

    d may guarantee absolute truth, because truth is always found by scientific means

7 In qualitative research, methodological congruency is:

    a the attempt to demonstrate cause and effect relationships by rigorous means

    b the fit, or correspondence, between foundational ideas and the activity phases of the research

    c interpretation, through theories, findings, results, insights, strategies and implications

    d the inherent contradictions in undertaking any kind of research into human experience

8 Collaborative group processes to sift through multiple interpretations of competing discourses to find tentative answers to complex socio-political questions involving social, historical, economic, political, cultural and personal determinants, are characteristic of:

    a qualitative critical methodologies

    b the scientific method

    c randomised controlled trials

    d qualitative interpretive methodologies

9 Qualitative interpretations will not all look alike and may be represented as:

    a numbers, statistics, theoretical propositions, findings, results and implications

    b reflective awareness, changed practice, multiple discourses and statistics

    c words, phrases, sentences, models, theories, action strategies and group summaries

    d results, insights, strategies, implications, reflective awareness and statistics

10 Interpretations influenced by postmodern thinking may feature:
  a reliability, congruency, coherence and validity research processes
  b multiple voices, difference, fragmentation and deconstruction
  c the truest meaning that can be derived from participants' accounts
  d critical questions at the transition from analysis to interpretation

Review topics

1 Explain why qualitative analysis usually precedes interpretation.

2 Discuss why qualitative interpretation is connected to assumptions about truth.

3 Discuss why there are so many different synonyms for qualitative interpretations.

4 Describe the nature of qualitative critical interpretations.

5 Discuss how affirmative postmodern approaches influence research interpretations.

Online reading

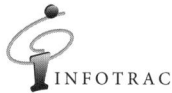

INFOTRAC® COLLEGE EDITION
When accessing information on interpreting qualitative research, use the following keywords in any combinations you require:

➤ action strategies
➤ analysis
➤ changed practice
➤ congruency
➤ critical
➤ deconstruction
➤ findings
➤ group summaries
➤ implications
➤ insights
➤ interpretive
➤ models
➤ multiple discourses
➤ postmodern
➤ reflective awareness
➤ results
➤ strategies
➤ theoretical propositions
➤ theories

References

Allen, D.G. 1995, 'Hermeneutics: philosophical traditions and nursing practice research', *Nursing Science Quarterly*, vol. 8, no. 4, 174–82.

Armishaw, J. & Davis, K. 2002, 'Women, hepatitis C, and sexuality: a critical feminist exploration', *Contemporary Nurse*, vol. 12, no. 2, 194–203.

Atkinson, P., Coffey, A., Delamont, S., Lofland, J. & Lofland, L. (eds) 2001, *Handbook of Ethnography*, Sage, London.

Beck, C.T. 2004, 'Birth trauma: in the eye of the beholder', *Nursing research*, vol. 53, no. 1, 28–35.

Bernstein, R. 1978, *The Restructuring of Social and Political Theory*, University of Pennsylvania Press, Philadelphia.

Cheek, J. 2000, *Postmodern and Poststructural Approaches to Nursing Research*, Sage, Thousand Oaks, California.

Colaizzi, P. 1978, 'Psychological research as the phenomenologist views it', in R.S. Valle & M. King (eds), *Existential Phenomenological Alternatives for Psychology*, Oxford University Press, New York.

Collins English Dictionary 1998, 4th Australian edn, HarperCollins Publishers, Glasgow.

Craig, D., Donoghue, J., Seller, M. & Mitten-Lewis, S. 2004, 'Improving nursing management of patients with diabetes using an action research approach', *Contemporary Nurse*, vol. 17, no. 1–2, 71–9.

Denzin, N. & Lincoln, Y. (eds) 2000, *Handbook of Qualitative Research*, 2nd edn, Sage, Thousand Oaks, California.

Fiveash, B. & Nay, R. 2004, 'Being active supports client control over care', *Contemporary Nurse*, vol. 17, no. 3, 192–203.

Gadamer, H.-G. 1975 trans., in G. Barden & J. Cumming (eds), *Truth and Method*, Seabury, New York.

Gibb, H. 2003, 'Rural community mental health nursing: A grounded theory account of sole practice', *International Journal of Mental Health Nursing*, vol. 12, no. 4, 243–50.

Glass, N. & Davis, K. 1998, 'An emancipatory impulse: a feminist postmodern integrated turning point in nursing research', *Advances in Nursing Science*, vol. 21, no. 1, 43–52.

Gubrium, J.F. & Holstein, J.A. (eds) 2002, *Handbook of Interview Research: Context and Method*, Sage, Thousand Oaks.

Habermas, J. 1981, *The Theory of Communicative Action: Reason and the Rationalization of Society*, Beacon, Boston.

Hardin, P. 2003, 'Shape-shifting discourses of anorexia nervosa: reconstituting psychopathology', *Nursing Inquiry*, vol. 10, no. 4, 209–17.

Kermode, S. & Brown, C. 1995, 'Where have all the flowers gone?: Nursing's escape from the radical critique', *Contemporary Nurse*, vol. 4, no. 1, 8–15.

Langridge, M. & Ahern, K. 2002, 'A case report on mixed methods in qualitative research', *Collegian*, vol. 10, no. 4, 32–6.

Maldonado, N., Efinger, J. & Lacey, C. 2003, 'Shared perceptions of personal moral development', *International Journal for Human Caring*, vol. 7, no. 1, 9–19.

McCann, T.V. & Clark, E. 2003, 'A grounded theory study of the role that nurses play in increasing clients' willingness to access community mental health services', *International Journal of Mental Health Nursing*, vol. 12, no. 4, 279–87.

Meyer, D. & de Oliveira, D. 2003, 'Breastfeeding policies and the production of motherhood: a historical-cultural approach', *Nursing Inquiry*, vol. 10, no. 1, 11–18.

Peters, K. 2003, 'In pursuit of motherhood: the IVF experience', *Contemporary Nurse*, vol. 14, no. 3, 258–70.

Rankin, J. 2003, '"Patient satisfaction": knowledge for ruling hospital reform – an institutional ethnography', *Nursing Inquiry*, vol. 10, no. 1, 57–65.

Reason, P. & Bradbury, H. (eds) 2001, *Handbook of Action Research: Participative Inquiry and Practice*, Sage, London.

Rew, L. 2003, 'A theory of taking care of oneself grounded in experiences of homeless youth', *Nursing Research*, vol. 52, no. 4, 234–41.

Richardson, L. 1992, 'The collective story: postmodernism and the writing of sociology', in P. Rosenau (ed.), *Post-Modernism and the Social Sciences: Insights, Inroads and Intrusions*, Princeton University Press, New Jersey.

Rosenau, P. 1992, *Post-Modernism and the Social Sciences: Insights, Inroads and Intrusions*, Princeton University Press, New Jersey.

Strauss, A.L. 1975, *Chronic Illness and Quality of Life*, C.V. Mosby Co., St Louis.

Sundelof, E.-M., Hansebo, G. & Ekman, S.-L. 2004, 'Friendship and caring communion: the meaning of caring relationship in district nursing', *International Journal for Human Caring*, vol. 8, no. 3, 13–20.

Taylor, B.J., Bulmer, B., Hill, L., Luxford, C., McFarlane, J. & Stirling, K. 2002, 'Exploring idealism in palliative nursing care through reflective practice and action research', *International Journal of Palliative Nursing*, vol. 8, no. 7, 324–30.

Watson, J., Turnbull, B. & Mills, A. 2002, 'Evaluation of the extended role of the midwife: the voices of midwives', *International Journal of Nursing Practice*, vol. 8, no. 5, 257–64.

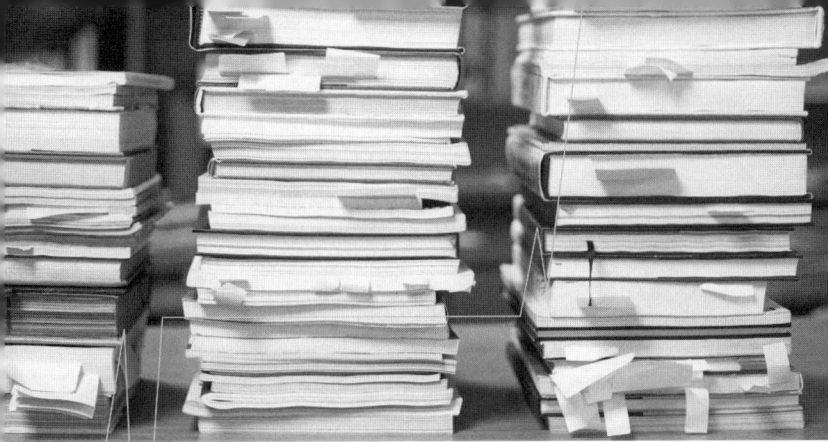

CHAPTER 18

DISSEMINATING THE FINDINGS

CHAPTER OBJECTIVES

The material presented in this chapter will assist you to:

- understand the reasons for preparing a research report
- identify the intended recipients of the research report
- write a research report
- identify the elements of a quantitative and a qualitative report
- submit a research report
- give a conference or seminar presentation
- prepare and present a poster
- prepare a journal article
- prepare a monograph.

Introduction

The **research report** is a formal account of the research project. It is the major means by which you disseminate essential information about your research project. It can be either in written form, in which case it becomes a permanent record, or it can be an oral report to a group of colleagues at a seminar or conference.

Students who are taking units at either undergraduate or graduate level, in which they are required to write a research report as a part of learning about the research process, will find the material in this chapter useful. Many undergraduate courses have a unit on research. Some of these focus mainly on proposal writing and the consumption of research, while others take students through the whole research process, including writing a report. In addition, many postgraduate courses have a research component. Honours students and higher degree students will find the material in this chapter useful as a starting point for writing their theses. Students who are studying units for which there is no written research report will still find this chapter useful for learning to assess other research reports.

Similarly, if you are a research officer in a clinical setting and you need some hints or reminders on how to go about writing a report, the practical advice in this chapter will help you. The emphasis is on student research reports because they are a common student exercise and part of the process of learning about research. Even so, the advice has the potential to be of use for anyone needing to write a credible research report. Researchers may also present seminars, reports at conferences, and **posters**. Researchers may publish research reports in journals after some adaptations. For example, student assignments in their original form are seldom suitable for publication due to their content, length and organisation. Assignments need to be adjusted to suit the format of the journal if they are to be successful in being published. Therefore, some mention is made of journal writing in this chapter. There are publications that specialise in teaching about writing for journals, for example, Greenwood (1998) and Plawecki and Plawecki (1998). Anyone doing a thesis should find the rudiments of report writing in this book helpful, but should also obtain specialist books in thesis writing such as Anderson and Poole (1998) and Walters (1999).

If carrying out research comprises a part of your employment, you have a responsibility to share the findings of your research with colleagues. There are a number of reasons for this. First, a report is essential because research that is not reported is meaningless and does not contribute to building a body of knowledge. Second, the findings may be useful to colleagues to help them make their practice more effective. Third, the findings may be useful in helping others plan their research more effectively. Finally, a research report allows your peers to evaluate the quality of your research. In return for fulfilling your responsibility, you will have the reward of helping other people, recognition by your colleagues and assistance with your career development.

EXERCISE

What are the main reasons you need to know how to write a research report? What form will your report take? Locate a publication cited above on journal and thesis writing and pursue your exploration further.

The research report

The most important purpose of a research report is to communicate key aspects of the project to the research consumer. Readers will probably be reading your report so that they can replicate your study, to do their own literature review, to plan a new study or to help find a solution for a clinical practice problem. In all of these situations, readers will be evaluating your study for validity and usefulness. To do this, they need to be able to determine how your study was conducted.

Research reports are presented in different media, have different lengths and serve different purposes. First, there are written reports, such as classroom project reports, **peer-reviewed journal articles** and theses or dissertations. These are intended to be read. Second, research findings may be presented as oral reports, such as seminar reports and conference papers. These convey information spoken to an audience, and are therefore an auditory or audiovisual experience.

A classroom research report is usually submitted as an assignment of about 2000 to 3000 words. It follows a standard format for a research report, as detailed in the 'Written report' section of this chapter.

A journal article will normally be between 3000 and 5000 words long. The main purpose of a journal article is to disseminate the results of the research to a large target audience. Journal articles often take a year between submission and publication. There is very little opportunity for direct comments to the researcher after publication; however, there is feedback built into the review process that precedes publication. Journal articles have the potential to reach the whole profession or specialty group. If you are involved in writing up a paper, either for a classroom assignment or a journal article, there are numerous writings on the topic to help you. Examples are an article by Greenwood (1998) and books by Day (1998) and Dees (1999).

A dissertation is a long, detailed discourse, and need not be a research report. A thesis is a research dissertation submitted for an honours degree or a higher degree such as a master's degree or a doctorate. The words 'thesis' and 'dissertation' tend to be used interchangeably, with the word 'thesis' preferred in Australia. The purpose of a thesis is to test the student's ability to demonstrate proficiency in the research process. A thesis for a master's degree will usually be at least 25 000 words long. A doctoral thesis will be much longer, up to 100 000 words. A thesis may only ever be read by a limited number of people who have an interest in the topic. If you are writing a thesis, you should obtain at least one specialist book in thesis writing. Examples are: *Assignment and Thesis Writing* (Anderson & Poole 1998) and *How to Write Health Sciences Papers, Dissertations and Theses* (Thomas 2000).

The purpose of conference and seminar papers is to communicate work in progress or completed results to a specific target group of interested persons. Papers allow personal communication with colleagues about your work, and allow for critical feedback. Conference papers are normally distributed to the conference delegates, and others who may be interested in purchasing them. Seminar papers may be distributed to those attending the seminar.

A poster is a presentation on poster board, usually at a conference, with the researcher in attendance to answer questions. You can prepare the poster yourself from stencilled letters or other printing. If you can afford it, you can have almost any stage of the poster prepared professionally. The text can be prepared from a computer program such as PowerPoint. The poster can be screen-printed in very large font on the board by a printery.

The final product can be professionally laminated. You can compose the poster from a series of A4 pages linked by arrows, which are far more portable than a full-sized poster.

A poster presentation is strongly visual; however, the visual information is supplemented by discussion between the presenter and the viewer. With the proliferation of research there has been an increasing tendency to use the poster as a medium for presenting research since many can be presented in one session. Posters also allow researchers to present work in progress or completed work. They are a good way to begin presenting research because they are a lot less intimidating than presenting a paper before a class or a conference. Posters are very small in comparison to any other medium. Posters are usually kept by the presenter. You can learn more about poster preparation in articles by McCann, Sramac and Rudy (1999), Cantrell and Bracher (1999) and Jackson and Sheldon (2000). There is even a whole book on poster presentation (Gosling 1999).

In the future, it is to be expected that the limited dissemination of conference papers and minor reports will change because of the ability to post many communications on the World Wide Web. Even theses are becoming available electronically. However, the large volume of a thesis will ultimately restrict the audience for it.

EXERCISE

Differentiate between a research report written and presented as an assignment, a journal article, a thesis, a conference presentation and a poster. What are the advantages and disadvantages of these presentations?

The written report
The target audience

Before beginning to write the report, consider the target audience. Whether you are writing for a lecturer, a thesis examiner or a journal editor, there will be expectations on their part as to the structure and content of the report. A lecturer will probably be most interested in whether or not the student has shown a comprehension of the research process. A thesis examiner will be interested in whether the student has demonstrated proficiency in the subject and in planning and executing research and interpreting the findings in their scientific context. A journal editor will be looking for evidence that the content of the report is suited to the journal's readership. For example, a clinical research journal will want clinical implications.

If a journal readership is your target, it is first necessary to select a journal that is aimed at that group. You can find out about the journals in a database such as CINAHL. In deciding which journal to target, consider its style, its readership and the type of article it publishes. For example, if your report is very specialised in content, you should aim at a journal that specialises in that content so that the information you have to present reaches an appropriate audience. You may also want to consider the demographics of the readership – if your article is nationally focused, you will do better to target a national journal. Depending on the quality of the report, you may choose to target a refereed (peer-reviewed) or a non-refereed journal.

If you are intending to pursue a career in academia, check your national research policies, which are reflected in the way your university attracts research funds. For example, in New Zealand and Britain research quality measures have been in place for some time. Australia is moving rapidly into a system of Research Quality Framework (RQF). This means that researchers in academia need to pursue publishing options in the journals with the greatest quality and impact factors, for example, international peer-reviewed journals with a high rating for status and prestige as publications.

EXERCISE

Ask a librarian to help you locate a list of the most prestigious peer-reviewed journals in your disciplinary area. Locate a copy of the journal rated number one and scan the articles to see if you can ascertain the nature of the publications. For example, are they quantitative, qualitative and/or mixed methodology research reports?

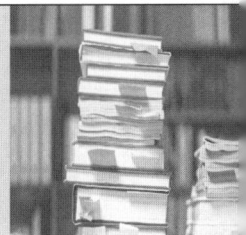

Guidelines

Whatever the target readership of your research report, you must obtain and follow any guidelines for the preparation of research reports. If you are writing for a classroom project, you should follow any guidelines that you have been given, as marks may be allocated for presentation and referencing. Many universities have guidelines for thesis presentation, which you should obtain if you are doing a thesis or research project as part of a graduate diploma, honours degree or higher degree. Most university calendars state the rules for presentation of theses for a research degree. They address type of paper, margins, line spacing, binding, number of copies, and so forth. These should be followed exactly. If you are writing for a journal, make sure you acquire a copy of their guidelines for authors and follow them exactly. These will concern referencing and presentation of the article. It is also worth photocopying several articles and analysing the approach that successful authors have used.

Planning and writing your report

When you have assembled the guidelines, you should plan your writing approach. It is wise to make an outline that is as detailed as possible. The outline can include the major topics and subtopics. Then write the sections of the report according to the format below, or whatever variation is specified by the guidelines. You will probably need to revise the report several times, polishing it as you go. If possible, have someone critique the report.

The style of writing for a research report is generally the same as for a research proposal. This can be read in more detail in Chapter 6; however, the major points will be reviewed here. The style should be concise, clear and coherent. One of the greatest scientific discoveries of all time, that of the molecular structure of deoxyribonucleic acid (DNA) was reported in an elegantly written one-page letter to the journal *Nature* (Watson & Crick 1953). Your style should suit your target audience. A report of quantitative research is usually written in the formal scientific style to convey objectivity. A report of qualitative research may sometimes be written in the personal style in situating the researcher within the research, but adhere to formal writing conventions in the literature review, methods, processes and methodology sections. Use good English that is appropriate for your audience, and avoid jargon and sexist language. Avoid the passive voice wherever possible. The tense is less of a problem in a research report than in the proposal because the report will mainly be in the past tense. The exception is statements of everyday knowledge, which are written in the present tense.

Structure of the report

In this chapter, we are giving you material on how to write both quantitative and qualitative research reports, with examples of both.

Common initial elements of quantitative and qualitative reports

The research report has three major components: the **preliminaries**, the **body of the report** and the **supporting materials**, presented in that order. The preliminaries introduce the report, the body contains the main information and the supporting materials contain the references and appendixes.

A sample format for a research report is as follows:

Sample format of a research report

Preliminaries
   Title page
   Required forms*
   Acknowledgements*
   Abstract
   Table of contents*
   List of tables*
   List of figures*
   Executive summary†
Body of report
   Introduction
   Literature review
   Methodology
   Results
   Discussion
Supporting materials
   References
   Appendixes

   Key: * *denotes applicable only to thesis or long report*
            † *denotes applicable only to long report*

Figure 18.1   Sample format of a research report

For a student research assignment, it is not necessary to use the components marked in Figure 18.1 with the symbol *. It is also not necessary to divide the content into chapters; the body of the report can all be one section. Begin each section on a new page. For a thesis or longer report, it is customary to use separate chapters for the introduction, methodology, results and discussion. If the literature review is long, it may merit a chapter on its own.

Headings and subheadings should be used within the document, as shown in Chapter 6. Headings for tables and figures should also follow a system. Usually tables and figures are numbered from 1. If using the chapter system and there are many tables and figures in various chapters, the number of the chapter can be used as a prefix. For example, tables in Chapter 1 would be labelled Table 1.1, etc., while those in Chapter 3 would be labelled 3.1, etc. The headings are usually indented in the table of contents and they may be indented in the text.

EXERCISE

Locate two examples of research articles listed in the reference list of any chapter of this book. What is the report format like? What is the order of the main headings, for example, title, abstract, aims, objectives, significance, and so on? Do the ideas flow well between sections? Can you comprehend the research methods, processes and outcomes now that you have read the articles? If not, why not?

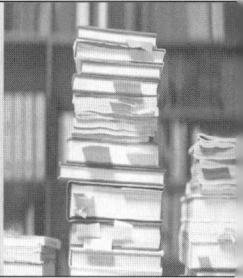

Components of the report

Preliminaries

The first part of the report is the 'preliminaries' or pages that precede the body of the report. A short report will need only a title page and an abstract. Great care and attention should be given to the title and abstract. In this day of electronic databases, the title will appear in lists of documents in many searches and the abstract will be accessed by many of those generating the search. It becomes the showcase for your work since it will be what determines whether researchers access the full paper. A longer report will require additional preliminaries such as a table of contents including a list of tables and a list of figures, both with page numbers to help the reader locate the tables and figures easily. A thesis will require additional papers to be inserted, such as a statement that the thesis is entirely the work of the candidate and a list of acknowledgements.

The title page

The title page should be similar to a title page of a research proposal, which was discussed in Chapter 6. The title page gives the title of the proposal, as well as the author's name, position and qualifications. The author's postal and email addresses should be given, as well as telephone and fax contact numbers. The date should be placed somewhere on the page; this can be done easily as a footer if you are using a word processor.

Elements of a quantitative report

Preliminaries

The title

The title of the report should be a mini report, or thumbnail sketch, of the work, conveying the essence of the report while stimulating interest in the study. The title can be either a statement or a question and should reflect the major theme of the report and the type of investigation, which can be achieved by using key words. Students often err on the side of excessive length when developing titles for theses, as they try to convey everything about the project, but an acceptable title will be a concise statement or question of no more than 15 to 20 words. Sometimes the agency for which you are writing will have restrictions on the length of the title. For a journal article, it is important to use key words that can be indexed so that the article can be retrieved by researchers. It is best to avoid expressions such as 'An investigation of . . .' or words similar to those. That is self-evident and simply takes up space. 'The influence of . . .' or 'The effect of . . .' in a short report are both unexciting and are therefore unlikely to catch the interest of the reader. Strangely enough, it is often best to compose the title last, because it must reflect the most up-to-date material in the report. An example of a title that piques the interest of the reader is: *How do perioperative nurses cope with stress?* This research by Gillespie and Kermode (2004) will be the quantitative example used in this section.

The abstract

The abstract is a succinct and accurate description of the project you have conducted, an introduction to your research report which gives the reader a summary of the project, highlighting its major themes. A well-written abstract will give a potential reader a good thumbnail sketch of the project. The abstract is one of the most important parts of the report because, essentially, it is a marketing device. It is the 'hook' that entices readers to select your research (Evans 1994). The abstract helps the person doing a literature search to make a decision about acquiring your article.

Abstracts are sometimes submitted for consideration of the presentation of a paper at a research meeting or conference. Abstracts may be published in conference programs to help delegates decide what part of the conference to attend. In fact, the abstracts may be the only parts of the conference proceedings that are published.

As with the title, the abstract can also be written near the end, or last. It should summarise the objectives, methodology, major findings and implications of the project. It should be concise, with a word limit of 250 to 300 words; in other words, no more than one page. Its major purpose is to help readers decide whether or not to read the entire report. The abstract is usually located between the title and the actual report. In writing an abstract, consider what you as the reader would want to know about this project. The abstract should not require the reader to refer to other supporting materials to understand it.

The abstract should include the problem statement, the theoretical framework, if one was used, an explanation of the design of the study, including the sample and data collection methods, and the major findings and any conclusions. Finally, if appropriate, it should conclude with any recommendations.

An example of an abstract is:

In recent years there has been broad discussion on the nature of stressors experienced by members of 'high risk' occupations and professions, for instance, nursing and emergency workers, whose role is to support others through traumatic scenarios (Lam et al, 1999:23). Perioperative nursing is a major specialisation in nursing practice in which there is an increased risk of exposure to traumatic events (Schwam, 1998:645). Moreover, the cumulative nature of critical events, if left undealt with will potentiate attrition among nurses in the perioperative environment (Michael and Jenkins, 2001:39). This triangulated study using self-administered questionnaires focused on how theatre nurses coped with contextual stressors in the work milieu. A purposive sample of 46 registered and enrolled nurses who worked at a major Brisbane hospital were asked to describe a recent stressful workplace event, and rate it using Horowitz's (1993) Impact of Event Scale (IES). Results indicated that nurses with the least general theatre experience, demonstrated the highest negative impacts. 25% of females demonstrated avoidance tendencies when stressed, while 83% of males used problem-solving strategies. Reactions following trauma among the nurses were predominantly negative, and included feelings of frustration and self-doubt. These findings support the eminent need for hospital organisations to take a more person-centred approach when dealing with workplace stress.

The abstract for a research article is very similar to the abstract for the original research proposal, but with the addition of the results.

EXERCISE

Judge the extent to which the quoted abstract above achieves the characteristics of an acceptable abstract, as described in this section.

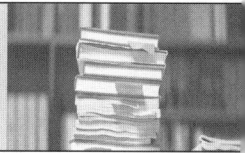

Body of the report

The body of your report should be a straightforward description of the problem, the methodology and the findings, plus the interpretation of those findings. There should also be an assessment of the significance and the adequacy of the study design, and recommendations for further research. There are four major sections in the body of the research report: the introduction, or 'why I did it'; the methodology, or 'what I did'; the results – 'what I found'; and the discussion – 'what it means' (Tornquist 1986). The introduction and methodology sections in the body of the research report are similar to the sections of the research proposal with the same titles. There may be minor variations in format required for different purposes, but these sections are fairly standard.

The introduction and literature review

The purpose of the introduction section is to acquaint the reader with the problem, background and purposes of the study. The introduction goes from the general to the specific, and sets the scene for your research question or problem. In fact, it includes your problem statement/research question and it should answer the questions: 'What problem was investigated?' and 'Why was it done?' The introduction to your research report is similar to the introduction section of your research proposal, except that the significance of the study is discussed in the discussion section. The introduction emphasises the study's importance and sets it in a context of previous work in the area. If it is a quantitative project, the introduction section contains a review of theoretical and empirical literature and the hypotheses. An acceptable quantitative research report will contain in its introduction an adequate review of the literature. As in the research proposal, the review of the literature comprises the review of both theoretical and empirical literature and it is normally constructed in much the same way as the review for the proposal. However, you will probably prune the literature review now to be congruent with what findings you wish to report. For example, if one part of your findings turned out to be unusable for some reason, and you decide to eliminate it from the report, you would delete the literature now redundant. When writing for a journal, you need to prune the literature review to include only the few most relevant studies, because of space restrictions. It should emphasise the findings and include a critique only where it was relevant to your methodology. Even more drastic reductions may be necessary for a conference paper or a poster. For these purposes, the aim is not to demonstrate your ability to review the literature, but to provide a brief summary of the relevant findings so that the reader can place your work in the context of previous work and so that you can interpret how your findings fit into the overall work on the subject. In a thesis, the review of the literature may occupy a separate chapter.

An example of an introduction and literature review is:

Veccio (1995) defines *stress* as 'the physical and psychological reactions experienced by an individual when confronted by a threatening situation'. Stress has the potential to become an inhibitive force and as such can diminish an individual's performance and satisfaction in work (Healy & McKay, 2000). These problems can become apparent when people are unable to invoke coping mechanisms which assist them to deal with the stressor in a constructive way. Conversely, stress is a necessary element of human activity, something which can energise and motivate people towards a higher performance (Lazarus and Folkman, 1984). Workplace stress is an important health issue as long-term exposure can lead to psychological trauma (Keane et al, 1985; Farrington, 1997).

Michael and Jenkins' (2000, 2001) research into the perioperative specialty attests that perioperative nurses are repeatedly exposed to stressful situations in the course of their working day. There is extensive literature to indicate that traumatic experiences are an existential and inescapable part of much of the perioperative nurse's work (Fox, 1999; Rohleder, 1993; Schwam, 1998; Shapiro, 1986). The perioperative nurse is confronted daily with a variety of impelling scenarios, such as verbal abuse and conflict with peers and doctors, dealing with new technologies as well as shocking motor vehicle accidents (Michael & Jenkins, 2001).

Occupational stress has been explained by using a number of competing paradigms, with various approaches placing different emphasis on the significance of the origins and effects of stress. Seyle (1976) and Hinkler (1979) defined stress in terms of physiological responses to the 'stressor', or as a reaction to disturbing or noxious agents or environmental demands. An alternative approach to these perspectives, which has gained notable acceptance, views stress as a dynamic and reciprocal relationship between an individual and his/her environment (Lazarus & Folkman, 1984). This perspective is in alignment with the person-environment fit theory, otherwise known as the *transactional approach* to stress. It recognises that work environments vary in the amount of quantitative workload they impose. This conceptual model views stress as a part of a process that involves a complex set of relationships between the working context, the capacities and behaviours of the worker to meet these environmental demands, and the worker's perception to meet these demands (Chiriboga, Jenkins and Bailey, 1983; Harris, 1989; Lazarus and Folkman, 1984). This transactional paradigm has provided the conceptual framework on which this study is based, as it best illustrates the interdependent relationship shared between the individual and his/her environment.

Lazarus and Folkman (1984) maintain that coping per se encompasses realistic expectations and flexible thoughts and actions. Within the transactional paradigm, coping thoughts and actions are invariably context driven, therefore in order to understand the ways in which an individual copes, it is important to define the situational stressor. The more narrowly defined the context, the easier it is to use a particular coping thought or behaviour as a contextual demand. Coping, as a process, involves continual appraisal and reappraisal within the context of the shifting person-environment relationship (Lazarus and Folkman, 1984). This shifting may be the result of coping directed outward at modifying the environment, or directed inward to alter the meaning of the event or increase personal understanding about the event.

For example, the nurse whose patient dies in both unexpected and traumatic circumstances (such as intra-operative death) may cope differently than if perhaps the same patient's death was imminent and fully expected (Frasier, 1990; Lazarus and Folkman, 1984). Clearly, one of the contextual variables in this scenario may well be in the lack of time for the nurse to anticipate his/her own personal grief, and that of the patient's relatives. Moreover, this unanticipated stressor conflates the environmental imbalance experienced by the nurse in this scenario and makes heavy demands on the nurse's ability to cope. Ultimately, this may adversely affect the nurse's workplace performance (Farrington, 1997).

The introduction and literature review sets the scene for the report and justifies the study. It provides a theoretical rationale for the importance or significance of the study.

EXERCISE

Judge the extent to which the quoted literature review above achieves the characteristics of an acceptable literature review, as described in this section.

The design

The design section describes in detail the framework, methods and procedures that were used in the study. Again, the design section of the report will be very similar to that of the proposal, assuming that there have not been many changes, but it will be written in the past tense.

The principle of this section is that it should describe your framework, methods and processes in enough detail to allow another researcher to replicate your study (that is, to conduct another study using the same approach that you have used), so it must include the design, setting, participants, sampling, instruments and procedures for the study and it should answer the questions: 'On whom was the research carried out?', 'How?', 'When?' and 'Where?' It is important to report the methodology accurately and completely because it helps the reader to evaluate its validity and the researcher's interpretation of the findings. It also facilitates comparison with other studies on the subject (Gething 1995).

When writing this section, you should make a statement about the design of the study, and explain why that design was appropriate to the research question. Quantitative designs were discussed in Chapter 7, and qualitative designs in Chapters 12 and 13.

The research question or hypothesis should be included as a description of what the purpose of the study was. It should show the relationships between the variables, stated in measurable terms. If appropriate, the independent and dependent variables should be identified and stated in measurable terms.

Next, the setting for the research should be given, showing where it took place. In a report it is not appropriate to give the names of agencies in which you carried out the research, unless they have given their permission to be identified.

The participants should be described next. State the characteristics of the group from which the participants were selected and where they were found, and give your rationale for selecting this particular group of participants. You should give the ideal size of sample, how you arrived at this figure, and the size you ended up with.

State the type of sample that you used, as discussed in Chapter 8. If it is a convenience sample, there will not be much to say except the basis of the convenience; for example, they were the patients on a ward. If it is a random or a stratified random sample, say how the sample was drawn from the population. Indicate any steps that you took to prevent bias in the sample. Describe the criteria for participant selection and give the rationale for the criteria. You should give the details of how the participants were recruited – by letter, by telephone or through personal contact.

Once you have described your sampling procedures, you should state the number of groups and the number of participants in each group, and how they were allocated to the groups. Any special procedures, such as matching participants on criteria, should be addressed.

In the instruments and materials section, you should describe the instruments or materials that you used, including any questionnaire or tool. It is not necessary to explain any standard tests, but you should explain any unconventional techniques, tests or instruments. If an instrument is new, you should include details of how it was developed and tested before use. If it has been used before, you should give the details of its origin, how much it has been used before, and its reliability and validity. You should describe any questionnaire that you used or state its name if it is well known. If your report is a thesis or a student research project, include a copy of the questionnaire in an appendix; however, this is not necessary for a journal article.

If you used a physical instrument, it should be named if it is well known, or described if it is unusual or new. You should say how the instrument is scored or measured, for example, on a Likert scale. You can use diagrams or photographs of an instrument to avoid long descriptions and to stimulate interest. You should say why the instrument was suitable for the acquisition of reliable, valid data. These concepts were discussed in Chapter 8.

In the procedures section, you describe the procedures that were used in the study. If it was an experiment, you describe how an experimental treatment was applied. You state how, when and where you collected the data, in enough detail to allow someone to replicate your procedures, including such procedures as participant observation, questionnaire administration, and application of an instrument or experimental treatment. Describe any calibration of the instruments or any training given to data collectors. For questionnaire administration, describe how you distributed the questionnaires, how they were returned to you, and whether the respondents were anonymous or identified.

You should say when you carried out your data collection procedures and how long they took. Any particulars concerning the exact time the procedures were carried out should be included if they were important to the design of the study.

In the data analysis section, you should describe briefly how you recorded your data and your procedures for managing them. These include coordination of data management if a multiple site is involved, and data entry into the computer, including coding of data.

Next, you should describe your data analysis in relation to your research question or hypotheses. You should say whether you analysed the data by hand or computer, and if the latter, you should name the data analysis package and which procedures you used. You should state which statistical tests you carried out to test each hypothesis.

It is not necessary in a research report to go into a great deal of detail about the ethical considerations. However, you should state that permission was given by the relevant ethics committees and name them. The reader will thus be assured that reasonable ethical procedures were in place. You should discuss briefly any procedures that were in place to protect participants from harm. In a short report this can be integrated with the appropriate parts of the report, such as the procedures section.

If you did a pilot study, give a brief description here. You should describe any changes in the methodology that resulted from the pilot study, and justify them.

An example of a research design section is:

Design
Subjects were invited to participate in this cross-sectional study from a major hospital in Brisbane. The accessible population consisted of 75 practising perioperative nurses, who worked either full time or part time. Purposive sampling was utilised based on the researcher's belief that the subjects chosen were typical of the perioperative population as a whole (Polit and Hungler, 1999). This group was judged to be particularly knowledgeable as regarding the existing issues that affect perioperative practice, and therefore, were 'experts' in their chosen specialty.

The research instrument used in this study was a self-administered survey questionnaire.

Sample
Inclusion Criteria of Sample:
- Aged 21 years or above;
- Both genders were eligible to participate;

- Registered or enrolled in Queensland;
- Be practising at the time as a perioperative nurse at a major metropolitan institution; and,
- Be employed at the time of the study on a full-time or part-time basis at the hospital under study.

Ethical Considerations

At the time the study was presented to potential subjects, issues of anonymity and confidentiality were explained verbally. All potential subjects had been assured of the right of discontinuation or withdrawal from the study at any time. The study was approved by the University ethics committee under the National Health and Medical Research Council (NH&MRC) guidelines.

Instruments

Horowitz's (1993) 15-item Impact of Event Scale (IES) is a self-report instrument which is derived from statements most frequently used to describe episodes of distress by persons who had experienced life changes. Items are rated on a 4-point Likert scale indicating the subject's degree of agreement or disagreement to each statement. Development of this scale allows these behaviours to be classified using either of the two major response sets, which fall into 'avoidance' or 'intrusion' behaviours, thus affirming this instrument's ability to assist in the identification of post-traumatic stress disorders (Horowitz et al, 1979). 'Avoidance' behaviours include denial of the meaning and consequences of the event, as well as awareness of emotional numbness. 'Intrusion' behaviours are characterised by disturbing images and thoughts, troubled dreams, intense sweeping emotions and repetitive responses.

Clinical Application of the IES

The IES has been widely used in clinical and research settings, with well-documented reliability in the subscales of 'intrusion' and 'avoidance' ($r = 0.77$ and 0.86 respectively) (Horowitz et al, 1979; Horowitz, 1993; Weiss, 1996).

Respondents were also asked to identify significant social and emotional supports to whom s/he turns to when they are faced with a stressful workplace situation (colleague, partner or friend), and whether or not they would attend debriefing (yes/no response). Demographic data of subjects including age, years of perioperative nursing experience, education and gender were included on a separate demographic data sheet.

Data analysis

Statistical analysis of the quantitative data was conducted using Statistical Product and Services Solutions (SPSS version 10). While preliminary analyses included a series of unpaired *t-tests* to compare the differences between two groups (males versus females), there were negligible differences in the mean values between the two groups (Polit and Hungler, 1999). Preliminary analysis of the IES using analysis of variance (ANOVA) to test for significant differences among three sub-groups based on independent variables such as age, education and years of perioperative experience demonstrated little statistical difference between or within each sub-group.

Preliminary analysis of data at nominal level data were conducted using chi square (χ^2) analysis to compare for differences in coping behaviours between genders, however, these results were unremarkable. The IES had been analysed using descriptive statistics in relation to the independent variables (age, gender, experience and education). Although gender was examined as an independent variable, other independent variables were tested, however, did not demonstrate notable statistical differences. Nominated Support Persons were analysed to determine what percentage of nurses used each type of support (colleague, friend or partner).

EXERCISE
Judge the extent to which the quoted research design above achieves the characteristics of an acceptable research design, as described in this section.

The results

The results section is where you present your findings, the outcomes of all of your hard work. This section presents an account of what your investigation found. The results comprise the text and supporting illustrations, such as tables, graphs, charts, photographs and models derived from the data.

The researcher has the responsibility of deciding which results should be reported. In a student report or thesis, it is customary to present all findings, whether or not they are important or significant. However, for other reports, pruning to key findings will be necessary to meet criteria for presentation time or journal space. It is never appropriate to elect to present only findings that support your hypotheses or beliefs.

Researchers often err on the side of over-reporting. They do this for three reasons – because they believe that every finding is equally important, because they think that if they have gone to the trouble of doing the procedure it must be reported, and because of their inability to sort the wheat from the chaff (Brown 1995). A report that is full of irrelevant detail can obscure the important findings. The aim is to make the key findings stand out.

The results tell a story, but should be presented in order of their importance, since people tend to read the first bit of a section more carefully and may skip over the following parts (Brown 1995). In a quantitative report, the results can be structured around the hypotheses. If your report is of a qualitative project, you present the findings as a narrative, focusing on the themes that have emerged. It is customary to interpose quotations from the interviews or journals to embellish or clarify the themes.

The results should be presented in such a way as to address the research question. You never present the raw data or your analysis of them in the results section; you present your analysis of the findings and the statistical significance, if it is a quantitative project.

If you have many results on several subtopics, use appropriate headings and present all the results on each subtopic together, even mixing qualitative and quantitative if you are using both approaches. You will have to decide whether to present the quantitative or the qualitative data first.

For quantitative results, the statistical tests should be reported with the appropriate result, giving the test, the result of the test, and the probability value. Some journals or bodies require that the degrees of freedom are also presented. The statistical test is usually presented in brackets after the result has been reported. Note that the letters representing the statistical test, for example, '*t*' and the probability '*p*' should be given in italics. In the past, the *p* value used to be expressed in terms of greater or less than the level of significance, which was usually 0.05. Thus, *p* = <0.05 meant that the result was significant, while *p* = >0.05 meant that it was not. Today, the exact *p* values should be given since computers can now generate them. The exact reporting of the *p* value allows the reader to see how close to significance the results were. If the computer gives a *p* value of 0.0136, the number should be rounded off to two decimal places, i.e. 0.01.

Experimental and quasi-experimental research reports should include a statement of whether or not an hypothesis was supported with each result. This will include a statement about the null hypothesis and the research hypothesis. The possibilities are: (1) that the null hypothesis was rejected, in which case the research hypothesis was supported; (2) the null hypothesis was not rejected, in which case the research hypothesis was not supported; and (3) the null hypothesis was rejected but the findings were in the opposite direction from that predicted by the research hypothesis, which was not supported.

Supporting illustrations

Various devices can be used to present results in ways other than using words. Photographs, diagrams, models, flow charts, graphs and tables are all alternative ways of presenting information. Tables are called tables; all the rest are collectively called figures. Tables and figures are called illustrations. Judicious use of illustrations will provide variety and enhance clarity. Illustrations are also concise and, therefore, economical methods of presenting information in ways that are reader-friendly. However, it is important not to overuse these devices. Never use a table or figure when you can say the same thing in one or two sentences. Reserve illustrations for the presentation of more complex data. The old saying that a picture is worth a thousand words is certainly true for figures and graphs: they should be used instead of a thousand words, but not instead of 10 or 20.

Illustrative devices should be introduced in the text before they are presented. Give each illustrative device a caption and a number. Put the caption of a table at the top of it, and the caption of a figure below it. The caption should inform the reader about the findings in the table or figure, but should not include the name of the statistical test. For short reports, the figures and tables may be numbered consecutively throughout, but for reports and theses that have chapters, it is useful to use the number of each chapter as part of the numbering system.

Tables were discussed in Chapter 10. When using tables, avoid giving too much detail; keep in mind what information you want your reader to extract and build the table to make the extraction as easy as possible (Brown 1995). Many researchers make the mistake of expecting the numbers to speak for themselves. They also make the mistake of falling in love with the numbers in their data and forgetting that they are a means to an end rather than an end in themselves (Brown 1995). Round the numbers off to the level of their significance. There is no virtue in using three decimal places if your data are not accurate to three decimal places. For example, if your number is 572 out of 1000, or 57.2 per cent, but the standard deviation is 10 per cent, your figure is accurate only to 57 per cent at best and 60 per cent is really close enough. All numbers should be rounded off to the same number of decimal places, and the decimal points should be under each other in a column. This is easy to do by using the centring tab function on the word processor, or the table function. Make sure that your columns and rows have top and side headings. If inferential statistics were used, the results of these tests should be presented at the bottom of the table. You can see an example of a table in the 'Results' section of our sample report, following.

A figure is a pictorial representation instead of a numerical one. It may be a photograph, model, flow chart or graph. Most journals have requirements concerning the presentation of photographs. Graphs are the most commonly used figures in a research report, and they may be hand-drawn, but these days most computers come equipped with a program that will generate graphs from your data. When preparing graphs, it pays to frame the graph, use visually prominent symbols, place labels for the values outside the graph and choose a scale that is appropriate for the data.

A graph will usually compare findings for groups, or within a group. For example, it may compare the results of two groups on the dependent variable. Most modern statistical computer programs will generate graphs, but graphs can also be made using graph paper, or pen and ink drawings on plain paper. When preparing graphs, the dependent variable is usually on the X or horizontal axis and the independent variable on the Y or vertical axis. The axes should be labelled. You can see examples of different types of graphs in Chapter 10. Different types of graphs are useful for different purposes, and the results that you want to show should be considered when you are selecting a type of graph. Tests of significance can be reported at the bottom of the figure, or in the text.

The simplest graph is a line graph. Line graphs will have a connecting line between points, as is used in a temperature, pulse and blood pressure chart. Only a few lines or curves should be shown on a line graph.

A histogram, or bar graph, is commonly used. This demonstrates the manner in which the number or percentage of instances of the dependent variable occurs in different groups. The bars can go either from side to side, or from top to bottom. It is helpful to give numerical labels to the bars if your computer program will generate them. Pie graphs are used to show a percentage breakdown, and are useful for describing a group on a variable. A regression graph will show the scattergram with a line drawn to show the relationship between X and Y.

The information in figures and tables should not just be repeated in the text. The narrative should concentrate on interpreting the table or figure. However, the reader should be able to interpret the figure or table without the text.

The tests of significance and other data analysis particulars are included in the results section, along with the actual result. Some people prefer to put the data analysis only in the results section, but wherever it is put, it should be comprehensive, giving the reader enough detail to understand exactly what you did.

The results section is purely for the presentation of the findings. It is inappropriate to discuss your opinions of the meaning of the data here. These comments should be saved for the discussion section.

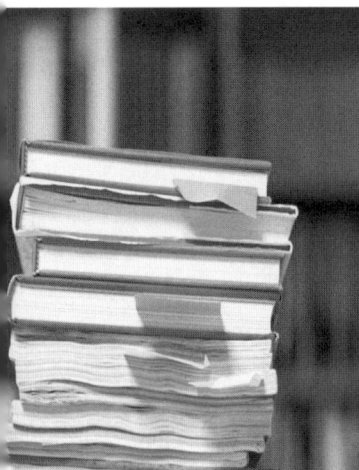

Table 18.1 Frequency of held nursing positions and primary roles

Main Roles	Scrub		Scout		Anaesthetic		PACU		TOTAL	
Current Position	(n)	%	(n)	%	(n)	%	(n)	%	(n)	%
Enrolled Nurse	0	0	0	0	5	100	0	0	5	100
Registered Nurse	17	57	8	27	0	0	5	17	30	100
Clinical Nurse	8	73	0	0	1	0	2	18	11	100

An example of a results section is:

Out of a potential 75 respondents, 46 theatre nurses participated (60%). Various traumatic experiences were reported by the respondents who were predominantly female (87%, 13% male), working assorted positions and multi-skilled in a range of perioperative roles (Table 18.1). The mean age of the sample was 39.8 $(SD = 4.1)$ years old.

Traumatic Clinical Events

While there was a selection of traumatic events reported, the utility of qualitative analysis allowed the coding of contextual data into five major themes; *practice issues, patient death, conflict/abuse, lack of material/human resources* and *patient condition* (Holloway, 1997). Described events fell into one of the five categories, with a further classification of who was principally involved with the perioperative nurse during the incident (Tables 18.2 and 8.3 respectively).

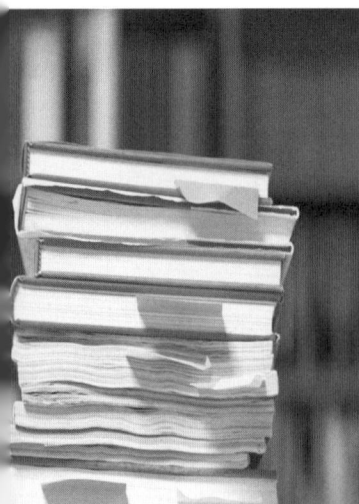

Table 18.2 Frequency of clinical events

Event Type	(n)	%
Practice issue	15	32.6
Patient death	9	19.6
Conflict/abuse	13	28.3
Lack of human/ material resources	16	34.7
Patient condition	11	23.9

Table 18.3 Frequency of person/s involved in critical incident

Event Theme	Person/s involved								Categories						
	EN		RN		CN		NPC		Doctor		Patient		Other		Total
	(n)	%	(n)	%	(n)	%	(n)	%	(n)	%	(n)	%	(n)	%	(n)
Patient issues	-	-	4	26.6	-	-	-	-	3	20	3	20	5	33.3	15
Practice death	2	22.2	5	55.5	2	22.2	-	-	-	-	-	-	-	-	9
Conflict/abuse	-	-	5	38.4	-	-	1	7.7	6	45.1	-	-	1	7.7	13
Lack of human/ material resources	-	-	2	12.5	-	-	-	-	12	75	1	6.25	1	6.25	16
Patient condition	-	-	1	9.2	-	-	-	-	5	45.5	5	45.4	-	-	11
Total (n)	(n) 2		(n) 18		(n) 2		(n) 1		(n) 26		(n) 9		(n) 7		

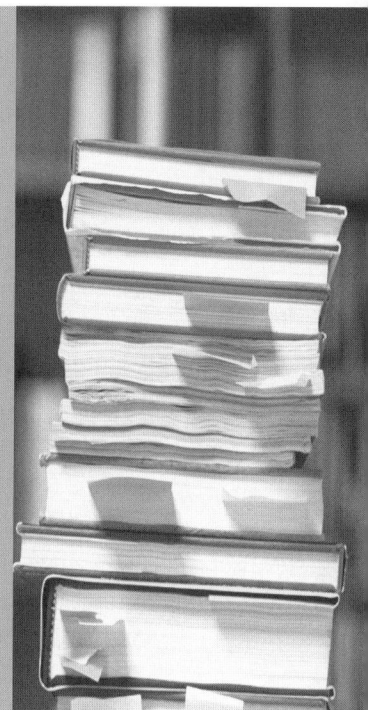

Observed Coping Patterns

The IES (Horowitz, 1993) identifies 'intrusion' (uninvited feelings, images and ideas) and 'avoidance' (consciously recognised avoidance of certain feelings, ideas or situations) as the two primary domains of measurement of symptomatic response to a traumatic event. While the mean totals for males and females on the 'intrusion' sub-scales were statistically insignificant, the mean total scores based on gender for the 'avoidance' sub-scales demonstrated that a higher percentage of females used avoidance strategies when coping with stressful workplace events (males – Mean = 14.88 SD = 8.5; females – Mean = 17.94 SD = 7.5). While other demographic characteristics were examined in relation to the IES using descriptive statistics, the results were non-significant.

Group Differences

The raw scores were calculated for each subject on the IES items (with a minimum score = 15, and a maximum score = 60, based on a Likert scale of 1–4 for each item). The aggregated scores for each sub-group were based on the individual's years of experience.

Mean aggregates for each sub-group demonstrated that nurses with 1–5 years general perioperative experience reported the highest event impact, compared to the 6–10 year and greater than 10 year sub-groups. Curiously, the sub-groups with greater than 10 years theatre experience posted the second highest mean aggregate scores on the IES.

Social Support

While many respondents identified more than one category of support persons, 58.7% nominated 'work associate' as a primary support during a stressful workplace event. Sadly,

15.2% of the group indicated that they did not utilise any social support, and identified the 'no-one' category. When asked if respondents would use a debriefing service, 52.2% stated in the affirmative, while 47.8% indicated they would decline.

Clearly, a much higher proportion of the female participants (57.5%) would attend some form of debriefing, as compared with the males. Generally, the percentages for 'yes/no' responses regarding the utilisation of debriefing among the females were more representative of the group totals in this area (52.2% 'yes' and 47.8% 'no' response).

EXERCISE

Judge the extent to which the quoted results section above achieves the characteristics of an acceptable results section in a research report.

The discussion

The discussion section is the last section of the body of the report, and should explain the importance and relevance of your findings. This is where you get a chance to demonstrate your ability to interpret the meaning of the findings. In this section, you highlight the most important findings, interpret them in relation to issues raised in the introduction section and place the results in the context of the theory and research on the topic (Gething 1995).

In quantitative studies, you discuss the meaning of the findings for the research question or research hypotheses. In the results section you will have given the actual statement about whether or not the null hypotheses have been rejected, and research hypotheses have been supported. You now reiterate briefly the result and interpret its meaning for the reader. If your research hypothesis is supported, this is quite easy. However, if it is not supported, you are left with the task of explaining why not. This is usually either because of flaws in your design or because the prediction was not valid. When this happens, the temptation to throw it all in the bin can be strong, but do not despair. Sometimes negative findings are just as important as positive findings and can have just as significant an impact on practice. Borderline findings can stimulate further research, as can reports with a design flaw, which can prevent other researchers from making the same mistakes. In any case, as a student, your job is to learn to report the results, and the process of writing the report is more important than the product. It is how you interpret the results that counts, not the actual findings. You will not be marked down for insignificant results, but you will be failed for not submitting a report at all.

When interpreting the findings of your study, be sure to distinguish between statistical significance and clinical significance. Results cannot be clinically significant if they are not statistically significant. However, results are sometimes statistically significant but not clinically significant. This happens when the 'p' values are less than 0.05 (or whatever level of significance has been set) but the difference between the means of the two groups is low. This can occur because, as the sample size increases, the difference required for statistical significance decreases. In other words, with large numbers of participants, the difference required to reach statistical significance is small. In order to reach clinical significance, a difference should be at least 10 per cent and preferably 20 per cent. For example, suppose that you compared the dependent variable of the tidal volumes of two groups on two different types of pillows. A normal tidal volume is 500 ml. Unless you got a difference of more than 50 ml between the mean tidal volumes of each group, the result would not be clinically significant, although with a large enough sample it may have been statistically significant.

You must relate your results to the research that you have discussed in your literature review. This means that you will compare what you found to what was found by previous researchers. Your findings may agree or disagree with theirs, or they may agree with some and not with others. This does not need to be done as a separate section; it can be integrated with your interpretation of the findings. This is one of the hardest parts of the research report to write, and the one that most students do least well.

You should also relate your research to the theoretical or conceptual framework. If you were testing a theory, you should state whether your findings support, modify or refute the theory. If, however, a theoretical framework was used as a conceptual framework without testing the theory, you should describe how your findings are related to the theory.

The statement on the significance of the study follows. It should show why this study was worth doing. It should answer the question: 'So what?' It should show how the results of this study advance knowledge or practice in nursing and/or health. If there are possible applications of the results of this study, state them. At the end of the discussion section you can present conclusions and make recommendations for further research and/or clinical implementation of the findings.

An example of a discussion section is as follows:

The findings of this study suggest that perioperative nurses have been frequently, and in some cases, excessively exposed to various traumatic incidents as a part of their daily work.

Group Vulnerability

Of real concern was the large number of reported incidents that culminated in the verbal abuse of nursing staff, which was perpetrated by registrars and consultants (28.3%). The profound and often overt impact of such an experience will, in many cases lead to psychological distress, including diminished feelings of worthiness, self-doubt, and a significant amount of loss of respect for colleagues and peers (Michael and Jenkins, 2001). Reported feelings of inadequacy, incompetence and self-blame were described in relation to incidents which culminated in patient death.

Similar sentiments as well as indignity and contempt were conveyed when the perioperative nurse was a victim of abuse. Following an incident of verbal abuse by a surgeon, one nurse respondent reflected

'*I coped well at the time but felt like crying when I went to the tearoom and no-one else was there . . .I had a nightmare about operating and having a mis-count. The following day I was unable to scrub due to major stress levels.*'

Webb (2002) warns that if these insidious issues are left undealt with, then these nurses will leave the profession.

There is convincing evidence that the impact of described events have the most profound effect on the least experienced perioperative nurses (Michael and Jenkins, 2000). This is likely to be attributed to the steep learning curve associated with becoming clinically competent in this area of nursing (Lively, 2000). The sub-group with greater than 10 years experience surprisingly demonstrated relatively high event impacts despite this degree of clinical expertise. Presumably, this reflects the role expectations this group holds as senior nurses.

Coping Outcomes

The IES scores for the 'avoidance' subscale indicates that females experienced moderate symptoms of avoidance behaviours compared with the males' mild usage of these behaviours as a way of coping with stressful events. It can not be extrapolated from these results that coping behaviours are gender-dependent.

Disconcerting, is the skewed perception held among some of the nurses in this enquiry, that to seek counsel post-event is a sign of the nurse's inability to cope, as reflected by almost 48% of respondents who answered 'no' in terms of attending debriefing. Debriefing responses based on gender revealed that only 16% of males would utilise a debriefing service, compared with 57% of females. It would appear that the majority of female perioperative nurses surveyed believe that debriefing can be used as a social resource for better coping, a concept supported by Farrington (1997). Conversely, the widely held belief of the male respondents is that debriefing alone may be inadequate to address their immediate needs, a notion concurred in Lam et al's (1999) discourse.

Future Research

Although the findings reported in this study are the result of the sample from one hospital sample, they should serve as a timely warning to hospital managers, perioperative nurses, and the nursing profession in general. There are several areas for future research originating from the issues that have been identified and discussed in this enquiry:

- To replicate the study at multiple sites with different samples of perioperative nurses;
- To conduct in-depth enquiries into each of the major stressors identified in this study; and,
- To investigate the reasons for, and incidence of employee attrition rates among perioperative nurses.

Conclusions

The tentative findings of this limited work appear to suggest that the impact of described traumatic workplace events had the greatest impact on the least experienced theatre nurses. Coping strategies such as avoidance, which may temporarily reduce emotional distress is merely a palliative and ineffective approach with few, if any adaptive outcomes. While this enquiry does not necessarily provide qualified support for Lazarus and Folkman's (1984) *transactional model*, it does nonetheless go some way to giving countenance to this concept. It would appear that situational agents are significant determinants of coping strategies and need to be considered when examining how perioperative nurses cope with stress.

EXERCISE

How does the results section of a research report differ from the discussion section?

In many quantitative studies it is appropriate to spell out the perceived limitations of your research so that readers do not mistakenly use or interpret your findings. In the era of evidence-based practice this is important in terms of being able to generalise findings from one study to a whole population. An example of a statement about limitations is:

Study Limitations

While it was the researcher's intention to deliberately select participants who possessed a requisite knowledge of issues that affected perioperative nurses, the use of a non-probability sampling technique has limited the extent to which this pilot study can be validated externally (Polit and Hungler, 1999). Arguably, there is always the possibility that not every component of the perioperative population has been adequately represented within this sample. In terms of the generalisibility of the findings of this study, they are restricted to the particular hospital where the study was conducted, and may not necessarily represent the larger population of theatre nurses.

Although the overall reliability for the IES (Horwitz, 1993) is high (r = 0 86 to 0 92), the small sample size of 46 subjects in this study limited the use of parametric statistical analysis. Essentially, a larger sample size would have permitted analysis within and between sub-cells to be statistically meaningful (Polit, 1996). Presumably, the sensitivity of the IES increases as the sample size increases, thus allowing a higher level of analysis.

A further limitation of self reported data in stress and coping is the assumption that the respondents are able to define their stressors (Wegmann, 1992). In reality some stressors are taboo, and recall of others may cause discomfort and therefore are not readily recalled. Moreover, an individual's perception of a particular stressor will vary according to his/her life experiences and the environment (Lazarus and Folkman, 1984). While the use of a mixed method design has in some way addressed these substantive issues, there will undeniably be human variation (mood and affect) in the ways the questionnaires were interpreted and answered (Wegmann, 1992).

In Chapter 6 we covered the rudiments of referencing, but you should follow the referencing system recommended by your institution or publisher. Whatever system is used, it is important to be accurate, particularly in a report that is going to be disseminated. Sloppiness in referencing will give the reader the impression that the research was sloppy, too. Even worse, errors in the journal name, volume number or issue number may prevent the reader from locating the reference, which negates a major reason for giving references. In a study of the accuracy of references in nursing journals, the researchers found minor errors in one-fifth to one-third of references, and major errors that prevented location of the article in 2.5 per cent of references (Foreman & Kirchhoff 1987). The use of a reference manager such as EndNote will help to prevent mismatches between the in-text citations and the reference list. The references section of the article we have been following is:

References
Chiriboga, D., Jenkins, G. & Bailey, J. 1983. Stress and coping among hospice nurses: Test for an analytic model. *Nursing Research* 32(5): 294–300.
Connelly, L., Folt, M., Hoffart, N. & Taunton, R. 1997. Methodological triangulation in a study of nurse retention. *Nursing Research* 48(5): 299–302.

Farrington, A. 1997. Strategies for reducing stress and burnout in nursing. *British Journal of Nursing* 6(1): 44–51.

Fox, R. 1999. Organ procurement: what is our role and what do we need to know? *ACORN Journal* Spring: 19–22.

Frasier, S. 1990. Survivors recollections of helpful and unhelpful emergency nurses' activities surrounding the sudden death of a loved one. *Journal of Emergency Nursing* 16(1):13–17.

Harris, R. 1989. Reviewing nursing stress according to a proposed coping-adaption framework. *Advances in Nursing Science* 11(2):12–28.

Healy, C. & MacKay, M. 2000. Nursing stress: the effects of coping strategies and job satisfaction in a sample of Australian nurses. *Journal of Advanced Nursing* 31(3)681–8.

Hinkler, L. 1979. The concept of stress in the biological and social sciences. In: Lipowski, D. & Whybrow, C. (eds) *Psychomotor medicine: current trends and clinical implications*. Oxford University Press, New York.

Holloway, I. 1997. *Basic concepts for qualitative research*. Blackwell, London.

Horowitz, M. 1993. Stress-response syndromes: A review of post-traumatic stress and adjustment disorders. In: Wilson, J. & Raphael, B. (eds) *International handbook of traumatic stress syndromes*. Plenum Press, New York.

Horowitz, M., Wilner, B. & Alvarez, M. 1979. Impact of Event Scale: A measure of subjective stress. *Psychomotor Medicine* 41(3):209–18.

Keane, A., Duccette, J. & Adler, D. 1985. Stress in ICU and Non ICU nurses. *Nursing Research* 34(4):231–7.

Lam, L., Ross, K., Cass, D., Quine, S. & Lazarus, R. 1999. The impact of work-related trauma on the psychological health of nursing staff: a cross-sectional study. *Australian Journal of Advanced Nursing* 16(3):14–20.

Lazarus, R. & Folkman, S. 1984. *Stress, appraisal and coping*. Springer Publishing, New York.

Lively, M. 2000. Morale within operating room departments. *British Journal of Perioperative Nursing* 10(3):144–52.

Michael, R. & Jenkins, H. 2000. Work-related trauma: the experiences of perioperative nurses. *Collegian* 8(2):19–26.

Michael, R. & Jenkins, H. 2001. The impact of work-related trauma on the well-being of perioperative nurses. *Collegian* 8(2):36–40.

Polit, D. & Hungler, B. 1999. *Nursing research: principles and methods*. Lippincott, Philadelphia.

Rohleder, I. 1993. Stress in the operating room. *ACORN* June:11–14.

Schwam, K. 1998. The phenomenon of compassion fatigue in perioperative nursing. *AORN* 58(2): 642–8.

Seyle, H. 1976. *The stress of life*. McGraw-Hill, New York.

Shapiro, P. 1986. Coping with death in the OR. *Today's OR Nurse* 8(7):17–20.

Veccio, R. 1995. *Organisational behaviours*. 3rd Edn. Harcourt Brace, Fort Worth.

Webb, Y. 2002. Nursing the nurses: why staff need support. *Nursing Times* 98(16):36–7.

Wegmann, J. 1992. Measuring coping. In: Stromborg, M. (ed.) *Instruments for clinical nursing research*. Jones & Bartlett, Boston.

Weiss, M. 1996. Measuring coping using the IES. In: Stamm, B. (ed.) *Measurement of stress, trauma and adaption*. Sidran Press, Lutherville.

If you are writing a report for an organisation that demands a particular referencing style, be sure to follow it. If you are free to choose, you can decide whether the space and lack of interruption of flow of the document that the Vancouver system provides is more important than the reader-friendliness of the Harvard system.

Appendixes are used to include material that is too cumbersome for the main text, for example questionnaires. Use appendixes wisely to avoid filling the report with unnecessary detail and interrupting the flow of the main text, but include only material that supports or expands on the information in the body of the text. Examples of things that are best put in an appendix are questionnaires, tools or tests, diagrams of instruments, consent forms and letters of support. Some disciplines may require, for a thesis, that the actual raw data be included in an appendix. Start each appendix on a new page, and index them alphabetically.

Putting it together

The mechanics of assembling the report are the same as for a proposal, which can be found in Chapter 6. It is important to use an appropriate heading system, which can also be found in that chapter. You will also need to construct a table of contents and for a long report the table of contents should include a list of tables and a list of figures. The table of contents should use the same system as the headings in the text. Make sure that all parts of the report are included and that you submit the required number of copies.

The presentation of a research report is similar to that of a proposal, using A4-size, good-quality, white bond paper. If possible, use a word processor with a legible 12-point font. Use double-spacing, particularly for class assignments, so that the lecturer can write between the lines. Make sure the pages are numbered correctly. If it is a longer report, some form of temporary or permanent binding will be required. Check again with your guidelines to make sure that you have conformed to them.

Before submitting the report, you should check it thoroughly for errors. It is vital to check the grammar and spelling, using the spellchecker and grammar checker on the word processor, if you have one. Particularly check that the numbers in the tables and figures are accurate and that your numbering of pages and captions is correct. This is especially important if you have been moving tables and figures around in the document. It is essential to check that your references are correct. It is crucial to proofread the document before submitting it in order to catch other errors, including word errors that the spellchecker will not pick up.

Writing the report of a qualitative project

An acceptable qualitative report will contain all of the features of an acceptable quantitative report, in terms of attention to the preliminaries, such as the title page, and the research summary or abstract. It will also pay the same amount of attention to clarity of presentation and thoroughness in setting out carefully all of the history and outcomes of the project.

Qualitative reports differ from quantitative reports in that they represent vast differences in methodologies within interpretive, critical and postmodern perspectives.

EXERCISE

Locate one research article from the reference lists at the end of Chapters 12 and 13. How does the representation of the methodological approaches differ, e.g. compare a research article which is interpretive to one reflecting a critical approach?

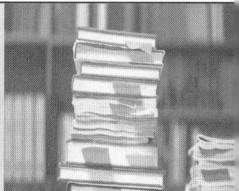

In order to step you through the fundamentals of writing a qualitative report, this section describes a project undertaken with mental health nurses. In each of the subsections, questions will be raised, the written answers to which will form the report. Exceptions to the norm and other hints and ideas will be also included, so that you can see that qualitative reports not only differ from quantitative reports, they may also differ from other qualitative reports.

In the following example (Taylor & Barling 2004), the description of preliminaries of the report will not be reiterated. To refresh your memory of these ideas refer to the section in this chapter on common initial elements of quantitative and qualitative reports.

Preliminaries

The title

Identifying Sources and Effects of Carer Fatigue and Burnout for Mental Health Nurses: A Qualitative Approach.

The aims and objectives

These are the same as those written for the proposal, but with the sentences converted to the past tense. Therefore, they read:

> This project aimed to: identify work related problems to assist Mental Health Nurses to locate the sources and effects of carer fatigue and burnout; set up a dialogue between the participants and the identified sources of stress in the workplace to address the identified problems; and make recommendations to Mental Health Division of an Area Health Service to prevent and manage stressors in the practice of Mental Health Nursing.

The literature review

The literature review for the report will be an amalgam of the literature presented in the proposal, plus that which has come to light since the project began. In some projects, such as grounded theory, the literature review may be done partially or completely after the data collection and analysis. Other collaborative and participatory approaches, such as action research, may review literature as thematic concerns emerge throughout the research processes.

The literature review is important, because it alerts you to disagreements, gaps, silences and contradictions in research findings, giving you confidence in claiming that your project is significant in its focus and findings. The literature review can also show the extent to which other researchers have made similar conclusions, thereby fortifying the impact of your project's implications. In your report writing, it is important to check that the literature review contains all of the elements of an acceptable literature review as described in this chapter and in Chapter 3. Ensure that your literature review has these features, but be assured that it takes a lot of practice to write a comprehensive and strongly argued literature review. For example:

> Carer fatigue or burnout is an acknowledged danger for health workers. Carer fatigue is like 'haemorrhaging of yourself for others' (O'Mahoney 1983 in Farrington 1997). The syndrome of emotional exhaustion, depersonalisation and reduced personal accomplishment describes a

cognitive and emotional state that people in the caring profession experience or witness in their colleagues. Burnout shares several common features: decreased energy, decreased self esteem, output exceeding input, a sense of helplessness/hopelessness, being unable to perceive alternative ways of functioning, cynicism, negativism, and a feeling of self depletion (Farrington 1997).

Mental Health Nursing as a discipline has always been associated with stress and burnout. In a Stress League Table of National Health Service professionals in the UK (Rees & Smith 1991), community Mental Health Nurses shared the top position with speech therapists. Ward based Mental Health Nurses and general nurses were in joint third position. A survey of Mental Health Nurses by Nolan (1995) revealed 37% of the sample fell within in the range of caseness as measured by the General Health Questionnaire (GHQ). Caseness is a term used to describe the likelihood of psychiatric pathology as measured by the GHQ. This is a similar finding of the Clayburg study with 41% of Community Mental Health Nurses (CMHN) and 28% of ward based Mental Health Nurses scoring within the range of caseness (Leonard et al 1995). Low self-esteem is associated with burnout. In a survey of 245 Mental Health Nurses 20% were identified with low self esteem.

Brown et al (1994) and Fagin et al (1995) administered the Maslach Burnout Inventory and General Health Questionnaire (GHQ) to CMHN and ward based Mental Health Nurses with the following results. Community Mental Health Nurses were experiencing high levels of psychological distress, high levels of emotional exhaustion for both CMHNs and ward based nurses, and moderate levels of depersonalisation. The ward nurses were more likely to score higher on the depersonalisation and personal accomplishment scale. The researchers concluded that ward based staff were experiencing more alienation from and lack of empathy towards their consumers and greater levels of frustration and hopelessness at work.

Stress has been associated with intense involvement and interaction of psychiatric nurses with patients suffering from severe mental illness (Melchior et al 1996). Thomas (1999) identified various challenges related to Mental Health Nursing, related to the nature of nursing acutely disturbed patients in an unpredictable environment with criticism from some staff members when seeking to maintain professional standards of care.

The Clayburg study of Mental Health Nurses (Carson et al 1995, Fagin et al 1995, Leonard et al 1995) compared the stressors of CMHN and ward based Mental Health Nurses. The stressors for CMHN included not having the facilities in the community to which consumers can be referred, knowing there are likely to be waiting lists before consumers can get access to the service, having to deal with suicidal consumers alone, not having enough time for study and personal improvement, trying to keep up good quality care, having too many interruptions when trying to work in the office, visiting unsafe areas, feeling there is not enough hospital backup, working with consumers with a known history of violence, and coping with changes at the work base. In contrast, the ward based nurses identified inadequate staffing cover in potentially dangerous situations, dealing with changes in the health service and hospital closures, low morale and poor atmosphere within the organisation, not being notified of changes before they occur, knowing that individual patient care is being sacrificed because of lack of staff, lack of consultation from management about influential structural changes, having to work with colleagues who do not do their share of the workload, the worry there might be further budget cuts, and not having sufficient financial resources to attend training courses or workshops. Similar themes emerged in studies by McLeod (1997), Hopkinson (1998), Alexander (1998), Carson (1997) and Leary (1995).

The stressors associated as contributing to burnout cannot be isolated from the present social and political context of change that is occurring within mental health systems in most western countries. A survey conducted (Sammut 1997) to determine psychiatric nurse satisfaction with acute psychiatric services following the closure of acute psychiatric beds, indicated a significant drop in morale. Deterioration in working conditions, poor communication and support from doctors, a considerable increase in patient turnover with shorter length of stay, crowding, greater levels of disturbed patient behaviour, increase in violent incidence and lack of help in an emergency were factors associated with the low morale. Butterworth (1995:360) identified changes in the mental health system effecting the profession of Mental Health Nursing leading to professional frustration and burnout. Changes included placement of patients in community settings creating role diffusion for psychiatric nurses, understaffed units in institutions, large consumer load in the community, and making nursing standards difficult to maintain.

Research suggests specific branches of nursing have their own unique stressors (Farrington 1995, Leiter and Harvie 1996, McLeod 1997, Wheeler 1998a). In a series of articles on stress in nursing (Wheeler 1997a,b,c,d, Wheeler 1998a,b) it was concluded that stress is experienced by nurses working in a variety of disciplines and is a phenomenon that requires further analysis and research. In a study of nurses' and midwives' stress levels, over 50% reported moderate to severe stress levels (Wheeler and Riding 1994). Between 1990 and 1992, 153 nurses, midwives and health visitors killed themselves in the UK, demonstrating that nursing is one of the most stressful occupations with nurse suicide the highest rate for female suicide (Farrington 1997). The literature demonstrates the serious problems associated with carer fatigue and burnout in nurses generally and Mental Health Nurses particularly. The proposed research will contribute in a practical sense to the area by identifying and addressing the problems identified as sources of stress in the everyday work lives of Mental Health Nurses, which contribute to carer fatigue and burnout.

EXERCISE

What is meant by a critical review of the literature? Has the previous example managed a critical review? If not, why not?

Body of the report

The research plan, including methodology, methods and processes

The body of a qualitative report contains sections on the methodology, methods and processes. The definitions for each of these sections, as they apply specifically to qualitative research, were given in Chapter 6.

Some questions to answer when writing the methodology section of the report are:

- What theoretical assumptions about the way knowledge is generated underlie the methods?
- What is the basic nature and intent of the chosen methodology?
- How did the methodology relate to this project?
- What were the main references to the methodological literature?

In a report of a project which is a thesis, the methodology may take part or all of a chapter. This is important to remember when using examples such as this to structure your own report. The research report must be appropriate to the audience.

At this point, you may also choose to insert a small section which outlines some key assumptions of qualitative research approaches. This will depend on the needs of the audience reading the report. If you think there is a chance that they will be relatively uninformed about qualitative research, it might be advisable. For example:

Methodology

Given the collaborative nature of the research interest, the methodology of choice was a qualitative approach informed by the therapeutic practices of Michael White and David Epston (1990), who use storying or self narrative. In mental health, the relevant discourses that inform practice create the framework to interpret and create meaning from experience. Accordingly, burnout as a phenomenon for mental health professionals is the result of professional experiences interpreted within the dominant story of emotional stress and fatigue.

Ethical requirements

It is important to report on the ways in which the ethical rights of the participants were safeguarded throughout the project. The report should address the following questions about ethical requirements.

- From which committees was ethical clearance obtained?
- What were the ethical considerations?
- How were informed consent, privacy and anonymity honoured?
  For example:

Ethical Implications

Ethical clearance was obtained from the University ethics committee and the Area Health Service ethics committee.

The researchers ensured the ethical integrity of the project by the following measures:

Research participants had the right to consent freely and without coercion. They were offered the right to refuse to participate, or to withdraw at any time, without penalty or coercion of any kind.

Measures taken to ensure that research participants had the capacity to understand the research project were to ascertain that each participant comprehended English, and to provide the services of an interpreter should this have been necessary.

The forms given to participants were relative to their comprehension. Participants received detailed explanations, verbally and in writing, of what the research involved, the aims and the processes of the research, and participants' commitments in it. Nurses were the only participants in this research, so the Plain Language Statement and the Consent Form were written relative to their comprehension, bearing in mind that nurses are professionals conversant with language used in higher education institutions and health care settings. Even so, any words and sentences that may have caused confusion were paraphrased into simple English so that the meaning was clear and unambiguous. The project was also explained in plain language verbally by the researchers. Participants had opportunities to ask questions, make comments and voice any concerns that they may have had concerning the project at the outset and throughout the duration of the project.

As this research encouraged nurses to share their practice issues, likely risks were that the privacy and confidentiality of patients and allied health workers may have been breached and that nurses may have felt vulnerable in sharing their experiences, leading to embarrassment or possible emotional catharsis, such as tearfulness or anger.

With respect to risks associated with emotional catharsis, the interviewer offered support to participants. No member became emotionally upset beyond the ability of the interviewer to support them, but had they become so, he or she would have been offered professional counselling.

Nurses are educated in the need for patient confidentiality and they practice it daily in their work. Even so, the researcher ensured that privacy and confidentiality measures were instituted and maintained. Interview transcripts were devoid of information, which could identify patients, relatives and staff.

Pseudonyms were used and identifying material was omitted or renamed to protect the identities of people within the written transcripts of the stories. Reports and published material describe the participants' accounts and interpretations according to the issues they raised and the practice improvements they caused, rather than to identify specific people, places and situations. All data collected in the course of the research are secured in a locked storage compartment for five years and the responsibility for the safety and security of it resides with the researchers.

The forms indicated a clear explanation of the benefits of the project, which were to improve mental health nursing practice. Benefits to participants included the identification of practice issues and the lessening of carer fatigue and burnout. The risks of the project were breaches of confidentiality and emotional catharsis, and these risks were communicated to participants at the outset of the project and repeated as often as necessary so that participants remembered the need for patient confidentiality and the availability of group and professional support.

Participants were informed verbally and in writing that they are at liberty to withdraw from the project at any time, without penalty or coercion of any kind.

As this project involved nurses who were healthy, consciously aware adults, they were able to consent for themselves.

EXERCISE

In the previous example, from which committees was ethical clearance obtained? What were the ethical considerations? How were the ethical requirements for informed consent, privacy and anonymity honoured?

Methods and processes

The actual methods and processes used in the project must be reported. If these varied from those proposed, this should be noted. Some questions that may guide the writing of this section are:

- How were participants enlisted into the project?
- How were their rights honoured?
- What was the sequence of the research methods?
- What interpersonal processes were involved in undertaking the methods?

If there was no variation from the research intentions, parts of this section may be inserted by changing the sentences to the past tense. For example:

Accessing Participants

Full ethical clearance processes preceded the commencement of the project. The research was for a 12 month period, from January to December 2001. Twenty experienced Registered Nurses were invited to participate through a snowballing method of recruitment, beginning with Mental Health Nurses working in a local mental health unit. Convenience sampling was used to target intentionally those research participants who are interested in identifying sources of carer fatigue and burnout in their work as Mental Health Nurses.

Justification of Numbers

The number of participants was congruent with the assumptions of qualitative research, which emphasise the context-dependent quality of process, experience, and language. Therefore, this project did not seek high numbers to generalise results or use them for predictive purposes, rather it sought to qualify the richness of the participants' experiences. Also, in research of this nature, the process is as important as the potential outcomes, because the focus is on what people learn as they experience the research itself.

Selection Criteria

The participants included Registered Nurses working as Mental Health Nurses who:
- identified with and were willing to speak of their experiences of carer fatigue;
- spoke English, or who could provide an English interpreter; and
- lived within a 100 kilometre radius of the local area.

The recruitment invitation sought participants experiencing carer fatigue, rather than burnout. It was anticipated that some nurses may not have identified with the term 'burnout' due to the connotation of being 'worn out' completely by work stress, whereas they may have been more willing to acknowledge varying degrees of carer fatigue.

Data Collection

Data collection was via semi-structured interviews which used questions reflecting the first stage of White and Epson's (1990) method of narrative therapy, in which relative influence questioning is used to externalise the problem. The relative influence questions were confined to 'mapping the influence of the problem'. The questions related to the effect of burnout in Mental Health Nursing across various interfaces through the dominant story of emotional stress and fatigue. For example, the interviewer began: *'Thank you for agreeing to be part of this research. In joining this project you have indicated that you are experiencing carer fatigue in your work as a Mental Health Nurse. This research invites you to tell us about your experiences.'*

After the establishment of the aims and processes of the research, participants were encouraged to share their experiences through practice stories. The questions included:

What are some of the issues in your Mental Health Nursing practice, that influence your experience of carer fatigue?

What have you noticed about your experience of carer fatigue in your own behaviour, feelings and attitudes?

How has the experience of carer fatigue influenced your role as a mental health nurse?

What are some of the ways you have sought to manage the experience of carer fatigue?

What kinds of work structures and processes would help you to manage and prevent carer fatigue?

The participants were given time to tell their stories. If a participant was having difficulty in maintaining the flow of the account, some prompts were given, such as:

'*What happened then?*'

'*Who was involved?*'

'*What was your part in the situation?*'

'*How did that make you feel?*'

The interviewer was PhD-prepared with previous experience in undertaking sensitive content interviews. At the beginning of the interview, biographical data were collected relating to the person's age, level of appointment and years of experience. Each participant was interviewed initially for approximately one hour, to allow sufficient time to identify the influences of carer fatigue. No follow-up interviews were required as a means of data validation, as sufficient time was given to the validation process during the initial interview. The interviews were audiotaped for later verbatim transcription. As no participants were uncomfortable with having the conversation recorded, note-taking was unnecessary.

EXERCISE

In the previous example, how were participants enlisted into the project? How were their rights honoured? What was the sequence of the research methods? What interpersonal processes were involved in undertaking the methods?

Analysis and interpretation

The report provides a description of how the analysis and interpretation of data was done. This is the part of the report that may differ from other qualitative projects. The reader must be able to see how you went about organising and making sense of the data, so be sure to set this section out carefully and clearly.

The report should also make the analysis and interpretation phases transparent by documenting them in the report. This means that the report should faithfully reflect the roles and contributions of all the people in the research to analysis and interpretation. The report should also provide excerpts of actual dialogue between researchers/co-researchers/participants as sources of data to assist in validating interpretations and to act as a decision trail for readers.

Some questions which may guide you in writing up the analysis and interpretation phase of the project are:

- Whose writing informed the choice of analysis?
- What were the steps in the analysis?
- Who did the analysis? That is, was it done by an individual or by a group?
- How did the individual/group go about doing the analysis?
- How were the data organised when they reached analysed form?
- What were the sub-themes/collective themes/competing discourses?
- Who made the interpretations?
- How were the interpretations made?
- What interpretations were made?
- How were the interpretations validated?

Responses to these questions will differ considerably, depending on whether the report is describing a qualitative interpretive or qualitative critical project. The report should be organised into sections or chapters in which the analysis and interpretation can be demonstrated. The report should demonstrate how individuals' accounts relate to those of other participants and, if it is appropriate to the methodology chosen, the report should discuss common themes that emerged from the data analysis and interpretation phases. For example:

Data Analysis

Data analysis and interpretation occurred at two levels: during the interview and later through data analysis methods. During the interview insights arose directly out of the conversation facilitated by the invitation to share practice narratives. These insights were identified directly by the participants and were recorded as part of the audiotaped data, allowing incorporation into the second level of analysis. After reading and re-reading the transcriptions, analysis proceeded using a computer-assisted thematic analysis procedure (Taylor, 1998), in relation to the project's aims. Themes and sub-themes were identified, which gave insights into what was being communicated about nurses' experiences, which formed the basis of the recommendations to the Mental Health Division of the Area Health Service.

Professor Taylor undertook the computer-assisted thematic analysis procedure in August 2002. The specific process used was:

- The interviews were transcribed onto computer disk.
- Pseudonyms were used and other identifying material was changed to protect identities.
- Each interview was analysed separately to locate sources and effects of carer fatigue.
- As each story contextualised participants and their work settings, for further participant protection, numbers were then assigned to replace pseudonyms in interview analyses.
- The subthemes from each participant's story were collated into common themes.

After the analysis, the decision was taken by Professor Taylor and Ms Jan Barling not to publish individual's contextual information and analyses, as a further means of protecting the identities of participants already self-identifying as experiencing carer fatigue and burnout.

The Collective Analysis

The sources of work related problems for Mental Health Nurses that contributed towards their experiences of carer fatigue and burnout for these participants were:

Employment insecurity and casualisation of the work force
Issues with management and the system
Difficulties with the nature of the work
Inadequate resources and services
Problems with doctors
Aggressive and criminal consumers
Undervaluing consumers and nurses
Physical and emotional constraints of the work setting
Nurse-nurse relationships and horizontal violence

The effects of stress are exemplified in the theme: *Dealing with and reacting to the effects of stress*

Example of the Themes

In a qualitative report, themes are often justified by participants' words. The project report of this research filled a lengthy chapter of the report, so only a brief example of the detailed analysis is as follows.

Employment Insecurity and Casualisation of the Work Force

Participants described their concerns about employment insecurity. For example:

Participant 1 described working two days a week, but in the last 12 months had secured a permanent contract position. Participant 1 said the contract was due to expire within two weeks and s/he was unsure what would happen after that. S/he had applied for another job, but s/he said:

Being in a rural area, jobs are really difficult to find and I don't think I'll get it because there's been a person working in that position already. That adds to the stress.

Participant 5 described a lack of choices about where to practice Mental Health Nursing locally.

Because we have been there for so long in mental health, we don't actually want to go back up to the general wards either. We have long since shifted away from that scene. Some of the newer trained graduates will get back there and keep their skills up. As an alternative to Mental Health Nursing, general nursing is not an option.

EXERCISE

Answer yes or no to the following questions. In the previous example, does the report explain:

- Whose writing informed the choice of analysis?
- What the steps were in the analysis?
- Who did the analysis?
- How the analysis was done?
- How the data were organised when they reached analysed form?
- What the sub-themes/collective themes/competing discourses were?
- Who made the interpretations?
- How the interpretations were made?
- What interpretations were made?
- How the interpretations were validated?

Discussion and insights/recommendations/suggestions/conclusions

This part of a qualitative report can be labelled variously, depending on what the project has aimed to achieve through its methods and processes. Some qualitative reports will offer suggestions, while others will offer recommendations. It all depends on the justification they have for offering them.

The final stage of the report documents any pertinent discussions of the findings and offers suggestions and/or recommendations for nurses and nursing practice. Projects may conclude the research by offering suggestions for practice, education and research. At times, however, and in line with the lack of certainty in qualitative research related to the relativity of 'truth', tentative statements are made, for example:

> All of the themes in the research reflect the sources of stress and how stress affects nurses as people in their work environments. It is interesting that the localised themes of the 20 participants in this project reflect findings in national and international literature relating to mental health care generally and Mental Health Nursing specifically (Barling, 2001; Clinton and Hazelton, 2000a-d).
>
> At a national level, sources of carer fatigue and burnout in Mental Health Nursing have been identified by Clinton and Hazelton (2000a-d), who were commissioned by the National Mental Health Working Group of the Australian Health Minister's Advisory Council to undertake a 'scoping study of Mental Health Nursing in Australia', because of 'widespread concern about the Mental Health Nursing workforce in Australia' (Clinton and Hazelton, 2000a:2). After consulting with a wide range of national and international literature, consumer organisations and other stakeholders, the researchers concluded that two dominant themes emerged:
>
> (i)   Mental Health Nurses report high levels of stress. Stress and burnout arise from the pace of change in mental health services, the perception that the personal safety of the nurse is under threat in acute units and in the community, and from the perceived over-bureaucratisation of mental health services.
>
> (ii) Nurse education is in need of reform. There is clear evidence that insufficient attention is given to preparing Bachelor of Nursing graduates for beginning practice in Mental Health Nursing. Furthermore, the attitudes of some Mental Health Nurses deter students from pursuing a career in the field of mental health (Clinton and Hazelton, 2000d:160).

The first theme reflects issues participants described in our research, particularly difficulties with the nature of the work, aggressive and criminal consumers, physical and emotional constraints of the work setting, employment insecurity and casualisation of the workforce, issues with management and the system, and inadequate resources and services. It is very possible also, that some of the nurses' stressors in our research related directly to a lack of educational preparation in mental health nursing, although many of the participants were qualified, experienced clinicians, who suffered mainly from a lack of recognition by others in the health care team of what they knew and how they practised.

Because of a lack of research in Mental Health Nursing research at a national level, Barling (2001) reviewed international studies and found that the issues were similar to those identified by Clinton and Hazelton (2000a-d). From literature sources highlighting international research findings, Barling (2001) compiled lists of work stressors related to community and acute admission ward Mental Health Nursing. The organisational, environmental and professional stressors associated with community Mental Health Nursing were similar to those identified in acute admission ward nursing. Although there has been no attempt to differentiate between acute inpatient and community mental health work contexts in our research, all of the stressors compiled from international literature by Barling (2001) were identified by Mental Health Nurses in our study, and some participants' accounts of these are located in this article.

In relation to the effects of workplace stress, the findings of our research reflect burnout syndrome (Barling, 2001). Participants spoke of emotional exhaustion, depersonalisation and reduced personal accomplishment manifesting variously in tiredness and insomnia, setting boundaries and limits, trying to cope by various means, thinking of other career options and specific personal problems.

Conclusion

This research offers descriptions of stressors and effects of stress that are not new, in that while they were generated from 20 Mental Health Nurses in a local area, they reflect national and international research findings. The fact that this research has yet again resurfaced long-standing issues in Mental Health Nursing attests to the entrenched nature and effects of stress in the workplace and the seeming futility of research projects to affect tangible and enduring people and environment changes. While this research offers possibilities for change, it also reiterates the powerful nature of entrenched work cultures and organisations that seem to be impervious to positive change, even in the face of real costs, in human terms, to the nurses involved.

The report of this research reflects the severe degree of carer fatigue and burnout in Mental Health Nurse participants and the attempts they have made already to set up a dialogue between themselves and the sources of their workplace stress. The participants' willingness to be part of this research attests to their intentions to acknowledge their stress and to try to do something about it. Many of the participants expressed their concern that involvement in this research would make them vulnerable to reprisals from those people and forces that oppress them already and compound their carer fatigue and burnout. Every attempt has been made to honour participants' privacy and anonymity, and to conceal the identities of the people and places mentioned in their accounts. Therefore, the nature of this research by its ethical limitations, cannot create directly, a frank and open dialogue between particular nurses and the unique sources of their stress, but it can point to these problems and issues from a place of relative safety. As noted in the research objectives, recommendations were made to the local area health service, but they are not listed in detail here, as they are specific to that area and their inclusion in this report risks breaches in confidentiality. However, as a general guide for readers of this publication, recommendations included strategies for decreasing mental health nurses' work stress by setting up regular forums for open, direct communication of issues between all parties, and ensuring respect for mental health nurses' practice knowledge and skills through representation on relevant committees and promotion to senior roles in the career structure.

Qualitative reports will differ in their concluding parts, depending on the particular approaches they have taken. The report should demonstrate that the final discussion and conclusions are congruent with the overall plan, methods and processes of the research.

The references for this qualitative research report example are:

Alexander, J., Lichtenstein, R., Joo Oh Hyuan & Ullman, E. 1998. A causal model of voluntary turnover among nursing personnel in long-term psychiatric settings. *Research in Nursing & Health* 21:415–27.

Barling, J. 2001. Drowning not waving: Burnout and mental health nursing. *Contemporary Nurse* 11(2-3):247–59.

Brown, D., Carson, J., Fagin, L., Bartlett, H. & Leary, J. 1994. Coping with caring. *Nursing Times* 9,45:53–5.

Butterworth, T. 1995. The current status and future challenges of psychiatric/mental health nursing. *International journal of Nursing Studies*. 32,4:353–65.

Carson, J. 1997. Self-esteem and stress in Mental Health Nursing. *Nursing Times* 93,44: 55–8 October.

Carson, J., Brown, D., Fagin, L., Leary, J. & Bartlett, H. 1996. Do larger case loads cause more stress in community? *Mental Health Nurses' Journal of Clinical Nursing* 5,2:133–4 March.

Carson, J., Leary, J., De Villiers, N., Fagin, L. & Randall, J. 1995. Stress in mental health nurses: comparison of ward and community staff. *British Journal of Nursing* 4,10: 579–81.

Clinton, M. & Hazelton, M. 2000a. Scoping mental health nursing education. *Australian and New Zealand Journal of Mental Health Nursing* 9:2–10.

Clinton, M. & Hazelton, M. 2000b. Scoping the Australian mental health nursing workforce. *Australian and New Zealand Journal of Mental Health Nursing* 9:56–64.

Clinton, M. & Hazelton, M. 2000c. Scoping practice issues in the Australian mental health nursing workforce. *Australian and New Zealand Journal of Mental Health Nursing* 9:100–9.

Clinton, M. & Hazelton, M. 2000d. Scoping the prospects of Australian mental health nursing. *Australian and New Zealand Journal of Mental Health Nursing* 9:159–65.

Fagin, L., Brown, D., Bartlett, H., Leary, J. & Carson, J. 1995. The Claybury community psychiatric nurse stress study; is it more stressful to work in the hospital or the community? *Journal of Advanced Nursing* 22,2:347–58.

Farrington, A. 1995. Stress and Nursing. *British Journal of Nursing* 4,10:574–8.

Farrington, A. 1997. Strategies for reducing stress & burnout in nursing. *British Journal of Nursing* 6,1:44–50.

Hopkinson, P., Carson, J., Brown, D., Fagin, L., Bartlett, H. & Leary, J. 1998. Occupational stress and community mental health nursing: what CPNs really said. *Journal of Advanced Nursing* 27: 707–12.

Leary, J., Gallagher, T., Carson, J., Fagin, L., Bartlett, H. & Brown, D. 1995. Stress and coping strategies in community psychiatric nurses: A Q methodological study. *Journal of Advanced Nursing* 21,2:230–7.

Leiter, M. & Harvie, P. 1996. Burnout among mental health workers: A review and a Research Agenda. *International Journal of Social Psychiatry* 42,2:90–101.

Mcleod, T. 1997. Work stress among community psychiatric nurses. *British Journal of Nursing* 6,10:569–73.

Melchior, M., Philipsen, H., Abu Saad, H., Halfens, R., Van de Berg, A. & Gassman, P. 1996. The effectiveness of primary nursing on burnout among psychiatric nurses in long-stay settings. *Journal of Advanced Nursing* 24:694–702.

Nolan, P. 1995. A measurement tool for assessing stress among Mental Health Nurses. *Nursing Standard* 9, 46:36–9 August.

Rees, D. & Smith, S. 1991. Work stress in occupational therapists assessed by occupational stress indicator. *British Journal of Occupational Therapy* 54,8:289–94.

Sammut, R. 1997. Psychiatric nurses satisfaction: the effects of closure of a hospital. *Journal of Advanced Nursing* 26:20–4.

Thomas, M., Beaven, J., Blacksmith, J., Ekland, E., Hein, J., Osborne, O. & Reno, J. 1999. Meaning of state hospital nursing 1: Facing challenges. *Archives of Psychiatric Nursing* X111, 1:48–54.

Wheeler, H. 1997a. A review of nurse occupational stress research 1: Coping and making meaning. *British Journal of Nursing* 6,11:642–5.

Wheeler, H. 1997b. Nurse occupational stress research 2: definition and conceptualisation. *British Journal of Nursing* 6,12:710–13.

Wheeler, H. 1997c. Nurse Occupational Stress research 3: a model of stress for research. *British Journal of Nursing* 6,16:944–9.

Wheeler, H. 1997d. Nurse occupational stress research 4: The prevalence of stress. *British Journal of Nursing* 6,21:1256–60.

Wheeler, H. 1998a. Nurse occupational stress research 5: sources and determinants of stress. *British Journal of Nursing* 7,1:40–3.

Wheeler, H. 1998b. Nurse occupational stress research 6: methodological approaches. *British Journal of Nursing* 7,4:226–9.

Wheeler, H. & Riding, R. 1994. Occupational stress in general nurse and midwives. *British Journal of Nursing* 3,10:527–34.

White, M. and Epston, D. 1990. *Narrative Means to Therapeutic Ends*. Adelaide, Dulwich Centre.

We hope you found this worked example of a research report helpful. Remember that you can use this outline for forming drafts of the research report. You will need to go back over the drafts to correct grammar, to reword ideas, and to undertake other editorial tasks that ensure a high-quality report. It is a good idea to locate and study research reports so that you can see how they have been prepared. Do not hesitate to borrow from other researchers ideas that appear to work well, but only after verifying that they are appropriate for your research.

Presenting a report at professional meetings
Oral presentations

From time to time, a researcher may need to present an oral presentation of the report to an audience, for example the whole research class, a seminar or a conference. A researcher may also have to present a paper at a conference or seminar. Consider the audience. The oral report should be dynamic and interesting. The audience will not normally have access to the written paper at the time of the presentation, so clarity is essential. An acceptable presentation seldom results from just reading a written paper, as the ways of conveying information by writing and speaking are different. It is boring to have to listen to a speaker read from a paper.

Visual aids can be useful to add interest to oral presentations. Use overhead transparencies, or if you are going to a conference, it is worth having professional slides made. If you have access to the software program PowerPoint or its equivalent, you can design professional-looking slides and transparencies. These are written using the Outline View (see Figure 18.2).

The Outline View is then converted to slides (see Figure 18.3). You can also use PowerPoint to give a slide show using your computer in conjunction with a data beam that projects the presentation from the computer onto a big screen. A laptop computer is

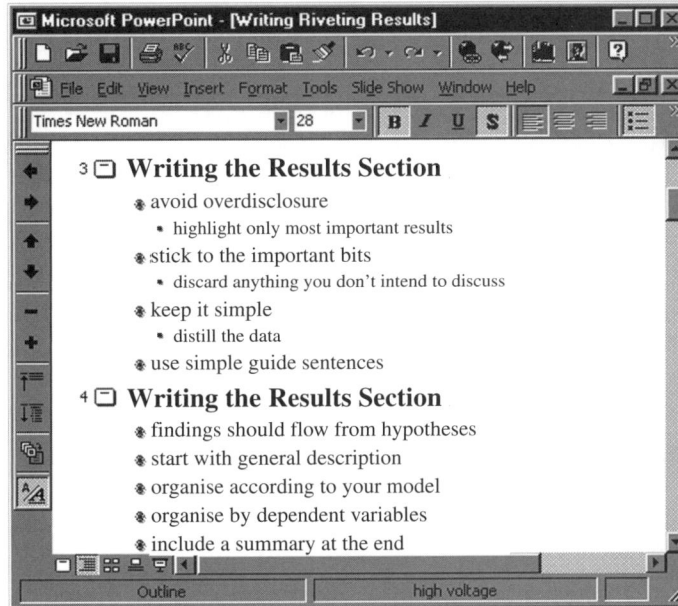

Figure 18.2 PowerPoint: Outline View

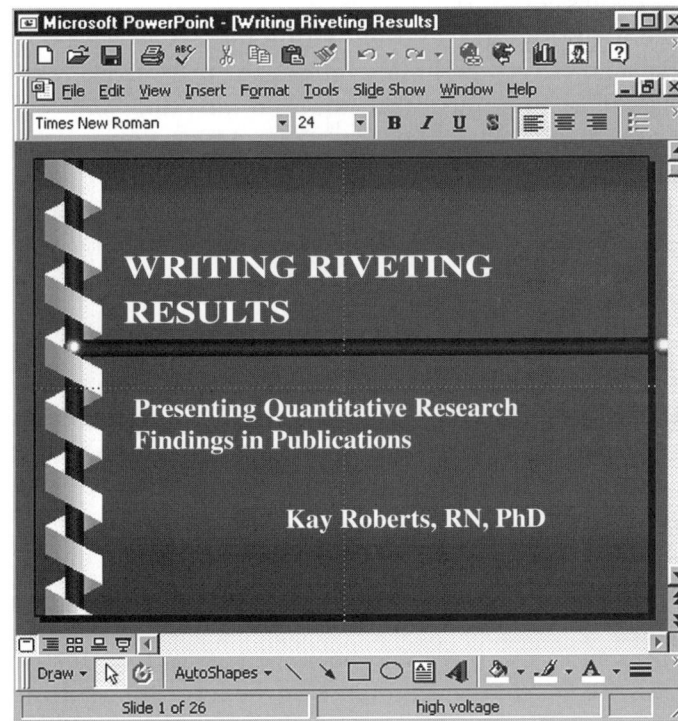

Figure 18.3 A PowerPoint slide

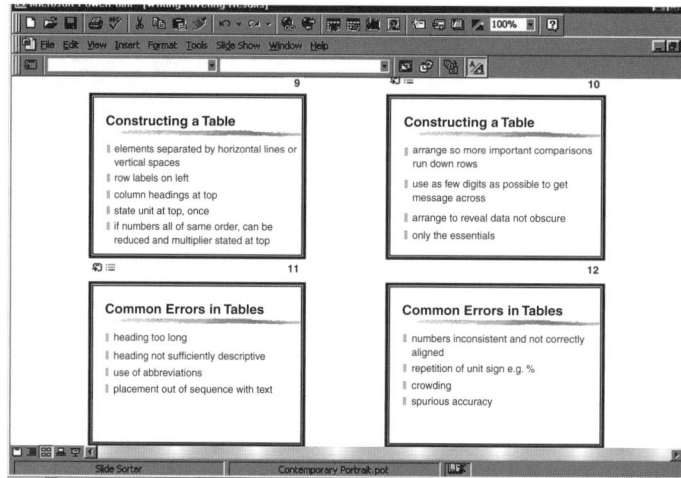

Figure 18.4 Handouts for the audience generated from PowerPoint slides

particularly useful for this purpose because of its portability. These slide shows are very effective because they use professionally designed layouts with dramatic colour schemes and allow for gradual introduction of points on the slide. PowerPoint presentations are becoming the norm at professional conferences.

The presenter controls the presentation with a mouse. PowerPoint presentations can be embellished with special effects, including interesting transitions between slides and separate introduction of individual points. You can even introduce musical effects and hypertext links to Internet sites.

You can also generate handouts for the audience that reproduce varying numbers of your transparencies to the page, with space for note-taking if you wish. See Figure 18.4.

Finally, you can generate a set of notes for yourself that have one panel to the page that takes up only half of the page. On the other half, you can type brief notes in a large bold font that will help you to remember supporting information during your presentation of the paper. See Figure 18.5.

The major errors made with these media are having too much information on the slide or transparency and having the printing too small. The latter is usually a consequence of the former. The printing should be in a large font. PowerPoint resists these errors. The material on slides should be oriented horizontally rather than vertically since the screen is wider than it is high (Day 1998). Consider the size of the room when composing your overheads or slides. If possible, check out the readability of the print from the back of the room. Make sure that your slides and transparencies are numbered and are in the correct order and the correct orientation (no upside-down slides!).

For most oral presentations, there will be some sort of time restriction: most presentations will not exceed 30 to 45 minutes, and may be as short as 10 minutes. Therefore, you will need to be selective about what to include and you will need to plan the allocation of the time, including an allowance for questions. Another option is to provide a

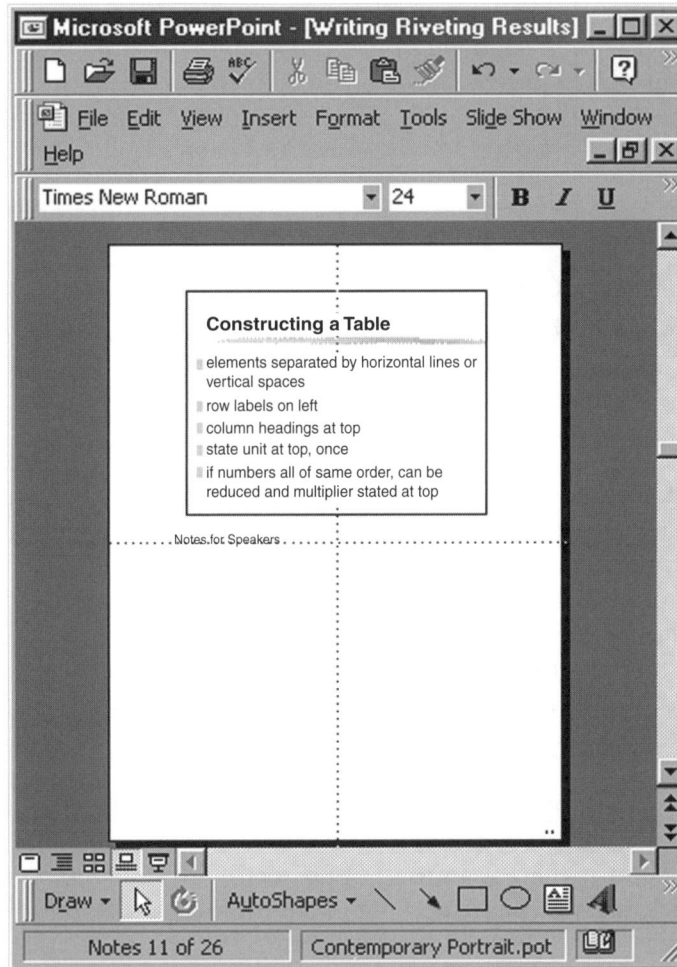

Figure 18.5 Speaker's notes generated from PowerPoint slides

handout and just do the highlights. Handouts give the person something to take away and can include graphics to support the written report. Sometimes people give the abstract as a handout.

The presentation should be organised and logical, following a similar format to that of a written report. However, the audience will be far more interested in the results and implications than in the literature review and methodology, so give a brief introduction to the purpose of the study and any previous findings, then focus on the results and the implications. Do not include a lengthy account of the methods or extensive citations of the literature (Day 1998).

Preparation is essential for an oral presentation. You will need a copy of the full report, preferably double-spaced in larger print to allow easy and unobtrusive reading. If you are confident and know the topic well, a good method is to write the main headings on cards in large print or use PowerPoint speaker notes and speak to them. This allows you to make more eye contact with the audience. You can keep the written paper handy in case you get stuck. It is also useful to practise giving your paper to colleagues, friends or relatives. This gives you feedback and allows you to gauge the timing, and to practise using any equipment. Try to anticipate any questions or criticisms and have a reply ready.

Posters

A poster is usually presented at a poster session of a conference. Originally, poster sessions were developed to meet a need for catering for more presentations than could be accommodated on a conference program. The way the system works is that people offer (or are asked to submit) abstracts of presentations, then invitations are issued to deliver a paper or present a poster. At one time posters were seen as a type of rejection of an abstract (Day 1998). However, now they are an important part of a conference program, with large areas set aside for poster presentations. Some types of material, for example, the results of complex research studies, can be presented more effectively in a poster than in an oral presentation (Day 1998).

The purpose of the poster presentation is to communicate the major points of the research project to a number of people who then have the opportunity to talk to the researcher about it. Usually there is a group of posters, with the presenters in attendance by their posters. The delegates walk around the room looking at the posters, and stopping to talk to the researchers whose posters interest them. The researchers can then discuss the finer details of their projects with the delegates.

It is important to have a poster that will attract the attention of the delegates. Posters can result in publicity for the research and also in the presenter acquiring valuable ideas from colleagues. Guidelines for the presentation of posters can be obtained from the conference presenters. You should adhere strictly to these guidelines when developing your poster.

You can prepare a poster yourself using large sheets of cardboard. Printing can be done either by hand, using felt-tipped pens or paint, or you can print the text on the computer printer and attach it to the cardboard. If you are not constrained by financial considerations, you can do the poster on a computer program and have it printed professionally by a graphics company.

The poster should contain the title of the project, the name of the researcher, the purpose of the study, the research question, the method, the results, the conclusions and the implications.

The poster should have visual appeal and impact. It should get across the main points without being wordy. If it is too heavy with words, you might as well give delegates a copy of your research report. Remember, 'less is more'. The most common mistake is to have too much information on the poster. There should be very little text in a poster, with much of the space occupied by illustrations (Day 1998).

The poster should be able to be read easily at a distance of about 1.5 metres and should attract people to stop at your display. Letters should be at least 2.5 cm high, or 24-point font. Information using bullet points is easier to read than paragraphs. Be sure to lay the poster out carefully and proofread it. You may want to use arrows to direct the reader to read the poster in a logical sequence. Remember that any material below knee level will not be readable. The contrast of colours should be pleasing, but avoid too many colours as it may overwhelm the viewer. Creative presentation is important – try attaching a three-dimensional visual aid.

Care should be taken with transporting a poster to a conference: you should pack it in a tube and carry it with you during the journey. If you check it in with your luggage when you are travelling by air, it may become lost. Store it in the overhead compartment and remember to retrieve it at your journey's end.

If you are invited to present a poster at a conference, you can find more detail about the content and format of poster construction in the following publications: Cantrell and Bracher (1999), Gosling (1999), Jackson and Sheldon (2000), Maltby and Serrell (1998), McCann, Sramac and Rudy (1999) and Russell, Gregory and Gates (1996).

Writing for a wider audience

One of the most lamentable situations that can happen to research findings is that they are not communicated adequately to the wider audience beyond the span of the research report. Research is intended for public consumption, so that it can be scrutinised and have beneficial effects. An important feature of scholarship is in inviting open discussion and critique of original work, to verify the usefulness or otherwise of the new information. Whereas research is open to anyone who shows interest in it, it makes the most sense to target people most directly associated with it. Effective ways of doing this are through journal articles and **monographs**.

Writing a journal article

If you have not written a journal article before, you may be thinking that it is beyond your ability. If this is what you are thinking, please reconsider. Journals are media for communication. In nursing and health care there are many opportunities to choose a journal which is best able to communicate the results of your research. Wander into the journal section of your library and take some time to browse. You will find many journals representing different areas of your discipline. One of them is sure to suit you as a means of disseminating your research.

While you are looking through the journals that seem to suit you best, notice the format and style of the journal. Locate the section about notes for contributors. It may be on the inside front or back cover. This is a practical guide by the editor of the journal as to what is expected of you in preparing a manuscript for submission. Make a photocopy so that you can study it carefully and use it to guide you in writing your article.

The original research report that documents the whole of the research will need to be adjusted to suit the requirements of the journal. You will notice that there are word limits for the categories of articles. As you will be putting your research forward, you would be best advised to prepare your research as a feature article, which will undergo a review process. Do not let this concern you too much. You have managed to do the research and to present the report, so this is just another step in your evolution as a researcher.

Prepare the manuscript according to what it is you want to put forward in the article. For example, you may want to present a synopsis of the entire project or you may want to extract certain themes or sections from the project and elaborate on them. If you want to present a synopsis of the entire project, your challenge will be to represent the project overall faithfully, while keeping to the word limit. This will mean that you will have to make decisions about what you will leave out of the manuscript. Make sure that the essential features of the project remain intact according to the particular approach you have taken. If you are unsure what these features are, consult a reference on critique of research, for example, this book. This will tell you what other people will be looking for when they read your research.

If you choose to extract certain parts of the project for further elaboration, you need to spend some time deciding on how you will do this. Be clear about the focus of the article you want to write. Ensure that it fits the content of the journal in which you are intending to publish. When you extract the section from the research report, read it carefully. It will most probably need a new introduction, a certain amount of extra work in the body of the text, and an appropriate conclusion.

When the writing phase is over, it is important to check the manuscript for spelling and grammatical errors. Check to see that it follows the referencing conventions of the journal and that it is set out clearly with headings and subheadings. Ideas should flow between sections, and the discussion and conclusions section should be well substantiated. When you think that you have the manuscript ready, give it to some colleagues to read for content, grammar, flow of ideas, fit for the selected journal and so on. You will then adjust the manuscript according to their feedback. Make sure you have added the other details as specified such as a title page, contact details and so on. Ensure that you have complied with the journal's requirements for content and format.

Always print your article in a large, easy-to-read font, for example, 12-point Times Roman, and in double line spacing. Photocopy the required number of copies, including one for your files. Send them with a covering letter to the editor and then wait for feedback. It is a good idea to date the copy and note to which journal you sent it before filing it.

When the letter arrives from the journal editor, it may suggest some changes. Feedback from reviewers will be supplied to assist you in adjusting the manuscript. Alternatively it may be flawless and ready to publish as is, but this seldom happens, even to very experienced writers. The journal will then probably ask you for a copy of your article on disk, or to be submitted by email. The worst case is that the letter may inform you that the manuscript is not suitable for publication in that particular journal. If so, do not despair. Life is like that. You can't always get it right the first time. Consider resubmitting the manuscript to a more suitable journal. With a few changes you may find it fits another journal's requirements – but ensure you meet the next journal's specifications. If you want to publish, the trick is not to take rejections too much to heart. Above all, don't give up!

If you want to learn more about publishing in journals, an excellent starting point for further reading is an article by Greenwood (1998). Another article you may care to access was written by journal editors (Plawecki & Plawecki 1998).

Writing a monograph

Definitions for a monograph differ, but there is usually agreement that a monograph is smaller than a book. It is usually presented as a soft-cover A5-size (half A4) document containing approximately 50 pages. It is usual for academic organisations to have their own printing facilities, and to publish their own monographs.

If you are thinking that you would like to try to have your work published in a monograph, your first port of call might be to an academic in the university or other tertiary institution. Ask this person whether the university has a monograph series for researchers. If the answer is yes, the rest of the inquiries will be up to you as to how you go about securing approval to submit a manuscript. Do not put a lot of work into a monograph unless you know it is appropriate for the publication series and that it will be reviewed for publication.

Preparing a monograph appears to be a larger task than preparing for submitting a journal article; however, in some ways it could be easier. For instance, the word limit will be larger, so there will be less challenge in presenting the research intact. Check with someone who understands copyright to ensure that you can cut and paste large sections of your thesis or research reports. You may find that much of the work you have already done can be transferred to the monograph manuscript. It will then be a matter of setting out a table of contents that gives the manuscript a good flow of ideas. Having done this, you will know where the areas for further elaboration lie, and these will be your main foci for writing.

As in any case of writing for publication, ensure that you follow the requirements of the publisher. Present the manuscript in its best possible version, after it has been thoroughly checked and rechecked by you and other willing readers. Send it to the publisher with a covering letter and wait for feedback.

Be prepared to make adjustments as directed by the publisher. If the manuscript is not appropriate for publication by that publisher, try working on the draft again and submitting it elsewhere. Remember, a rejection is not a comment about you as a person; it is a comment about a piece of written work and what the publisher wants.

Summary

In this chapter we have discussed the importance of a research report as a vehicle for disseminating the findings of the project and demonstrating professional accountability. We have also shown how to construct a research report. The mechanisms were outlined for presenting a research report orally and by poster to professional meetings. Ideas were also given about how to prepare a manuscript for submission for publication as a journal article or a monograph.

Main points

- A research report is a formal account of a research project and the major means of disseminating essential information about it. The report can be formal or informal, oral or written.
- Researchers have a responsibility to share findings so as to help build a useful body of knowledge, to help their colleagues practise more effectively, to help others plan research more effectively and to allow peer review.
- The purpose of a research report is to communicate key aspects of the project to research consumers so they can: replicate your study, do their own literature review, plan a new study or help find a solution for a clinical practice problem.
- When writing a report, consider your target audience and write to it after obtaining guidelines for content and presentation.
- In planning and writing the report, make an outline, write a draft and revise it, have someone critique it and rewrite it until it is the best you can do.
- The writing style generally is the same as for a research proposal – concise, clear and coherent, with good English usage and written in the past tense.
- The structure of the report is the same as for the proposal, with preliminaries, introduction, methodology and methods, but with the addition of results, discussion and conclusions.
- The results section should present the results concisely, with the judicious use of illustrations such as graphs and tables.
- The discussion section highlights the most important findings, explains their significance and relevance, interprets them in relation to issues raised in the introduction section and places them in the context of theory and previous research.
- The conclusions section draws conclusions derived from the findings, and includes recommendations for implementing the findings, for further research and for theory development.
- Supporting materials include references and appendixes.
- A qualitative report has many similarities with a quantitative report, including a research plan that covers methodology, methods and processes. The findings tell a story, using themes and sub-themes, with quoted material as appropriate. The discussion section presents insights, recommendations, suggestions and conclusions.
- In developing oral presentations, consider the audience, be dynamic and interesting, use visual aids, prepare and practise, and keep to time during the presentation.
- Posters communicate the major points of the research project to colleagues who have an opportunity to talk to the researcher. In preparing a poster, adhere strictly to the guidelines, and pay attention to creating visual appeal and impact.
- When writing a journal article, select the target journal, obtain and follow its author guidelines, prepare the manuscript, send it with a covering letter to the editor and wait for feedback.

Case study

Carmel was introduced in Chapter 14. If you have not been following Carmel's case study, go to the end of Chapters 14 to 17 and review her story so far. Carmel used a collaborative research approach with 10 other experienced nurses working in acute care settings. She set up a participatory action research (PAR) group and they met for one hour per week for 16 weeks in all. The group identified a thematic concern of the use of power in the health care organisation, so they undertook a literature review of organisational power in hospitals. The PAR group analysed their own practice stories collectively in group meetings. Possible interpretations of the practice stories were made through in-depth discussion, in order to make sense of nurses' experiences of power in their workplaces. The PAR group developed an action plan for identifying the detrimental effects of power in the workplace and how nurses might respond to this kind of power assertively. The time has now come to write the research report.

1   What are the possible means of disseminating the research information?
2   Describe the process for writing a qualitative research report.
3   What must Carmel and the other co-researchers do when preparing the research report as a peer-reviewed journal article?

Multiple choice questions

1   The major means by which essential information is disseminated about a research project is a research:
   a   article
   b   report
   c   email
   d   presentation
2   The usual length of a peer-reviewed article is:
   a   3000 to 5000 words
   b   unlimited
   c   the same as a thesis
   d   100 000 words
3   A long, detailed discourse, submitted for an honours degree or a higher degree, such as a master's degree or a doctorate, is a:
   a   presentation
   b   monograph
   c   poster
   d   thesis

4 Which of the following is part of the body of a research report? The:
    a abstract
    b references
    c literature review
    d appendices

5 In a quantitative research report, the design describes in detail the research:
    a aims, objectives and background
    b context, literature and objectives
    c abstract, literature and procedures
    d framework, methods and procedures

6 In relation to a research report involving humans, ethical considerations are described:
    a only for quantitative projects
    b for all research projects
    c only for qualitative projects
    d for potentially harmful designs

7 For quantitative results, the statistical tests should be reported:
    a with the appropriate result, giving the test, the result of the test, and the probability value
    b in subjective language that allows for possible differences in interpretations
    c as findings in a narrative, focusing on the various themes that have emerged
    d in their entirety, unedited, whether or not they are important or significant

8 Qualitative reports vary from one another because:
    a they do not have to be as careful as quantitative research in reporting their methods and findings
    b creativity in thinking, researching and writing is encouraged in all qualitative approaches
    c they represent vast methodological differences in interpretive, critical and postmodern perspectives
    d qualitative researchers do everything they can to make their reports as interesting as possible

9 Some qualitative research reports provide excerpts of actual dialogue between researchers/co-researchers/participants in order to:
    a demonstrate that they are aware of the assumptions of postmodern perspectives
    b assist in validating interpretations and to act as a decision trail for readers
    c reflect faithfully the roles and contributions of all the people in the research
    d make the reports as interesting as possible for readers of the research findings

10 At a professional conference, an effective way to present a concise version of your research, while making yourself available for delegates' questions and comments is by a:
    a poster
    b thesis
    c monograph
    d brochure

Review topics

1   Who are the possible recipients of a research report?
2   What are the common features of a qualitative and quantitative report?
3   Discuss how you would prepare a research project article for peer-review.
4   Describe the preparations required for giving a successful conference presentation of your research.
5   Discuss why a monograph of your research report may be advisable.

Online reading

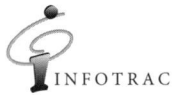

INFOTRAC® COLLEGE EDITION

When accessing information about writing and disseminating research information use the following keywords in any combinations you require:

➤ **conference presentation**
➤ **journal**
➤ **monograph**
➤ **poster**
➤ **qualitative**
➤ **quantitative**
➤ **research report**
➤ **seminar**
➤ **writing**

INFOTRAC

References

Anderson, D. & Poole, M. 1998, *Assignment and Thesis Writing*, 3rd edn, John Wiley & Sons, Brisbane.

Brown, R. 1995, *Key Skills for Writing and Publishing Research*, Write Way Consulting, Brisbane.

Cantrell, J. & Bracher, L. 1999, 'How to design and present a poster', *Advancing Clinical Nursing*, vol. 3, no. 2, 91–2.

Day, R. 1998, *How to Write and Publish a Scientific Paper*, 5th edn, Cambridge University Press, Cambridge.

Dees, R. 1999, *Writing the Modern Research Paper*, Allyn & Bacon Inc., Needham Heights.

Evans, D. 1995, *How to Write a Better Thesis or Report*, Melbourne University Press, Melbourne.

Evans, J. 1994, 'The art of writing successful research abstracts', *Neonatal Network*, vol. 13, no. 5, 49–52.

Foreman, M. & Kirchhoff, K. 1987, 'Accuracy of references in nursing journals', *Research in Nursing and Health*, vol. 10, 177–83.

Gething, L. 1995, *How to Manage Research Effectively*, The Sydney Nursing Research Centre, The Faculty of Nursing, The University of Sydney, Sydney.

Gillespie, B. & Kermode, S. 2004, 'How do perioperative nurses cope with stress?', *Contemporary Nurse*, vol. 16, no. 1, 20–9.

Gosling, P. 1999, *Scientist's Guide to Poster Presentations*, Kluwer Academic/Plenum Publishers, New York.

Greenwood, J. 1998, 'The "write advice" or "how to get a journal article published"', *Contemporary Nurse*, vol. 7, no. 2, 84–90.

Jackson, K. & Sheldon, L. 2000, 'Demystifying the academic aura: preparing a poster', *Nurse Researcher*, vol. 7, no. 3, 70–3.

Maltby, H. & Serrell, M. 1998, 'The art of poster presentation', *Collegian*, vol. 5, no. 2, 36–7.

McCann, S., Sramac, R. & Rudy, S. 1999, 'The poster exhibit: guidelines for planning, development, and presentation', *Dermatology Nursing*, vol. 11, no. 5, 373–9.

Plawecki, H. & Plawecki, J. 1998, 'Writing for publication: understanding the process', *Journal of Holistic Nursing*, vol. 16, no. 1, 23–32.

Russell, C., Gregory, D. & Gates, M. 1996, 'Aesthetics and substance in qualitative research posters', *Qualitative Health Research*, vol. 6, no. 4, 542–52.

Taylor, B. & Barling, J. 2004, 'Identifying sources and effects of carer fatigue and burnout for mental health nurses: a qualitative project', *International Journal of Mental Health*, vol. 13, 117–25.

Thomas, S. 2000, *How to Write Health Sciences Papers, Dissertations and Theses*, Churchill-Livingstone, Edinburgh.

Tornquist, E. 1986, *From Proposal to Publication*, Addison-Wesley, Menlo Park, California.

Walters, D. 1999, *The Readable Thesis: Clear & Effective Writing*, Avocus Publishing, Inc., Gilsum.

Watson, J. & Crick, F. 1953, 'Molecular structure of nucleic acids: a structure for deoxyribose nucleic acid', *Nature*, vol. 171, 773–8.

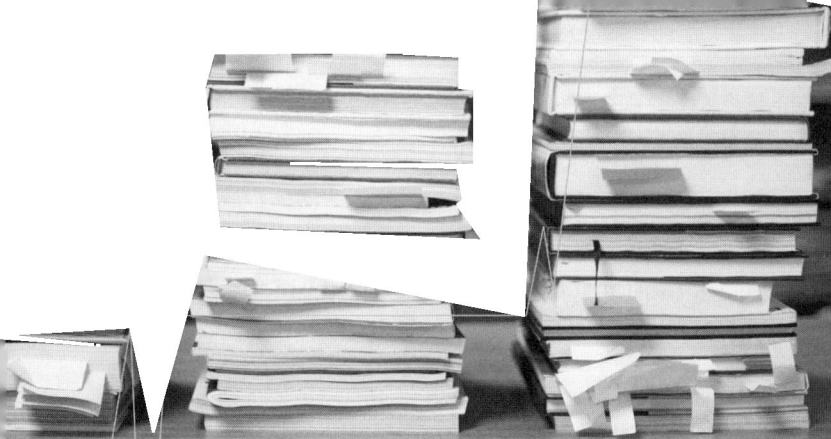

CHAPTER 19

USING RESEARCH IN PRACTICE AND EDUCATION

CHAPTER OBJECTIVES

The material presented in this chapter will assist you to:

- discuss the links between research, practice and education
- describe evidence-based practice
- examine the reasons it is difficult to get research into practice
- describe strategies for improving research uptake in practice settings
- describe strategies for educating evidence-based clinicians.

Introduction

This is the last chapter of this book, so it focuses on using research in practice and education. In writing this chapter we have made certain assumptions: that evidence-based practice (EBP) bases current practice on research, that it is not always easy for clinicians to use research in their practice, and that teachers need to use research in their work to show clinicians how to become researchers and consumers of research.

With these assumptions in mind, this chapter offers you strategies for getting research into practice, such as through national governance, the establishment of effective change measures, and **clinical guidelines**. Policy and procedure manuals are also described as means to ensure that research finds its way into practice. Clinicians need research that is easy and accessible. Some ideas to ensure ease and accessibility include creating a **research culture** in clinical settings, enhancing research–practice links, and undertaking collaborative research.

If research is to be used in clinical settings, education is needed that prepares clinicians for research-based practice. This chapter offers ideas for helping teachers prepare evidence-based clinicians and for enhancing their own teaching effectiveness. The suggestions do not claim to be complete, nor exclusive of other possibilities.

Research and practice

Perhaps the most powerful influence in promoting the use of research in clinical practice is the introduction of evidence-based practice. As outlined in Chapter 1, evidence-based practice bases current practice on research. Evidence-based practice is 'the conscientious, explicit and judicious use of current best evidence in making decisions about the healthcare of patients' (Sackett et al. 1997, p. 2) and it also involves patients' values (Sackett, Straus & Richardson 2000). Dawes (2005, p. 4) suggests that evidence-based practice 'aims to provide the best possible evidence at the point of clinical (or management) contact'.

> ### EXERCISE
> Do clinicians use research in their practice? Think about your professional group and discuss with colleagues the extent to which you consider clinicians use research in their practice.

Health professions are claiming that their practices are based on research (Courtney 2005; Clifford & Clark 2004; Dawes et al. 2005), however, their claims need to be justified. For example, even though nursing strives to be a research-based profession it still does not conduct enough research, nor heed and apply research findings in all its spheres of practice, education and management. There is also a timelag between development and implementation of research, and theory derived from research is not immediately applied to the everyday work, concerns and issues of clinical nursing practice.

This seems not to be the case for the practice of medicine. Evidence-based practice has been established in medicine for decades and only more recently has evidence-based practice moved its influence into allied health areas. The US medical profession began to develop evidence-based medicine after a study reported that few current medical procedures had been shown by clinical trials to be effective. The evidence-based medicine movement was also stimulated by evidence of substantial variation in clinical practice patterns, increased financial pressure and the difficulty that clinicians have in incorporating rapidly evolving evidence into their practice.

The medical profession has set up an international initiative to facilitate the retrieval and synthesis of literature relevant to evidence-based practice. The **Cochrane Collaboration** is based in Oxford, England, and comprises specialised databases of systematic reviews to promote evidence-based practice. These reviews are disseminated through medical journals, CD-ROM and the Internet. There are Cochrane Centres in various countries, including Canada, the United Kingdom, the USA and Australia. Evidence-based medicine has grown rapidly in the United Kingdom, Canada and the USA. Evidence-based practice is a growth industry that has almost become a medical specialty on its own. It even has its own journal, *Evidence-Based Medicine*.

However, some notes of caution have been sounded. Naylor (1995) suggests that the culture of the clinician influences decisions about the value of the evidence and that there is a large area of practice for which current data are insufficient. What evidence there is may be skewed since researchers are more likely to publish positive than negative results. Also, the establishment of evidence-based practice does not mean that every clinician must know every research finding to provide good care. It is also possible that there is still an inadequate amount of published research and that what is available is not being heeded and applied in clinical settings.

EXERCISE

Ask your co-workers how they define evidence-based research and if they think it is applied completely in their clinical settings.

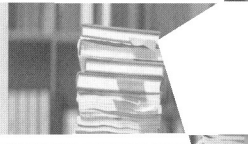

Research and education

Research books, such as the one you are reading right now, are geared towards teaching you about research. Books and journal articles comprise the main teaching tools when teachers are conveying the essentials of research paradigms, methods and processes. These tools give you the basics in knowledge and skills required to locate a project within a paradigm of knowledge generation and validation, and to then match that paradigm with congruent methods and processes for undertaking the project. If you refer to Chapter 1, you will see the introduction to these teaching strategies. After Chapter 1, this entire book sets out in a logical flow of information all that you need to become a beginning researcher educated in quantitative and qualitative approaches.

As you no doubt realise, there is a lot more to knowing and doing research than can be conveyed in a single book. Undergraduate degrees in tertiary education organisations set up comprehensive research programs, at honours, postgraduate diploma and degree, master's and PhD levels. Such programs are studded with generic and specialised information relative to the level of education and geared specifically to fine-tune research knowledge and skills.

As well as these tertiary institutions, other educational sites where research is offered include professional development and clinical education programs within hospitals and health departments, and professional bodies, such as colleges of nursing, medicine, surgery, and so on. Research is a subject taught in many places for different purposes. In relation to health care, research education must have clinical relevance to be of use to patients for whose 'good' it espouses to serve.

In the United Kingdom, Australia and New Zealand, the increased focus on research in health care has come about since the 1980s, the time when practice disciplines such as physiotherapy, nursing and midwifery moved to the tertiary sector and the impetus for evidence-based practice was first being felt in health care generally. As Clifford (2004) noted:

> For most professionals, with few exceptions — for example disciplines such as medicine, dentistry and psychology — the emphasis was on skill acquisition and in general little time was spent on developing the thought processes required to take a more analytic approach to work or the critical thinking skills that underpin research . . . Traditional healthcare education more commonly presented information to students as a series of facts to be acquired with little exploration of how these facts had been come by. Interest in research began to expand with increased affiliation with the higher education sector in the later 1980s and early 1990s (p. 7).

Getting research into practice

While there seems to be a general consensus that evidence-based practice is necessary in health care, there does not seem to be an equal degree of confidence and conviction in ensuring that the evidence actually finds its way into practice. Zeitz and McCutcheon (2003, p. 272) ask a very pertinent question: 'Rather than focusing on EBP as the solution to the development of best practice, is it not time to change the focus to real strategies that will assist in achieving best practice?' The authors argue that getting research into practice involves 'the creation of rigorous, relevant evidence, the valuing of clinical expertise and the changing of cultures' in which clinicians 'develop and practice' (Zeitz & McCutcheon 2003, p. 272). After all, what is the use of clinical research if it is not applied in practice?

EXERCISE

Why is it difficult to get clinicians to use research in their practice?

Busy clinicians have many pressures competing for their attention and if they are to base their practice on recent research there must be practical strategies in place in the clinical context to ensure that EBP happens. If clinicians ignore, avoid or otherwise obstruct EBP, no research-based practice changes will happen. Various research uptake and change strategies are discussed in literature, including national governance (Griffiths & Clark 2004), the establishment of effective change measures (Dawes et al. 2005) and clinical guidelines (Osborne & Webster 2005).

National health imperatives

In the United Kingdom, as a means of national governance, **national health imperatives** often originate in the National Health Service (NHS) through research and development initiatives. These are transmitted in the form of government funding through the Medical Research Council (MRC) to medical and allied health practices throughout the nation. Research governance applies high standards of research to clinical areas and ensures an ongoing and focused interest in EBP (Griffiths & Clark 2004).

A similar process happens in Australia, in that the Federal Government has a health portfolio and the Minister for Health takes advice from key leaders in the health field. The government also connects with health researchers through peak bodies on an organisational level, such as through the National Health and Medical Research Council (NHMRC) and key university and medical departments. The government funding goes to high priority health care areas. EBP is a high priority, so researchers and developers apply an EBP focus to their work and ensure that the outcomes are reflected in current practice.

Connected to national governance is the imperative that health research benefits the population and has marketability internationally. This means that the research projects funded through government-sponsored agencies are usually those projects of immense importance, such as cures for diseases and innovative diagnostic and treatment advances. This places medical researchers in ideal positions to pursue their research while serving the altruistic good of society. Unsurprisingly, the positive effects of medical research are rewarded with the highest proportion of government funding for further projects. Therefore, change reaches clinical areas when medical and health research findings are introduced into practice 'for the good of the patient'.

Effective change measures

Research can also find its way into practice by the establishment of effective change measures. Dawes et al. (2005) suggest that it is important to be aware of how change happens in individuals and organisations, and the levels of change from micro to macro that are negotiated as the culture of the workplace adapts gradually to research-based changes. They also describe ways to bring about effective change, such as for opinion leaders to make personal contact with clinicians in their workplaces to influence them to be willing to drop their practice fads and traditions in favour of embracing and establishing evidence-based changes.

Davies (2005) reminds us that change

can take place at [the] macro and micro level of health care, at the national and local level, at the strategic level and the operational level . . . It is important that health care practitioners clarify at the outset the level at which they are operating, the types of innovation that are appropriate and feasible at that level, and the systems, individuals and groups that they are likely, and unlikely, to be able to influence (pp. 225–6).

Clinical guidelines

It is at the level of basic clinical practice that evidence-based practice needs to be fostered. Clinicians have problems in applying research – lack of evidence, lack of time to acquire the evidence, and a lack of research skills and experience to evaluate the evidence critically. Even if clinicians can acquire and appraise evidence, they may have difficulty in recalling it at the time it is required. This situation has led to the development of clinical practice guidelines or evidence-based protocols.

Clinical guidelines are systematically developed statements to assist clinician and patient decisions about appropriate health care for specific clinical circumstances (Field & Lohr 1992). Clinical practice guidelines normally comprise a set of statements related to a specific condition or patient problem. They are prepared by a committee of experts who translate the evidence into formulas for practice. Clinicians then implement the guidelines rather than distilling the research findings and making decisions based on the evidence. The latter half of the 1990s saw the development of hundreds of sets of clinical guidelines.

Essentially, a clinical guideline will appear in hard copy as a sheet of paper in a procedures or clinical guidelines book or folder, or in electronic form on a database in a computer file. It is a helpful, practical and sequential guide for clinicians in how to go about a clinical procedure safely and effectively. For example, a clinical guideline may be about caring for a patient with confusion, or undertaking the care of a patient receiving chemotherapy. If clinicians accept well-prepared and researched clinical guidelines, the research-based information within them can find its way into practice.

In Australia, the NHMRC has set up a preferred process for clinical practice guideline development. The Joanna Briggs Institute issues regular clinical practice guidelines in the form of Best Practice Sheets. Practice matters covered so far include pressure sores, falls in hospitals and management of peripheral intravascular devices. The Joanna Briggs Institute has a website at http://www.joannabriggs.edu.au.

Problems with clinical guidelines

On the surface, it would seem that clinical guidelines are the best way of ensuring that research gets into practice. However, clinicians

> will criticize new guidelines for novelty, old ones for age, complicated guidelines for complexity, brief guidelines for simplicity, broad guidelines for lack of specificity, narrow ones for depth, visual guidelines for over-simplicity and written guidelines for verbosity (Dowswell, Harrison & Wright 2001, p. 122).

Another issue with clinical guidelines is the extent to which clinicians feel they have been imposed on their practice. For example, when non-nursing groups impose guidelines on nursing it can be problematic. They may try to encourage nurses to practise using a non-nursing framework and rate randomised clinical trials (RCTs) as the highest form of evidence and expert opinion as the lowest form. Enshrining clinical trials as the highest form of evidence demotes qualitative research, which is also very important in answering nursing questions. Clearly, clinicians should develop their own clinical practice guidelines and decide what evidence they deem is appropriate for sound practice. This requires clinicians to break down the barriers preventing the implementation of research in the clinical setting, upgrade their skills concerning the consumption and practice of research, and identify research priorities.

A problem with clinical guidelines is that they address only discrete parts of care and may be inappropriate for complex problems. This approach supports a reductionist view of patients and dismisses other holistic considerations of them as people. Therefore, clinicians need to set up some criteria for judging the quality of clinical practice guidelines and to remain open to broader views of caring for people beyond the scripted guidelines for practice.

Another issue surrounding clinical practice guidelines is whether they will have the expected impact. After all, practitioners are slow to adopt other research, so why would they adopt clinical practice guidelines? For example, a study of medical practitioners' attitudes to clinical practice guidelines (Gupta, Ward & Hayward 1997) showed that most general practitioners had positive views about the concept of clinical practice guidelines developed from evidence. However, most considered that guidelines were developed by experts, who did not understand general practice. Fewer than half thought that they would improve client outcomes, and only half indicated that the guidelines had changed their practice.

It may come as no surprise then, that the best laid plans of change agents can go awry when faced with the culture of a workplace resistant to evidence-based change. Even so, the predominance of EBP in health care and the concerted and sustained efforts by governments and leaders in research and development will ensure that more and more research finds its way quickly into practice and creates a new and effective EBP culture.

Policy and procedure manuals

Policy and procedure manuals play an important part in establishing the ways in which health professionals work. These documents are found in hospital wards and departments in accessible areas for clinicians to read quickly and easily. Policy and procedure manuals are written according to the latest thinking in the particular practice discipline. The presence and use of these manuals by staff may in fact be essential in ensuring the organisation retains its accreditation as a health care facility. Therefore, much emphasis is placed on maintaining policy and procedure manuals with up-to-date information that staff can use in practice and refer to if and when problems arise.

For information in policy and procedure manuals to be clinically relevant and contemporary, the documents must reflect best practice principles. The best practice professionals can give is in turn based on the latest research evidence. Therefore, practice procedures are based on directives and policies from the respective health departments that are operationalised at clinical level clinically, legally and ethically. As explained in Chapter 1, this evidence is derived from research projects reported in refereed journal articles, which have been subjected to a systematic review process. The process involves developing the review protocol, asking answerable questions, finding the evidence, appraising the evidence and judging the applicability of the evidence (Pearson & Field 2005).

Obvious disadvantages of policy and procedure manuals are that they are only as effective as the information within them and the extent to which clinicians put that information into practice. The information within these manuals must be generated from the most recent and best research, as determined by a systematic review process. To be transparent in the process, manuals should cite the authors of the research and provide full referencing details for clinicians to access and read the research projects in full.

EXERCISE

Locate the policy and procedural manuals in your workplace. Are they research-based? Are the research projects fully referenced in the manuals?

There are many barriers to clinicians putting research into practice and they are described in this chapter. Even so, the culture of hospitals places great faith and reliance in the use of succinct information in policy and procedure manuals. If information is accessible and easy to read, there is a very good chance that busy clinicians will pay heed to it. Some strategies for ensuring clinicians use research in practice are described in this chapter.

Easy and accessible clinical research

Sometimes, the best options also turn out to be the simplest. For example, clinicians would possibly be more interested in research if they felt it was easy and accessible for them. Myths have been perpetuated about research, along the lines that only the cleverest people can do it. Clinicians may believe that doing research is reserved for the people who do not stay in practice, but leave for the 'ivory towers' of academia, or the weekends-off ease of health research departments. This section suggests some means of breaking down the myths about research to encourage clinicians to undertake projects themselves and/or to cooperate with others in creating practice-based research projects. Some ideas shared in this section include practical strategies for creating a research culture in clinical settings, research–practice links, and types of collaborative research that can be undertaken easily.

Creating a research culture in clinical settings

Health funding to health care organisations can include the establishment of research positions, such as joint appointments between the health sector and universities, and/or research and professional development roles conducted solely within the health care organisation. Project-based funding is also available through the respective health departments. Regardless of the means by which these research positions are established, they will only be effective if they meet the needs of clinicians and improve clinical practice.

A research culture refers to a group of people who are conversant with the fundamentals of research methods and processes and are confident in promoting and sharing the practice and application of research. Such conversancy and confidence only comes with regular exposure to doing research and to understanding and applying its outcomes. If research activity is local and logical, it can be learned and done by any clinician with a mind to pay attention.

Practical measures for creating a research culture in clinical settings are as many and as broad as the imagination and the research budget can stretch. For example, researchers can involve wards and departments in manageable projects of clinical relevance to daily work. Management can give staff time off from work to attend hospital-organised research talks and seminars, and/or to attend relevant national and international professional conferences. Clinicians can work on losing their cringe about research activity as being what 'only the cleverest' do, by becoming conversant with research language through professional development seminars and conferences, and by talking about research often and openly in familiar places, such as ward meetings and tearooms.

Research (theory)–practice links

One of the biggest challenges for health professionals is to put theory into practice. Theory comes from research, because theory is knowledge and research creates and validates knowledge. If we assume that research and theory are inextricably linked, all that remains is to ensure that research (theory) and practice also become linked just as firmly. The debates of the 1980s covered the area of the theory–practice gap and it comes as no surprise that this was also the decade in which the education of practice disciplines, such as midwifery, nursing and physiotherapy, entered tertiary settings. It is not our intention to breathe life once again into those old debates; essentially, it was recognised that the translation of theory into practice was not as good as it could be, and that certain strategies could be helpful in strengthening theory–practice links.

For example, in our practice discipline of nursing in Australia, the 1980s witnessed the establishment of nursing units, joint appointments, faculty practice and postgraduate research degrees for nurses. Nursing units were established in hospitals and health agencies to provide primary nursing care and to research the effectiveness of that care. Joint appointments were set up, funded between universities and clinical organisations, to undertake research and establish that evidence in practice. Faculty practice was established to ensure that teachers of nursing had clinical relevance to teach from experience, being up to date with clinical policies, procedures and practices. Postgraduate research degrees previously taken in other disciplines such as education, psychology and sociology were taken in nursing.

There are many incentives and strategies for clinicians to use research in their practice. Clinical research can be made easy and accessible by using the research (theory)-practice links described already and by other simple and effective means. For example, sharing research information in ward discussions, seminars and conferences can strengthen practice links. University researchers can become involved in clinical research, not only through their own research interests, but also in supervising undergraduate and postgraduate degrees focusing on clinical issues.

Collaborative research

Collaborative research processes can be oriented to the needs of clinicians. Chapter 1 introduced the idea of research collaboration within the multidisciplinary health team. The easiest and most accessible clinical research involves clinicians researching their own practice to answer their own clinical problems. In the process, clinicians may choose to gain academic recognition through attaining research awards for their practice-centred research.

Any research project can become collaborative if it is undertaken in partnership with other professionals within and across practice disciplines. Examples of collaborative research projects include Anderson, McAllister and Moyle (2002), Craig et al. (2004) and Taylor et al. (2002).

Any research project can reflect collaboration if it is done with cooperation and sharing of the workloads and responsibilities. Any number of variations are possible in using quantitative, qualitative or mixed methods approaches. The whole idea of collaborative research is open to whatever can be arranged between interested parties in the clinical and academic settings.

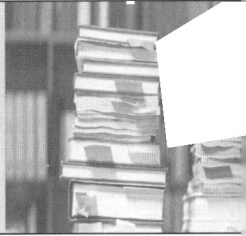

EXERCISE

Some ideas for making clinical research easy and accessible include practical strategies for creating a research culture in clinical settings, research–practice links, and types of collaborative research that can be undertaken easily.

What other possibilities can you imagine for making clinical research easy and accessible?

Educating evidence-based clinicians

This section describes some means for educating evidence-based clinicians, thus increasing the likelihood that research will be put into practice. Ideas are offered for helping teachers prepare evidence-based clinicians and for enhancing their own teaching effectiveness. The suggestions are by no means complete, nor are they exclusive of other possibilities.

Preparing evidence-based clinicians

If you find yourself in a teaching role, the following suggestions may help you in promoting evidence-based practice. Starting with the assumptions that clinical practice is complex, that changes occur rapidly, and that clinicians need to be up to date with the latest research, there are many simple strategies for teachers to prepare evidence-based clinicians for practice.

Teaching evidence-based care

One way to encourage clinicians to read and use research is to model those behaviours in education. Teachers model evidence-based behaviours when citing research sources and using researchers' names and projects. Later on, these behaviours may be highly influential in the ways that clinicians become familiar with and operationalise research in their daily practice.

Teachers can enlist simple teaching measures on a regular basis, such as always teaching from research, and listing the researchers whose work underlies clinical procedures and theories relating to practice. Researchers' work should be fully referenced with name, initials, date, title, journal article, volume, number and pages. Full referencing details connect the procedure or theory directly to research and enable students to pursue further reading. Consistent referencing of practice to research strengthens the connection, so that the link becomes strong and expected. It follows that clinicians grounded in evidence-based education will transplant the expectations of evidence into clinical practice, and demand up-to-date procedures validated by systematic review processes to substantiate clinical decisions.

Encouraging honours and postgraduate research degrees

Research knowledge and skills take time to develop. Rarely would an undergraduate degree provide sufficient preparation in research knowledge and skills as to prepare a clinician to undertake independent research. Teachers can become involved in career trajectory advice and actively encourage undergraduates to pursue further research programs. Students may feel they are unable to 'do' research or be unaware of the possibilities that a research degree holds for them in the future.

Research becomes easier and more accessible when it is experienced as 'do-able'. Clinicians with research degrees are needed in practice, not only to undertake research in practice but also to demystify research to their peers. If research is seen as easy and accessible, it follows that it will be feared less and respected more, thereby receiving acceptance with clinicians. Clinicians who respect and understand research will be more likely to use the latest research in their work. Thus, educators who encourage students to undertake honours and postgraduate research degrees are likely to be highly influential in increasing research uptake and impact in practice.

Encouraging research skills

Teachers encourage students to become researchers and research consumers by teaching practical skills, such as questioning and critical thinking, database skills, critical literature review skills and reflective practice.

Fostering an inquiring mind underpins the passion for research, which is based on the love of questioning. Critical thinking (Bandman & Bandman 1995; van Hooft, Gillam & Byrnes 1995; Wilkinson 1996) is often aligned with questioning skills. Critical thinking is integrated into professional undergraduate curricula, for example, most Australian undergraduate nursing curricula claim to teach critical thinking and to enable those skills in nurses.

Critical thinking is not just about rationality and emotional detachment for intellectual pursuits. Van Hooft, Gillam and Byrnes (1995, pp. 6–7) are keen to define the first important element of critical thinking as rational thinking, yet they emphasise that it is practical as well as theoretical – that it is conducive to dialogue and that it includes empathy and sensitive perception. They also describe critical thinkers as committed, self-aware and sympathetic to the commitments of others. The addition of practicality, dialogue, empathy and sensitivity in critical thinking, and self-aware and altruistic features in critical thinkers, places a huge responsibility on teachers who espouse to embody and teach the benefits of critical thinking. Therefore, questioning and critical thinking need to be practised at every opportunity and teachers need to work actively in building in these skills into teaching and learning exercises. Once harnessed, questioning and critical thinking skills integrate easily into research methods and processes and enable clinicians to become more effective researchers and consumers of research in their practice.

Database skills are essential in keeping up with the latest research literature. Teachers need to emphasise the usefulness of information technology (IT) skills connected directly to research. Some of these skills were described in Chapter 2.

Once procured through database and library searches, students need skills in undertaking critical literature reviews. By being built into academic essay writing and research units of instruction, literature review skills can be enhanced through repeated practice. Literature review skills were described in Chapter 4 of this book.

In a similar fashion to critical thinking, reflective practice has been promoted in health professions for some time. Reflective practice involves systematic questioning and focuses itself on practice (Taylor 2006). Teachers can become reflective practitioners in their teaching and clinicians can become reflective practitioners in their work. Researchers need to reflect on their practice of research, in order to constantly develop expertise. Teachers can encourage reflective practice skills and connect those skills to research (for example, Freshwater 1999; Glaze 2001; Handcock 1999; Johns 2000, 2003).

Enhancing teaching effectiveness

Clinical research can also be made easier and more accessible when teachers enhance their teaching effectiveness. Some suggestions for teaching research more effectively include membership of research agencies, engaging in research with clinicians, supervising research, examining research theses, reviewing journal articles and writing for publication.

Membership of research agencies

Teachers can ensure they keep up to date with research directions and results by engaging actively in research agencies. Research organisations include health committees at national level, such as the NHMRC (see Chapter 1) and National Health Service (NHS). Other agencies may be connected to evidence-based practice, such as the Joanna Briggs Institute in Australia, or the Centre for Evidence Based Nursing-Aotearoa (CEBNA), and the New Zealand Guidelines Group in New Zealand. Membership of these agencies may be by invitation, ballot or other means. These peak research bodies are influential in dictating research directions and/or uptake, so teachers/researchers attaining membership are in the front line for influencing the ease and accessibility of evidence-based practice.

Engaging in research with clinicians

Practice-based research is of prime relevance to clinicians. Many tertiary and professional teaching organisations have an expectation that employees will engage in research. This being the case, the best way to foster research–practice links is to engage in research with clinicians. The basis for the projects will be determined to some extent by the relationship between the teacher/researcher and the clinical agency. There may be possibilities in supporting the knowledge and skills of the clinical researcher already employed, of establishing collaborative links with clinicians to assist them in researching their own practice, and/or of supervising practice-based research projects so clinicians gain a tertiary award.

Engaging in other research-related work

Other means of ensuring that teachers become more effective in using research in their teaching and in teaching research include examining research theses, reviewing journal articles, and writing for publication. All of these research-related activities form the basis of role responsibilities as an academic and/or research agency professional. It is not the task of this book to teach teachers how to undertake these activities. Rather this section emphasises the importance of such research-related activities in ensuring teachers are effective in using research in their teaching, and credible as teachers of research in the eyes of their students. It is possible that credible teachers impress students, who then become clinicians, who are more involved in research-related activities, thus increasing the chance that clinicians will use research and research-related activities in their practice.

EXERCISE

Some ideas for educating evidence-based clinicians have been suggested in this section. What other possibilities can you imagine for educating evidence-based clinicians?

Summary

This chapter focused on using research in practice and education. The assumptions within the chapter were that evidence-based practice bases current practice on research, that it is not always easy for clinicians to use research in their practice, and that teachers need to use research in their work to show clinicians how to become researchers and consumers of research.

Strategies were suggested for getting research into practice, such as national governance, the establishment of effective change measures, and clinical guidelines. Policy and procedure manuals were also described as important in establishing the ways in which health professionals work. The chapter made the point that for clinicians to use research it must be easy and accessible. Some ideas to ensure ease and accessibility included creating a research culture in clinical settings, research–practice links, and types of collaborative research.

Part of the equation for uptake of research in clinical settings is the education that prepares clinicians for research-based practice. This chapter offered ideas for helping teachers prepare evidence-based clinicians and for enhancing their own teaching effectiveness. The suggestions did not claim to be complete, nor exclusive of other possibilities.

This is the last chapter of this book, so it is now time to wish you well as a researcher or consumer of research. Our steadfast hope is that this book assists you in understanding research paradigms, methods and processes, and equips you in part for undertaking and using research.

Main points

- The assumptions within this chapter are that evidence-based practice bases current practice on research, that it is not always easy for clinicians to use research in their practice, and that teachers need to use research in their work to show clinicians how to become researchers and consumers of research.

- Evidence-based practice has been established in medicine for decades and has only more recently moved its influence into allied health areas.
- In the United Kingdom, Australia and New Zealand, the increased focus on research in health care has come about since the 1980s, the time when practice disciplines such as physiotherapy, nursing and midwifery moved to the tertiary sector and the impetus for evidence-based practice was first being felt in health care generally.
- While there seems to be a general consensus that evidence-based practice is necessary in health care, there does not seem to be an equal degree of confidence and conviction in ensuring that the evidence actually finds its way into practice.
- Research can find its way into practice by the establishment of effective change measures.
- If clinicians accept well-prepared and researched clinical guidelines the research-based information within them can find its way into practice.
- For information in policy and procedure manuals to be clinically relevant and contemporary, the documents must reflect best practice principles, based on the latest research evidence.
- Practical measures for creating a research culture in clinical settings are as many and as broad as the imagination and the research budget can stretch.
- The easiest and most accessible clinical research involves clinicians researching their own practice to answer their own clinical problems.
- Starting with the assumptions that clinical practice is complex, that changes occur rapidly, and that clinicians need to be up to date with the latest research, there are many simple strategies for teachers to prepare evidence-based clinicians for practice.
- Some suggestions for teaching research more effectively include membership of research agencies, engaging in research with clinicians, supervising research, examining research theses, reviewing journal articles and writing for publication.

CASE STUDY

Carmel was introduced in Chapter 14. If you have not been following Carmel's case study, go to the end of Chapters 14 to 18 and review her story so far. Carmel set up a participatory action research (PAR) group and they identified a thematic concern of the use of power in the health care organisation. The PAR group developed an action plan for identifying the detrimental effects of power in the workplace and how nurses might respond to this kind of power assertively. The research report has been written and the group are preparing a research publication in a peer-reviewed journal. The task now is to encourage other nurses to use the action plan in their practice.

1   Can Carmel claim the PAR research findings can guide practice?
2   Is the research an example of evidence-based practice, in the strictest sense of the word? Explain your answer.

Multiple choice questions

1 The conscientious, explicit and judicious use of current best evidence in making decisions about the health care of patients is:
   a evidence-based practice
   b best practice
   c practice-based evidence
   d clinical excellence

2 In the United Kingdom, Australia and New Zealand, the increased focus on research in health care has come about since the:
   a 1960s
   b 1970s
   c 1980s
   d 1990s

3 In the United Kingdom, as a means of national governance, health imperatives often originate in the:
   a Research Governance Board (RGB)
   b National Health Service (NHS)
   c National Health and Medical Research Council (NHMRC)
   d Medical Research Council (MRC)

4 Clinicians have problems in applying research because of a lack of:
   a time
   b evidence
   c research skills
   d all of the above

5 For information in policy and procedure manuals to be clinically relevant and contemporary, the documents must:
   a be written by a researcher who is up to date with the latest research findings
   b be updated every time the hospital accreditation is being undertaken
   c be forwarded to the health agency by the national health department
   d reflect best practice principles and be based on the latest research evidence

6 Any research project can become collaborative if it is:
   a given funding by a national external grants source
   b undertaken in partnership with other professionals
   c overseen by an experienced quantitative researcher
   d approved by a health service to access patients

7 Teachers model evidence-based behaviours when:
   a citing research sources and using researchers' names and projects
   b using stories from people's experiences of health and illness
   c using regularly updated documents from clinical agencies
   d inviting survivors of life-threatening diseases to talk to a class

8 Teachers encourage students to become researchers and research consumers by teaching practical skills, such as:

    a   questioning and critical thinking

    b   database skills

    c   reflective practice

    d   all of the above

9 In tertiary and professional teaching organisations where there is an expectation that employees will engage in research, the best way to foster research-practice links is to:

    a   encourage research degrees

    b   create a research culture

    c   contact a research institute

    d   engage in research with clinicians

10 In relation to educating evidence-based clinicians, it is possible that credible teachers impress students, who then become clinicians, who:

    a   practise according to the norms of the setting in which they find themselves

    b   contact the teacher every time they are not sure if a practice is safe and correct

    c   are more involved in research-related activities and evidence-based practice

    d   leave practice to undertake teaching of research and evidence-based practice

Review topics

1 Is your practice discipline a research-based profession? Discuss.

2 Describe the relationship of practice, research and education in relation to the potential for evidence-based practice.

3 Discuss three strategies for getting research into practice.

4 Discuss the perceived problems with clinical practice guidelines.

5 Discuss four strategies for educating evidence-based clinicians.

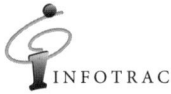

References

Anderson, C., McAllister, M. & Moyle, W. 2002, 'The postmodern heart: a discourse analysis of a booklet on pacemaker implantation', *Collegian*, vol. 9, no. 1, 19–23.

Bandman, E.L. & Bandman, B. 1995, *Critical thinking in nursing*, 2nd edn, Appleton and Lange, Norwalk.

Clifford, C. 2004, 'Chapter 1 Introduction', in C. Clifford & J. Clark (eds), *Getting Research into Practice*, Churchill Livingstone, Edinburgh.

Clifford, C. & Clark, J. (eds) 2004, *Getting Research into Practice*, Churchill Livingstone, Edinburgh.

Courtney, M. (ed.) 2005, *Evidence for Nursing Practice*, Elsevier Churchill Livingstone, Sydney.

Craig, D., Donoghue, J., Seller, M. & Mitten-Lewis, S. 2004, 'Improving nursing management of patients with diabetes using an action research approach', *Contemporary Nurse*, vol. 17, no. 1–2, 71–9.

Davies, P. 2005, 'Changing policy and practice', in Dawes, M. 2005, 'Evidence-based practice', in M. Dawes, P. Davies, A. Gray, J. Mant, K. Seers & R. Snowball, *Evidence-Based Practice: A Primer for Health Care Professionals*, 2nd edn, Elsevier Churchill Livingstone, Edinburgh, 223–40.

Dawes, M. 2005, 'Evidence-based practice', in M. Dawes, P. Davies, A. Gray, J. Mant, K. Seers & R. Snowball, *Evidence-Based Practice: A Primer for Health Care Professionals*, 2nd edn, Elsevier Churchill Livingstone, Edinburgh, 1–10.

Dawes, M., Davies, P., Gray, A., Mant, J., Seers, K. & Snowball, R. 2005, *Evidence-Based Practice: A Primer for Health Care Professionals*, 2nd edn, Elsevier Churchill Livingstone, Edinburgh.

Dowswell, G., Harrison, S. & Wright, J. 2001, 'Clinical guidelines: attitudes, information, processes and culture in English primary care', *International Journal of Health Planning and Management*, vol. 16, 107–24.

Field, M.J. & Lohr, K.N. 1992, *Guidelines for Clinical Practice. From Development to Use*, National Academy Press, Washington DC.

Freshwater, D. 1999, 'Clinical supervision, reflective practice and guided discovery: clinical supervision', *British Journal of Nursing*, vol. 8, no. 20, 1383–9.

Glaze, E. 2001, 'Reflection as a transforming process: student advanced nurse practitioners' experiences of developing reflective skills as part of an MSc program', *Journal of Advanced Nursing*, vol. 34, 639–47.

Griffiths, M. & Clark, J. 2004, 'Managing the local agenda: planning to get research/evidence-based care into practice', in C. Clifford & J. Clark (eds), *Getting Research into Practice*, Churchill Livingstone, Edinburgh, 61–82.

Gupta, L., Ward, J. & Hayward, R. 1997, 'Clinical practice guidelines in general practice: a national survey of recall, attitudes and impact', *Medical Journal of Australia*, vol. 166 (20 January), 69–72.

Handcock, P. 1999, 'Reflective practice – using a learning journal', *Nursing Standard*, vol. 13, no. 17, 37–40.

Johns, C. 2000, 'Working with Alice: a reflection', *Complementary Therapies in Nursing and Midwifery*, vol. 6, 199–303.

Johns, C. 2003, 'Easing into the light', *International Journal for Human Caring*, vol. 7, no. 1, 49–55.

Naylor, C. 1995, 'Grey zones of clinical practice: some limits to evidence-based medicine', *Lancet*, vol. 345 (1 April), 840–2.

Osborne, S. & Webster, J. 2005, 'Development and use of evidence-based guidelines', in M. Courtney (ed.), *Evidence for Nursing Practice*, Elsevier Churchill Livingstone, Sydney, 183–97.

Pearson, A. & Field, J. 2005, 'The systematic review process', in M. Courtney (ed.), *Evidence for Nursing Practice*, Elsevier, Churchill Livingstone, Sydney.

Sackett, D.L., Richardson, W.S., Rosenbery, W. & Haynes, R.B. 1997, *Evidence-Based Medicine: How to Practice and Teach EBM*, Churchill Livingstone, New York.

Sackett, D.L., Straus, S.E. & Richardson, W.S. 2000, *Evidence-Based Medicine: How to Practice and Teach EBM*, 2nd edn, Churchill Livingstone, New York.

Taylor, B.J. 2006, *Reflective Practice: A Guide for Nurses and Midwives*, 2nd edn, Open University Press, UK.

Taylor, B.J., Bulmer, B., Hill L., Luxford, C., McFarlane, J. & Stirling, K. 2002, 'Exploring idealism in palliative nursing care through reflective practice and action research', *International Journal of Palliative Nursing*, vol. 8, no. 7, 324–30.

van Hooft, S., Gillam, L. & Byrnes, M. 1995, *Facts and Values: An Introduction to Critical Thinking for Nurses*, Maclennan & Petty, Sydney.

Wilkinson, J.M. 1996, *Nursing Process: A Critical Thinking Approach*, Addison-Wesley Nursing, Menlo Park.

Zeitz, K. & McCutcheon, H. 2003, 'Evidence-based practice: To be or not to be, this is the question!', *International Journal of Nursing Practice*, vol. 9, no. 5, 272–9.

GLOSSARY

abstract
A succinct and accurate description of the project, including the problem statement, the theoretical framework, an explanation of the design of the study, including the sample and data collection methods, the major findings, conclusions, and, if appropriate, any recommendations.

active deception
Deliberately withholding some information or giving false information about a study to secure people's participation.

affirmative postmodernism
A less pessimistic approach to postmodernism, which does not abandon the author completely, but reduces the author's authority, so that researchers can focus on humans as subjects, and human existence remains open to constant questioning as possibilities.

agent or agency
In postmodernism, a person and institution assumed to have authority and power, by virtue of his/her/its knowledge and skills.

analysis
Reviewing research data systematically with the intention of sorting and classifying them into representational groups and patterns.

anonymity
The concealment or obscuring of the identity of the participants.

applied research
Knowledge applied to specific situations.

author
In postmodernism, a person who creates a text, or is responsible for an outcome, for example, researchers are authors of research projects.

basic research
Developing fundamental knowledge and testing theory.

beneficence
The ethical principle of 'doing good', relating to only doing good for research participants.

body of report
Contains the main information of a research report, including the introduction, literature review, methodology, results and discussion.

bracketing
The process derived from mathematics, whereby researchers' presuppositions are put to one side (in brackets) to be attended to separately, so they do not impose meaning on the research.

causal relationships
Those which establish 'cause and effect' between variables. They can only be inferred from an experimental design.

clinical guidelines
Systematically developed statements to assist clinician and patient decisions about appropriate health care for specific clinical circumstances (Field & Lohr 1992).

clinical significance
The meaningfulness of your findings to clinical practice. It can be determined using

confidence intervals, odds ratios and risk calculations.

Cochrane Collaboration
An international initiative to facilitate the retrieval and synthesis of literature relevant to evidence-based practice.

comparative design
Compares the characteristics of one group to another group.

computer etiquette
Consideration of other researchers when using a computer.

concept
An abstract generalised idea that describes a phenomenon or a group of related phenomena.

confidentiality
A human right for private matters to remain secret, so the researcher has the responsibility to keep data confidential so that individuals are not compromised.

congruency
In qualitative research, the fit or correspondence between foundational ideas and the activity phases of the research, such as the project's assumptions, aims, objectives, methods and processes.

constant comparative analysis
A flexible and open-ended feature of grounded theory, in which the researcher works with the data from the beginning of the project in a process of analysis to constantly compare all new data that emerge from participants' accounts of their experiences, to identify similarities in codes and categories.

contexts
The particular features of the research setting that need to be taken into account when planning, undertaking and reporting a research project.

correlational design
Examines whether one variable is influencing another variable.

culture
A way of life for a group of people, interpreted through their symbols, beliefs, customs, language and life patterns.

data
Numbers and/or words collected by the researcher in order to answer the research question.

data mining
The extraction of existing data from web-based sources, which can be used to answer particular research questions.

deconstruction
A postmodern method of analysis that tears a text apart, not with the arrogant intention of improving, revising or offering a better text, but rather to reveal contradictions in claiming (overtly or covertly) to offer 'truth'.

descriptive design
Uses numbers to describe a phenomenon.

descriptive statistics
Statistics which describe a phenomenon.

discourse
All that is written and spoken and invites dialogue or conversation.

discourse analysis
Interrogates knowledge and power inherent in spoken and written life texts.

emancipation
Freedom from something to something. Critical research approaches can assist in experiencing freedom from the bonds of taken-for-granted expectations and roles, to more knowledgeable, skilful and creative practice.

empirico-analytical research
Referred to as quantitative, is interested in observation and analysis by the scientific method.

empowerment
The process of giving and accepting power; in critical research the methods and processes are geared towards helping people to find their own power, to liberate them from their

oppressive circumstances and self-understandings.

epistemology
The study of knowledge and how it is judged to be 'true'. Whenever researchers raise questions about what they know, and how they know it is trustworthy, they are asking epistemological questions.

ethics
In nursing and health research, concerns moral questions and behaviour in conducting research.

ethnography
Provides a 'portrait of people' by describing and raising awareness of a group of people's cultural characteristics, such as their shared symbols, beliefs, values, rituals and patterns of behaviour.

evidence-based practice (EBP)
Current clinical practice based on the best, most recent research.

experimental design
The design used for establishing cause and effect relationships between variables. Provides conclusive evidence of causality.

explicit themes
Those themes that come up from the text easily, because they are part of the pattern of answers and insights within the text, and are relevant because their identity is connected clearly and directly to the research aims and objectives.

Foucauldian-style discourse analysis
A complex examination of text, because it requires 'careful reading of entire bodies of text and other organising systems (such as taxonomies, commentaries and conference transcriptions) in relation to one another in order to interpret patterns, rules, assumptions, contradictions, silences, consequences, implications, and inconsistencies' (Powers 1996, p. 211).

grand theories (narratives)
'Big stories' or statements that claim universal truth, and that can be applied in all like cases.

grounded theory
Starts from the 'ground' of an area of human interest and works up in an inductive fashion to make sense of what people say about their experiences, and to convert these statements into theoretical propositions.

hegemony
Ascendancy or domination of one power over another, so that power seems unassailable, and that the conditions are not only good, but also appropriate for the people over whom they have control.

historical research
Reconstructs from primary and secondary sources (with due attention to a rigorous research process) an accurate and 'truthful' record of events over time, thereby amending previous knowledge and discovering new knowledge in relation to specific eras and interests.

human research ethics committee (HREC)
Group of people constituted to conduct research surveillance in an institution.

hypothesis
A statement of what the researcher thinks is going to be the outcome of the investigation.

implicit themes
Lie hidden in the text, not always stated as a direct word or words, or even as an easily recognisable concept.

indexes
Databases by which disciplines list their articles in the most relevant journals by keyword headings.

inferential statistics
Statistics that allow us to make inferences about the population from which the data were collected, through a process of hypothesis testing.

informed consent
The agreement of the participant to take part in the research project after having been thoroughly briefed about the project and its possible outcomes.

instrumentation
The type of tool, device or approach that is used to make a measurement.

integrity
In research is expressed in a commitment to the search for knowledge honestly and ethically.

interpretation
Taking the forms of analysed information to another level or levels of abstraction, so that statements can be made about what they mean in light of the intentions, methods and processes of the research.

interpretations
In qualitative research reports, may be theories, findings, results, insights, strategies, implications, examples of reflective awareness and changed practice and so on, to reflect the assumptions and intentions of the research methodology.

interpretive qualitative research
Aims mainly to generate meaning, to explain and describe, in order to make sense out of areas of interest.

interval data
Data which can only be counted as whole numbers.

justice
The ethical principle that all participants have the right to be treated fairly and with respect and courtesy at every stage of the research process, from the design of the project to the reporting of findings.

laboratory setting
A place that is specially constructed for the purposes of research or controlled practice.

legal aspects, computers
The possibilities of committing civil or criminal offences when communicating by electronic means.

literature
The total body of writing that deals with the topic being researched, mainly comprising theoretical and research papers.

lived experience
The knowledge people have of things of interest, because they have experienced them through the daily activities of living their lives.

measurement
The process of determining a quantitative characteristic of some phenomenon, such as 'how big', 'how often' or how many'.

methodological congruency
The match of epistemological assumptions of a particular methodology to the research methods used to gather that type of knowledge.

methodology
The theoretical assumptions underlying the choice of methods and processes in generating and validating a particular form of knowledge.

methods
The means or strategies by which data are sought and analysed in a qualitative research project.

mobile methodologies
The potential of methodologies to move across 'paradigmatic' positions.

model
A structure that represents phenomena or concepts.

monograph
A small book, usually presented as a soft-cover A5-size (half A4) document containing approximately 50 pages, produced usually by academic/professional organisations to publish their research.

multiple methodologies
Combinations of methodologies that offer wider frames of reference with greater likelihood of generating more options for knowledge generation.

narrative analysis
Attempts to find meaning in stories through a variety of methods that best suit the research questions, aims and objectives.

narratives
Views or stories. Although postmodernists are opposed to grand/meta-narratives or world views based on claims to legitimise their 'truth', mini/micro/local/traditional narratives as stories making no truth claims are acceptable to postmodernists.

national health imperatives
Health research priorities that originate at national government level and are transmitted in the form of government funding to medical and allied health practices throughout the nation.

naturalistic setting
A place in which people carry out their activities of daily life.

nominal data
Data which are in the form of names or categories.

non-maleficence
The ethical principle of 'doing no harm'; in research it relates to the right of human participants to not be harmed as a result of participating in a study.

non-probability sample
One that does not attempt to represent the population.

ontology
The study of existence itself; whenever researchers are asking about the nature of the existence of something or someone, they are asking ontological questions.

ordinal data
Data that are in the form of names or categories.

p values
The probability of making an error in interpreting your findings because your sample, for some reason, does not accurately reflect the real population parameters.

paradigm
A broad world view or perspective that provides a comprehensive approach to particular areas of interest.

parametric data
Data that are collected on at least an interval level scale, and which are representative of the population from which they were collected.

peer-reviewed journal article
Has been judged by at least three peers to be of a standard high enough to be published in a professional journal.

phenomenology ('phenomen - ology')
The 'study of things' within human existence, by discovering, exploring and describing the essence of phenomena through attending towards them directly.

pilot study
A small-scale dress rehearsal for the main study.

population
A group whose members have specific common characteristics that you wish to investigate in your research study.

poster
At a conference is a succinct overview of research depicted on a cardboard sheet to communicate the major points of the research project to delegates, who then have the opportunity to talk to the researcher about it.

postmodern possibilities
Refers to the affirmative position that allows researchers as the authors of projects to collect data and offer tentative insights for readers' interpretations and discussion.

postmodernism
An approach that questions and rejects paradigmatic views and requires researchers to redefine their basic assumptions, intentions and roles, in order to make adjustments to their present ways of viewing and doing research.

praxis
Change through critical reflection on practice. In qualitative critical research it is facilitated through participatory, collaborative methods and processes.

preliminaries
Introduces the research report, and usually includes the title page and abstract, and sometimes includes forms, acknowledgements, a table of contents, lists of figures and tables, and an executive summary.

primary sources
Pieces of literature written by the author and which have the advantage of being the author's own ideas.

privacy
In the research context refers to the right of participants to decide which information they wish to disclose, particularly concerning their attitudes, beliefs, behaviours, opinions, and records such as diaries and other private papers.

probability sample
One that attempts to portray the target population in miniature by representing the broad characteristics of that population.

processes
How data collection and analysis methods are undertaken, involving the embodied values of researchers, such as respecting, being patient and thoughtful, honouring, acknowledging, and other ways of being mindful of the human nature of the research.

qualitative analysis
Attempts to find meaning by working carefully and systematically through participants' words, language and/or images using manual or computer-assisted means.

qualitative critical methodologies
Interpret meaning by aiming to bring about change and raised awareness by systematic political critique and attempting to expose control, oppression, power and domination.

qualitative interpretive research methodologies
Interpret meaning by exploring, explaining and describing things of interest in order to make sense out of them.

qualitative research
Research interested in questions that involve human consciousness and subjectivity, and which values humans and their experiences in the research process.

ratio data
Data that can be collected on a scale with infinitely small graduations of measurement, with an absolute zero.

readers
The observers, who are given the power of interpreting the text; thus postmodernists empower the reader over the author.

reading
Understanding and interpretation that in postmodern terms may be 'my reading', 'your reading' or 'a reading' without judgement of adequacy or validity of the said reading.

research
Literally means 'looking carefully again'; researchers are searching again for new or adapted knowledge to inform them about areas of interest, to begin or add to a body of knowledge.

research area
In qualitative approaches this is a broad or focused interest for research.

research culture
A group of people who are conversant with the fundamentals of research methods and processes and are confident in promoting and

sharing the practice and application of research.

research design
The framework by which a project will answer a particular research question.

research plan
A map or outline of the steps to be achieved in a research project.

research problem
Selected within the general area of a discipline, it is stated particular to that discipline as an issue that needs research inquiry.

research proposal
A formal, structured, written account of a plan for a research project, which argues why, how, where, when and at what cost it will be done.

research purpose
A general statement of purposes, aims, intentions and/or objectives of the study.

research question
A specific question about a problem or issue, which guides the study, to keep the research interest in focus.

research report
A formal account of a research project, presented variously as classroom project report, journal article, thesis, dissertation, or seminar and conference paper.

respect for human dignity
The ethical principle that affirms the rights of humans to self-determination; in research it relates to the right to decide whether to participate in a research project after full disclosure of information about the project.

review of the literature
To read, sort and analyse the literature, putting it into some kind of order, and critiquing individual research reports.

'rigour' or trustworthiness
The strictness in judgement and conduct that must be used to ensure that the successive steps in a project have been set out clearly and undertaken with scrupulous attention to detail, so that the results/findings/insights can be trusted by people with whom they resonate.

sampling
Extracting a sub-group from within a population in order to study this group through research.

scale of measurement
The level of precision associated with a measurement technique.

sceptical postmodernism
An extreme relativist view, which rejects authors' authority as writers, the human as subject, and the human construction of history, time, truth and language, thereby dismissing the possibility of research.

scientific misconduct
An act of deception/misrepresentation/fraud of one's own work, such as fabrication of data to report non-existent research, falsification of data by changing records, and irresponsible authorship such as plagiarism and false attribution of authorship.

secondary sources
Pieces of literature to which an author refers.

special participants
Persons who have a diminished ability to give informed consent, or are in a dependent relationship, and are therefore at risk of exploitation, for example, developmentally disabled people, confused elderly, mentally ill persons, children, elderly persons, wards of state and unconscious patients.

statistical significance
The probability that a finding is false. It is expressed as a p value.

subjectivity
That which comes from the individual's sensing of inner and external things.

supporting materials
In a research report, these contain the references and appendixes.

text
Everything, so that all events and phenomena are texts.

thematic analysis
A method for identifying themes, essences or patterns within text.

theoretical sensitivity
A beginning point in grounded theory for seeking some clarity on the nature of the research area to sensitise the researcher and give insights into what might be possible.

theory
An attempt to describe, organise or explain a phenomenon or group of phenomena of a discipline in a language appropriate to the discipline.

triangulation
Refers to the use of multiple references, such as data, investigators, theories, methods and methodologies, which converge in research projects to draw conclusions that may be more confidently claimed as being trustworthy.

unethical research
Instances of researchers harming participants in the name of research.

variable
A factor that varies in a quantitative project.

voice
The modern conception of the author's perspective, but postmodernists question the attribution of privilege or special status to any voice. Thus, a 'public voice' is more acceptable, making discourse broadly understandable.

ANSWERS TO MULTIPLE CHOICE QUESTIONS

Chapter 1:
1b, 2a, 3d, 4c, 5b, 6b, 7c, 8a, 9c, 10d
Chapter 2:
1b, 2a, 3c, 4d, 5a, 6c, 7d, 8b, 9a, 10c
Chapter 3:
1b, 2d, 3a, 4b, 5b, 6d, 7c, 8c, 9b, 10d
Chapter 4:
1d, 2b, 3a, 4b, 5c, 6b, 7c, 8d, 9b, 10c
Chapter 5:
1b, 2a, 3d, 4c, 5d, 6d, 7b, 8b, 9a, 10a
Chapter 6:
1a, 2b, 3a, 4d, 5c, 6a, 7c, 8d, 9c, 10d
Chapter 7:
1a, 2c, 3a, 4b, 5b, 6a, 7d, 8b, 9a, 10d
Chapter 8:
1d, 2d, 3c, 4a, 5b, 6d, 7d, 8a, 9b, 10b
Chapter 9:
1b, 2d, 3a, 4b, 5d, 6c, 7c, 8d, 9a, 10d
Chapter 10:
1d, 2b, 3c, 4a, 5d, 6a, 7c, 8b, 9b, 10a

Chapter 11:
1d, 2d, 3c, 4c, 5a, 6d, 7d, 8a, 9c, 10b
Chapter 12:
1a, 2b, 3d, 4c, 5a, 6d, 7a, 8d, 9c, 10b
Chapter 13:
1d, 2b, 3a, 4a, 5b, 6a, 7b, 8c, 9b, 10c
Chapter 14:
1b, 2d, 3c, 4b, 5b, 6c, 7a, 8c, 9d, 10b
Chapter 15:
1c, 2b, 3a, 4a, 5b, 6d, 7d, 8c, 9c, 10b
Chapter 16:
1c, 2a, 3a, 4d, 5c, 6a, 7b, 8d, 9a, 10c
Chapter 17:
1b, 2a, 3d, 4d, 5c, 6b, 7b, 8a, 9c, 10b
Chapter 18:
1b, 2a, 3d, 4c, 5d, 6b, 7a, 8c, 9b, 10a
Chapter 19:
1a, 2c, 3b, 4d, 5d, 6b, 7a, 8d, 9d, 10c

INDEX

Aboriginal and Torres Strait Islander
  peoples   120–2
abstracts   83
    of research proposals   137–8
    of quantitative research reports
    516–17
action research   66, 369–74
adjunct analytical methods   477
analysis and interpretation
    distinguish between   487–9
    methodology   9, 319–53, 445–78
    in research proposals   151–4
    in research reports   83, 88–9, 91, 528–33,
    541–2, 543–4
        qualitative research findings   487–502
        research proposals and   155–6
        see also data analysis; interpretive processes
analysis, of research reports   92
anonymity   115–16
ANOVA   297
appendixes, of research proposals   159–60
applied research   2
    see also research
approvals, for research proposal projects   134
archival searches   405
articles   79
    see also literature
artistic expression   406
assisted reproduction technology   119–20
associations in data   286–9
    findings of   305–13
    see also data analysis
assumptions   321
auditability   402

bar graphs   274
basic research   2
behavioural systems   21

Belmont Report   104
beneficence   104
Benner's Model of Skill Acquisition   20–1
books   77
    writing up your research as   553
bracketing   332
brainstorming   63
breast self-examination   23
budgeting   145–6, 157–8

carative factors   21
case studies   406–9
case-based samples   206
cases   269
causal relationships   306–8
central limit theorem   280–2
chi-square test   292–4
clarity   133
clinical practice guidelines   11–13, 564–6
clinical significance   309–11
cluster samples   204–5
codes of ethics   101–2
    see also ethics
cohort designs   192
collaborative research   3, 568
comparing for differences and associations
  286
computers
    backing up data   36
    etiquette   36–7
    legal aspects   37
    structure of   34–5
    systems for qualitative data analysis and
      management   473–5
    types of   35–6
    transcripts and data analysis   417, 464–8
    using in research   34–48
concept   15

conceptual frameworks 16–23
  using in research projects 23–4
conference proceedings 77–8
confidence intervals 309
confidentiality 118–19
confirmability 402
congruency 493, 494
congruent methods 396–7, 493, 494
constant comparative analysis 332–3
content analysis 219
contextuality 403
contingency tables 292–4
control groups 185–6, 187–8, 190–1
convenience samples 205–6
  see also sampling
correlation 286–9
  and significance 289–90, 305–8
correlational designs 175–6
  see also research design
counterbalanced design 192–3
  see also research design
credibility 402
critical ethnography 380–3
  see also ethnography
critical theory 364–6
critiques, of research reports 85–94
cross-sectional designs 191
culture and care 20

data analysis 256–61,271–99, 304–14,
  448–50
  evaluation 313
  introduction to 269–71
  see also qualitative data analysis;
    quantitative data analysis
data categorisation 333
data coding 333
data collection 3, 143, 153–4, 417
  and filing 37–8, 43–8, 55, 417
  qualitative 438–51
  quantitative 208–36, 245–64
  see also qualitative data collection;
    quantitative data collection
data mining 43–4
data preparation 304
data reduction 304–5
databases 37–41
deception 113–14
deconstruction 325–6

degrees of freedom 284–5
Delphi survey technique 230–1
descriptive research designs 173–5
  see also research design
descriptive statistics 272–4
  see also statistics
difference, findings of 305–13
direct and indirect measurement 209–10
discourse 366, 383–4
  analysis 470–3
discriminant analysis 297
discussion
  in research reports 528–33
  of research reports 92–3
dissertations 511
document preparation 46–7
  key ideas from initial literature
    reviews 83–4

education and research 561–2
  clinicians 569–72
effect modifiers 180
effective change measures 563–4
email 44
emancipation 365–6
empirico-analytical research see quantitative
  research
empowerment 366
epistemology 320
  postmodern influences on 323–4, 327
equivalent control group pre-test post-test
  design 187–8
ethics 91–2,99–125, 408
  codes of 101–2
  examples of lack of 99–101
  in health practices 123
  research proposals 144–5, 154–5
  research project writing and 537–8
  special cases 119–23
ethnography 344–5, 380–3
  see also critical ethnography
evidence-based practice 2–3, 10–13, 560
  relationship to theory and research 13–14
experimental designs 176–7
  quasi 189–93
  reliability 181–2
  true 185–7
  types of 182–94
  validity 177–81, 321, 322

experimental mortality   178
experimenter effect   180

factor analysis   296
factorial designs   189
feminisms   9, 374–9
fieldwork   409–10
findings, data analysis and   308–12, **322**, 487–502
    meaning of   312–14
fittingness   402
focus groups   410–12
Foucaldian thought   471–3
    see also discourse

germ warfare   100
goal attainment   20, 21
goodness in qualitative research   404
google   43
grand narratives   368, 383
    see also theory
graphical display   274–7
grounded theory   330–6
    see also theory
group work   412–13
guidelines
    clinical practice   11–13, 564–6
    ethical   101–2
    when writing research reports   513, 537–8

harm, to research participants   105–7
Hawthorne effect   180
Health Belief Model   22–3
health care, collaborative nature of   3
health practices, research ethics in   123
Health Promotion Model   23
heart removal   100–1
hegemony   366
hermeneutics   495–6
histograms   274
historical research   347–51
    see also research
history, and validity   178
human research ethics committees (HREC)   102–4, 121, 132
human rights, of research participants   104–23
hypothesis testing   280–6

hypothesising   63–5, 87–8
    statistical analysis and   306

images   425–6, 445, 478
    in research proposals   159
in vitro and *in vivo* measurements   210
indexes   37–8
indigenous research participants, ethics and   120–2
inferential statistics   283
information
    acquiring your own collection   82–3
    as data   218–19
    presenting in quantitative research reports   523–8
    reading and documenting   83–5
informed consent   108–12, *109, 111–12*
instrumentation   213–15
instruments and procedures
    effect on validity   179
    quantitative data collection   213–15
Internet and research   36–7, 43, 44–8
interpretive processes   492–4
    see also qualitative interpretive categories; qualitative interpretive methodologies; qualitative research interpretation
interviews   232–4, 413–18, 463, 465–70
IVF research ethics   119–20

Japanese wartime experiments   100, 105
Johnson's Behavioural Systems Model   21
journal articles   511, 551–3
journal keeping   418–19
journals   78–9

key ideas, documenting   84–5
King's Theory of Goal Attainment   20
knowledge   13–14, 319–20, **322**
    nature of   65
    power and   469–73
    research as means of generating   319–20
    researcher's and problem selection   58–9

Leininger's Model of Transcultural Care   20
Levine's conservation principles   17–18
libraries and their staff   76–7, 79–80
Likert scale   224
literature
    acquiring your own collection   82–3

as data source   333
   identifying relevant   74–6
   indexes   37–8, 42–3, 79
   interpreting results and   501
   searches   73–94, 419–20
   selecting   81–2
   sources of problems   55–7
   types of sources   77
   where to find sources   79–80
literature reviews   73–94, 419–20
   critiquing   87
   possible resources   76–7
   research proposals   139–41, 149–51
   research report   517–19, 534–6
   setting boundaries   75–6
   why do it?   73–4
lived experience   336, 439
logistic regression   297
longitudinal designs   191

manipulation of independent variable   186–7
maturation   178
mean   277–8
   testing for differences in   294–5
measurement   208–13, 269–71
   and validity   178–80
   data collection   208–13
   scales of   211–12
measurement-related error   212–13
measures of central tendency   277–80
median   278–9
member checks   421
mental health, staff knowledge of   55
Mercer's Theory of Maternal Role Attainment   21
meta-analysis   220
method
   action research   370
   computer based research and   37–48
   critical ethnography   380–1
   data analysis   459–68
   data collection, sampling and triangulation   200–36
   differentiating between processes and methodologies   394–6
   ethnography   344–5
   feminist   375
   grounded theory   331–3
   historical research   348–50

more than one variable and   295–6
   phenomenology   337–9
   qualitative research   394–430
   see also quantitative methods
methodology   9
   distinguish from methods and processes   394–6
   see also qualitative research methodology
Miligram obedience experiment   106
mixed findings   311
mixed methods   421–2
mobile methodologies   327–8
mode   279
models   14, 15
   grand   18–19
   middle-range   19–23
   of critiques   85
   using in research   16, 18–19
modernity   324
multi-centre and multi-site research, ethics and   122–3
multiple methodologies   327–8
multiple regression   296
multi-stage samples   205
mustard gas   100

narrative analysis   468–70
National Health and Medical Research Council (NHMRC)
   ethical research codes and guidelines   101–2, 107
   indigenous research participants, ethics and   121
     National Research Ethics Committee   102
     Principles of Ethical Conduct   104
national health imperatives   563
Nazi medical experiments   99–100, 105
Neuman's systems model   18–19
New Zealand Cancer Study   100, 105–6
Newman's Model of Health as Expanding Consciousness   21
non-equivalent control group designs   190–1
non-probability sampling   205–7

observation   215–18, 422–5
observational effects, and validity   180, 215–18
odds ratios   310
one group-pre-test post-test design   183–4

one-shot case study   182
one-tailed and two-tailed tests   285–6
ontology   320
    postmodern influences on   323–4, 327
oral presentations   546–50
Orem's self-care deficit nursing theory   14, 16–17

paradigms   9, 326
Parse's Theory of Becoming Human   21–2
participant observation   422–5
people
    as sources of help in research surveys   76–7
    as sources of problems   54–5
Peplau's Model of Psychodynamic Nursing   22
percentage   273
percentage distributions   273–4
phenomenology   336–42
phenomenon   15
photography   425–6, 445, 478
pie charts   274–5
pile on the kitchen table method   463
pilot study   218, 261–2
placebo effect   179
plain language, informed consent and   109
policy and procedure manuals, research and   566
population, defining   142, 144, 201
posters   511–12, 550–1
postmodernism   323–5
    alternative influences for qualitative methodologies   325–7
    and research approach   66, 364–86, 440
    and research interpretation   496–7
    compared with poststructuralism   367–9
poststructuralism   364, 366–9, 472–3
post-test only control group design   188
potential for change   440
power   471–3
practice and research   560–1
pre-experimental designs   182–5
preliminaries   515–17, 534–6
pre-test post-test design   183–4, 187–8
Preventive Health Behaviour Model   22–3
primary sources   77
principle of justice   115–23
Principles of Ethical Conduct   104
privacy   116–18

probability sampling   203
probability   280–98
processes
    distinguish from method and methodology   394–6
    interpretive   492–4
    research problems and   63
    synthesizing research results   494–502
professionalism   4
professions, defined   4

Q-sort   231–2
qualitative critical methodologies   325–7, 364–86, **442**, 492
    action research   369–74
    compared with poststructuralism   366–7
    critical ethnography   380–3
    feminisms   374–9
    interpretation and   499–500
    theoretical assumptions of   365–6
qualitative data
    forms of   438–9
    usefulness of   439–40
qualitative data analysis   448–50, 456–78
    adjunct analytical   477
    approaches to   456–68
    computer assisted   464–8
    computer systems   473–5
    confidence   459
    copies of data   458, 462
    discourse   470–3
    examples of completed   475–7
    get your thinking together   463–4
    images   478
    interpretation and   487–9, 495–7
    manual approaches   462
    methods appropriate to intentions   460
    narrative   468–70
    organizing system   458–9
    orientation of the researcher   458
    presenting in reports   540–3
    questions in transition   494
    review aims   462
    themes   461, 542
qualitative data collection   438–51
    computers   448–50
    management of   446–50
    preparing for   441–3
    presenting in reports   539–40

strategies for   443–8
qualitative interpretive categories   492–4
qualitative interpretive methodologies   492
   assumptions of   321, 365–6
   combining   329–30
   differences between interpretive and
    critical   325, 492
   ethnography   344–5, 380–3
   flexible approaches to   327–8
   grounded theory   331–3
   historical research   348–50
   phenomenology   337–9
   postmodern influences   325–7, 364–86
   result interpretation and   497–8
qualitative research   7–10
   coming of age of   457
   context and participants   399–400, 439
   critical   8–9, 364–86
   critiquing   90–3
   data handling   45, 153–4
   differences from quantitative   321–3
   ethics   154–5, 408, 537–8
   defining an area and identifying
    intentions   65–6
   interpretive   8–9, 319–53
   literature reviews   74–5, 149–51
   methods   405–30
   method and processes   152–4
   orientation of the researcher   458
   rigour in   400–5
qualitative research findings   487–502
   as relative interpretation   490–1
   in relation to methodologies   491–2
   presenting in reports   533–46
   synthesizing results   494–502
qualitative research interpretation   487–502
   analysis and   487–9, 495–7
   hermeneutics and   495–6
   literature and   501–2
   postmodernism and   496–7
   processes for synthesizing results   494–502
   preconditions for   493
   presenting in reports   543–5
   reasons for questions in transition   494
   relevance   501
   scope of   491
   what do they look like?   500
qualitative research methodology   320–53
   critical   364–86

ethnography   343–4, 380
feminisms   375–6
grounded theory   330–6
historical research   348
phenomenology   336–42, 384
research report presentation and   536–7
qualitative research methods   405–27
   alone or combinations   397–8
   choosing congruent   396–7
   mixed   421–2
   research contexts and participants
    399–400, 439
   report presentation and   539–40
qualitative research proposals, elements
  of   147–58
qualitative research reports   533–46
   body of, what they contain   536–43
   examples of presentation style   537–8,
    539–44
quantitative data analysis   271–99, 304–14
quantitative data collection   208–36, 245–64
   access to site and participants   247–9
   management of data   256–61
   managing equipment and materials   252
   managing and processing   253–61
   pilot study   261–2
   preparing for   246–7
   process of   251–6
   questionnaires   252–3
   recruitment and preparation of partici-
    pants   249–51
   researchers and collectors   251
   staff   249
quantitative methods   200–36
quantitative research   5–7
   critiquing   86–90
   differences from qualitative   321–3
   research problems and   56–7
   stating an hypothesis and identifying
    variables   63–5
quantitative research proposals
   elements of   135–46
   literature reviews   139
quantitative research reports
   assembling   533
   body of, what it contains   517–33
   example of presentation style   521–33
   statement of limitations   531
quasi-experimental designs   189–93

questionnaires   220–32, 234, 246–7, 252–3
quota samples   206–7

random assignment to groups   186
random samples   203–4
range   279
reference management   47, 531, 545–6
references, filing and storing   39–40, 55
relative truths   490
relevance of interpreted results   501
reliability   181–2, 214, 403
reports *see* research reports
research
    clinical guidelines and   564–6
    databases and indexes   37–41, 77
    easy and accessible to practitioners   567–8
    encouraging honours and postgraduate
      degrees   570
    engaging in work related to   571–2
    ethics guidelines   101–2
    getting it into practice   562–9
    literature searches and   73–94
    managing and analysing data   45–7
    meaning of   2
    policy and procedure manuals   566
    professionalism and   4
    paradigms   5–10
    relationship to theory and practice   13–14
    skills, encouraging   570–1
    using computers in   34–48
    using in practice and education   560–72
    see also qualitative research; quantitative
      research
research agencies   571
research conditions   **322**
research culture, in clinical settings   567
research design   133, 141–4, 173–95
    in research report   519–23
    major types   173–7
research findings   47
    interpreting   487–502
research gaps   56
research group   412–13
research outcomes   **322**
research plans   91, 151–4, 536–7
research priorities, identifying   57–8
research problem
    budget for and cost-benefit   61–2
    criteria for selecting   58–62

finding   54–8
priorities, identifying   57–8
process   63
resources available and   60–2
sources and strategies for, finding
    them   54–8
stating it   62–3
research project
    presenting   477
    reorienting   494
research proposals   132–66
    common elements of   159–60
    content of   135
    design   141–4
    elements of   135–58
    ethical considerations   104, 144–5
    funding   164
    obtaining approvals   164–5
    preliminary steps   133–5
    qualitative   147–58
    quantitative   135–46
    referencing   159, 531
    writing it   160–4
research question   148–9, **322**
    formulating   53
    potential nursing and health   335–6,
      341–2, 347, 351, 374, 379, 383
    stating it   62–3
research reports   78, 510–56
    common elements   514–16
    critiques of   83–5
    ethical considerations   125
    guidelines   513
    qualitative   90–3, 514–16, 533–46
    quantitative   85–90, 514–33
    lengths and types of   511–12
    planning and writing   513–14
    presentations   477, 546–51
    structuring   514–16
    target audience   512–13
    written   512–46
    see also qualitative research reports;
      quantitative research reports
respect for human dignity   108–14
results
    dissemination of   145, 156
    presenting in reports   523–8
    qualitative interpretive   494–502
rigour   400–5

Rogers's theory of unitary human
  beings   19–20
Roy's adaptation model   18

sample size and power calculations   207–8
samples, representativeness testing   282–3
sampling   142, 144, 202–8, 332
science   5–6
scientific method   326
scientific misconduct   124–5
scientific research
    reliability   181–2
    validity in   177–81
searches
    computer   38–9
    literature   73–94, 419–20
    setting boundaries   75–6
secondary sources   77
selection effects   179
self-report   220
seminar papers   511
serendipitous findings   311–12
setting for study   142, 143, 200–1
significance
    level of   284, 308–13
    statement of   139, 148
single patient trials   193
skills   20–1
snowball samples   206
Solomon four-groups design   188–9
special participants   112–13
spreadsheets   45
standard deviation   279–80
statement of limitations   531
static group comparison   184–5
statistical significance   309–11
statistical software   46
statistics   272–80
    creating complex   296–7
storytelling   426–7
stratified samples   204
subjectivity   439–40
sum   272–3
systematic reviews   11

t-tests   290–2

tables   275–7
Tamoxifen breast cancer study   100
target audience, of research report
   512–13
teaching evidence-based care   569–72
testing effect   178
tests   296–8
thematic analysis
    computer assisted   464–8
    manual   459–64
theoretical memos and diagrams   333
theoretical sampling   332
theoretical sensitivity   332
theory   14–16
    grand   16, 326, 368
    grounded   330–6
    middle-range   20–3
    qualitative research methodology   320–53
    relationship to research and practice
      13–14, 16–23
    research problems   65–6
theory-practice links   567–8
theses   78, 476, 511
time series design   192
timeframes   145, 156–7
title page   515, 516, 534
transcripts   417, 463, 465
triangulation   235–6, 403
true experimental research designs   185–7
Tuskegee Syphilis Study   99
two-way and three-way ANOVAs   297
type 1 and type 11 errors   283–4

unethical research conduct, examples   99–101
   see also ethics

validity   178–81
variability, measures of   279
variables   269
    statistical methods involving more than
      one   295–6
visual analog scales   225

Watson's model (carative factors)   21
words, as qualitative data   438, 445, 459
work plans   145